MW00838143

PROGRESS IN CATHETER ABLATION

Developments in Cardiovascular Medicine

VOLUME 241

Progress in Catheter Ablation

Clinical Application of New Mapping and Ablation Technology

Edited by

Liong Bing Liem

Associate Professor of Medicine, Stanford University,
Director, Experimental Cardiac Electrophysiology,
Stanford University Medical Center,
Stanford, California, U.S.A.

and

Eugene Downar

Professor of Medicine, University of Toronto,
Director, Invasive Cardiac Electrophysiology,
Toronto General Hospital,
Toronto, Ontario, Canada

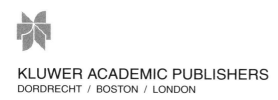

KLUWER ACADEMIC PUBLISHERS
DORDRECHT / BOSTON / LONDON

A C.I.P. Catalogue record for this book is available from the Library of Congress.

ISBN 1-4020-0147-9

Published by Kluwer Academic Publishers,
P.O. Box 17, 3300 AA Dordrecht, The Netherlands.

Sold and distributed in North, Central and South America
by Kluwer Academic Publishers,
101 Philip Drive, Norwell, MA 02061, U.S.A.

In all other countries, sold and distributed
by Kluwer Academic Publishers,
P.O. Box 322, 3300 AH Dordrecht, The Netherlands.

Printed on acid-free paper

Printed in the Netherlands.

Dedicated to our families,

James Saylor and Tina Carriere

Table of Contents

Part III. Newer Ablation Approaches and Modalities

Part IV. Arrhythmia Surgery

Part V. Future Perspective

* Production of Color Plates was sponsored partly by a generous grant from Endocardial Solutions Inc., Saint Paul, Minnesota, USA.

Preface

Catheter ablation is widely accepted as an effective and safe form of therapy for cardiac arrhythmia. In many instances this curative procedure is considered as the first line of therapy if not the ultimate treatment of choice. With the use of radiofrequency (RF) modality; which has revolutionized the technology from a barotraumatic, potentially injurious procedure using high-voltage, direct-current (DC) shock to a safe and relatively painless one; catheter ablation procedure now carries a very low risk and is extremely effective for certain types of arrhythmia. Its efficacy rate in curing supraventricular tachycardia involving an accessory pathway or dual atrioventricular nodal pathways has been near perfect and its application for certain types of atrial and ventricular arrhythmia have also been very satisfactory.

However, conventional RF ablation has several well known limitations, most notably is its ability to only produce relatively small, point lesions; rendering it effective only for an arrhythmia with a small and/or a superficial target. It was soon recognized that the technology would not likely to have significant utility in arrhythmia with a more widespread target such as atrial fibrillation or those which involve scarred and deep myocardial tissue such as ventricular tachycardia. Indeed, the application of conventional RF technology in these complex but common arrhythmia has yielded unsatisfactory results. Ablation of ventricular tachycardia, even with meticulous mapping, has accomplished only moderate success and ablation of atrial fibrillation was rarely attempted. It was soon recognized that in order to achieve a reasonable success rate in curing or controlling the more complex arrhythmia, further improvement in catheter ablative technology was needed.

Fortunately, the frustration from the interim failures has not dampened the pursuit for a cure of complex arrhythmia. The enthusiasm from the past great success with RF ablation and the demand for a better therapy for the complex but common arrhythmia has carried forward the progress of catheter ablation technology. In the past few years, there has been a significant progress in the development of better mapping and ablative techniques. Such progress has resulted in a steady improvement in the success of ablation of more complex atrial and ventricular tachyarrhythmia as well as our knowledge about their anatomy and pathophysiology. However, the enthusiasm for finding the ideal tools for the cure of complex arrhythmia has also resulted in proliferation of changes in catheter designs, mapping apparatus, and heat energy sources. The clinician of nowadays technology is faced with a wide and often confusing choices of new instruments and methods of ablation. There are few, if any, comparative studies involving the various new tools; nor there is any compilation of data on any specific new discovery. It is timely to provide ourselves with a review of available data on the progress of newer technology in order to enhance our knowledge and to concentrate our effort into the development of an ultimate practical and yet effective methodology.

The purpose of this publication is, therefore, to provide a forum in which the authors can present their experience, even if only in its preliminary stage, in the respective field or technology. Following a review of current understanding in some critical anatomical and electrophysiological aspects of complex arrhythmia in Part I, various technological advancements in mapping and ablation are presented. Progress in mapping is presented in Part II, starting with chapter discussing refinement in the utility of current electrode catheters progressing to the various newly released mapping systems, including electroanatomical mapping, tracking system and multi-site acquisition methods. In Part III, various ablation techniques and alternative energy sources are discussed. The contemporary issue of focal atrial fibrillation ablation is covered in various aspects, including a review of its progress. In Part IV, some aspects of arrhythmia surgery for atrial fibrillation, which is becoming an important form of management of the entity, are reviewed. Finally, closing statements are presented, from the point of view of both the electrophysiologist and the arrhythmia surgeon.

The authors are selected based on their interest and expertise on the subject. Each topic is presented in a concise form and with relevance to the development of newer technology. For example, the review of the mechanism of cardiac arrhythmia includes the discussion on the anatomical and pathological issues as they relate to the concept of catheter ablation. In some instance, the presentation may be short and preliminary because an in depth investigation of the technology may have not been accomplished as yet. The introduction of an idea with a relatively sound substantiation is the element of this publication and hence many of its content may be more speculative rather than comprehensive in nature. Furthermore, the authors are encouraged to provide their opinion on the issues. It is, of course, understood that the opinions presented can not be expected to be representative of the general opinion; its inclusion is merely intended to stimulate further investigation. A thorough and solid presentation of certain technology would be beyond the scope of this rapid publication; yet it is intended to incorporate the complete progress of all aspects of ablation technology such that it would provide the reader with a global and comparative view.

Undoubtedly the technology will continue to progress at its rapid pace and other, new development would continue to emerge. It is, therefore, hoped that this form of publication would continue to be updated and any suggestion or criticism is welcomed.

L. Bing Liem
Eugene Downar

Contributing Authors

Walter L. Atiga, MD
Assistant Professor of Medicine
University of Pittsburgh
Pittsburgh, Pennsylvania, USA

Boaz Avitall, MD, PhD
Professor of Medicine
Director,
Cardiac Electrophysiology
University of Illinois at Chicago
Chicago, Illinois, USA

Antonius Baartscheer, PhD
Investigator
Experimental and Molecular Cardiology
Group
Academic Medical Center
University of Amsterdam
Amsterdam, The Netherlands

A. L. Bartorelli, MD
Director
Interventional Cardiology
Institute of Cardiology
University of Milan
Milan, Italy

Anton E. Becker, MD, PhD
Professor, and Head of the
Department of Cardiovascular Pathology
Academic Medical Center
University of Amsterdam
Amsterdam, The Netherlands

Ronald D. Berger, MD, PhD
Associate Professor of Medicine
Johns Hopkins University
Baltimore, Maryland, USA

Dany Berubé, PhD
Director,
Research and Education
AFx, Incorporated
Fremont, California, USA

Tim R. Betts, MB, ChB, MRCP
Fellow
Wessex Cardiothoracic Center
Southampton General Hospital
Southampton, UK

Hugh Calkins, MD
Professor of Medicine
Director,
Arrhythmia Service
Clinical Electrophysiology Laboratory
Johns Hopkins University
Baltimore, Maryland, USA

Eric K. Y. Chan, PhD
Vice President, Product Development
CARDIMA, Inc.
Fremont, California, USA

Mau-Song Chang, MD
Professor of Medicine
National Yang-Ming University
Director,
Taipei Veterans General Hospital
Taipei, Taiwan

Shih-Ann Chen, MD
Professor of Medicine
National Yang-Ming University
Director,
Cardiac Electrophysiology Laboratory
Taipei Veterans General Hospital
Taipei, Taiwan

Sung H. Chun, MD
Assistant Professor of Medicine
Stanford University School of Medicine
Associate Director,
Cardiac Arrhythmia and Electrophysiology
Stanford, California, USA

Ruben Coronel, MD, PhD
Experimental Cardiologist
Experimental and Molecular Cardiology
Group
Academic Medical Center
University of Amsterdam
Amsterdam, The Netherlands

André d'Avila, MD
Assistant Physician
Heart Institute (InCor)
University of São Paulo Medical School
São Paulo, Brazil

Jacques M. T. de Bakker, PhD
Professor of Experimental Cardiac
Electrophysiology
Experimental and Molecular Cardiology
Group
Academic Medical Center
University of Amsterdam
Amsterdam, the Netherlands

Paolo Della Bella, MD
Director,
Clinical Electrophysiology Laboratory
Institute of Cardiology
University of Milan
Milan, Italy

Angelo A. V. De Paola, MD
Director,
Cardiology Division
Clinical Cardiac Electrophysiology
Paulista School of Medicine
Federal University of São Paulo
São Paulo, Brazil

Yu-An Ding, MD
Professor of Medicine
National Yang-Ming University
Chairman,
Cardiology Department
Taipei Veterans General Hospital
Taipei, Taiwan

Eugene Downar, MB, ChB
Professor in Medicine
University of Toronto
Director,
Invasive Cardiac Electrophysiology
Toronto General Hospital
Toronto, Ontario, Canada

Marc Dubuc, MD, FRCPC
Associate Professor of Medicine
Director,
Clinical Electrophysiology Service
Montreal Heart Institute
Montreal, Quebec, Canada

N. A. Mark Estes, III, MD
Professor of Medicine
Tufts University School of Medicine
Director,
Cardiac Arrhythmia Center
New England Medical Center
Boston, Massachusetts, USA

Rafaelle Fanelli, MD
Chief of Cardiology
Casa Sollievo della Sofferenza
San Giovanni Rotondo, Italy

Roberto L. Farias, MD
Fellow,
Clinical Cardiac Electrophysiology
Paulista School of Medicine
Federal University of São Paulo
São Paulo, Brazil

David M. Fitzgerald, MD
Associate Professor of Medicine
Director,
Cardiac Electrophysiology
Wake Forest University School of Medicine
Winston-Salem, North Carolina, USA

Caroline B. Foote, MD
Assistant Professor of Medicine
Tufts University School of Medicine
Co-Director,
Cardiac Arrhythmia Center
New England Medical Center
Boston, Massachusetts, USA

Bruce N. Goldreyer, MD
Clinical Professor of Medicine
University of Southern California
Director
Clinical Cardiac Electrophysiology
San Pedro Peninsula Hospital
San Pedro, California, USA

Rosa Gouveia, MD
Pathology Specialist
Hospital de Santa Cruz
Lisbon, Portugal

Gerard M. Guiraudon, MD
Professor of Surgery
London Health Science Center
London, Ontario, Canada
Director of Clinical Trials
University of Ottawa Heart Institute
Ottawa, Ontario, Canada

Joachim Hebe, MD
Assistant Medical Director,
Department of Cardiology
Head of Electrophysiology
St. Georg Hospital
Hamburg, Germany

Munther K. Homoud, MD
Assistant Professor of Medicine
Tufts University School of Medicine
Co-Director,
Cardiac Arrhythmia Center
New England Medical Center
Boston, Massachusetts, USA

Ming-Hsiung Hsieh, MD
Instructor of Medicine
National Yang-Ming University
Division of Cardiology
Chung Shan Medical and Dental College
Hospital
Taichung, Taiwan

John D. Hummel, MD
Cardiac Electrophysiologist
Riverside Methodist Hospital
Mid Ohio Cardiology Consultants
Columbus, Ohio, USA

George J. Juang, MD
Fellow
Cardiac Electrophysiology
Johns Hopkins University
Baltimore, Maryland, USA

Paul Khairy, MD, FRCPC
Cardiology Fellow
Montreal Heart Institute
Montreal, Quebec, Canada

Michael Knaut, MD
Cardiovascular Institute
University of Dresden
Dresden, Germany

Bradley P. Knight, MD
Assistant Professor of Medicine
University of Michigan
Ann Arbor, Michigan, USA

L. Bing Liem, DO
Associate Professor of Medicine
Director,
Experimental Cardiac Electrophysiology
Acting Director,
Cardiac Arrhythmia and Electrophysiology
Stanford University
Stanford, California, USA

Mark S. Link, MD
Assistant Professor of Medicine
Tufts University School of Medicine
Co-Director,
Cardiac Arrhythmia Center
New England Medical Center
Boston, Massachusetts, USA

Laszlo Littman, MD
Director of Electrophysiology
Laser and Applied Technologies Laboratory
Carolinas Heart Institute
Charlotte, North Carolina, USA

Ana P. Martins, MD
Director,
Pathology Department
Hospital de Santa Cruz
Lisbon, Portugal

Stéphane Massé, MSc
Professional Engineer
Toronto General Hospital
Toronto, Ontario, Canada

João Q. E. Melo, MD
Director
Cardiovascular Surgery
Hospital de Santa Cruz
Lisbon, Portugal

Scott C. Millard, BS
University of Illinois at Chicago
Chicago, Illinois, USA

Fred Morady, MD
Professor of Medicine
Director,
Cardiac Electrophysiology Laboratory
University of Michigan
Ann Arbor, Michigan, USA

John M. Morgan, MD
Consultant Cardiologist &
Electrophysiologist
Wessex Cardiothoracic Center
Southampton General Hospital
Southampton, UK

Rainer Moosdorf, Prof., Dr.
Department of Cardiovascular Surgery
Philipps-University of Marburg
Marburg, Germany

Andrea Natale, MD
Professor of Medicine
Ohio State University
Director,
Electrophysiology Laboratory
The Cleveland Clinic Foundation
Cleveland, Ohio, USA

Douglas Packer, MD
Professor of Medicine
Mayo Clinic Foundation
Rochester, Minnesota, USA

Ennio Pisano, MD
Staff Cardiologist
Casa Sollievo della Sofferenza
San Giovanni Rotondo, Italy

Domenico Potenza, MD
Staff Cardiologist
Casa Sollievo della Sofferenza
San Giovanni Rotondo, Italy

Johannes. M. E. Rademaker, MD, PhD
Investigator
Experimental and Molecular Cardiology
Group
Academic Medical Center
University of Amsterdam
Amsterdam, The Netherlands

Almino C. Rocha Neto, MD
Fellow,
Clinical Cardiac Electrophysiology
Paulista School of Medicine
Federal University of São Paulo
São Paulo, Brazil

David L. Ross, MD
Department of Cardiology
Westmead Hospital and University of
Sydney
Westmead, New South Wales, Australia

Walid Saliba, MD
Staff Cardiologist
Cleveland Clinic Foundation
Cleveland, Ohio, USA

Pietro Santarelli, MD
Staff Cardiologist
Casa Sollievo della Sofferenza
San Giovanni Rotondo, Italy

Teresa Santiago, MSc
Science Researcher
Hospital de Santa Cruz
Lisbon, Portugal

Mauricio Scanavacca, MD, PhD
Assistant Physician
Heart Institute (InCor)
University of São Paulo Medical School
São Paulo, Brazil

Stephan Schüler, MD
Professor
Cardiovascular Institute
University of Dresden
Dresden, Germany

Robert A. Schweikert, MD
Staff Cardiologist
Cardiac Electrophysiology and Pacing
Cleveland Clinic Foundation
Cleveland, Ohio, USA

Elias Sevaptsidis, DCS
Engineering Technologist
Toronto General Hospital
Toronto, Ontario, Canada

Mei-Hao Shi, MD, MSc
Senior Technician
Toronto General Hospital
Toronto, Ontario, Canada

Eduardo Sosa, MD, PhD
Director,
Cardiac Arrhythmia Unit
Heart Institute (InCor)
University of São Paulo Medical School
São Paulo, Brazil

Stefan G. Spitzer, MD
Director
Department of Electrophysiology and
Pacing
Institute of Cardiovascular Research
Dresden, Germany

Robert Splinter, PhD
Research Scientist
Laser and Applied Technologies Laboratory
Carolinas Heart Institute
Charlotte, North Carolina, USA

Robert H. Svenson, MD
Medical Director
Laser and Applied Technologies Laboratory
Carolinas Heart Institute
Charlotte, North Carolina, USA

Craig Swygman,
Cardiac Arrhythmia Center
New England Medical Center
Boston, Massachusetts, USA

Ching-Tai Tai, MD
Associate Professor of Medicine
National Yang-Ming University
Division of Cardiology
Taipei Veterans General Hospital
Taipei, Taiwan

George P. Tatsis, MS
Administrative Director
Laser and Applied Technologies Laboratory
Carolinas Heart Institute
Charlotte, North Carolina, USA

N. Trevisi, MD
Staff Cardiology
Institute of Cardiology
University of Milan
Milan, Italy

Chin-Feng Tsai, MD
Instructor of Medicine
National Yang-Ming University
Division of Cardiology
Chung Shan Medical and Dental College
Hospital
Taichung, Taiwan

Arvydas Urbonas, MD
Research Associate
University of Illinois at Chicago
Chicago, Illinois, USA

Dalia Urboniene, MD
Research Associate
University of Illinois at Chicago
Chicago, Illinois, USA

George F. Van Hare, MD
Associate Professor of Pediatrics
Director,
Pediatric Arrhythmia Center
Stanford University
Stanford, California, USA

Jessica T. Vermeulen, MD, PhD
Experimental Cardiologist
Experimental and Molecular Cardiology
Group
Academic Medical Center
University of Amsterdam
Amsterdam, The Netherlands

Paul J. Wang, MD
Associate Professor of Medicine
Tufts University School of Medicine
Associate Director,
Cardiac Arrhythmia Center
New England Medical Center
Boston, Massachusetts, USA

Menashe B. Waxman, MD
Professor in Medicine
University of Toronto
Toronto, Ontario, Canada

David Wilber, MD
Professor of Medicine
Director,
Electrophysiology Laboratories
University of Chicago
Chicago, Illinois, USA

N. Parker Willis, PhD
Chief Technologist
Cardiac Pathways Corporation
Sunnyvale, California, USA

Fred H. M.Wittkampf, PhD
Investigator
The Heart Lung Institute
Department of Cardiology
University Medical Center
Utrecht, The Netherlands

Part I

Challenges in Catheter Ablation

Chapter 1

THE ARRHYTHMOGENIC SUBSTRATE IN ISCHEMIC AND NON-ISCHEMIC CARDIOMYOPATHIES

Structural and Functional Basis of Ventricular Arrhythmias

Ruben Coronel, Antonius Baartscheer, Johannes M.E. Rademaker, Jessica T. Vermeulen, Jacques M.T. de Bakker
Experimental and Molecular Cardiology Group, Academic Medical Center, University of Amsterdam, Amsterdam, The Netherlands

INTRODUCTION

For the mechanistic study of arrhythmias in clinical practice the terms "arrhythmogenic substrate", "initiating factor" and "modulating factors" have been introduced.[1] We define the substrate as "a pre-existing condition that forms a prerequisite for the induction of an arrhythmia". For example in the Wolff-Parkinson-White syndrome the substrate is formed by the accessory bundle and removal of the bundle is curative.[2] In clinical cardiology the "substrate" is studied by invasive electrophysiology, whereas the "initiating factor" is primarily the subject of non-invasive electrophysiologic studies. Although this approach has proved valuable in the study of the substrate in AV-reentrant arrhythmias it fell short in the mechanistic evaluation of ventricular arrhythmias.[1] In ventricular myocardium, multiple mechanisms may underlie the inducibility of a sustained arrhythmia.

In spite of this, the "triangle of Coumel" (Figure 1) has helped to channel thought in research on arrhythmogenic mechanisms. If defined as above, the substrate transcends the meaning of a structural alteration but may also reflect a functional change of the myocardium. Also, a "substrate" can be present temporarily in the same manner as the initiating factors (the "triggers"). This has led to the awareness that an arrhythmia occurs only if there is concurrence of the trigger and the substrate and that shifting of one or the other in time may result in increased or decreased arrhythmogenesis e.g. in acute myocardial ischemia (Figure 2).[3]

L. Bing Liem and E. Downar (eds.), Progress in Catheter Ablation, 3-11.

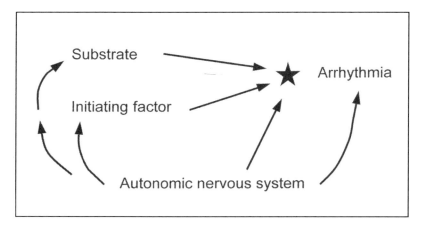

Figure 1

In line with this thought is the application of specific interventions to reduce the number of triggers (premature ventricular beats) and thereby reducing mortality caused by sudden cardiac death.[4] We surmise that the CAST (Cardiac Arrhythmia Suppression Trial) study failed because the effective reduction of the number of triggers coincided with an increased severity of the substrate, leading to an increased rather than a decreased number of sudden cardiac deaths.

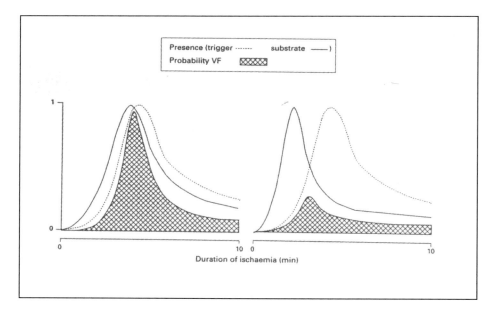

Figure 2

The mere documentation of the spontaneous occurrence of arrhythmias in the course of time does not enable a mechanistic discrimination between trigger and substrate. Only the conclusion may be drawn that both nuclear factors are present at the same time and the association with other –modulating- factors may be described (e.g. cellular uncoupling, pharmacological interventions).[5,6] By providing a trigger (e.g. premature beats, increase in heart rate, introduction of a long RR interval) the inducibility of the arrhythmia defines the changing presence (or the severity) of the arrhythmogenic substrate.[7]

In this chapter we will discuss the arrhythmogenic substrates in two conditions: (1) The infarcted heart (where changes in tissue architecture primarily define a *structural* substrate), and (2) heart failure (where changes in cellular electrophysiologic parameter define a *functional* substrate). We reason that the former substrates are "ablatable", the latter (at least at present) more amenable to implantation of an automatic defibrillator.

1.   THE INFARCTED HEART: THE *STRUCTURAL* SUBSTRATE FOR ARRHYTHMOGENESIS

Survivors of acute myocardial infarction often experience severe life-threatening arrhythmias months or years following infarction.[8-11] These arrhythmias often take the form of sustained monomorphic or polymorphic tachycardia. Surgical resection of the arrhythmogenic "substrate" in these patients has been directed by intraoperative activation mapping. The aim of activation mapping was to identify the (sub)endocardial site where earliest cardiac electrical activity was recorded during induction of the relevant tachycardia. Although the success of these ablative procedures were variable and the use of guiding by mapping has been debated,[12-17] mapping techniques have helped to gain insight in the activation patterns during ventricular tachycardia.

Figure 3 (next page) shows an example of activation maps obtained during mapping in an explanted perfused heart obtained from a patient with drug resistant ventricular tachycardia following myocardial infarction.[18] A balloon electrode with 64 electrodes was introduced into the left and right ventricular cavities and the arrhythmia was induced with programmed stimulation. The figure shows the activation pattern of the left ventricular subendocardium (upper left panel) during one cycle of a monomorphic ventricular tachycardia. The shaded area represents the infarcted myocardium. Lines indicate isochrones. At the reference time (t=0) the activity seems to originate from the posterior part of the left ventricular free wall and spreads in a centrifugal pattern towards the rest of the heart. The activity apparently terminates after about 220 msec (arrow indicates sequence of activation). However, at the sites overlying the scar tissue indicated by *e* and *f* (right panel) small diastolic potentials could be recorded distinctly indicative of local activity (small arrows). This activity seems to bridge the gap between the end of gross ventricular activation at 220 msec and the tachycardia cycle length (270 msec). The right ventricular subendocardium shows a focal activation pattern.

The observation of diastolic electrical activity in tissue adjacent to the apparent "focal" origin of the tachycardia wave and immediately preceding earliest ("gross") activity supports the notion of a reentrant pathway through isolated surviving fibers spanning the infarcted tissue. Indeed, the correlative histologic and electrophysiologic study on the same heart as in Figure 3 demonstrated a close correlation between surviving myocardial fibers and local electrical activity.[18] A full reconstruction of the activation pattern of an infarcted human papillary muscle demonstrated "zig-zag" conduction: large conduction delays were recorded over small distances. The calculated conduction velocity along the tortuous pathway in these isolated myocardial fibers, however, was normal.[19]

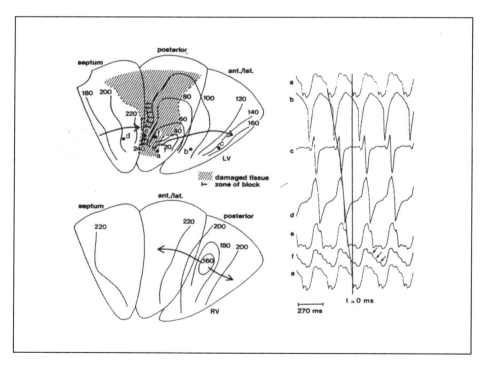

Figure 3

After mapping-guided ablative therapy either the reentrant pathway may be completely interrupted leading to disappearance of the arrhythmogenic substrate, or one of the often multiple exit points of the reentrant circuit may be ablated. In the latter case ablation does not lead to a complete "cure" and the arrhythmia may take another path to complete its reentrant circuit. This is probably the reason why surgical resection of a large area of endocardial tissue overlying the scar, <u>not</u> guided by electrophysiological mapping was very effective in the destruction of the arrhythmogenic substrate.[12] This implies that more localized ablation techniques like radio frequency catheter ablation are less effective, unless they are repeated several times to cover a larger area.

2.   HEART FAILURE: THE *ELECTROPHYSIOLOGICAL* SUBSTRATE FOR ARRHYTHMOGENESIS.

The surviving myocardial tissue of infarcted hearts demonstrates adaptational changes to the loss of contractile proteins. These changes are reflected by hypertrophy.[20-24] When these compensatory changes fail, heart failure ensues. Mortality associated with heart failure is high and in about 50% of the cases death is unexpected and probably arrhythmic.[25]

In the early phases of heart failure the incidence of sudden cardiac death is higher than in later stages of heart failure.[26] The mechanism of arrhythmogenesis during heart failure is presently not fully understood but various animal models of heart failure have demonstrated electrophysiologic remodelling of non infarcted tissue from individuals with heart failure,[27,28-34] both remote from the infarcted area[35] and directly overlying the infarct scar.[36]

2.1   A Rabbit Model of Heart Failure

A rabbit model of heart failure induced by a combined pressure and volume overload (by aortic banding in combination with aortic insufficiency) has been described by Bril et al.[37] In this model spontaneous ventricular arrhythmias develop in the course of weeks to months after induction of heart failure.[29] In addition, sudden death in this particular model occurs in about 30% of the animals. Trabecula harvested from similar animals with overt "clinical" signs of heart failure (ascites, pulmonary edema, increased relative heart weight, increased left ventricular end diastolic pressure) demonstrated several electrophysiological alterations especially after provocation with an altered "failure like" composition of the superfusate (with decreased potassium concentration and in the presence of noradrenalin).[27]

Like in other models of heart failure[38] action potential duration was prolonged, but only at longer -unphysiological- cycle lengths.[27] The implication of this is that a higher propensity for triggered activity induced by early afterdepolarizations (EADs) is not likely to be expected, unless EADs are induced by long pauses. Although early afterdepolarizations were never directly observed [27] long sinus pauses have been shown to precede VTs in about 30 % of the intact animals.[29]

Figure 4 shows an example of the ECG of a rabbit with pressure/volume overload induced heart failure. Heart failure was induced at day 0 and developed over the following weeks/months. The ECG at 3 weeks following heart failure induction (panel A) shows a pause followed by a single ventricular premature beat (VPB). Panel B shows the ECG from the same rabbit 28 weeks following induction of heart failure. A pause is followed by a short run of VT. Thirty-two weeks after heart failure induction (panel C) a pause is followed by a VPB and a VT. This figure illustrates that the complexity of arrhythmogenesis increases with the development of heart failure, probably in concert with the formation of the arrhythmogenic substrate.[29]

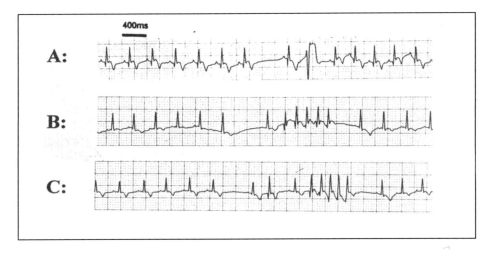

Figure 4

Delayed afterdepolarizations could be induced in about 50% of the preparations from rabbits with heart failure (as well as in 50% of isolated human myocardium from patients undergoing heart transplantation because of heart failure) following a period of burst pacing.[27] Indeed, Rademaker[29] has demonstrated that an acceleration of the rhythm preceded the occurrence of a VPB in most of the cases.

Vermeulen et al. have recently shown that in isolated myocytes from hearts with similarly induced heart failure calcium-aftertransients followed a period of burst pacing and that these Ca^{2+}-aftertransients sometimes were of the same amplitude as a normal Ca^{2+}-transient. These phenomena only occurred in myocytes obtained from animals from which the ECG showed ventricular arrhythmias and were absent in animals without ventricular arrhythmias.[39] These results suggest that the heart failure specific electrophysiological changes in ventricular myocardium (remodelling) are disperse rather than localized.

It is remarkable that the cellular electrophysiologic alterations induced by heart failure have been studied on isolated tissues or myocytes that were randomly selected from the failing heart.[35] Only in recent publications attention has been paid to the differential effect of heart failure induced remodelling on the various layers of ventricular myocardium.[34,40] The corresponding arrhythmogenic substrate, therefore, is more amenable to systemic (pharmaceutical) or cardiac (automatic implantable defibrillator), rather than localized interventions.

CONCLUSIONS

In ischemic as well as non-ischemic cardiomyopathies the heart undergoes structural alterations as well as functional changes. In the above we have argued that both aspects may underlie the formation of an arrhythmogenic substrate. In addition, both forms of arrhythmogenic substrate may be present in the same heart. This is particularly evident in the heart of a patient with an ischemic cardiomyopathy where the infarcted tissue may form a substrate for reentry (see section 2) and the remodelled normal myocardial may form the substrate for a premature beat (see section 3). An example of one of many possible sequences is given here: Depending on the appropriate trigger (e.g. a sinus pause) a premature beat may occur in the functionally remodelled hypertrophied myocardium (in this case caused by an early afterdepolarization). If the suitable substrate for reentry is available (surviving myocardial fibers traversing the infarcted tissue), this premature beat may in turn act as a trigger and initiate ventricular tachycardia. Thus, in one heart one set of conditions may cause the initiation, the other maintenance of the arrhythmia.

Selection of the appropriate antiarrhythmic therapy depends on the type of substrate encountered. A structural substrate is more suited for ablative procedures whereas a –more dispersed- functional substrate demands systemic interventions like antiarrhythmic drug therapy or the implantation of an automatic defibrillator.

Acknowledgement: The authors wish to express their gratitude to dr. J.R. de Groot for critical reading the manuscript.

REFERENCE LIST

1. Coumel P: The management of clinical arrhythmias. An overview on invasive versus non-invasive electrophysiology. Eur Heart J 1987;8:92-99
2. Wellens HJJ, Janse MJ, van Dam RT, van Capelle FJL, Meijne NG, Mellink HM, Durrer D: Epicardial mapping and surgical treatment in W.P.W. syndrome type A. Am Heart J 1974;88:69-78
3. Coronel R: Heterogeneity in extracellular potassium concentration during early myocardial ischaemia and reperfusion. Implications for arrhythmogenesis. Cardiovasc Res 1994;28:770-777

4. The Cardiac Arrhythmia Suppression Trial (CAST) Investigators. Preliminary report: effect of encainide and flecainide on mortality in a randomized trial of arrhythmia suppression after myocardial infarction.. N.Engl.J.Med. 1989;321:406-412

5. Smith IV WT, Fleet WF, Johnson TA, Engle CL, Cascio WE: The 1B phase of ventricular arrhythmias in ischemic in situ porcine heart is related to changes in cell-to-cell coupling. Circulation 1995;92:3051-3060

6. Manning AS, Coltart DJ, Hearse DJ: Ischemia and reperfusion-induced arrhythmias in the rat. Effects of xanthine oxidase inhibition with allopurinol. Circ Res 1984;55:545-548

7. Coronel R, Wilms-Schopman FJG, Janse MJ: Profibrillatory effects of intracoronary thrombus in acute regional ischemia of the in situ porcine heart. Circulation 1997;96:3985-3991

8. Bigger T: Why patients with congestive heart failure die: arrhythmias and sudden cardiac death. Circulation 1987;75:IV-28-IV-35

9. Goldstein S, Brooks MM, Ledingham R, Kennedy HL, Epstein AE, Pawitan Y, Bigger JT: Association between ease of suppression of ventricular arrhythmia and survival. Circulation 1995;91:79-83

10. Kennedy HL, Brooks MM, Barker AH, Bergstrand R, Huther M, Beanlands DS, Bigger JT, Goldstein S: Beta-blocker therapy in the cardiac arrhythmia suppression trial. Am J Cardiol 1994;74:674-680

11. Willems AR: Determinants of mortality in late ventricular tachycardia or fibrillation after myocardial infarction. Eur Heart J 1988;9:266 (Abstract)

12. Thakur RK, Guiraudon GM, Klein GJ, Yee R, Guiraudon CM: Intraoperative mapping is not necessary for VT surgery. Pacing.Clin.Electrophysiol. 1994;17:2156-2162

13. Guiraudon GM, Thakur RK, Klein GJ, Yee R, Guiraudon CM, Sharma A: Encircling endocardial cryoablation for ventricular tachycardia after myocardial infarction: experience with 33 patients. Am.Heart J. 1994;128:982-989

14. Van Hemel NM, Kingma JH, Defauw JA, Vermeulen FE, Mast EG, Ernst JM, Ascoop CA: Left ventricular segmental wall motion score as a criterion for selecting patients for direct surgery in the treatment of postinfarction ventricular tachycardia. Eur.Heart J. 1989;10:304-315

15. Ostermeyer J, Borggrefe M, Breithardt G, Podczek A, Goldmann A, Schoenen JD, Kolvenbach R, Godehardt E, Kirklin JW, Blackstone EH, et, al: Direct operations for the management of life-threatening ischemic ventricular tachycardia. J.Thorac.Cardiovasc.Surg. 1987;94:848-865

16. Platia EV, Griffith LS, Watkins LJ, Mower MM, Guarnieri T, Mirowski, Reid PR: Treatment of malignant ventricular arrhythmias with endocardial resection and implantation of the automatic cardioverter-defibrillator. N.Engl.J.Med. 1986;314:213-216

17. Lawrie GM, Wyndham CR, Krafchek J, Luck JC, Roberts R, DeBakey ME: Progress in the surgical treatment of cardiac arrhythmias. Initial experience of 90 patients. JAMA 1985;254:1464-1468

18. De Bakker JMT, Coronel R, Tasseron S, Wilde AAM, Opthof T, Janse MJ, Van Capelle FJL, Becker AE, Jambroes G: Ventricular tachycardia in the infarcted, Langendorff-perfused human heart: Role of the arrangement of surviving cardiac fibers. J Am Coll Cardiol 1990;15:1594-1607

19. de Bakker JM, van Capelle FJ, Janse MJ, Tasseron S, Vermeulen JT, de, Jonge N, Lahpor JR: Slow conduction in the infarcted human heart. 'Zigzag' course of activation. Circulation 1993;88:915-926

20. Belichard P, Pruneau D, Brown NL, Salzmann JL, Rouet R: Hypertrophie myocardique hypertensive et troubles du rhythme: deux origines probables. Arch Mal.Coeur.Vaiss. 1989;82:1303-1308

21. Conrad CH, Brooks WW, Hayes JA, Sen S, Robinson KG, Bing OHL: Myocardial fibrosis and stiffness with hypertrophy and heart failure in the spontaneously hypertensive rat. Circulation 1995;91:161-170

22. Dunn FG, Pringle SD: Sudden cardiac death, ventricular arrhythmias and hypertensive left ventricular hypertrophy. J Hypertens. 1993;11:1003-1010

23. Messerli FH, Soria F: Ventricular dysrhythmias, left ventricular hypertrophy, and sudden death. Cardiovasc Drug Therapy. 1994;8:557-563
24. Weber JR: Left ventricular hypertrophy: Its prevalence, etiology, and significance. Clin Cardiol 1991;14:13-17
25. Hofmann T, Meinertz T, Kasper W, Geibel A, Zehender M, Hohnloser S, Stienen U, Treese N, Just H: Mode of death in idiopathic dilated cardiomyopathy: a multivariate analysis of prognostic determinants. Am.Heart J. 1988;116:1455-1463
26. Kjekshus J: Arrhythmias and mortality in congestive heart failure. Am J Cardiol 1990;65:42I-48I
27. Vermeulen JT, McGuire MA, Opthof T, Coronel R, de Bakker JMT, Klopping C, Janse MJ: Triggered activity and automaticity in ventricular trabeculae of failing human and rabbit hearts. Cardiovasc Res 1994;28:1547-1554
28. Vermeulen JT, Tan HL, Rademaker H, Schumacher CA, Loh P, Opthof T, Coronel R, Janse MJ: Electrophysiologic and extracellular ionic changes during acute ischemia in failing and normal rabbit myocardium. J Mol Cell Cardiol 1996;28:123-131
29. Rademaker, H. Arrhythmogenesis during the development of heart failure in rabbits. 1-127. 1997. Amsterdam, Ponsen & Looijen, Wageningen.
30. Pye MP, Black M, Cobbe SM: Comparison of in vivo and in vitro haemodynamic function in experimental heart failure: use of echocardiography. Cardiovascular Research 1996;31:873-881
31. Pye MP, Cobbe SM: Arrhythmogenesis in experimental models of heart failure: the role of increased load. Cardiovascular Research 1996;32:248-257
32. Belichard P, Savard P, Cardinal R, Nadeau R, Gosselin H, Paradis P, Rouleau JL: Marked different effects on ventricular remodeling result in a decrease in inducibility of ventricular arrhythmias. J Am Coll Cardiol 1994;23:505-513
33. Aronson R, Ming Z: Cellular mechanisms of arrhythmias in hypertrophied and failing myocardium. Circulation 1993;87:76-83
34. McIntosh MA, Cobbe SM, Smith GL: Heterogeneous changes in action potential and intracellular Ca2+ in left ventricular myocyte sub-types from rabbits with heart failure. Cardiovasc Res 1999;in press
35. Tomaselli GF, Marban E: Electrophysiological remodeling in hypertrophy and heart failure. Cardiovasc Res 1999;42:270-283
36. Pinto JMB, Boyden PA: Electrical remodeling in ischemia and infarction. Cardiovasc Res 1999;42:284-297
37. Bril A, Forest MC, Gout B: Ischemia and reperfusion-induced arrhythmias in rabbits with chronic heart failure. Am J Physiol 1991;261:H301-H307
38. Hart G: Cellular electrophysiology in cardiac hypertrophy and failure - Review Article. Cardiovasc Res 1994;28:933-946
39. Vermeulen JT, Baartscheer T, Schumacher CA, Belterman C, Fiolet JWT, Coronel R, Janse MJ: Ventricular arrhythmias in failing hearts are related to calcium aftertransients. Circulation 1998;98:I-679(Abstract)
40. Prestle J, Dieterich S, Preuss M, Bieligk U, Hasenfuss G: Heterogeneous transmural gene expression of calcium-handling proteins and natriuretic peptides in the failing human heart. Cardiovasc Res 1999;43:323-331

Chapter 2

ANATOMY AND ELECTROPHYSIOLOGY OF THE AV JUNCTION AND CORONARY SINUS
A Practical Guide for the Interventionist

David L. Ross
Department of Cardiology, Westmead Hospital and University of Sydney, Westmead, New South Wales, Australia

INTRODUCTION

Familiarity with the regions and characteristics of the AV node and coronary sinus is essential for the daily practice of modern clinical electrophysiology. Despite huge advances in knowledge in recent years, there remain significant gaps in understanding such as, for example, the precise anatomy and cellular electrophysiology of dual AV junctional ("nodal") pathways or the precise sites and mechanisms of slowing of conduction responsible for the property of decremental conduction that is so characteristic of the AV node.

1.   THE ATRIOVENTRICULAR (AV) JUNCTION

1.1   Anatomy

The atrial septal region is often misunderstood. There is only a relatively small area at and above the foramen ovale where the right and left atrial septal myocardium are in direct continuity. Below this area the right and left atrial muscle diverge to form the posterior septal or pyramidal space. The relations of this space were elegantly described in the pioneering publications of Sealy, Cox and colleagues in the early days of WPW surgery[1-4] and beautifully illustrated by Macalpine using meticulous dissection and photography.[5] The anterior apex of the space is formed by the central fibrous body at the conjunction of the

13

L. Bing Liem and E. Downar (eds.), Progress in Catheter Ablation, 13-28.

tricuspid, mitral and aortic valve annuli. The planes of the tricuspid and mitral valve annuli diverge as they extend posteriorly from the central fibrous body, with the mitral annulus located more superiorly. This means that the lower right atrial endocardium of the posterior septal space overlies the superior process of left ventricle. This part of the muscular ventricular septum is superior to the tricuspid annulus. The posterior interventricular groove at the junction of right and left ventricular walls extends into the floor of the posterior septal space with right ventricular myocardium forming the right posteroseptal floor of the space. Atrio-ventricular or ventriculo-atrial accessory connections in the posterior septal space usually arise from or insert into the superior left ventricular process of the interventricular septum. Right posteroseptal atrioventricular connections may insert directly into true right ventricular myocardium. Septal walls of the right and left atrium fuse at the superior apex of the posterior septal space just below the foramen ovale.

From its orifice just above the tricuspid valve, the coronary sinus runs horizontally across the posterior floor of the space to enter the posterior left atrio-ventricular groove. The compact AV node is located in the anterior third of the floor of the posterior septal space.[6,7] Its anterior extension penetrates the central fibrous body to become the bundle of His which descends through the membranous septum to bifurcate at the crest of the muscular interventricular septum into right and left bundle branches. The AV nodal artery is usually a branch of the distal right coronary artery or occasionally a dominant circumflex and runs anteriorly along the floor of the posterior septal space to penetrate the compact node. The posterior septal space is filled with fat interspersed with irregular strands of myocardium, fibrous tissue and neural elements. The tendon of Todaro is a linear fibrous strand extending from the Eustachian valve posteriorly to the central fibrous body anteriorly. It is a subendocardial structure that varies from a well-marked "tendon" to a few thin strands of collagenous tissue. An anatomical triangle termed the triangle of Koch is formed by the tendon of Todaro superiorly, the corresponding tricuspid annulus inferiorly and the os of the coronary sinus (see Figure 1 below). The anterior insertion of the tendon of Todaro is a reliable locator of the central fibrous body and allows inference of the likely position of the AV node at the apex of the triangle of Koch. The apex of the triangle of Koch is the site of the most proximal His bundle electrogram from an electrode catheter lying across the tricuspid annulus along the course of the His Purkinje system.

This space is much larger than is generally appreciated. The distance from the central fibrous body to the junction between the posterior septal space and the right free wall is 30 ± 4mm and from the central fibrous body to the junction of the posterior septal space and the left free wall is 29 ± 3mm. The length of the posterior epicardial border of the posterior septal space is 34 ± 5mm.[8] The distance from the inferior margin of the CS os to the adjacent tricuspid annulus is 13 ± 3mm.[9]

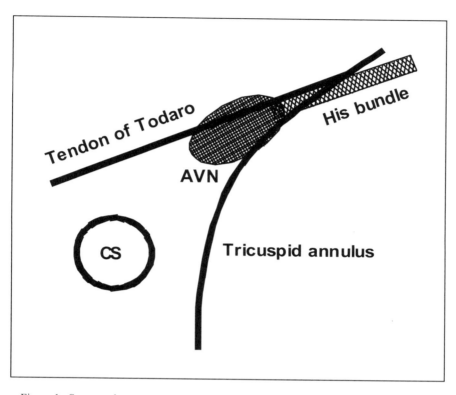

Figure 1. See text above

1.2   AV Nodal Electrophysiology, Transitional AV node and Atrionodal Connections

AV nodal cells are characterised by slow channel dependent depolarisation with resting membrane potential approximately –60mV. The predominant channels involved in Phase 0 depolarisation are calcium and slow sodium channels. These cells show decremental conduction with prematurity, which is the hallmark of AV nodal tissues. There is a gradation of cellular characteristics from atrial myocardium through transitional AV node to compact node then finally to the His bundle. The location of cells responsible for delay in the AV node was studied using cobalt deposition to label individual cells from which AV nodal action potentials were recorded.[10,11] The majority of such cells were in the compact node but there was significant dispersion to the posterior transitional zone. The precise routes of conduction from atrium to AV node and the precise cellular sites of delay and conduction block remain obscure. Gap junctions in AV nodal tissues are relatively small and sparse. The predominant connexins are 45 and 40.[12] Unlike the sinoatrial node, connexin 43 is also detectable but in small quantities. In the bundle of His and Purkinje system, connexins 40, 43 and 45 are abundant.[12]

Sympathetic agonists and enhanced sympathetic tone shorten conduction times and decrease refractoriness in the AV node. Vagal agonists and enhanced parasympathetic tone depress AV nodal conduction and prolong refractoriness. Calcium channel and beta adrenergic antagonists generally inhibit AV nodal conduction. Adenosine given in 6-24mg boluses intravenously is a potent inhibitor of the AV node; usually (but not always) causing total block in the AV node for 1-5 seconds. This is particularly useful in the electrophysiology laboratory for inducing temporary block or slowing of AV nodal conduction. Esmolol is a short acting beta blocker that is occasionally useful for producing more sustained inhibition of the AV node during electrophysiological studies than is feasible with adenosine.

Histological reconstructions show several relatively broad areas of apparent connections between atrium and the AV node. Right atrial endocardium inserts into the superior surface of the AV node extending from its posterior extent as far anteriorly as the point where the compact node penetrates the central fibrous body and becomes His bundle. Other connections come from the left atrium to the left margin of the AV node, including bundles of myocardium coursing immediately posterior to the aortic root. Scattered bundles of myocardium, which appear to arise from the coronary sinus, traverse the fat of the posterior septal space to join the posterior margin and superior surface of the AV node. There is considerable inter-individual variation in the presence or absence or extent of the various atrionodal connections. As noted in the opening paragraph, the precise routes of conduction through this complex structure at a 3 dimensional cellular level are unknown.

1.3   Types of AV Nodal Conduction

Normal conduction is characterised by smoothly progressive prolongation of AH interval with prematurity prior to block. In most normal humans the AH interval with the earliest conducted premature beat is prolonged by at least 100ms compared to baseline. The AV nodes of patients in whom the resting AH interval was abnormally short (<60ms) and who achieved less than 100ms maximum prolongation with atrial extrastimuli were labelled as manifesting "enhanced AV nodal conduction".[13] However, others did not find this definition to detect a specific subgroup and concluded that it described just one end of the spectrum of normal AV nodal conduction.[14]

A sudden increment in AH interval with prematurity producing 2 discontinuous AH versus AA curves indicates the presence of dual pathways.[15] The fast pathway of the dual pathways complex may have entirely normal AV nodal characteristics or may resemble enhanced AV nodal function.

Occasionally there are several discontinuities in AA versus AH curves suggestive of 3 or more AV nodal pathways.[16] Multiple AV nodal pathways may be present in the antegrade direction, retrograde direction, or both. Various combinations of these pathways may participate in tachycardia circuits. Thus some authors term the usual slow antegrade pathway, fast retrograde pathway form of AV node reentry as slow-fast tachycardia. The usual "atypical" form of AV node reentry is fast-slow AV node reentry. Some unusual forms of AV node reentry use different "slow" pathways for both antegrade and retrograde limbs of the tachycardia circuit and are termed slow-slow tachycardias. The tissues or connections responsible for slow pathway conduction are unknown. Tchou and colleagues have performed experiments separating the anterior and crista terminalis inputs to the AV node which suggest that these different inputs are a possible cause of dual AV nodal pathways.[17]

High frequency components of atrial electrograms in the region of the triangle of Koch have been considered to be slow pathway potentials and used to guide RF ablation of AV nodal reentrant tachycardia.[18] Others have described low frequency deflections following atrial electrograms that they also attributed to slow pathway potentials and used to guide RF ablation for AV nodal reentry.[19] However, similar high and low frequency potentials may be found in the triangle of Koch in most normal humans and animals without AV node reentrant tachycardia, suggesting that they are due to the complex anatomy of the area rather than specific markers for the slow pathway. McGuire and colleagues studied this question in pigs and dogs and concluded that the high frequency deflections following low frequency potentials in the posterior segment of the triangle of Koch were due to normal activation of muscle bundles adjacent to the CS os and not specialised slow pathway conduction and that AV junctional cells extending along the postero-septal tricuspid annulus with electrophysiological characteristics similar to AV nodal cells were probably responsible for slow pathway conduction.[20,21]

1.4   Catheter Recording From the AV Junction Area

Deflectable multipolar catheters (octa or decapolars are satisfactory) are useful for recording stable, clear, proximal His bundle electrograms. This arrangement permits several simultaneous bipolar His bundle electrograms to be recorded which enables antegrade versus retrograde depolarisation of the His bundle to be seen at a glance (this is useful for diagnosing atrio-fascicular tachycardias) and usually permits good low atrial electrograms adjacent to the His bundle region to be recorded which show whether atrial activation during retrograde conduction is earliest anteriorly or posteriorly in the triangle of Koch. Direct pacing of the His bundle is occasionally useful to study conduction via the His Purkinje system versus an accessory pathway. Retrograde His bundle potentials are often visible at the onset of QRS in the drive chain with ventricular pacing if good recordings of the His bundle potential are achieved in sinus rhythm as described above. If not, they often become apparent after the QRS with premature extrastimuli. This is due to retrograde conduction block in the right bundle branch with VA conduction then proceeding over the longer route via the left bundle branch.[22]   Pacing of the high right ventricular septum as described by Jackman can be useful for demonstrating retrograde His potentials during ventricular pacing when these are obscured by adjacent ventricular electrograms during standard right ventricular apical pacing and for distinguishing retrograde nodal from septal accessory pathway conduction.[23]

1.5   Variations in AV Junctional Anatomy

There is considerable normal variation in the size and shape of human AV nodes. Some are long and narrow, others short and wide. The density of atrial connections at various parts of the node also varies considerably. Some nodes have excrescences of nodal type tissue into the central fibrous body which appear to be blind ends surrounded by fibrous tissue and not connected to neighbouring atrium or ventricle. The amount of fat in the posterior septal space varies from minimal to extensive. Patients with AV canal defects have abnormal posterior displacement of the AV node to the right posteroseptal region between the os of the coronary sinus and the crest of the ventricular septum at the lower margin of the septal defect.[24]   The bundle of His runs anteriorly in the crest of the ventricular septum at the inferior margin of the defect. The AV node is said to be located normally in Ebstein's anomaly but there is usually right bundle branch block and a relatively high incidence of first degree AV block due to impaired conduction in the AV node suggesting disease induced damage or an abnormal structure. The septal and posterior tricuspid leaflets are those most commonly displaced in Ebstein's anomaly but the junction of the septal and anterior leaflets is usually at or near the central fibrous body which the His bundle penetrates in the usual place.[25]

Rare cases have been reported of RF lesions in the posterior segment of the triangle of Koch creating complete AV block suggesting an abnormal location of the AV node in the absence of associated congenital heart disease.[26]

1.6   Lessons From Surgical Dissections in the Perinodal Region

In patients with AV junctional reentrant tachycardia (AV nodal reentrant tachycardia) surgical section of atrial connections to the anterior segments of the AV node modified but did not usually abolish antegrade slow AV junctional pathways at late EP study but did modify retrograde conduction by lengthening retrograde HA intervals to a minor degree.[27]   This dissection usually abolished the usual type of AV node reentrant tachycardia. As with catheter RF ablation, single AV junctional echoes were often still inducible during antegrade slow pathway conduction but sustained AV junctional reentrant tachycardia (AV node reentry) was not inducible even with large doses of isoprenaline and atropine.

Surgical section of the posterior connections to the AV node for the more unusual form of AV junctional reentry where the atrial exit during tachycardia is posterior to the AV node (posterior AV junctional reentry) was usually successful in abolishing this type of tachycardia. As above, this dissection modified but did not usually abolish the antegrade slow pathway at late EPS but did usually modify VA conduction markedly. However, VA conduction was usually still demonstrable during isoprenaline infusion even if absent in the baseline state.

Detailed studies of the electrophysiology and histopathology of these dissections in dogs confirmed that they usually achieved section of the desired atrionodal connections although there was often some degree of associated damage to the AV node itself.[28,29]

In some patients with both anterior and posterior AV junctional reentry, both anterior and posterior connections to the AV node were dissected with successful abolition of both forms of tachycardia yet preservation of AV conduction. This indicates that additional connections to the AV node are present which maintain atrionodal continuity outside the areas dissected. Since this type of surgery involved dissection of the right atrial endocardium from the surface of the AV node to expose the posterior septal space, plus selective dissections of the inputs to the anterior segment of the AV node derived from the tissue of the posterior septal space and left atrial derived myocardium running to the AV node posterior to the aortic root, plus dissection of connections running from the coronary sinus towards the posterior margin of the AV node, the residual connections most likely run from the left atrium through the left margin of the posterior septal space to the left margin of the AV node. In other cases, posterior AV junctional reentrant tachycardia recurred after previous successful surgery for anterior AV junctional reentry and vice versa. This suggests that different tissues and circuits are responsible for these two types of AV nodal reentry although they probably share parts of their circuits.

Cox and colleagues performed cryoablation to the posterior approaches to the AV node and were able to abolish antegrade slow pathway conduction.[30,31] These lesions were in a similar area to that targeted nowadays for catheter RF ablation for AV junctional reentry.[18] A case report of the histopathological findings in a patient, in whom RF ablation successfully ablated antegrade slow pathway conduction and rendered tachycardia no longer inducible, confirmed that the lesion was located at the posterior approaches to the node rather than affecting the compact AV node itself.[32]

1.7   Accessory Ventriculoatrial Connections With Long Conduction Time

These are unusual accessory ventriculo-atrial connections that are usually but not always located in the posterior septal region. They have conduction times that are 2-3 times as long as the standard type of accessory pathway with VA intervals in tachycardia of 250ms or longer. Tachycardia is often frequently recurrent or incessant and initiated by almost any beat (sinus or ectopic) that activates the heart. These pathways are relatively disorganised long sinuous bundles running through the posterior septal space giving them their characteristic properties of long conduction times and decremental conduction.[33] These pathways can be ablated selectively by catheter or surgical techniques with preservation of normal AV nodal conduction. Dual antegrade AV nodal pathways and reentry in the region of the AV node may occur in association with this type of accessory pathway although presumably unrelated.

1.8   Nodoventricular Fibres and Atrioventricular Fibres

True nodo-ventricular fibres or Mahaim fibres have been reported to exist[34] and be amenable to surgical section.[35] However, the majority of tachycardias labelled as nodoventricular or Mahaim tachycardias are caused by connections between right atrial myocardium and the right ventricle well distant from the tricuspid annulus, in clear distinction from the usual type of accessory pathway that inserts into the ventricle close to the AV ring. These connections are now termed atrio-fascicular connections and have been shown to originate from the right atrium near the tricuspid annulus, usually anterolateral or lateral and well away from the AV node. They have decremental properties suggestive of AV nodal characteristics, often have a pathway potential between atrial and ventricular electrograms suggestive of a His bundle type electrogram, and insert distally into either the right bundle branch or the distal right ventricle. This latter feature suggests insulation of the distal pathway from surrounding ventricle prior to the insertion site in a similar manner to the His-Purkinje system. In other words, these unusual pathways have the characteristics of a duplicate AV conduction system. VA conduction is usually poor or absent over such pathways but is intact in rare cases.[36] Rarely, the atrial origin of these pathways may arise in the postero-septal area. Catheter RF ablation of atriofascicular connections is usually possible near the AV junction at the site where the His-bundle-like accessory pathway potential was recorded.

1.9   Role for Arrhythmia Surgery in the AV Junctional Area in the Era of Catheter Ablation

Although almost all of the common forms of supraventricular tachycardia can be cured by catheter RF ablation with repeat attempts if initially unsuccessful, there are occasional cases which are refractory to the full range of current technology. These cases are usually septal or right free wall accessory pathways or atriofascicular fibres. The usual reason for failure is that the pathway is deeper within the posterior septal space, out of range of RF lesions delivered by catheter to the endocardial surfaces of the space (right or left atrial endocardium or within the coronary sinus and its septal branches). Some of these pathways are amenable to catheter ablation using irrigated RF ablation catheters to produce deeper lesions. However, surgery remains a valuable option in refractory cases and is preferable to accidental or deliberate creation of complete AV block by excessive catheter ablation.

2.   CORONARY SINUS

2.1   Anatomy

The coronary sinus arises at the junction of the medial and inferior walls of the right atrium just above the tricuspid annulus and slightly inferior to the Eustachian valve at the junction of the inferior vena cava and the right atrium. There is often a funnel shaped cavity leading to the orifice of the coronary sinus demarcated by the Thebesian valve. This valve is usually attached posteriorly and inferiorly to the os, thereby deflecting the coronary sinus effluent superiorly along the septal surface of the right atrium when viewed in the LAO projection. The middle cardiac vein, otherwise known as the posterior interventricular vein, arises from the CS in the septal segment and runs inferiorly in the epicardium of the posterior interventricular groove. A circumflex tricuspid annular branch often joins the middle cardiac vein prior to its entry to the CS. There are often 1-2 additional small septal venous branches arising from the CS and running towards the left margin of the ventricular septum. A number of lateral left ventricular branches arise from the CS within the left atrioventricular groove. The distal coronary sinus becomes the anterior interventricular vein and runs parallel to the left anterior descending coronary artery over the anterior ventricular septum.

The vein of Marshall is the vestigial remnant of the left superior vena cava. It is a small vein that runs superiorly and obliquely across the posterior wall of the left atrium from its origin in the mid CS. This vein has been catheterised selectively using very small Cardima catheters.   Some authors have found arrhythmias to arise in this vein.[37]

The valve of Vieussens is located in the body of the CS usually distal to the origin of the oblique vein of Marshall. It is often a well-formed valve that can impede passage of catheters to the distal CS.

2.2   Connections Between Coronary Sinus and Adjacent Atrium

Myocardium extends along the wall of the CS.   Antz and colleagues demonstrated the functional presence of a direct left atrial to CS connection in a dog by surgically isolating the CS os.[38] Chauvin et al studied the anatomical connections between the CS and neighbouring atrium in man and found a wide range of connections ranging from 1-2 strands to a "widely intermingled continuum" of fibres.[39]

2.3   Dimensions

In adult hearts the CS is on average 73±10mm long as measured from the os to the origin of the anterior interventricular vein. The length of CS from its os to left margin of the posterior septal space is 23±4mm.[8] The distance from the central fibrous body to the nearest margin of the CS os is 17±3mm and from the lower margin of the CS os to adjacent tricuspid annulus 13±3mm.[9]

2.4   Anomalies of the Coronary Sinus

The most commonly encountered anomalies of the CS in electrophysiological practice are persistent left superior vena cavae draining into the CS and diverticulae within the posterior septal space.

A persistent left superior vena cavae usually enters the body of coronary sinus in the left AV groove. Venous catheters via the left arm then enter the CS directly and pass from the mid CS to proximal CS, in the reverse direction compared to normal CS cannulation. The proximal CS is usually dilated due to the extra flow and prominent on echocardiography.

CS diverticula extend from the CS into the crest of the ventricular septum either as blind sacs or connected to normal venous structures.[40] When diverticulae are associated with an AV accessory pathway, they are often refractory to the usual approaches with RF ablation to the posterior septum. Conduction proceeds from the atrium to the myocardium of the CS, then to the myocardium in the wall of the diverticulum, then inserts into the ventricle distally. Surgical dissection of the neck of the aneurysm usually interrupted pre-excitation.[40] RF ablation to the neck of the aneurysm is also usually successful.[41]

Rare anomalies include unroofing of the CS in the left atrium establishing direct drainage to that structure and various forms of arterio-venous malformations.

2.5   Course of Coronary Sinus in the Left Free Wall Relative to the Mitral Annulus

The CS tends to be displaced in the direction of the left atrium rather than lie exactly at the mitral annulus. Several authors have studied the relations of these structures.[42,43] The distance from the mitral annulus varies along its course.[43] The sites of closest apposition are usually in the proximal and distal CS with maximal deviation in the mid section. The site of widest deviation from the mitral annulus is usually in the posterolateral left free wall. This is important in mapping of left free wall pathways. Endocardial sites at the true annulus are usually earlier than the adjacent coronary sinus.

2.6   Does Coronary Sinus Anatomy vary With the Various Arrhythmias?

There is a clinical impression that the CS os is larger in patients with AV nodal reentrant tachycardia than others. Doig et al found the os and proximal CS to be more dilated than control patients.[44] Other workers performed a large series of angiograms in patients with supraventricular tachycardia and failed to find a significant correlation.[45]

2.7   Coronary Sinus Catheterisation and Angiography

The CS may be catheterised easily in most cases via either SVC or IVC approaches. A superior approach via antecubital, subclavian or internal jugular access was the initial method of choice and is still frequently used. However, the femoral approach proved to be effective too and has the advantages of minimising the number of access sites and has a lower complication rate compared to subclavian or internal jugular access.

Catheters with at least 10 electrodes are desirable for mapping the CS because they span a larger distance than quadpolar catheters and enable clear bracketing of an accessory pathway or detection of multiple left free wall pathways. Decapolar catheters are not more difficult to use than quadpolars for CS cannulation.

Entrance into the coronary sinus is facilitated nowadays by deflectable catheters. However, there are still occasions where it is difficult to cannulate the CS or pass a multipolar electrode catheter distally. Strategies to deal with this problem include initial cannulation with an ablation catheter to mark the route then subsequent passage of a decapolar catheter. This will often pass surprisingly easily alongside the other catheter. Catheters specifically designed to enter the CS are available commercially. An alternative and effective approach is use of a shaped long sheath. The sheath can usually be placed easily in the proximal CS and used for angiography as well as passage of an electrode catheter.

A relatively common clinical occurrence is an electrode catheter crossing the atrial septum to the left atrium via a patent foramen or unsuspected atrial septal defect. The catheter then usually follows an unusual course for the coronary sinus, does not usually have atrial and ventricular electrograms of similar size, and can often be advanced out a pulmonary vein beyond the cardiac silhouette.

In some individuals there is a relatively well developed inferomedial fossa of the right atrium at the base of the atrial septum posterior to the CS.[5] Catheters placed in an inferomedial fossa in the LAO view may appear quite a distance leftward and are not in the right ventricle in the RAO view. This can suggest that they have entered the CS but encountered an obstruction even though the CS has not been entered at all.

Angiography of the CS is necessary to show the true location of the CS os and the distal anatomy. Non-angiographic estimation of the location of the CS os by observing the plane of the septum from the lie of His and RV catheters in the LAO projection, or observing the site of prolapse when the catheter is advanced or anatomical landmarks like the vertebral bodies are relatively inaccurate.[46] There is often a pronounced curve to the septum so that the CS os is much further leftwards than suspected. CS angiography may be done by direct cannulation with an angiographic catheter or long sheath or purpose built CS electrode catheters with an angiographic lumen plus or minus a proximal balloon to enable better opacification. It may also be opacified in the venous phase of a left coronary angiogram.

2.8   Distal Cannulation of Coronary Sinus

Placing an electrode catheter in the distal CS to bracket the location of distal left free wall pathways is sometimes difficult. The usual sites of obstruction are at the Valve of Vieussens or a relatively sharp angulation in the distal CS as it passes under the base of the left atrial appendage. Distal placement may be easier via the IVC approach to the CS. Biplane CS angiography to define valves and branches helps in difficult cases. Deflectable catheters are also useful. Small diameter catheters such as those manufactured by Cardima may permit cannulation of the very distal CS.

2.9   Electrophysiology of Coronary Sinus

Since the CS lies close to the atrioventricular junction, the typical electrogram of the proximal CS has both atrial and ventricular electrograms of good size. More distally the relative sizes of atrial versus ventricular electrograms varies depending on the relative distances of the CS from adjacent atrium and ventricle which may vary as described above. Bipolar pacing within the CS usually captures local atrium but may pace the ventricle directly, especially in more distal locations. High output pacing in the distal CS commonly causes simultaneous pacing of both atrium and ventricle. The speed of conduction along the CS is fast, approximately 1metre/sec. This is faster than expected for atrial myocardium. In the presence of accessory pathways, unusual electrograms and accessory pathway potentials may be present. Jackman designed a catheter with 3 sets of 4 orthogonal electrodes to facilitate detection of accessory pathway potentials.[47] Multiple left free wall pathways or eccentric pathways may produce complex electrograms in the CS recordings.

2.10   Radiofrequency Ablation in the Coronary Sinus

Initially there were concerns whether this would be safe based on rupture of the CS caused by DC ablation in the CS. However, Huang and colleagues found in dogs that it was safe although there was some local thrombus formation acutely and occasionally sclerosis of neighbouring coronary arteries at late study.[48] Haissaguerre and colleagues confirmed the safety of this approach in humans.[49] RF ablation in the CS is often required for posterior septal pathways and may be needed for epicardial left free wall pathways. Coronary sinus occlusion has been reported as a complication of extensive RF within the CS but appears to be rare and not particularly symptomatic. Occasionally, occlusion of the distal right coronary artery with consequent myocardial infarction is induced by RF ablation in the proximal CS or middle cardiac vein.

Epicardial mapping and RF ablation of ventricular tachycardia via left ventricular veins is discussed elsewhere in this book.

CONCLUSIONS

Many important clinical arrhythmias involve the AV junction and coronary sinus. Increased knowledge and new technology have vastly improved our capacity to diagnose and treat these arrhythmias but much work remains to improve the technology and remove gaps in understanding of this crucial area of clinical electrophysiology.

REFERENCES

1. Sealy WC, Gallagher JJ. The surgical approach to the septal area of the heart based on experiences with 45 patients with Kent bundles. J Thorac Cardiovasc Surg. 1980;79:542-551.
2. Sealy WC, Mikat EM. Anatomical problems with identification and interruption of posterior septal Kent bundles. Ann Thorac Surg. 1983;36:584-595.
3. Sealy WC. Kent bundles in the anterior septal space. Ann Thorac Surg. 1983;36:180-186.
4. Cox JL, Ferguson TB, Jr. Surgery for the Wolff-Parkinson-White syndrome: the endocardial approach. Semin Thorac Cardiovasc Surg. 1989;1:34-46.
5. McAlpine WA. Heart and Coronary Arteries. 1 ed. Berlin: Springer-Verlag; 1975.
6. Truex RC, Smythe MQ. Reconstruction of the human atrioventricular node. Anat Rec. 1967;158:11-19.
7. Becker AE, Anderson RH. Morphology of the human atrioventricular junctional area. In: Wellens HJJ, Lie KI, Janse MJ, eds. The Conduction System of the Heart. Philadelphia: Lea and Febiger; 1976:263-286.
8. Davis LM, Byth K, Ellis P, McGuire MA, Uther JB, Richards DA, Ross DL. Dimensions of the human posterior septal space and coronary sinus [see comments]. Am J Cardiol. 1991;68:621-625.
9. McGuire MA, Johnson DC, Robotin M, Richards DA, Uther JB, Ross DL. Dimensions of the triangle of Koch in humans. Am J Cardiol. 1992;70:829-830.
10. Anderson RH, Janse MJ, van Capelle FJ, Billette J, Becker AE, Durrer D. A combined morphological and electrophysiological study of the atrioventricular node of the rabbit heart. Circ Res. 1974;35:909-922.
11. Janse MJ, Van Capelle FJL, Anderson RH, P T, Billette J. Electrophysiology and structure of atrioventricular node of the isolated rabbit heart. In: Wellens HJJ, Lie KI, Janse MJ, eds. The system of the heart. Philadelphia: Lea and Febiger; 1976:296-315.
12. Davis LM, Rodefeld ME, Green K, Beyer EC, Saffitz JE. Gap junction protein phenotypes of the human heart and conduction system [see comments] [published erratum appears in J Cardiovasc Electrophysiol 1996 Apr;7(4):383-5]. J Cardiovasc Electrophysiol. 1995;6:813-822.
13. Gallagher JJ, Sealy WC, Kasell J, Wallace AG. Multiple accessory pathways in patients with the pre-excitation syndrome. Circulation. 1976;54:571-591.
14. Jackman WM, Prystowsky EN, Naccarelli GV, Fineberg NS, Rahilly GT, Heger JJ, Zipes DP. Reevaluation of enhanced atrioventricular nodal conduction: evidence to suggest a continuum of normal atrioventricular nodal physiology. Circulation. 1983;67:441-448.
15. Denes P, Wu D, Dhingra RC, Chuquimia R, Rosen KM. Demonstration of dual A-V nodal pathways in patients with paroxysmal supraventricular tachycardia. Circulation. 1973;48:549-555.
16. Lee KL, Chun HM, Liem LB, Lauer MR, Young C, Sung RJ. Multiple atrioventricular nodal pathways in humans: electrophysiologic demonstration and characterization. J Cardiovasc Electrophysiol. 1998;9:129-140.
17. Tchou PJ, Cheng YN, Mowrey K, Efimov IR, Van Wagoner DR, Mazgalev TN. Relation of the atrial input sites to the dual atrioventricular nodal pathways: crossing of conduction curves generated with posterior and anterior pacing [see comments]. J Cardiovasc Electrophysiol. 1997;8:1133-1144.
18. Jackman WM, Beckman KJ, McClelland JH, Wang X, Friday KJ, Roman CA, Moulton KP, Twidale N, Hazlitt HA, Prior MI, et al. Treatment of supraventricular tachycardia due to atrioventricular nodal reentry, by radiofrequency catheter ablation of slow-pathway conduction. N Engl J Med. 1992;327:313-318.
19. Haissaguerre M, Gaita F, Fischer B, Commenges D, Montserrat P, d'Ivernois C, Lemetayer P, Warin JF. Elimination of atrioventricular nodal reentrant tachycardia using discrete slow potentials to guide application of radiofrequency energy [see comments]. Circulation. 1992;85:2162-2175.

20. McGuire MA, de Bakker JM, Vermeulen JT, Moorman AF, Loh P, Thibault B, Vermeulen JL, Becker AE, Janse MJ. Atrioventricular junctional tissue. Discrepancy between histological and electrophysiological characteristics. Circulation. 1996;94:571-577.
21. McGuire MA, de Bakker JM, Vermeulen JT, Opthof T, Becker AE, Janse MJ. Origin and significance of double potentials near the atrioventricular node. Correlation of extracellular potentials, intracellular potentials, and histology. Circulation. 1994;89:2351-2360.
22. Akhtar M, Gilbert C, Wolf FG, Schmidt DH. Reentry within the His-Purkinje system. Elucidation of reentrant circuit using right bundle branch and His bundle recordings. Circulation. 1978;58:295-304.
23. Hirao K, Otomo K, Wang X, Beckman KJ, McClelland JH, Widman L, Gonzalez MD, Arruda M, Nakagawa H, Lazzara R, Jackman WM. Para-Hisian pacing. A new method for differentiating retrograde conduction over an accessory AV pathway from conduction over the AV node. Circulation. 1996;94:1027-1035.
24. Thiene G, Wenink AC, Frescura C, Wilkinson JL, Gallucci V, Ho SY, Mazzucco A, Anderson RH. Surgical anatomy and pathology of the conduction tissues in atrioventricular defects. J Thorac Cardiovasc Surg. 1981;82:928-937.
25. Lev M, Gibson S, Millar RA. Ebstein's disease with Wolff-Parkinson-White syndrome: report of a case with histopathologic study of possible conduction pathways. Am Heart J. 1955;49:724.
26. Schaffer MS, Silka MJ, Ross BA, Kugler JD. Inadvertent atrioventricular block during radiofrequency catheter ablation. Results of the Pediatric Radiofrequency Ablation Registry. Pediatric Electrophysiology Society. Circulation. 1996;94:3214-3220.
27. Ross DL, Johnson DC, Denniss AR, Cooper MJ, Richards DA, Uther JB. Curative surgery for atrioventricular junctional ("AV nodal") reentrant tachycardia. J Am Coll Cardiol. 1985;6:1383-1392.
28. McGuire MA, Yip AS, Robotin M, Bourke JP, Johnson DC, Dewsnap BI, Chard R, Uther JB, Ross DL. Surgical procedure for the cure of atrioventricular junctional ("AV node") reentrant tachycardia: anatomic and electrophysiologic effects of dissection of the anterior atrionodal connections in a canine model. J Am Coll Cardiol. 1994;24:784-794.
29. McGuire MA, Robotin M, Yip AS, Bourke JP, Johnson DC, Dewsnap BI, Grant P, Uther JB, Ross DL. Electrophysiologic and histologic effects of dissection of the connections between the atrium and posterior part of the atrioventricular node. J Am Coll Cardiol. 1994;23:693-701.
30. Holman WL, Ikeshita M, Lease JG, Ferguson TB, Lofland GK, Cox JL. Alteration of antegrade atrioventricular conduction by cryoablation of peri-atrioventricular nodal tissue. Implications for the surgical treatment of atrioventricular nodal reentry tachycardia. J Thorac Cardiovasc Surg. 1984;88:67-75.
31. Cox JL, Holman WL, Cain ME. Cryosurgical treatment of atrioventricular node reentrant tachycardia. Circulation. 1987;76:1329-1336.
32. Gamache MC, Bharati S, Lev M, Lindsay BD. Histopathological study following catheter guided radiofrequency current ablation of the slow pathway in a patient with atrioventricular nodal reentrant tachycardia. Pacing Clin Electrophysiol. 1994;17:247-251.
33. Critelli G, Gallagher JJ, Monda V, Coltorti F, Scherillo M, Rossi L. Anatomic and electrophysiologic substrate of the permanent form of junctional reciprocating tachycardia. J Am Coll Cardiol. 1984;4:601-610.
34. Gmeiner R, Ng CK, Hammer I, Becker AE. Tachycardia caused by an accessory nodoventricular tract: a clinico- pathologic correlation. Eur Heart J. 1984;5:233-242.
35. Gallagher JJ, Selle JG, Sealy WC, Colavita PG, Fedor JM, Littmann L, Svenson RH, Zimmern SH. Variants of pre-excitation: update 1989. In: Zipes DP, ed. Cardiac electrophysiology: From cell to bedside. Philadelphia: W. B. Saunders; 1990:480-490.
36. Kreiner G, Heinz G, Frey B, Gossinger HD. Demonstration of retrograde conduction over an atriofascicular accessory pathway. J Cardiovasc Electrophysiol. 1997;8:74-79.
37. Hwang C, Wu TJ, Doshi RN, Peter CT, Chen PS. Vein of marshall cannulation for the analysis of electrical activity in patients with focal atrial fibrillation. Circulation. 2000;101:1503-1505.

38. Antz M, Otomo K, Arruda M, Scherlag BJ, Pitha J, Tondo C, Lazzara R, Jackman WM. Electrical conduction between the right atrium and the left atrium via the musculature of the coronary sinus. Circulation. 1998;98:1790-1795.

39. Chauvin M, Shah DC, Haissaguerre M, Marcellin L, Brechenmacher C. The anatomic basis of connections between the coronary sinus musculature and the left atrium in humans. Circulation. 2000;101:647-652.

40. Guiraudon GM, Guiraudon CM, Klein GJ, Sharma AD, Yee R. The coronary sinus diverticulum: a pathologic entity associated with the Wolff-Parkinson-White syndrome. Am J Cardiol. 1988;62:733-735.

41. Lesh MD, Van Hare G, Kao AK, Scheinman MM. Radiofrequency catheter ablation for Wolff-Parkinson-White syndrome associated with a coronary sinus diverticulum. Pacing Clin Electrophysiol. 1991;14:1479-1484.

42. Shinbane JS, Lesh MD, Stevenson WG, Klitzner TS, Natterson PD, Wiener I, Ursell PC, Saxon LA. Anatomic and electrophysiologic relation between the coronary sinus and mitral annulus: implications for ablation of left-sided accessory pathways. Am Heart J. 1998;135:93-98.

43. Yamanouchi Y, Igawa O, Hisatome I. Activation mapping from the coronary sinus may be limited by anatomic variations. Pacing Clin Electrophysiol. 1998;21:2522-2526.

44. Doig JC, Saito J, Harris L, Downar E. Coronary sinus morphology in patients with atrioventricular junctional reentry tachycardia and other supraventricular tachyarrhythmias. Circulation. 1995;92:436-441.

45. Weiss C, Cappato R, Willems S, Meinertz T, Kuck KH. Prospective evaluation of the coronary sinus anatomy in patients undergoing electrophysiologic study. Clin Cardiol. 1999;22:537-543.

46. Davis LM, Byth K, Lau KC, Uther JB, Richards DA, Ross DL. Accuracy of various methods of localization of the orifice of the coronary sinus at electrophysiologic study. Am J Cardiol. 1992;70:343-346.

47. Jackman WM, Friday KJ, Yeung-Lai-Wah JA, Fitzgerald DM, Beck B, Bowman AJ, Stelzer P, Harrison L, Lazzara R. New catheter technique for recording left free-wall accessory atrioventricular pathway activation. Identification of pathway fiber orientation. Circulation. 1988;78:598-611.

48. Huang SK, Graham AR, Bharati S, Lee MA, Gorman G, Lev M. Short- and long-term effects of transcatheter ablation of the coronary sinus by radiofrequency energy. Circulation. 1988;78:416-427.

49. Haissaguerre M, Gaita F, Fischer B, Egloff P, Lemetayer P, Warin JF. Radiofrequency catheter ablation of left lateral accessory pathways via the coronary sinus. Circulation. 1992;86:1464-1468.

Chapter 3

ANATOMY OF THE TRICUSPID CAVO ISTHMUS

Anton. E. Becker

Department of Cardiovascular Pathology, Academic Medical Center, University of Amsterdam, Amsterdam, The Netherlands

INTRODUCTION

The past decade has shown an almost explosive growth in electrophysiologic studies and catheter ablation procedures for cardiac arrhythmias. In the wake of this all a pressing need was felt to understand the underlying anatomy. Particularly so since some of the more frequent supraventricular tachyarrhythmias use reentrant circuits determined by preexistent anatomic pathways. One example, to be elaborated in this chapter, is atrial flutter. The typical situation is that of a counter clockwise reentrant circuit bordered on the one side by the tricuspid valve annulus and, on the other side, by the terminal crest.[1,2] Crucial for the genesis of a reentrant circuit is the presence of a delay-producing zone. The latter is generally accepted to be confined to the right atrial inferior wall between the entrance of the inferior caval vein, guarded by the Eustachian valve, and the tricuspid valve annulus immediately inferior to the os of the coronary sinus.[3,4] Cosio and coworkers[5] used radiofrequency catheter ablation in this particular zone to treat patients with common atrial flutter. They introduced the term "inferior vena cava-tricuspid isthmus". Since then the concept that this area serves as an electrophysiologic isthmus has been generally acknowledged and the term used often is shortened to either "tricuspid cavo isthmus", "posterior isthmus" or "flutter isthmus". It should be noted though that the term "posterior isthmus" was introduced because the tricuspid cavo isthmus was considered to be posterior to the os of the coronary sinus and the triangle of Koch. However, the right atrial wall between the Eustachian valve and the tricuspid valve annulus is not posterior, but rather inferior to Koch's triangle and, hence, is better termed "inferior isthmus". A right anterior oblique projection immediately will clarify this point. Indeed, the true anatomic relationships are

L. Bing Liem and E. Downar (eds.), Progress in Catheter Ablation, 29-38.

much more accurately expressed using the attitudinal approach to topography, by taking the body coordinates as points of reference, rather than the intrinsic cardiac coordinates, such as the cardiac long and short axes, which regrettably is common practice in electrophysiology.[6-8]

The following paragraphs will provide an account of the anatomy of the tricuspid cavo isthmus.

1.   BASIC ANATOMY

The general outline of the architecture of the tricuspid cavo isthmus has been well described recently by Cabrera and associates.[9]   From a practical viewpoint there are three distinct anatomic parts to be considered (Figure 1). First, a part that borders immediately upon the tricuspid annulus, composed of muscle with a smooth endocardial surface; this zone is known as the vestibule of the tricuspid valve. This particular smooth walled part of the tricuspid cavo isthmus is uniformly present in all hearts; thus far I have not seen an exception to this statement.

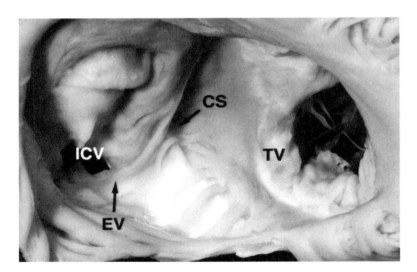

Figure 1.   Opened right atrium with transilluminated inferior wall in a simulated right anterior oblique position.   The tricuspid cavo isthmus is situated between the tricuspid valve (TV) annulus anteriorly and the Eustachian valve (EV) guarding the orificeof the inferior caval vein (ICV) posteriorly.   The isthmus is inferior to the os of the coronary sinus (CS). The isthmus contains a smooth walled part, the vestibule of the tricuspid valve, a trabeculated part, known as the sinus or recess, and the Eustachian valve.

The second and adjoining part, on the other hand, is highly variable in texture. It is part of the inferior right atrial wall, known as the sinus or recess, and often presents as a pouch-like expansion, which occasionally can be alsmot aneurysmal-like. This part extends between the Eustachian valve, guarding the orifice of the inferior caval vein, posteriorly and the vestibule, alluded to above, anteriorly. Hence, the area is anterior to the Eustachian valve and, therefore, should not be termed sub-Eustachian. In fact, as already emphasized, those in favor of an iconoclastic approach should use sub-Thebesian, since it is inferior to the os of the coronary sinus guarded by the Thebesian valve rather than sub-Eustachian. The floor of the sinus part consists of muscle bands, basically pectinate muscles, constituting the terminal postero-inferior ramifications of the terminal crest. The overall course of these pectinate muscles is anterosuperiorly, generally abutting upon the vestibular component and the adjoining site of the os of the coronary sinus. The thickness of the pectinate muscles varies considerably from one individual to the other and usually the atrial wall in between these muscle bundles is very thin. The arrangement of these bundles, moreover, may vary considerably, as will be discussed below. Furthermore, the width of the tricuspid cavo isthmus is markedly variable; Cabrera and coworkers[9] measured in their heart specimens an average width of 31∇4 mm, with a range of 19 to 40.

The third and final constituent of the tricuspid cavo isthmus is the Eustachian valve. It presents usually as a concentric flap, which guards the orifice of the inferior caval vein anteriorly. The transition between the sinus part of the isthmus and the Eustachian valve is not always distinct, since the muscular component of the sinus often extends also into the valve. Again, there is marked individual variability, as with the other parts of the isthmus, which will be dealt with separately.

It is of note, albeit beyond the context of this chapter, that the inferior right atrial wall, which constitutes the sinus part of the isthmus, largely overlies left ventricular myocardium, which swings in from the back to contribute to the formation of the ventricular septum, and is closely related to the so-called posteroseptal space. Occasionally, therefore, this area may serve as the target site for catheter ablation of accessory atrioventricular pathways with a left ventricular insertion.

2.   TRABECULAR ARRANGEMENTS

The detailed anatomy of the trabecular architecture of the right atrial inferior wall, the area designated above as the sinus part, together with the Eustachian valve, has been described recently from our own institution by Waki and coworkers.[10]   These authors examined 50 randomly selected heart obtained at autopsy from patients without atrial tachyarrhythmias. Within the setting of the basic trabecular arrangement alluded to above, considerable variability was noted, in fact to an extent that in not one heart was the arrangement of muscle bundles the same. Because of these differences an accurate classification was not feasible, other than a grouping into hearts with a more or less parallel arrangement of trabeculae and those in which the muscular arrangement showed abundant cross overs and interlacing trabeculae. The former trabecular pattern was designated as "uniform", whilst the latter was termed "non-uniform".

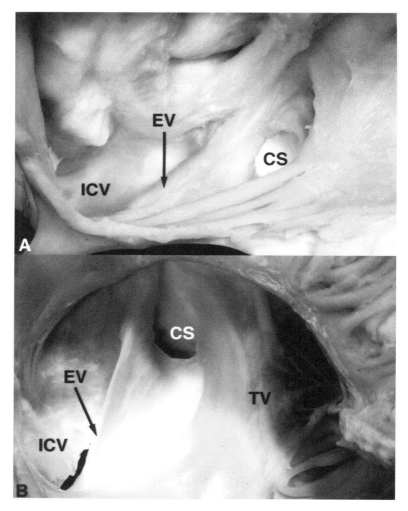

Figure 2. Examples of a so-called uniform trabecular allignment in the tricuspid cavo isthmus; specimens oriented and labelled as in Figure 1. (A) shows a solid muscular floor of the isthmus; (B) shows a large (transilluminated) fibrous part which extends into the inferolateral part of the Eustachian valve, next to smaller "defects". Reprinted with permission from reference 10.

It appeared that only a minority of the 50 heart specimens (13 of 50) presented with a uniform trabecular pattern (Figure 2). In three of the 13 hearts there was a solid myocardial floor without "muscular defects" between the trabeculae (Figure 2A). The remaining 10 hearts showed well aligned pectinate muscles separated by areas without appreciable myocardium; the occurrence of such "defects", or electrically silent zones, was usually more pronounced posterioly, towards the site of the inferior caval vein, and the areas varied in size from small to very large (Figure 2B). In all these cases the Eustachian valve contained a muscular extension from the terminal crest, although in 5 of these the most inferolateral part of the valve was fibrous without muscle (Figure 2B).

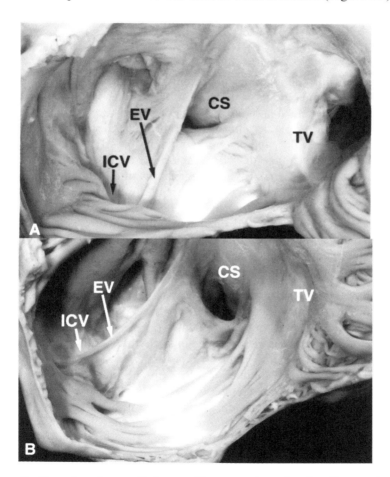

Figure 3. Examples of a so-called non-uniform muscular trabecular alignment in the tricuspid cavo isthmus; specimens oriented and labelled as in Figure 1. (A) shows a few relatively large (transilluminated) fibrous parts between the muscular trabeculae; (B) shows a multitude of such "defects." Note that non-uniformity is particular outspoken in the area adjoining the os of the coronary sinus. Reprinted with permission from reference 10. See also Color Plate 1.

The vast majority of the 50 heart specimens presented a non-uniform trabecular pattern (37 of 50) (Figure 3). The crossovers and interlacing trabeculae were generally most pronounced in the area immediately inferior to the os of the coronary sinus. In only 7 of the 37 hearts the pouch contained a solid muscle layer; the remaining 30 hearts showed a trabecular meshwork with a multitude of "defects", often with considerable variation in size (Figure 3A, B). In only 3 of these 30 hearts was the Eustachian valve almost completely fibrous.

3.   ANATOMY IN PERSPECTIVE OF ELECTROPHYSIOLOGY

It appears that the anatomy of the inferior right atrial wall known as the tricuspid cavo isthmus, often designated as the "flutter isthmus" because of the potential to produce the area of slow conduction necessary for a reentrant circuit, contains a highly variable muscular trabrecular architecture. Indeed, as demonstrated by Waki and coworkers[10] an orderly and nicely parallel arrangement of the pectinate muscles in this zone occurs in a minority of hearts only, whereas the vast majority contains a non-uniform muscular trabecular arrangement. The latter, moreover, particularly conspicuous in the area immediately inferior to the coronary sinus os. These observations are the more noteworthy since they are based on the examination of 50 randomly selected hearts obtained at autopsy from patients without atrial tachyarrhytmias. The question thus arises to what extent these observations affect current electrophysiological concepts pertaining to the genesis of atrial flutter?

There is no doubt that an area of slow conduction is a necessary part of a macro-reentrant circuit. And, many studies have pointed to the inferior right atrial wall as the crucial zone. Incremental pacing from the low lateral right atrium and coronary sinus os, during sinus rhythm, produced rate-dependent conduction delay in the low right atrial isthmus.[11] Atrial pacing, moreover, resulted in unidirectional conduction block in the area of the tricuspid cavo isthmus, which induced either counter clockwise or clockwise atrial flutter. These observations led to the conclusion that the low right atrial isthmus has slow conduction properties and, therefore, is critical to the development of atrial flutter in humans. Others have demonstrated in humans that the type of flutter induced depends on the site of induction.[12] Counter clockwise flutter was induced from the smooth right atrium and clockwise flutter was induced from the trabeculated right atrium. However, irrespective of the type of flutter the site of unidirectional block always occurred in the low right atrial wall, between the inferior caval vein and the tricuspid annulus, inferior to the os of the coronary sinus. The critical role of this particular site of the right atrial wall in atrial flutter was further endorsed by Feld and associates, [13] showing that patients with type 1 atrial flutter had a significantly slower conduction velocity in the "flutter isthmus" than patients without atrial flutter.

How does the anatomy of the tricuspid cavo isthmus fit into these electrophysiologic concepts?

It is tempting, given the concept of anisotropic conduction, to consider the non-uniform trabecular arrangement as important.[14,15] It is well accepted that conduction velocity in the longitudinal direction of muscle fibers is faster than the velocity perpendicular to the alignment of muscle fibers. Indeed, the normal action potential shows abrupt slowing and the extracellular wave front changes its shape at sites of muscle bundle branches or at junction of two separate muscle bundles. Spach and associates[14,15] considered these phenomena as caused by discontinuities of effective axial resistivity. This concept then becomes highly relevant when put in perspective of the anatomic observations, since a non-uniform trabecular arrangement in the tricuspid cavo isthmus is the rule rather than the exception. One can easily envision that this arrangement underlies non-uniform anisotropic conduction and, therefore, may lead to conduction delay. Moreover, progressive electrical uncoupling of side-to-side fibers has been shown to occur with advancing age;[16] a phenomenon which most likely relates to an age-dependent increase in endomysial collagen. The latter phenomenon may be further aggravated by volume loading and dilating, as is often the case in patients with atrial flutter, thus inducing progressive electrical uncoupling. This could also provide the explanation for the findings reported by Feld and associates[13] that conduction in the tricuspid cavo isthmus is slower in patients with atrial flutter compared to those without.

The question nevertheless remains why not all human beings develop atrial flutter, since after all the vast majority will possess a non-uniform trabecular arrangement in the inferior right atrial wall. Indeed, one may easily envision that any condition initiating an ectopic beat may induce a macro-reentrant atrial tachyarrhythmia because of the natural occurrence of a zone of normal conduction delay within the inferior right atrial wall. At the same time, inspection of the architecture of the pectinate muscles, as they originate from the terminal crest to produce the typical anatomy of the lateral wall of the right atrium, will reveal that non-uniformity in the trabecular arrangement is very common and certainly dominates normal anatomy. In other words, although electrophysiologic data very much point to the tricuspid cavo isthmus, a much larger anatomic area could be incriminated if we accept that non-uniform anisotropic conduction provides the background for the genesis of atrial arrhythmias. It could be worthwhile to keep this notion in mind when exploring the genesis and, in particular, the perpetuation of atrial tachyarrhythmias.

The above considerations also provide an alternative approach to attempts to understand the mechanisms that underlie atrial flutter. As indicated by Waki and co-workers,[12] the question "is there a particular anatomic substrate in the flutter isthmus that produces delay?" may well be redirected to "what has changed so that the normal potential for conduction delay in the flutter isthmus has become effective?".

From the point of view of the "ablationists" the anatomic characteristics of the sinus part of the tricuspid cavo isthmus are most relevant. It is presently well accepted that in order to interrupt the flutter circuit a linear ablation line is necessary. Arguments rage whether such a line of block should be produced between the Eustachian valve and the tricuspid valve annulus, inferior to the os of the coronary sinus, or whether the smooth vestibular part between the tricuspid valve and the os of the coronary sinus, known as the "septal isthmus", should be targeted. It is beyond the scope of this chapter to get involved in such a discussion. However, what does count is the fact that the muscular trabecular arrangement is highly variable, thus producing not only non-uniformity in the spatial arrangement of the muscle bundles, but also distinct irregularities in the endocardial surface lining. In addition, muscle bundles can be found throughout the isthmus, from the vestibular part up to the free edge of the Eustachian valve. Hence, in case of preference to create a line of block solely at the level of the vestibule, anterior to the os of the coronary sinus, one should be aware of the fact that a substantial number of individuals will contain muscular extensions from the terminal crest in the Eustachian valve, which run in an anterosuperior direction and cross the coronary sinus os posteriorly. In other words, from the morphologic viewpoint it is obvious that procedures to create a complete line of blockage have to overcome the difficulties of the complex and highly variable anatomy of the isthmus.

CONCLUSIONS

The tricuspid cavo isthmus is part of the right atrial inferior wall, delineated by the free edge of the Eustachian valve posteriorly, the tricuspid annulus anteriorly and the coronary sinus os superiorly. It contains a vestibular part, characterized by a smooth endocardial surface, a sinus part, often presenting as a pouch, which is highly trabeculated albeit most variable in architecture, and the Eustachian valve, which in the vast majority contains pectinate muscles. The pectinate muscles that constitute the muscular floor are derived from the terminal crest. In the vast majority of individuals these trabeculae show an outspoken non-uniform arrangement, with interlacing fibers and cross overs, particularly in the area close to the os of the coronary sinus. This arrangement may well be responsible for non-uniform anisotropic conduction and, therefore, a zone of conduction delay, considered crucial in the genesis of atrial flutter. Given the fact that non-uniform alignment is the rule rather than the exception, so that the normal anatomy of the pectinate muscles in the right atrium —and not only in the tricuspid cavo isthmus— could cater for sites that may generate conduction delay, and given the current concepts of the underlying mechanisms of atrial tachyarrhythmias in general, the key question to be addressed may need to be redirected to "what initiates the genesis of ectopic foci?"

REFERENCES

1. Kalman JM, Olgin JE, Saxon LA, Fisher WG, Lee RJ, Lesh MD. Activation and entrainment mapping defines the tricuspid annulus as the anterior barrier in typical atrial flutter. Circulation 1996;94:398-406.
2. Nakagawa H, Lazzara R, Khastgir T, Beckman KJ, McClelland JH, Imai S, Pitha JV, Becker AE, Arruda M, Gonzalez MD, Widman LE, Rome M, Neuhauser J, Wang X, Calame JD, Goudeau MD, Jackman WM. Role of the tricuspid annulus and the Eustachian valve/ridge on atrial flutter. Relevance to catheter ablation of the septal isthmus and a new technique for rapid identification of ablation success. Circulation 1996;94:407-424.
3. Olshansky B, Okumura K, Hess PG, Waldo AL. Demonstration of an area of slow conduction in human atrial flutter. J Am Coll Cardiol 1990;16:1639-1648.
4. Feld GK, Fleck RP, Chen PS, Boyce K, Bahnson TD, Stein JB, Calisi CM, Ibarra M. Radiofrequency catheter ablation for the treatment of human type I atrial flutter. Identification of a critical zone in the reentrant circuit by endocardial mapping techniques. Circulation 1992;86:1233-1240.
5. Cosio FG, Lopez-Gil M, Goicolea A, Arribas F, Barroso JL. Radiofrequency ablation of the inferior vena cava-tricuspid isthmus in common atrial flutter. Am J Cardiol 1993;71:705-709.
6. Cosio FG, Anderson RH, Kuck K-H, Becker AE, Borggrefe M, Campbell RWF, Gaita G, Guiraudon GM, Haissaguerre M, Rufilanchas JJ, Thiene G, Wellens HJJ, Langberg J, Benditt DG, Bharati S, Klein G, Marchlinski F, Saksena S. Living anatomy of the atrioventricular junctions. A guide to electrophysiologic mapping. A consensus statement from the Cardiac Nomenclature Study Group, Working Group of Arrhythmias, European Society of Cardiology, and the Task Force on Cardiac Nomenclature from NASPE. Circulation 1999;100:e31-e37.
7. Cosio FG, Anderson RH, Becker A, Borggrefe M, Campbell RW, Gaita F, Guiraudon GM, Haissaguerre M, Kuck KJ, Rufilanchas JJ, Thiene G, Wellens HJJ, Langberg J, Benditt DG, Bharati S, Klein G, Marchlinski F, Saksena S. Living anatomy of the atrioventricular junctions. A guide to electrophysiological mapping. A Consensus Statement from the Cardiac Nomenclature Study Group, Working Group of Arrythmias, European Society of Cardiology, and the Task Force on Cardiac Nomenclature from NASPE. Eur Heart J 1999;20:1068-1075.
8. Cosio FG, Anderson RH, Kuck K-H, Becker AE, Benditt DG, Bharati S, Borggrefe M, Campbell RWF, Gaita G, Guiraudon GM, Haissaguerre M, Klein G, Langberg J, Marchlinski F, Rufilanchas JJ, Saksena S Thiene G, Wellens HJJ. ESCWG/NASPE/P Experts Consensus Statement: Living anatomy of the atrioventricular junctions. A guide to electrophysiologic mapping. J Cardiovasc Electrophysiol 1999;10:162-170.
9. Cabrera JA, Sanchez-Quintana D, Ho SY, Medina A, Anderson RH. The architecture of the atrial musculature between the orifice of the inferior caval vein and the tricuspid valve: the anatomy of the isthmus. J Cardiovasc Electrophysiol 1998;9:1186-1195.
10. Waki K, Saito T, Becker AE. The right atrial flutter isthmus revisited – normal anatomy favors nonuniform anisotropic conduction. J Cardiovasc Electrophysiol 1999;11:90-94.
11. Tai CT, Chen SA, Chiang CE, Lee SH, Ueng KC, Wen ZC, Huang JL, Chen YJ, Yu WC, Feng AN, Chiou CW, Chang MS. Characterization of low right atrial isthmus as the slow conduction zone and pharmacological target in typical atrial flutter. Circulation 1997;96;2601-2611.
12. Olgin JE, Kalman JM, Saxon LA, Lee RJ, Lesh MD. Mechanism of initiation of atrial flutter in humans: site of undirectional block and direction of rotation. J Am Coll Cardiol 1997;29:376-384.
13. Feld GK, Mollerus M, Birgersdotter-Green U, Fujimura O, Bahnson TD, Boyce K, Rahme M. Conduction velocity in the tricuspid valve–inferior vena cava isthmus is slower in patients

with type I atrial flutter compared to those without a history of atrial flutter. J Cardiovasc Electrophysiol 1997;8:1338-1348.

14. Spach MS, Miller WT III, Dolber PC, Kootsey JM, Sommer JR, Mosher CE Jr. The functional role of structural complexities in the propagation of depolarization in the atrium of the dog. Cardiac conduction disturbances due to discontinuities of effective axial resistivity. Circ Res 1982;50:175-191.

15. Spach MS, Josephson ME: Initiating reentry: the role of nonuniform anisotropy in small circuits. J Cardiovasc Electrophysiol 1994;5:182-209.

16. Spach MS, Dolber PC. Relating extracellular potentials and their derivatives in anisotropic propagation at a microscopic level in human cardiac muscle. Evidence for electrical uncoupling of side-to-side fiber connections with increasing age. Circ Res 1986;58: 356-371.

Chapter 4

ARRHYTHMIAS FOLLOWING REPAIR OF CONGENITAL HEART DISEASE
Background and Scope of the Problem

George F. Van Hare
Department of Pediatric Cardiology, Stanford University School of Medicine, Palo Alto, California, USA

INTRODUCTION

When a child is born with congenital heart disease and requires surgical repair of the heart defect, most of the focus of the surgeon, cardiologist and parents is on obtaining as good a hemodynamic result as possible. For many defects, such as atrial or ventricular septal defects, atrioventricular canal defects, and tetralogy of Fallot, surgical results are excellent and one can expect to have a perfect or nearly perfect hemodynamic result, with complete closure of all septal defects, normal ventricular function, and normal valve function. With somewhat more complex defects, such as truncus arteriosus, double outlet right ventricle, and transposition of the great arteries, a modern surgical approach can also be expected to produce a normal or nearly normal hemodynamic situation, with an excellent long-term prognosis for the child. In even the most complex defects, including the single ventricle lesions, good results can also be obtained, prolonging life into adulthood and further. It is in this setting that one must consider the impact of late post-operative arrhythmias, both on the child who has undergone repair as well as on the parents of that child. It is extremely disappointing for the patient and the family to have an otherwise excellent hemodynamic result complicated by the occurrence of tachyarrhythmias, which can be annoying, debilitating, or even life threatening. Indeed, for many such patients, the late-appearing tachyarrhythmia is their only active cardiac problem.

Late post-operative arrhythmias contribute significantly to morbidity and mortality. Therefore, it is logical that every effort is made in patients with such arrhythmias to treat them and prevent their recurrence. Such treatments have included medical therapy with antiarrhythmic agents, implantation of anti-

L. Bing Liem and E. Downar (eds.), Progress in Catheter Ablation, 39-57.
© 2001 *Kluwer Academic Publishers. Printed in the Netherlands.*

tachycardia pacemakers, catheter ablation, and surgical ablation. Unfortunately, there are serious limitations to the effectiveness, applicability and safety both of antiarrhythmic drug therapy and of anti-tachycardia pacing. Not surprisingly, ablative techniques, which potentially offer a curative treatment, are favored, but such techniques have not been as successful as initially hoped. While one can expect an overall success rate of >90% for radiofrequency ablation in children with most types of heart rhythm disorders, the success rate is substantially lower for children with repaired congenital heart disease, and the recurrence rate following initially successful ablation is very high. It is hoped that the advent of new energy sources and mapping technology will advance the field of post-operative arrhythmia ablation.

In this chapter, the substrate for tachycardia will be discussed, as it is influenced both by the initial cardiac defect and by the subsequent surgical repair, and also how it evolves with the passage of time. Information about actual mapping and ablation techniques will be discussed in other chapters of this text.

Post-operative tachyarrhythmias tend to group themselves into four main groups, based on type of defect, type of tachycardia, and current success rates of radiofrequency ablation attempts. The first group, which will be termed "simple atriotomy-based atrial flutter" included patients who have had simple cardiac repairs such as atrial septal defects, ventricular septal defects, tetralogy of Fallot, atrioventricular canal defects, and related defects. The second group, which will be termed "intra-atrial reentry following atrial repair of transposition" included patients who have had either the Mustard or the Senning procedure. The third group, termed "intra-atrial reentry following the Fontan procedure" included patients who have undergone the various forms of the Fontan procedure, perhaps excluding those with the external conduit variety in which there is no atriotomy. Finally, a fourth group, called " ventricular tachycardia following tetralogy repair" includes tetralogy of Fallot patients, as well as those with related lesions such as certain types of double outlet right ventricle. For each group, the anatomic details which support the tachyarrhythmia and which are important in ablation will be discussed.

1.   ATRIAL ANATOMY AND ELECTROPHYSIOLOGY

As atrial flutter and nearly all types of post-operative IARTs seem to involve only the anatomic right atrium, the exact anatomy of the right atrium becomes important in understanding these arrhythmias. Therefore, a detailed knowledge of right atrial anatomy is essential for effective mapping and ablation of IART and atrial flutter.

During cardiac embryological development, the right atrium is thought to be derived from three sources.[1] The primitive right atrium forms adjacent to the tricuspid annulus and gives rise to the heavily trabeculated right atrial freewall and right atrial appendage. The sinus venosus is incorporated into the right atrium and provides the origin for the smooth-walled portion of the right atrium (sinus venarum) which exists between the cavae posterior to the primitive right atrial structures. Finally, septation of the primitive common atrium is accomplished by the formation of the atrial septum from septum primum and septum secundum. The ostium secundum is a foramen that forms in the septum primum, which is subsequently closed by the septum secundum, which forms a flap over this ostium to create the foramen ovale. The foramen ovale provides a route for right atrial blood to cross the left atrium in the fetal circulation. All along the junction between the primitive right atrium and the sinus venosus portion of the right atrium is the crista terminalis ("terminal crest"), which appears as a ridge along the inner surface of the right atrium. The crista terminalis runs from superior to inferior along the lateral wall of the right atrium. At its superior edge, near the superior vena cava-right atrial junction, is the sinus node pacemaker complex. As it arches inferiorly toward the inferior vena cava, it gives rise to the Eustachian valve ridge (EVR), which appears as more of a flap than a ridge. The EVR is a remnant of the primitive right sinoatrial valve, guarding the ostium between the sinus venosus and primitive right atrium. The EVR runs anterior to the inferior vena caval orifice and posterior to the posterior portion of the tricuspid valve annulus. As such, in the fetal circulation, the EVR acts to direct inferior vena caval (IVC) flow away from the tricuspid annulus and toward the foramen ovale. This feature provides one element of the separation between higher-oxygenated placental blood returning via the IVC to the left atrium, ventricle and upper body, from the lower oxygenated SVC return which enters the right ventricle, pulmonary artery and ductus arteriosus to the descending aorta and placenta. As the EVR arches toward the inferior atrial septum, it passes just superior to the ostium of the coronary sinus. It joins with the valve of the coronary sinus to form the tendon of Todaro, which inserts on the atrial septum near to site where the His bundle is recorded. With the coronary sinus ostium and the tricuspid annulus, the tendon of Todaro forms the triangle of Koch, and at the apex of this triangle, the compact atrioventricular node is found.

1.1　Typical and Reverse Typical Atrial Flutter

Classical atrial flutter is characterized by atrial rates of approximately 300 beats per minute with typical and very characteristic "saw-tooth" flutter waves visible on the surface electrocardiogram. This suggests the presence of nearly continuous atrial activity, due to the relative lack of a long atrial isoelectric interval. In typical atrial flutter, the flutter waves are prominent and are negative in leads II, III and AVF, suggesting inferior to superior atrial activation. While initially thought to represent reentry around the caval veins or around the tricuspid valve annulus, the work of multiple investigators has clearly established the actual circuit. Impulses emerge from an isthmus of atrial tissue between the inferior vena cava and tricuspid annulus to spread up the atrial septum, activating the atrium at the site of the His bundle recording, and then down the right atrial free wall the enter the isthmus again.[2]   This counterclockwise activation has recently been categorized as "typical" atrial flutter, while atrial flutter which utilizes the same circuit but in the clockwise order of activation has been categorized as "reverse typical" atrial flutter.[3]   In addition, further details have been provided recently, using techniques of entrainment pacing which depend on the demonstration of equivalence of the post-pacing interval (PPI) during entrainment and the tachycardia cycle length (TCL) to establish that any given site is in the circuit (PPI=TCL). These studies have demonstrated the importance of the crista terminalis and Eustachian valve ridge as sites of conduction block during atrial flutter.[4-6]   Conduction block is suggested by the demonstration that there are sites along the ridge where double potentials can be recorded.[5-8]   The importance of such areas of conduction block is strengthened by entrainment pacing, demonstrating that atrial myocardium on one or another side of the line of conduction block is part of the circuit. The critical nature of these lines of block is proven by radiofrequency ablation lesions that are designed to bridge from one line of block to another, with resultant abolition of the atrial flutter.[9-11] These criteria have been satisfied with both typical and reverse typical atrial flutter, and the features of the circuit now seem well characterized.

As previously described, the wave of activation leaves the region of the tricuspid valve-inferior vena cava isthmus to climb the inter-atrial septum and enter the heavily trabeculated right atrial freewall in the region of the superior vena cava. It then spreads down the right atrial freewall, with the crista terminalis behind and the tricuspid annulus in front, turning counter-clockwise around the tricuspid annulus when viewed from below (LAO view fluoroscopically). As the wave of activation turns posteriorly, it enters a "funnel", as described by Nakagawa,[6] created because the distance between the crista and the tricuspid annulus becomes progressively shorter. The wave is funneled to the isthmus between the inferior vena cava and tricuspid valve annulus, now with the annulus anterior and inferior, and the EVR (the extension of the crista terminalis) posterior and superior. It is important to note that at this site, the EVR bisects the isthmus between the IVC and tricuspid valve, and that it is the EVR, not the IVC, which provides the critical site of conduction block. As it enters the inter-atrial septum, the wave again spreads in a superior fashion along the septum for the next circuit. Atrial flutter can be effectively attacked using radiofrequency ablation either at the septal site of EVR insertion, by lesions which bridge from the tricuspid valve to the EVR,[6] or posteriorly, from the tricuspid annulus down to the IVC.[9]

2.   POST-OPERATIVE ARRHYTHMIA SUBSTRATES

2.1   Simple Atriotomy-Based Atrial Flutter

When performing surgery to repair a simple secundum atrial septal defect, the surgeon typically places a long incision in the right atrial freewall, which is oblique and runs from the right atrial appendage laterally down towards, but not to, the tricuspid annulus or IVC. Care is typically taken to avoid the sinus node, and this concern results in the crista terminalis not being incised. This incision gives adequate exposure for repair of atrial septal defects, and is also used for the atrial approach to repair of ventricular septal defects, either alone or as part of tetralogy of Fallot. The atrial septal defect itself is commonly closed using sutures, but for large defects, a patch may be employed.

This surgical approach clearly creates a long line of permanent conduction block, which is entirely in the trabeculated right atrium, anterior to the crista terminalis. This anatomy potentially creates a tunnel of atrial tissue between the crista and the atriotomy, and another between the atriotomy and the tricuspid annulus. Such tunnels can easily be imagined as the required protected zones of conduction, mediating IART. Numerous patients have now been reported who exhibit "incisional" IART in which the atriotomy seems to act as the critical barrier,[12] and in such patients, radiofrequency application from the atriotomy to either the IVC, tricuspid annulus, or SVC has been successful in terminating tachycardia and preventing re-induction.

Because the atrial structures that support typical atrial flutter are also present, and because such patients often have the other risk factors for the development of flutter (atrial dilation, fibrosis, etc.), post-operative patients may also have typical atrial flutter. Furthermore, as has become apparent in patients with otherwise structurally normal hearts, such IART and flutter circuits can run in either direction (counter-clockwise or clockwise). This potential variability creates the possibility for several distinct P-wave morphologies and atrial cycle tachycardia cycle lengths. Finally, in patients who have undergone patch closure of a secundum atrial septal defect, the patch itself has been reported to be a possible site of conduction block, mediating tachycardia.[9]

Patients may, of course, have several reentrant circuits. One commonly observes typical atrial flutter, and after successful ablation, a second IART with a longer or shorter tachycardia cycle length and non-involvement of the flutter isthmus, or indeed of any structure posterior to the crista terminalis. The slower cycle length of such IARTs may be due to conduction that is confined to the heavily trabeculated atrial freewall, in which atrial conduction may be slower, or alternatively may reflect slow conduction due to fibrosis.

2.2   Intra-atrial Reentry Following Atrial Repair of Transposition

The Senning and Mustard procedures are similar operations meant to address the hemodynamic abnormality in transposition, by directing systemic return to the left ventricle and pulmonary artery, and directing pulmonary venous return to the right ventricle and aorta.[13,14] While very successful, these operations are for the most part no longer done, in part because of the success of the arterial switch procedure, and in part due to the high incidence of atrial arrhythmias and increased risk of sudden death. However, there has recently been interest in the so-called "double switch" procedure as a strategy for managing patients with L-transposition (congenitally corrected transposition) and in the procedure, a Senning atrial baffle is constructed.[15] Therefore, this surgical substrate may not, in fact, disappear. In the Mustard procedure, after a long atriotomy anterior to the crista terminalis and resection of the atrial septum, a baffle is constructed and sewn into place around each caval vein, through the isthmus between the IVC and tricuspid annulus, and to the posterior wall of the left atrium, so that caval flow is direct to the mitral annulus.[14] Pulmonary venous flow travels around the baffle and finds the tricuspid annulus. It is important to note that the baffle, where it is sewn into place along the tricuspid annulus, has the same function as the EVR in fetal life, that is to prevent IVC flow from reaching the tricuspid valve. Furthermore, surgical technique is directed at avoiding injury to the sinus node, so the crista terminalis is not disturbed. Finally, various approaches are used to avoid atrioventricular block, and often these lead to the coronary sinus being incorporated into the pulmonary rather than systemic venous atrium.[16] These details leave the entire right atriotomy, as well as the isthmus of atrial tissue between the EVR and tricuspid annulus, in the new pulmonary venous atrium. The one exception is the situation in which the coronary sinus drainage is the systemic venous atrium, in which a catheter can reach the flutter isthmus from the IVC.

In most respects, the Senning procedure is similar electrophysiologically to the Mustard procedure. The Senning procedure was designed to use mostly atrial tissue rather than artificial material to construct the baffle.[13] In order to accomplish this, two atrial incisions are made. The first is in the right atrium, longitudinal, parallel and anterior to the crista terminalis. The second, in the left atrium, is parallel to the first and between the right pulmonary veins and interatrial septum. A U-shaped incision in the atrial septum is made, just above the coronary sinus, leaving the flutter isthmus intact. This flap of atrial septum is sewn to the back of the left atrium, to the left of the left pulmonary veins. The flap of right atrial freewall is sewn into place near or at the site of the EVR, preventing IVC flow from crossing the tricuspid valve. The left atrial incision is closed by sewing to the other edge of the right atrial incision. As in the Mustard procedure, both the flutter isthmus and the right atriotomy are part of the new pulmonary venous atrium.

Typically, and predictably based on the above, one commonly finds two types of IART in such patients. First, typical atrial flutter is usually present, utilizing the usual anatomic structures as barriers to support reentry. Second, true "incisional" IART is often found, and is confined to the anatomic trabeculated right atrium, with the wave of activation passing between the lower limit of the atriotomy and the tricuspid annulus. Patients have been studied who exhibited a sudden shift from one tachycardia, involving the flutter isthmus, to a second tachycardia, not involving this isthmus but instead involving the atriotomy, resulting from successful RF ablation at the flutter isthmus. Such a phenomenon may be an indication of true "figure of eight" reentry, with ablation of one, but not both, limbs of the figure of eight. Because most of these critical structures are in the new pulmonary venous atrium, the approach for ablation is not straightforward, and often, the arrhythmia must be approached either via a leak or separation in the baffle, or by a retrograde trans-aortic approach.[17]

One can speculate that the presence of a suture line at the site of the EVR in such patients might cause fibrosis and conduction delay, perhaps dramatically increasing the likelihood that atrial reentry will occur.

2.3   Intra-atrial Reentry Following the Fontan Procedure

The Fontan procedure has changed many times since its development as a palliative procedure for patients without two functional ventricles, as a way of relieving ventricular volume overload and of normalizing arterial saturations.[18] Initially, it was thought that the right atrium could be used as an effective pumping chamber, provided that pulmonary artery pressures were low (atriopulmonary connection). Largely as a result of an extremely high incidence of atrial arrhythmias after such procedures, as well as concerns about hydrodynamic energy loss in the system and pulmonary venous obstruction, this approach has been abandoned in favor of approaches that bypass the heart entirely (total cavo-pulmonary connection via the lateral tunnel or via an external conduit).[19] Within each of the two categories, many modifications exist. Despite the approach of total cavopulmonary connection, atrial arrhythmias continue to be observed, and surgical details are critical in planning mapping and ablation procedures in such patients.

With the various forms of atriopulmonary connection, there is a long atriotomy placed. In patients who had a conduit from the right atrium to pulmonary artery, and those in whom the right atrial appendage was connected directly to the pulmonary artery or right ventricular outflow tract, this atriotomy was anterior to the crista terminalis. Often in such patients, patch augmentation of the right atrium was performed, using a piece of pericardium or other material incorporated into the closure. Invariably, closure of a large atrial septal defect was also necessary. As in the simpler situation of ASD repair (above) both typical atrial flutter as well as incisional reentry around the anterior atriotomy are possible and have been observed. In excellent multi-site mapping studies using basket catheters, slow conduction up the lateral wall has been demonstrated by Triedman, et al.,[20] and this configuration fits the concept of conduction in a long isthmus bounded by the atriotomy and the crista terminalis. Reentry around the ASD patch is also possible. Finally, patch closure of the tricuspid annulus has been occasionally performed in patients with single ventricle without tricuspid atresia, potentially creating areas of slow atrial conduction on the other side of the suture line.

Catheter ablation in the atriopulmonary connection type of Fontan has been quite disappointing, in contrast to the experience with atrial septal defect repair and with Mustard and Senning procedure patients.[12,17,21-23] It is uncertain why this is the case, but multiple tachycardia circuits and a high incidence of recurrence after initial success have been observed. It may be that with high atrial pressures, the resulting thickening of the atrial wall due to atrial hypertrophy prevents the development of full transmural lesions. Alternatively, sluggish blood flow may not allow adequate tip cooling, limiting energy delivery and resulting in ineffective lesions.

More recent innovations involving total cavopulmonary connection by the lateral tunnel technique are clearly associated with better hemodynamics and lower atrial pressures. Unfortunately, IART is still frequently observed in such patients. In order to exclude the atrium, the SVC is connected directly to the pulmonary artery, and a tunnel is created which directs IVC flow to the underside of the pulmonary artery. The baffle which accomplishes this is similar to that used in the Mustard or Senning procedure, with a line of sutures going through the region of the EVR and with the baffle directing IVC flow away from the tricuspid annulus. The long atriotomy used to construct the lateral tunnel is closed and this suture line is in the new pulmonary venous atrium. This anatomy creates the potential for reentry in the usual flutter circuit, as well as incisional IART involving the right atriotomy, which has been elegantly demonstrated in an animal model by Rodefeld and colleagues.[24] There is not yet sufficient experience with RF ablation in this particular anatomic substrate to comment on the effectiveness, but one would expect similar results to those reported for the Senning and Mustard procedures.

3.   VENTRICULAR ARRHYTHMIAS

3.1   Ventricular Tachycardia Following Tetralogy Repair

Ventricular tachycardia remains as one of the most difficult management problems in patients who have previously undergone surgical repair of tetralogy of Fallot and other related congenital heart defects. Typically, in such patients, surgery has taken place years or decades prior to the presentation of ventricular tachycardia or the occurrence of a fatal arrhythmic event. The actual etiology of sudden death in patients following tetralogy repair is still somewhat uncertain. However, because of the frequent occurrence of premature ventricular contractions, nonsustained and sustained ventricular in patients who have undergone complete repair of tetralogy of Fallot and related defects such as double outlet right ventricle,[25-31] ventricular tachycardia has been implicated in the etiology of sudden death in this patient group. Indeed, it is known that post-operative tetralogy of Fallot is the single most common condition seen in children between the ages of 1 and 16 years who have experienced sudden death.[32]

The majority of available information concerning patients with ventricular tachycardia and congenital heart disease pertains to tetralogy of Fallot, as compared with other forms of congenital heart disease. Ventricular arrhythmias do occur, but are much more rare, in patients with other lesions.[33] However, for the purposes of management, tetralogy of Fallot can be viewed as an archetype for other lesions, when patients with other lesions present with ventricular arrhythmias in the setting of ventriculotomy and/or right ventricular dysfunction.

Great controversy still exists regarding the role of various risk factors for the occurrence of ventricular arrhythmias and sudden death, the exact relationship between ventricular arrhythmias and sudden death, the role of electrophysiologic study and other procedures for risk stratification, and ultimately the appropriate management of post-operative patients with ventricular tachycardia. It is only recently that major advances in understanding the role of antiarrhythmic agents and implantable cardioverter-defibrillators in patients with coronary disease have been made, due to the conduct of large multi-center trials.[34-36] One can understand the much greater challenge of answering similar questions in this much smaller patient population. Indeed, Bricker has pointed out that sufficient numbers of post-operative patients may not be available to perform an adequately powered cohort study to sort out the various likely predictors of sudden death, even in a multi-center study.[37]

One must consider the changes in surgical technique that have taken place over the years to understand how patient age, age at repair, and method of repair may interact to increase the risk of arrhythmias. The first complete repair of tetralogy of Fallot was performed in 1954 by Dr. W.C. Lillehei.[38] Starting in the 1960's, complete repair of this defect became commonplace. While infants were corrected from the beginning, the mortality rate was high, and it was more usual for patients to undergo repair later, often as late as the second or even third decade of life. Starting in the 1970's, due to improvements both in surgical technique and post-operative care, some centers chose to perform primary repair in infancy, with good results, and this is now the current practice everywhere.

Patients with tetralogy of Fallot have a ventricular septal defect with some degree, usually severe, of right ventricular outflow tract obstruction, leading to chronic cyanosis. The placement of a systemic-to-pulmonary artery shunt as a palliative procedure adds the element of potential left ventricular volume overload. Correction of the defect involves patch closure of the ventricular septal defect with relief of right ventricular obstruction. In nearly all patients, this requires resection of a large amount of right ventricular muscle, and early in the experience, this was not done via an atriotomy with retraction of the tricuspid valve, but instead required a ventriculotomy. Finally, in tetralogy, the pulmonary annulus is typically smaller than normal. This has been approached by the placement of a transannular patch, which leads to chronic pulmonic insufficiency. Pulmonic insufficiency may be very severe if it is associated with downstream obstruction related to significant pulmonary arterial stenosis. It has been hypothesized that ventricular arrhythmias are due to the effect of years of chronic cyanosis, followed by the placement of a ventriculotomy, with elevation of right ventricular pressures due to inadequate relief of obstruction, and severe pulmonic regurgitation with right ventricular dysfunction and enlargement.[25,39-41] Such factors as wall stress and chronic cyanosis, coupled with the passage of time, may lead to myocardial fibrosis and result in the substrate for reentrant ventricular arrhythmias. This hypothesis is supported by histologic examination of the hearts of patients with tetralogy of Fallot who had died suddenly. These studies have shown extensive fibrosis.[42] The hypothesis is also supported by the observation of fractionated electrograms and late potentials, recordable from the right ventricle at electrophysiologic study, suggesting the presence of slow conduction.[43,44] While there is a 5% incidence of coronary artery abnormalities in tetralogy of Fallot, putting the left anterior descending coronary artery or other large branches at risk at the time of complete repair, such potential damage has never been implicated in the etiology of ventricular arrhythmias or of sudden death. Garson[45] has attempted to create an animal model of post-operative tetralogy of Fallot, in which a ventriculotomy was placed along with the placement of a pulmonary artery band to produce right ventricular systolic hypertension. It is notable that these animals did not have pulmonic insufficiency, and had not gone through a period of cyanosis. Such animals were observed to have frequent ventricular ectopy, and some had inducible ventricular tachycardia, for which the method of induction by programmed stimulation suggested a mechanism involving triggered activity rather than reentry.[45]

Careful electrophysiologic studies in patients with ventricular tachycardia following tetralogy surgery have supported the concept that the mechanism of tachycardia is macroreentry, which involves the right ventricular outflow tract, either at the site of anterior right ventriculotomy or at the site of a ventricular septal defect patch. Transient entrainment has been documented, with constant fusion at the paced cycle length and progressive fusion at decreasing cycle lengths. Furthermore, the evaluation of post-pacing intervals strongly suggests that sites in the right ventricular outflow tract are part of a macro-reentrant circuit.[46,47]

Early reports noted the frequent occurrence of premature ventricular contractions in patients who had previously undergone tetralogy of Fallot repair. Gillette, et al. identified premature ventricular contractions on routine electrocardiograms in 18% of patients.[25] With exercise testing, the incidence may increase, to around 20% in one study.[30] With Holter monitoring, the incidence of ventricular ectopy is reported to be as high as 48%.[48] In about half of these patients, ventricular ectopy is complex, defined as multiform beats, couplets or ventricular tachycardia. In the great majority of patients, this ventricular ectopy is entirely asymptomatic.

Many investigators have tried to correlate the incidence of ventricular ectopy with various factors, including age at presentation, age at time of repair, and various hemodynamic features. Four factors seem to be the most important: 1) age at initial repair; 2) time since repair; 3) presence of residual right ventricular obstruction; and 4) presence of significant pulmonic insufficiency. Older age at time of operation, especially beyond 10 years of age, was associated with nearly a 100% incidence of ventricular arrhythmias, regardless of follow-up interval, in Chandar's multi-center study.[48] In the same study, time since repair also predicted the occurrence of ventricular ectopy, which occurred in 4/4 patients followed for >16 years despite repair in infancy. Walsh, however, showed that in a group of patients repaired at less than 18 months of age, ventricular ectopy was rare on electrocardiogram (1%) but more common on Holter (31%) after an average of 5 years follow-up.[49]

Garson et al. in a study of 488 patients with repaired tetralogy of Fallot, showed that the incidence of ventricular arrhythmias was closely related to right ventricular hemodynamics.[50] The incidence of ventricular arrhythmias was significantly higher in those with a right ventricular systolic pressure > 60 mmHg, and in those with a right ventricular end-diastolic pressure > 8 mmHg, suggesting that residual right ventricular outflow tract obstruction as well as pulmonic insufficiency negatively influence outcome. They also found a relationship to age at surgery, but this was not as important as the follow-up interval. Zahka, et al., in a prospective study of 59 patients with tetralogy of Fallot repaired prior to 11 years of age, found that the degree of pulmonary regurgitation was by far the most important predictor of the frequency and severity of spontaneously occurring ventricular arrhythmias.[39] While the degree of residual right ventricular outflow tract obstruction was not a predictor in this study, significant residual obstruction was rare in their study group

Spontaneously occurring sustained ventricular tachycardia is, in fact, fairly uncommon among patients with repaired tetralogy, in distinction to the high incidence of ventricular ectopy. Chandar, et al., in their multi-center report, identified ventricular tachycardia on Holter monitoring in 9% of 359 patients, but few had sustained ventricular tachycardia clinically.[48] The best data in this regard comes from a report by Harrison, et al. of patients with repaired tetralogy of Fallot attending an adult congenital heart disease clinic.[51] Eighteen of 210 patients (8.6%) had either documented sustained ventricular tachycardia, syncope or near-syncope with palpitations and inducible sustained monomorphic ventricular tachycardia at electrophysiologic study. The origin of the ventricular tachycardia was determined to be in the right ventricular outflow tract by intra-operative mapping. Ventricular tachycardia was closely related to right ventricular hemodynamics, and in particular, right ventricular outflow tact aneurysms and pulmonic insufficiency. This finding is consistent with the earlier report by Zahka, et al.[39] which emphasized the importance of pulmonic insufficiency as a risk factor for ventricular ectopy..

The occasional but persistent observation of sudden, unexpected death in this group of patients with repaired congenital heart disease, along with the high incidence of spontaneously occurring ventricular arrhythmias, both simple and complex, has lead to the hypothesis that sudden death in such patients is due to ventricular tachycardia. In some patients, ventricular tachycardia has been observed to progress quickly to ventricular fibrillation. Attempts to prevent the occurrence of sudden death in the past have logically been directed at suppressing ventricular arrhythmias, either spontaneously occurring ventricular ectopy or inducible ventricular tachycardia at electrophysiologic study. During the 1970's and 1980's, it was the standard practice to perform electrophysiologic studies in a large proportion of patients who had undergone repair of tetralogy of Fallot or related congenital defects in an attempt to identify inducible sustained monomorphic ventricular tachycardia. Nearly all such patients were asymptomatic from the point of view of arrhythmias. Antiarrhythmic drug therapy was often prescribed based on the results of such studies. This approach has, for the most part, been abandoned, due to the lack of strong evidence supporting the proposition that sudden death can be prevented with this approach. Furthermore, the possibility of a proarrhythmic effect of the antiarrhythmic medications chosen for treatment has not been adequately dealt with.

The results of invasive electrophysiologic testing in a large number of patients with repaired tetralogy of Fallot are disturbing, in that ventricular tachycardia can be induced in a large proportion, nearly all of whom have never had a clinical episode of ventricular tachycardia. Kugler, et al.[52] reported the findings at electrophysiologic study in three asymptomatic adolescent patients, all of whom had inducible sustained monomorphic ventricular tachycardia, seeming to originate from the inflow-septal area of the right ventricle, and which was suppressible with propranolol. These early reports coupled with data suggesting a direct link between ventricular arrhythmias and sudden death, lead to the widespread use of invasive electrophysiologic testing in largely asymptomatic patients, with subsequent antiarrhythmic treatment, often with repeated electrophysiologic study to guide therapy. Subsequent examination of the results of this approach has not supported its utility, however. In a large multi-center review, Chandar et al. reported the experience with 359 post-operative tetralogy of Fallot patients who underwent invasive electrophysiologic testing.[48] Ventricular tachycardia could be induced in 17% of patients, but not in any patient who was asymptomatic and had a normal 24 hour electrocardiogram.

While late sudden death occurred in 5 patients, none of these patients had inducible ventricular tachycardia at electrophysiologic study. These results call into question the rationale behind aggressive diagnostic investigation of asymptomatic patients. They also call into question the notion that sudden death can be prevented by the identification and treatment of potentially life-threatening ventricular arrhythmias.

Recent data suggest that one can assess the risk of ventricular tachycardia from the surface electrocardiogram QRS duration. Gatzoulis et al. found that in a group of 48 well-studied post-operative tetralogy patients, those with a QRS duration ≥ 180 msec had a greatly increased risk of spontaneous ventricular tachycardia and/or sudden death.[40] Similarly, Balaji et al. showed that a QRS duration ≥ 180 msec predicts the finding of inducible sustained monomorphic ventricular tachycardia at electrophysiologic study.[53] The cause of this relationship is uncertain. Certainly, patients with tetralogy of Fallot who have been corrected usually have right bundle branch block with resulting QRS prolongation. Excessive QRS prolongation in such patients may be a marker for the degree of pulmonic insufficiency which results in right ventricular dilation. Alternatively, it may be a marker for the degree of right ventricular infundibular resection that was necessary at surgery.

The incidence of sudden death is, in fact, much lower than previously feared, and may in fact be falling. Early reports of sudden death following tetralogy of Fallot repair estimated the incidence at 2-3%.[26,27] Garson, et al. reported a somewhat higher incidence of 3.4% (8/233) but noted that the incidence was more than 30% among those patients with premature ventricular beats on a routine electrocardiogram.[50] This finding prompted great concern, in view of the frequent occurrence of ventricular ectopy in this patient group, as described above. Subsequent reports have shown consistently lower estimates of the risk of sudden death. Wren has reviewed the results of 14 studies of post-operative tetralogy of Fallot patients, and found a pooled incidence of 1.6% (49/3006) with a mortality rate of 0.14% per patient-year of follow-up.[54] The multi-center study of Chandar, et al.[48] showed a very similar incidence of 1.4% (5/359), despite the fact that all of these patients had undergone electrophysiologic study.

While the incidence of sudden death may have fallen due to earlier age at surgery and improvements in surgical technique, there is some evidence that it may increase at late follow-up. In a careful study of 490 survivors of tetralogy of Fallot repair at a single center, Nollert et al. constructed actuarial survival curves out to 36 years following surgery.[55] In this study, the yearly actuarial mortality rate during the first 25 years was 0.24%/year, but mortality increased dramatically after 25 years to 0.94%/year. Most mortality was due to sudden death. The mortality risk was also related to date of operation (highest before 1970), the degree of pre-operative polycythemia (highest with hematocrit > 48) and the use of a right ventricular outflow tract patch (highest with a patch). The last factor is most likely related to the presence of pulmonic insufficiency, as suggested above. The importance of polycythemia may not be a direct factor, but instead may be related to the degree and duration of preoperative cyanosis, which could conceivably contribute to myocardial fibrosis.

The treatment decision in patients with ventricular ectopy following correction of congenital heart disease may be directed at one or both of two goals: the prevention of sudden death, and the suppression of termination of symptomatic episodes of ventricular tachycardia. Treatment may involve antiarrhythmic medication, radiofrequency catheter ablation, surgical cryoablation, or implantation of a tiered-therapy device providing antitachycardia pacing and cardioversion/defibrillation.

It is difficult to know which patients deserve electrophysiologic study and/or treatment. When one considers that there are no prospective studies demonstrating that sudden death can be prevented in any group of post-operative patients by treatment of any type, it does not seem that one should recommend routine electrophysiologic study and treatment of asymptomatic patients with ventricular ectopy. While it seems likely that certain subgroups exist in whom carefully chosen antiarrhythmic therapy may exert a beneficial effect in lowering mortality, it is also quite possible that there are subgroups for whom the proarrhythmic potential of antiarrhythmic medications more than makes up for any beneficial effect, a result similar to that seen in the Cardiac Arrhythmia Suppression (CAST) trial.[34,35] Until such prospective, controlled trials are performed, therapy with drugs such as flecainide, quinidine, and sotalol cannot be recommended for most asymptomatic patients. An argument can be made for selecting certain patients for prophylactic treatment with beta blockers, as Garson[56] has suggested. Examples of such patients might include those with significant pulmonic regurgitation and/or residual right ventricular obstruction and complex ventricular ectopy. One can also argue that such patients should be considered for cardiac surgery to correct hemodynamic abnormalities, such as residual obstruction, especially branch pulmonary artery stenosis, and should also be considered for placement of a homograft valve to eliminate pulmonic insufficiency.

If the goal of therapy is to prevent recurrence of clinically documented ventricular tachycardia, then one might consider proceeding in a fashion similar to that with other forms of ventricular tachycardia. Electrophysiologic study for induction of ventricular tachycardia with subsequent drug testing is reasonable, bearing in mind that there very well may be some proarrhythmic risk to the use of certain medications, especially flecainide and propafenone. One might also use exercise testing as a means of inducing ventricular tachycardia in certain patients. The choice of a pharmacological agent for long-term treatment is then based both on the effect of suppression of the arrhythmia by the drug, and on its proarrhythmic potential. In the former consideration, investigators have reported some success with most class I agents, and especially quinidine, propafenone, and flecainide, as well as with beta blockers. The latter consideration, of proarrhythmia, is difficult to judge. There was a high incidence of documented proarrhythmia with flecainide and encainide in patients with structural cardiac disease, as reported by Fish, et al. in a pediatric series.[57] Furthermore, cardiac arrest and deaths occurred predominantly among patients with underlying heart disease. Sotalol is also known to be proarrhythmic, particularly in patients with significant ventricular dysfunction.[58] D-sotalol has been found to increase mortality in post-infarction patients with ventricular dysfunction (the SWORD trial).[59] These findings suggest that sotalol and the class 1c agents should be used with extreme caution in repaired tetralogy of Fallot patients with ventricular dysfunction. This, of course, leaves amiodarone, which has the advantage of very little reported proarrhythmia, even in patients with significant ventricular dysfunction. Concern over long-term side effects, such as pulmonary fibrosis, ocular abnormalities, thyroid dysfunction, transaminase elevations, and significant bradycardia, have been raised in children and young adults,[60-62] and the use of this agent in a young person means that there is a likelihood that the medication will be needed for several decades at least. These concerns naturally lead to consideration of nonpharmacological therapy.

If ventricular tachycardia is easily inducible and well tolerated hemodynamically, one may consider radiofrequency ablation. As most evidence supports the concept of macroreentry as the mechanism of such well –tolerated ventricular tachycardia, the use of entrainment pacing and mapping techniques is indicated. Investigators have reported successful procedures using radiofrequency energy.[63-68] Successful sites have included the area between the pulmonic annulus and outflow tract patch,[65] the isthmus of ventricular tissue between an outflow tract patch and the tricuspid annulus,[68] and the region of the ventricular septal defect patch.[63]

While well-tolerated ventricular tachycardia can be mapping in the electrophysiology laboratory, many patients have ventricular dysfunction and/or rapid ventricular tachycardia rates, and will not tolerate this. Several investigators have reported intra-operative mapping and ablation.[63,69-72] In particular, Downar et al. have used intra-operative mapping of the right ventricular outflow tract in the beating heart employing an endocardial electrode balloon and a simultaneous epicardial electrode sock array.[71] Ablation was carried out by cryotherapy lesions during normothermic cardiopulmonary bypass with the heart beating, or during anoxic arrest, with good success in 3 patients.

With the rapid changes recently in lead and generator technology, implantable cardioverter-defibrillators (ICDs) have become a more viable option for the treatment of patients with ventricular tachycardia following repair of congenital heart disease. Patients with repaired congenital heart disease made up 18% of patients with ICDs in the multi-center review by Silka, et al. of 125 pediatric patients.[73] Most reports to date have dealt mainly with devices attached to epicardial patches, but recent reports have included patients with transvenous systems.[74]

CONCLUSIONS

The field of catheter ablation in patients with arrhythmias following repair of congenital heart disease is ripe for innovation. Success in this endeavor will require the development of energy sources which allow for the formation of deep, transmural lesions, as well as lesions which are linear and which can be designed to bridge the gap between anatomic and surgically created obstacles to cardiac conduction. Success will also require an extensive understanding of both the preexisting cardiac anatomy as well as the details of the surgical procedures which have been performed, coupled with mapping systems which allow for detailed reconstruction of the conduction patterns which exist in these patients. Fortunately, the recent development of exciting new technology, both in new mapping systems as well as new energy sources, promises to accelerate progress in this field over the next several years.

REFERENCES

1. Moore KL. The Developing Human. Clinically oriented embryology. Philadelphia: W.B. Saunders Company; 1974.
2. Cosio FC. Endocardial mapping of atrial flutter. In: Touboul P, Waldo AL, eds. Atrial Arrhythmias. St. Louis: Mosby Year Book; 1990:229-240.
3. Saoudi N, Cosio F, Waldo A, Chen S-A, Iesaka Y, Lesh M, Saksena S, Salerno J. A new classification of atrial tachycardias based on electrophysiologic mechanisms. Eur Heart J. 2000:in press.
4. Olgin JE, Kalman JM, Fitzpatrick AP, Lesh MD. Role of right atrial endocardial structures as barriers to conduction during human type I atrial flutter. Activation and entrainment mapping guided by intracardiac echocardiography. Circulation. 1995;92:1839-1848.
5. Kalman JM, Olgin JE, Saxon LA, Fisher WG, Lee RJ, Lesh MD. Activation and entrainment mapping defines the tricuspid annulus as the anterior barrier in typical atrial flutter. Circulation. 1996;93:398-406.
6. Nakagawa H, Lazzara R, Khastgir T, Beckman KJ, McClelland JH, Imai S, Pitha JV, Becker AE, Arruda M, Gonzalez MD, Widman LE, Rome M, Neuhauser J, Wang X, Calame JD, Goudeau MD, Jackman WM. The role of the tricuspid annulus and the eustachian valve/ridge on atrial flutter: Relevance to catheter ablation of the septal isthmus and a new technique for rapid identification of ablation success. Circulation. 1996;93:407-424.
7. Feld GK, Shahandeh-Rad F. Mechanism of double potentials recorded during sustained atrial flutter in the canine right atrial crush-injury model. Circulation. 1992;86:628-641.
8. Olshansky B, Okumura K, R.W. H, Waldo AL. Characterization of double potentials in human atrial flutter: Studies during transient entrainment. J Am Coll Cardiol. 1990;15:833-841.
9. Lesh MD, Van Hare GF, Epstein LM, Fitzpatrick AP, Scheinman MM, Lee RJ, Kwasman MA, Grogin HR, Griffin JC. Radiofrequency catheter ablation of atrial arrhythmias. Results and mechanisms. Circulation. 1994;89:1074-1089.
10. Feld GK, Fleck P, Chen PS, Boyce K, Bahnson TD, Stein JB, Calisi CM, Ibarra M. Radiofrequency catheter ablation for the treatment of human type 1 atrial flutter: Identification of a critical zone in the reentrant circuit by endocardial mapping techniques. Circulation. 1992;86:1233-1240.
11. Klein G, Guiraudon G, Sharma A, Milstein S. Demonstration of macroreentry and feasibility of operative therapy in the common type of atrial flutter. Am J Cardiol. 1986;57:587-591.

12. Kalman JM, Van Hare GF, Olgin JE, Saxon LA, Stark S, Lesh MD. Ablation of "incisional" reentrant atrial tachycardia complicating surgery for congenital heart disease: Use of entrainment to define a critical isthmus of slow conduction. Circulation. 1996;93:502-512.
13. Senning A. Surgical correction of transposition of the great vessels. Surgery. 1959;45:966.
14. Mustard WT, Keith JD, Trusler GA, Fowler R, Lidd L. The surgical management of transposition of the great vessels. J Thorac Cardiovasc Surg. 1964;48:953-.
15. Karl TR, Weintraub RG, Brizard CP, Cochrane AD, Mee RB. Senning plus arterial switch operation for discordant (congenitally corrected) transposition. Ann Thorac Surg. 1997;64:495-502.
16. Ebert PA, Gay WA, Engle MA. Correction of transposition of the great arteries: Relationship of the coronary sinus and postoperative arrhythmias. Ann Surg. 1974;180:433-438.
17. Van Hare GF, Lesh MD, Ross BA, Perry JC, Dorostkar PC. Mapping and radiofrequency ablation of intraatrial reentrant tachycardia after the Senning or Mustard procedure for transposition of the great arteries. Am J Cardiol. 1996;77:985-991.
18. Fontan F, Baudet E. Surgical repair of tricuspid atresia. Thorax. 1971;26:240.
19. Jonas RA, Castaneda AR. Modified Fontan procedure: Atrial baffle and systemic venous to pulmonary artery anastomotic techniques. J Cardiac Surg. 1988;3:91.
20. Triedman JK, Jenkins KJ, Saul JP, Lock JE, Colan SD, Walsh EP. Right atrial mapping in humans using a multielectrode basket catheter. PACE. 1995;18:800 (Abstract).
21. Treidman JK, Saul JP, Weindling SN, Walsh EP. Radiofrequency ablation of intra-atrial reentrant tachycardia after surgical palliation of congenital heart disease. Circulation. 1995;91:707-714.
22. Balaji S, Johnson TB, Sade RM, Case CL, Gillette PC. Management of atrial flutter after the Fontan procedure. Journal of the American College of Cardiology. 1994;23:1209-1215.
23. Case CL, Gillette PC, Douglas DE, Liebermann RA. Radiofrequency catheter ablation of atrial flutter in a patient with postoperative congenital heart disease. Am Heart J. 1993;126:715-716.
24. Rodefeld MD, Bromberg BI, Schuessler RB, Boineau JP, Cox JL, Huddleston CB. Atrial flutter after lateral tunnel construction in the modified Fontan operation: a canine model. Journal of Thoracic & Cardiovascular Surgery. 1996;111:514-526.
25. Gillette PC, Yeoman MA, Mullins CE, McNamara DG. Sudden death after repair of tetralogy of Fallot. Electrocardiographic and electrophysiologic abnormalities. Circulation. 1977;56:566-571.
26. James FW, Kaplan S, Chou TC. Unexpected cardiac arrest in patients after surgical correction of tetralogy of Fallot. Circulation. 1975;52:691-695.
27. Quattlebaum TG, Varghese J, Neill CA, Donahoo JS. Sudden death among postoperative patients with tetralogy of Fallot: a follow-up study of 243 patients for an average of twelve years. Circulation. 1976;54:289-293.
28. Marin-Garcia J, Moller JH. Sudden death after operative repair of tetralogy of Fallot. British Heart Journal. 1977;39:1380-1385.
29. Deanfield JE, McKenna WJ, Hallidie-Smith KA. Detection of late arrhythmia and conduction disturbance after correction of tetralogy of Fallot. British Heart Journal. 1980;44:248-253.
30. Garson A, Jr., Gillette PC, Gutgesell HP, McNamara DG. Stress-induced ventricular arrhythmia after repair of tetralogy of Fallot. American Journal of Cardiology. 1980;46:1006-1012.
31. Shen WK, Holmes DR, Jr., Porter CJ, McGoon DC, Ilstrup DM. Sudden death after repair of double-outlet right ventricle. Circulation. 1990;81:128-136.
32. Garson A, Jr., McNamara DG. Sudden death in a pediatric cardiology population, 1958 to 1983: relation to prior arrhythmias. J Am Coll Cardiol. 1985;5:134B-137B.
33. Vetter VL, Horowitz LN. Electrophysiologic residua and sequelae of surgery for congenital heart defects. Am J Cardiol. 1982;50:588-604.
34. Preliminary report: effect of encainide and flecainide on mortality in a randomized trial of arrhythmia suppression after myocardial infarction. The Cardiac Arrhythmia Suppression Trial (CAST) Investigators [see comments]. N Engl J Med. 1989;321:406-412.
35. Effect of the antiarrhythmic agent moricizine on survival after myocardial infarction. The Cardiac Arrhythmia Suppression Trial II Investigators. N Engl J Med. 1992;327:227-233.

36. A comparison of antiarrhythmic-drug therapy with implantable defibrillators in patients resuscitated from near-fatal ventricular arrhythmias. The Antiarrhythmics versus Implantable Defibrillators (AVID) Investigators [see comments]. N Engl J Med. 1997;337:1576-1583.

37. Bricker JT. Sudden death and tetralogy of Fallot. Risks, markers, and causes [editorial; comment]. Circulation. 1995;92:158-159.

38. Lillehei CW, Varco RL, Cohen M, Warden HE, Gott VL, DeWall RA, Patton C, Moller JH. The first open heart corrections of tetralogy of Fallot. A 26-31 year follow-up of 106 patients. Ann Surg. 1986;204:490-502.

39. Zahka KG, Horneffer PJ, Rowe SA, Neill CA, Manolio TA, Kidd L, Gardner TJ. Long-term valvular function after total repair of tetralogy of Fallot. Relation to ventricular arrhythmias. Circulation. 1988;78:III14-19.

40. Gatzoulis MA, Till JA, Somerville J, Redington AN. Mechanoelectrical interaction in tetralogy of Fallot. QRS prolongation relates to right ventricular size and predicts malignant ventricular arrhythmias and sudden death [see comments]. Circulation. 1995;92:231-237.

41. Gatzoulis MA, Till JA, Redington AN. Depolarization-repolarization inhomogeneity after repair of tetralogy of Fallot. The substrate for malignant ventricular tachycardia? Circulation. 1997;95:401-404.

42. Deanfield JE, Ho SY, Anderson RH, McKenna WJ, Allwork SP, Hallidie-Smith KA. Late sudden death after repair of tetralogy of Fallot: a clinicopathologic study. Circulation. 1983;67:626-631.

43. Deanfield J, McKenna W, Rowland E. Local abnormalities of right ventricular depolarization after repair of tetralogy of Fallot: a basis for ventricular arrhythmia. American Journal of Cardiology. 1985;55:522-525.

44. Zimmermann M, Friedli B, Adamec R, Oberhansli I. Ventricular late potentials and induced ventricular arrhythmias after surgical repair of tetralogy of Fallot. American Journal of Cardiology. 1991;67:873-878.

45. Garson A, Jr. Ventricular dysrhythmias after congenital heart surgery: a canine model. Pediatr Res. 1984;18:1112-1120.

46. Kremers MS, Wells PJ, Black WH, Solodyna MA. Entrainment of ventricular tachycardia in postoperative tetralogy of Fallot. Pacing & Clinical Electrophysiology. 1988;11:1310-1314.

47. Aizawa Y, Kitazawa H, Washizuka T, Takahashi K, Shibata A. Conductive properties of the reentrant pathway of ventricular tachycardia during entrainment from outside and within the zone of slow conduction. Pacing & Clinical Electrophysiology. 1995;18:663-672.

48. Chandar JS, Wolff GS, Garson A, Jr., Bell TJ, Beder SD, Bink-Boelkens M, Byrum CJ, Campbell RM, Deal BJ, Dick Md, et a. Ventricular arrhythmias in postoperative tetralogy of Fallot. American Journal of Cardiology. 1990;65:655-661.

49. Walsh EP, Rockenmacher S, Keane JF, Hougen TJ, Lock JE, Castaneda AR. Late results in patients with tetralogy of Fallot repaired during infancy. Circulation. 1988;77:1062-1067.

50. Garson A, Jr., Randall DC, Gillette PC, Smith RT, Moak JP, McVey P, McNamara DG. Prevention of sudden death after repair of tetralogy of Fallot: treatment of ventricular arrhythmias. Journal of the American College of Cardiology. 1985;6:221-227.

51. Harrison DA, Harris L, Siu SC, MacLoghlin CJ, Connelly MS, Webb GD, Downar E, McLaughlin PR, Williams WG. Sustained ventricular tachycardia in adult patients late after repair of tetralogy of Fallot [see comments]. J Am Coll Cardiol. 1997;30:1368-1373.

52. Kugler JD, Pinsky WW, Cheatham JP, Hofschire PJ, Mooring PK, Fleming WH. Sustained ventricular tachycardia after repair of tetralogy of Fallot: new electrophysiologic findings. American Journal of Cardiology. 1983;51:1137-1143.

53. Balaji S, Lau YR, Case CL, Gillette PC. QRS prolongation is associated with inducible ventricular tachycardia after repair of tetralogy of Fallot. American Journal of Cardiology. 1997;80:160-163.

54. Wren C. Late postoperative arrhythmias. In: Wren C, Campbell RWF, eds. Paediatric Cardiac Arrhythmias. Oxford: Oxford University Press; 1996:251.

55. Nollert G, Fischlein T, Bouterwek S, Bohmer C, Klinner W, Reichart B. Long-term survival in patients with repair of tetralogy of Fallot: 36- year follow-up of 490 survivors of the first year after surgical repair [see comments]. J Am Coll Cardiol. 1997;30:1374-1383.

56. Garson A, Jr., Gillette PC, McNamara DG. Propranolol: the preferred palliation for tetralogy of Fallot. American Journal of Cardiology. 1981;47:1098-1104.
57. Fish FA, Gillette PC, Benson DW, Jr. Proarrhythmia, cardiac arrest and death in young patients receiving encainide and flecainide. The Pediatric Electrophysiology Group [see comments]. J Am Coll Cardiol. 1991;18:356-365.
58. Hohnloser SH. Proarrhythmia with class III antiarrhythmic drugs: types, risks, and management. Am J Cardiol. 1997;80:82G-89G.
59. Waldo AL, Camm AJ, deRuyter H, Friedman PL, MacNeil DJ, Pauls JF, Pitt B, Pratt CM, Schwartz PJ, Veltri EP. Effect of d-sotalol on mortality in patients with left ventricular dysfunction after recent and remote myocardial infarction. The SWORD Investigators. Survival With Oral d-Sotalol [see comments] [published erratum appears in Lancet 1996 Aug 10;348(9024):416]. Lancet. 1996;348:7-12.
60. Daniels CJ, Schutte DA, Hammond S, Franklin WH. Acute pulmonary toxicity in an infant from intravenous amiodarone. Am J Cardiol. 1997;80:1113-1116.
61. Celiker A, Kocak G, Lenk MK, Alehan D, Ozme S. Short- and intermediate-term efficacy of amiodarone in infants and children with cardiac arrhythmia. Turk J Pediatr. 1997;39:219-225.
62. Villain E. Amiodarone as treatment for atrial tachycardias after surgery. Pacing Clin Electrophysiol. 1997;20:2130-2132.
63. Ressia L, Graffigna A, Salerno-Uriarte JA, Vigano M. [The complex origin of ventricular tachycardia after the total correction of tetralogy of Fallot]. [Italian]. Giornale Italiano di Cardiologia. 1993;23:905-910.
64. Burton ME, Leon AR. Radiofrequency catheter ablation of right ventricular outflow tract tachycardia late after complete repair of tetralogy of Fallot using the pace mapping technique. Pacing & Clinical Electrophysiology. 1993;16:2319-2325.
65. Biblo LA, Carlson MD. Transcatheter radiofrequency ablation of ventricular tachycardia following surgical correction of tetralogy of Fallot. Pacing & Clinical Electrophysiology. 1994;17:1556-1560.
66. Goldner BG, Cooper R, Blau W, Cohen TJ. Radiofrequency catheter ablation as a primary therapy for treatment of ventricular tachycardia in a patient after repair of tetralogy of Fallot. Pacing & Clinical Electrophysiology. 1994;17:1441-1446.
67. Gonska BD, Cao K, Raab J, Eigster G, Kreuzer H. Radiofrequency catheter ablation of right ventricular tachycardia late after repair of congenital heart defects. Circulation. 1996;94:1902-1908.
68. Horton RP, Canby RC, Kessler DJ, Joglar JA, Hume A, Jessen ME, Scott WP, Page RL. Ablation of ventricular tachycardia associated with tetralogy of Fallot: demonstration of bidirectional block. Journal of Cardiovascular Electrophysiology. 1997;8:432-435.
69. Frank G, Schmid C, Baumgart D, Lowes D, Klein H, Kallfelz HC. [Surgical therapy of life-threatening tachycardic cardiac arrhythmias in children]. [German]. Monatsschrift Kinderheilkunde. 1989;137:269-274.
70. Lawrie GM, Pacifico A, Kaushik R. Results of direct surgical ablation of ventricular tachycardia not due to ischemic heart disease. [Review] [45 refs]. Annals of Surgery. 1989;209:716-727.
71. Downar E, Harris L, Kimber S, Mickleborough L, Williams W, Sevaptsidis E, Masse S, Chen TC, Chan A, Genga A, et a. Ventricular tachycardia after surgical repair of tetralogy of Fallot: results of intraoperative mapping studies. Journal of the American College of Cardiology. 1992;20:648-655.
72. Misaki T, Tsubota M, Tanaka M, Watanabe G, Watanabe Y, Iwa T. [Surgical treatment of ventricular tachycardia after radical correction of tetralogy of Fallot]. [Japanese]. Nippon Kyobu Geka Gakkai Zasshi   Journal of the Japanese Association for Thoracic Surgery. 1990;38:130-134.
73. Silka MJ, Kron J, Dunnigan A, Dick Md. Sudden cardiac death and the use of implantable cardioverter- defibrillators in pediatric patients. The Pediatric Electrophysiology Society. Circulation. 1993;87:800-807.
74. Wilson WR, Greer GE, Grubb BP. Implantable cardioverter-defibrillators in children: a single-institutional experience [In Process Citation]. Ann Thorac Surg. 1998;65:775-778.

Chapter 5

CATHETER MAPPING AND ABLATION TECHNOLOGY
Limitations of Conventional Method and Challenges of Newer Technology

L. Bing Liem
Cardiac Arrhythmia and Electrophysiology, Stanford University, Stanford, California, USA

INTRODUCTION

Radiofrequency (RF) ablation has become the standard method for the management of many types of cardiac arrhythmias. Its safety and efficacy have been well described and the final outcome of RF-based ablation is frequently so satisfying that many patients would prefer it over medical therapy. Consequently, RF ablation has been attempted in virtually all types of cardiac arrhythmias including those with much less-defined substrates such as atrial fibrillation and its limitations were soon realized. This chapter outlines the fundamental aspects of the relatively low efficacy of conventional RF ablation technology. Other chapters in this book describe further technical components of RF ablation and alternative solutions.

Radiofrequency ablation takes advantage of physical properties of resistive heating. Electrical voltage produced by the RF generator is impressed upon the tissue and causes electrical force emanating from the tip of an intracardiac catheter electrode positioned against the cardiac tissue. The electrical field passes through the body and returns to the generator through a large dispersive electrode placed on the skin. The electrical field at the tissue in contact with the catheter electrode is transformed into heat by resistive mechanism. This local heating is then dispersed to surrounding tissue by conductive mechanism. As such, deeper tissue is heated to a lesser degree than the endocardial surface. The drop in temperature in the deeper tissue is not linear. It is estimated that the temperature drops by a factor of four over distance from the surface. Because permanent tissue destruction requires a temperature in the range of $45\text{-}50^{0}$ C, effective ablation typically reaches a depth of 3 to 5 mm. Attempts at producing

L. Bing Liem and E. Downar (eds.), Progress in Catheter Ablation, 59-62.

deeper heating by delivering more power would usually result in overheating of endocardial surface and can cause charring.

The success of reaching deeper tissue is not only dependent on those basic physical properties of RF energy. Other variables, such as electrode-to-tissue contact and tissue geometry and pathology also play a big role. Thus, in the presence of good contact, transformation of electrical force into heat can be predicted because the delivery of power would more or less follow the expected pattern. Poor catheter-to-tissue contact, however, poses multiple problems. In such a situation, power delivery must adjust to the changes in impedance. Furthermore, intermittent contact would allow circulating blood to get trapped and form a coagulated layer, which would not only impede further RF delivery into tissue but could also pose the risk for thromboembolism. Temperature monitoring could lower such mishap by preventing overheating. Indeed, temperature monitoring has been found to be quite helpful in assisting safe and effective ablation when used as a continuous feedback for the control of the amount of delivered power. Thus, when set at the desired temperature of 50-70^0C, the closed feedback loop system would continuously adjust the delivered power to match the need for achieving that temperature. However, when there contact is inadequate, even delivery of full power would not overcome it and tissue temperature would reach below the desired 50^0C.

The dependence of effective RF ablation upon good contact also limits the utility of this method for the creation of linear ablation. With RF technology, linear ablation using stationary catheter would require delivery of RF energy over multiple electrodes simultaneously. Unless all electrodes are in contact with tissue to the same extent, RF delivery is likely to be uneven. Thus, to create linear lesion, the point-and-drag method is still frequently used. Several new methods are being employed to overcome uneven RF delivery with the multipolar catheter technique, as described in later chapters. If temperature from all electrodes can be monitored, an integrated system can be used to adjust power delivery to compensate for contact irregularities.

Another limitation to the use of conventional RF technology for the creation of linear lesion lies in its limited depth. While a 3-5 mm ablation depth may be sufficient in some instances, it would be unlikely to produce uniform transmural lesion in some areas of the heart with widely variable thickness, such as the trabeculated portion of the right atrium. Such trabeculation would also pose difficulty in obtaining uniform contact with the ablation catheter. Thus, even for its relatively thin tissue, the atria may require a form of heating that is more powerful in penetration and less dependent on tissue contact. Data from some animal studies using multipolar catheter prototypes show that transmural linear lesions can be achieved with RF energy (see later chapters) but clinical data are still scanty. The limited data are presented in later chapters in this book.

Based on the principles mentioned above, conventional RF ablation is also unlikely to produced deep lesions. Thus, for substrates such as ventricular reentry from myocardial scars, conventional RF would have low success rate. Indeed clinical data support such notion. However, recent progress with cooling and irrigation of the electrode has improved RF ablation ability in producing deep lesions (discussed in later chapters). The problem with ablation of tissue underneath myocardial scar has also been recognized and may be the key to the low success rate of catheter ablation for VT from chronic ischemic scar.

Alternative sources of energy are being tested. Cryoablation and ablation using laser and microwave energy have shown some promise but clinical data are still limited. Available data on the utility of these technologies are also presented later in this book. Advantages and limitations of alternative methods and energy sources are recognized and at the present stage, application of these newer methods are not as "user-friendly" as conventional RF ablation system. As a result, conventional RF remains the "standard" method in most instances. Conventional RF ablation is also utilized in complex arrhythmia because its application can be modified and tailored to the pattern of desired lesions. Thus, despite its limitations, point ablation remains the standard method for creating linear ablation within the atria and the orifice of pulmonary veins. The result of such application is also discussed in later chapters. While such method is feasible, it is highly impractical and frequently results in high utilization of fluoroscopy and radiation.

Mapping technology has also evolved significantly in the past several years. However, until recently, conventional mapping technique using single roving catheter had been the standard method. Such form of mapping indeed serves the purpose of simple ablation perfectly because single-site high-resolution mapping is typically needed. However, as the application of ablation technology was broadened to include arrhythmia with complex pattern, single point mapping has become inadequate. As mentioned in previous chapters, the pattern of ischemic VT can be quite complex and would likely need mapping with simultaneous multiple-point acquisition. Furthermore, such VT is frequently associated with rather precipitous hemodynamic destabilization and, therefore, mapping must be completed within a very short period of time. Mapping the arrhythmogenic substrate of arrhythmia in patients who has undergone repair of congenital heart disease also poses unique challenges. In such patients, mapping should also, ideally, provide anatomical data. Data acquisition using a single roving catheter would be very laborious and frequently incomplete.

Multiple-point acquisition mapping was first made available intraoperatively, as discussed in later chapters. Subsequently, basket catheters were designed for the same purpose during endocardial procedures. Such technology has indeed provided the operator with better mapping data that would not only assist in the ablation procedure but also in the understanding of the mechanism of the particular arrhythmia. A non-contact form of such mapping has also become available with even greater resolution. The use of such mapping may further assist in the elucidation of complex arrhythmia such as atrial and ventricular fibrillation.

Other newer forms of mapping have also become available recently. The electroanatomical reconstruction mapping provides the identification of catheter position relative to an estimation of cardiac anatomy and also reduces the need for fluoroscopy. Activation and voltage mappings can be acquired with great resolution but acquisition using this form of mapping still requires single point recording and may not be suitable for nonsustained arrhythmia. Similar "tracking" type of mapping is also available using ultrasonic referencing. With better visualization of the catheters, fluoroscopy use may be further reduced. However, the use of these mapping methods require familiarization with the specific apparatus and the degree of resolution still requires the skill of single catheter maneuver. Thus, in most cases, the operator would simply start with conventional mapping using a single catheter.

Thus, in this rapidly advancing field, limitations and challenges of old and new technology are also recognized. Data on recent and future technology are presented in subsequent chapters.

Part II

Newer Mapping Techniques

Chapter 6

UTILITY OF ORTHOGONAL ELECTRODES IN RADIOFREQUENCY ABLATION
Discriminate Near-Field Sensing

Bruce N. Goldreyer, MD
Clinical Professor of Medicine, University of Southern California and Director Clinical Cardiac Electrophysiology, San Pedro Peninsula Hospital, San Pedro, CA.

INTRODUCTION

The field of cardiac electrophysiology is barely thirty years old. From its inception, the understanding of cardiac arrhythmias was predicated upon the use of intracardiac electrograms recorded from the endocardial surface of the human heart with electrode catheters manipulated with the assistance of fluoroscopic equipment.[1] Although catheter materials, designs and the recent addition of steerability have gradually evolved and improved, the basic design of the electrodes used for electrogram recording has remained constant. Essentially, metal bands or ''rings' attached to the surface of cardiac catheters have been used to record bipolar electrograms either between two rings (bipolar signals) or between a ring and a remote electrode (unipolar signals).

It has long been recognised that whereas unipolar electrograms provide a means for assessing directionality, bipolar electrograms allow for more discriminate sensing.[2] Whereas electrode catheters of the 1960's and 70's employed rings with 1 cm inter-electrode distance, more modern catheters employ electrodes spaced at 2 to 5 mm distance in order to enhance their near-field sensing ability.

In the early 1980's attempts to develop a single pass pacemaker lead led to the development of a new and unique electrode sensing configuration. In studies of non-contacting electrodes, small 'dot' electrodes were affixed to the lead and oriented in the X, Y and Z-axis of the lead body. Because of their orientation, these electrodes were called: Orthogonal.[3] Early studies revealed that orthogonal

L. Bing Liem and E. Downar (eds.), Progress in Catheter Ablation, 65-77.
© 2001 *Kluwer Academic Publishers. Printed in the Netherlands.*

electrograms had characteristics, which were quite different from their unipolar and bipolar counterparts.

1.   ORTHOGONAL ELECTROGRAMS

The characteristics of orthogonal electrograms that render them so useful for clinical electrophysiology were not initially recognised and are a function of the manner in which orthogonal electrodes sense electrical events. While it was assumed that signals recorded in the X and Y planes would be reciprocally related, it was found that the amplitude of X and Y bipolar signals varied only as a function of proximity to the endocardial surface. Furthermore, X and Y electrode orientation always generated signals of greater amplitude and higher frequency content than those oriented in the Z direction or parallel the endocardial surface.[4] Being oriented circumferentially the electrodes were approximately perpendicular to the signal generator. The signal amplitude therefore was a function of the decrease in local electrical field and the bipolar signal amplitude and frequency content reflected the difference in signal between the pair as the cube of the distance from the signal generator.[5]

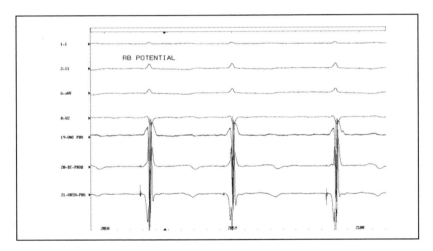

Figure 1. LOCALIZED ELECTROGRAM SENSING: Recorded are surface electrocardiographic signals reflecting leads I, II, avF, and V2, along with intracardiac signals recorded from the endocardial surface of the right ventricle adjacent to the right bundle branch. Note the extreme near field sensing demonstrated on the orthogonal electrode pair (ORTH PRO) as the right bundle potential is recorded.

It is this feature of orthogonal electrograms that render them so unique. Signals generated by sources remote to them are seen by the electrode pair as being the same and are 'cancelled.' The electrode configuration acts as a differential amplifier in and of itself. Near field signals are amplified and discrete, far field signals are rejected.[6]   In Figure 1, for example, localized depolarisation of the right bundle branch is amplified by the use of orthogonal electrodes as opposed to bipolar and unipolar signal sources.

2.   ORTHOGONAL ELECTRODES FOR INTRACARDIAC MAPPING

Because of their unique near field sensing capabilities, orthogonal electrodes were first employed in clinical cardiac electrophysiology by Jackman.[7]   In patients with WPW syndrome and left sided bypass tracts, a catheter with multiple sets of orthogonal electrodes was used for mapping accessory pathways from the coronary sinus. Local electrograms recorded from orthogonal electrodes could accurately localize not only areas of continuous atrial and ventricular electrical activity, they were near field enough to frequently record potentials from the accessory pathways themselves.

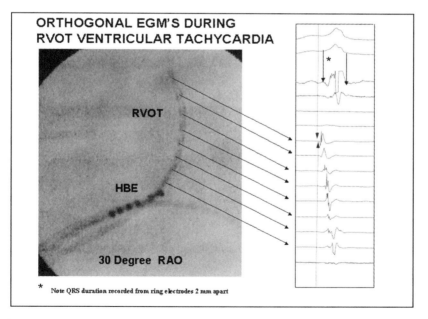

Figure 2. LINEAR MAPPING OF RVOT VENTRICULAR TACHYCARDIA: To the left of the figure is the X-ray position of a multipolar orthogonal catheter positioned in the right ventricular outflow tract (RVOT) as seen in the 30 degree RAO projection. A His bundle catheter with standard ring electrodes is seen in the right ventricular inflow tract. The arrows indicate electrograms recorded from orthogonal pairs. To the right of the figure, surface EKGs, two His bundle recordings and orthogonal electrograms recorded during sustained RVOT ventricular tachycardia are shown. The clear-cut linear activation sequence demonstrates that the tachycardia originates for an area adjacent to the distal most orthogonal electrodes.

Because of the extreme near field sensing, more recently, orthogonal electrodes have been employed on a variety of catheters used in the mapping and ablation of cardiac arrhythmias. Linear steerable catheters with multiple sets of orthogonal electrodes have been used to map not only the coronary sinus, but also the right ventricular outflow tract (Figure 2) and crista terminalis of the right atrium.

Orthogonal electrodes placed circumferentially along the course of 'halo-like' catheters have been used to map tricuspid annular activation in atrial flutter (Figure 3) and for the localisation of right sided accessory pathways.

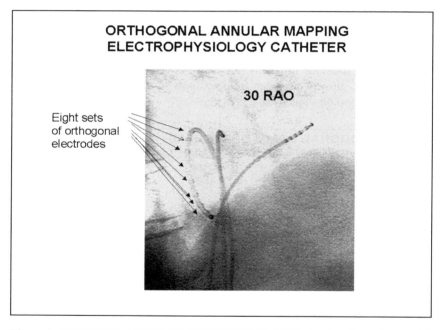

Figure 3. TRICUSPID ANNULAR ORTHOGONAL MAP: An annular catheter with multiple orthogonal sensors has been positioned around the tricuspid annulus. Recordings reflecting annulus activation may be made during the mapping and ablation of atrial flutter and right-sided accessory pathways.

3.   ORTHOGONAL ELECTROGRAMS FOR EVOKED RESPONSE SENSING AND DURING RF ENERGY APPLICATION

A catheter was recently developed for purposes of intracardiac mapping and ablation, which incorporated the use of orthogonal electrodes. This catheter (Figure 4) has a 4-mm distal tip for both pacing and the delivery of RF energy. Immediately behind the tip are two orthogonal electrodes for discriminate near field sensing. There follow, two standard rings, one just behind the orthogonal sensors for standard bipolar sensing and bipolar stimulation, and one 22 cm proximal to be used as an indifferent electrode for unipolar mapping.

Orthogonal electrograms may be differentially recorded during energy application again because of the unique sensing capabilities of orthogonal electrodes. Even 5 to 10 ma stimuli applied between the distal tip and ring are seen as 'far-field' and fail to obliterate the localized evoked response. Similarly, although specialised filters might be capable of rejecting the signals resulting from the application of RF energy between the catheter tip and a dispursive pad on the body surface, orthogonal electrodes, by their very nature, fail to record the delivery of RF energy. Thus, discrete electrograms may be recorded from tissue being ablated *during* the application of RF energy.

Specific examples of the use of orthogonal electrodes in clinical electrophysiology and radiofrequency ablation follow.

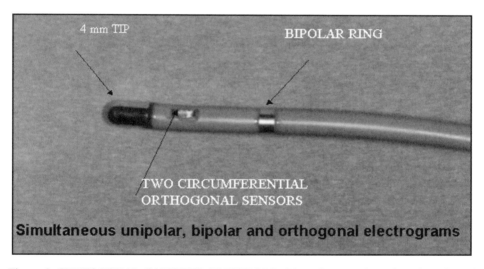

Figure 4. ORTHOGONAL CATHETER ELECTRODE CONFIGURATION: The orientation of the distal electrodes on an orthogonal mapping and ablation catheter is shown. A 4-mm distal tip with two circumferential orthogonal sensors, a distal ring and a ring 22-cm proximal provide the ability for simultaneous recording of unipolar, bipolar and orthogonal electrograms.

4.   ORTHOGONAL ELECTRODES IN AV NODAL REENTRANT TACHYCARDIA ABLATION

Using orthogonal electrodes may be of great benefit in AVNRT ablation for several reasons. Electrograms recorded during mapping of the slow pathway area may be used to localize target areas for ablation. In Figure 5, a 'slow-pathway' potential is recorded from an area along the tricuspid annulus inferior and posterior to the AV node. Despite controversy as to the etiology of these potentials, application of RF energy to these areas frequently result in the typical "junctional" rhythms characteristic of a successful slow pathway ablation.[8]

More importantly, however, are orthogonal electrograms recorded during the application of RF energy. These electrograms reveal catheter movement as well as document the relationship between atrial and ventricular activity seen during RF application.[9] As opposed to conventional catheters where electrogram recording is impossible during the RF delivery, with orthogonal sensors, electrograms reflecting movement of the catheter, for example, across the tricuspid annulus or into the coronary sinus would be immediately evident and the delivery of RF energy could be terminated.

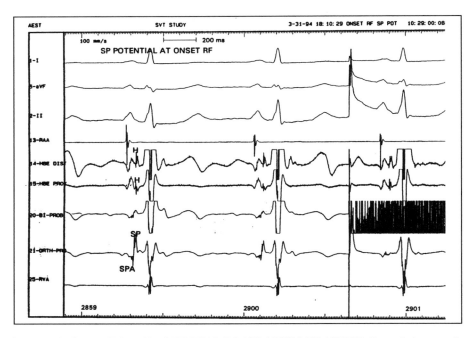

Figure 5. SLOW PATHWAY POTENTIAL IN ABLATION OF AVNRT: Recorded are surface ECG leads avF II, along with electrograms from the right atrial appendage (RAA), and distal and proximal His Bundle (HBE DIST and HBE PROX). Electrograms recorded from the bipolar (BI-PROB) and orthogonal electrodes (ORTH-PROB) and shown prior to and at the onset of RF delivery. A clear-cut slow-pathway potential (SP) is seen on the orthogonal electrodes prior to and after the initiation of RF delivery.

In Figure 6, typical recordings made during the application of RF energy to the AV nodal slow pathway area are displayed. Delay in the appearance of the local atrial signal during RF is the result of AV nodal 'heating' and heralds the fact that energy delivery should be terminated.

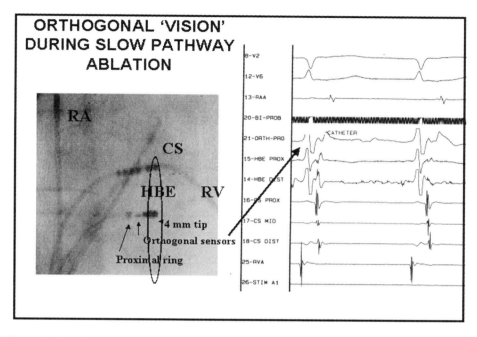

Figure 6. JUNCTIONAL RHYTHM DURING AVNRT RF: To the left is an AP radiograph demonstrating catheter position during RF delivery in a patient with AV nodal reentrant supraventricular tachycardia. Catheters are positioned in the right atrium (RA), Coronary sinus (CS), His bundle recording site (HBE) and right ventricle (RV). An orthogonal catheter is positioned in an area where 'slow pathway' potentials were recorded. The general position of the tricuspid annulus is indicated by the oval. To the right are electrograms recorded during the delivery of RF energy to the slow pathway area. The 'junctional' rhythms typical of successful slow pathway ablation are seen. From top to bottom are recorded surface ECG leads V2 and V6, along with electrograms recorded from the right atrial appendage (RAA), His bundle area (HBE) and the orthogonal electrode pair on the ablation catheter. Note that during RF delivery, a discrete electrogram is still recorded from the orthogonal electrode pair.

5.   ORTHOGONAL ELECTRODES IN THE ABLATION OF 'TYPICAL' ATRIAL FLUTTER

Mapping the tricuspid annulus during atrial flutter and establishing bi-directional isthmus block has allowed for the successful ablation of atrial flutter.[10] Catheters employing orthogonal electrodes are utilised the ablation of atrial flutter in two ways. By mapping the tricuspid annulus with orthogonal electrodes on a 'halo-like' catheter, a very discrete annular map with clearly discernible activation sequence is produced. Of more importance, however, is the use of orthogonal electrodes on the ablation catheter. By recording electrograms from the area immediately behind the ablation tip, the position of the tip is precisely localized even during RF delivery.

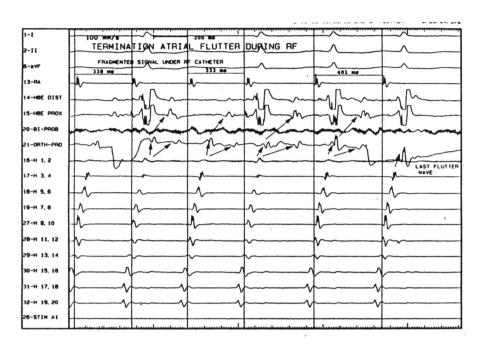

Figure 7. ORTHOGONAL EGM DURING RF IN ATRIAL FLUTTER: Recorded are surface ECG leads I, II and avF. Intracardiac electrograms from the right atrium (RA) and distal and proximal His Bundle (HBE DIST and HBE PROX) are also recorded. Electrograms from a standard Halo catheter are labelled with 'H'. Although the bipolar electrogram from the ablation catheter is obscured by the delivery of RF energy, orthogonal electrograms are clearly shown. The interval between the fragmented electrogram directly adjacent to the ablation tip becomes progressively prolonged (arrows) until atrial flutter terminates.

Typically, RF energy is delivered to the isthmus between the inferior margin of the tricuspid valve, the coronary sinus os, and the inferior vena cava. Only by recording electrograms during RF delivery can the position of the tip be determined with accuracy. Electrograms characteristics are dramatically dissimilar in different locations and these differences are immediately recognisable.

An interesting phenomenon seen during one atrial flutter ablation is shown in Figure 7. The local electrogram directly under the ablation tip shows fragmented activity. The interval between the initial and terminal portions of the signal becomes progressively prolonged, until finally, conduction block occurs and the flutter terminates.

6.   ORTHOGONAL ELECTRODES IN THE ABLATION OF WPW ACCESSORY PATHWAYS

Accessory pathway localisation is simplified by the use of orthogonal electrodes. Using linear or annular orthogonal mapping catheters in right and left sided WPW mapping, speeds the recognition of continuous atrial and ventricular activation and may in certain situations allow for the recording of accessory pathway potential.

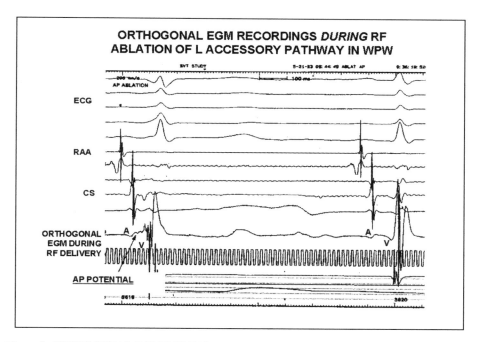

Figure 8. ORTHOGONAL EGM DURING AP ABLATION: Recorded from top to bottom are five surface ECG leads, an orthogonal electrogram from the right atrial appendage (RAA), three orthogonal electrograms recorded from the coronary sinus (CS) and an electrogram recorded from orthogonal electrodes positioned next to a left sided accessory pathway in a patient with WPW syndrome. RF energy is applied to the distal electrode. The ventricular pre-excitation seen during the first beat, is no longer present on the second.

An example of the successful ablation of a left sided accessory pathway is shown in Figure 8. As RF energy is delivered, the accessory pathway is successfully ablated in 2 beats. Again, the ability to record electrograms during RF application may be extremely useful in determining whether or not the catheter has moved during RF application. Unsuccessful RF deliveries *where there is no variation in signal* demonstrates that an inappropriate site was chosen. On the other hand, signal variation with failed energy delivery may be used to demonstrate that catheter movement rather than site location was at fault.

7.   ORTHOGONAL ELECTRODES IN RIGHT VENTRICULAR OUTFLOW TRACT VENTRICULAR TACHYCARDIA ABLATION

The choice of ablation sites in the treatment of RVOT ventricular tachycardia again is crucial.[11]   Whereas previously, the local electrograms from the ablation catheter recorded prior to energy delivery was used to find 'early' sites of activation compared to the surface ECG during tachycardia, orthogonal electrograms are particularly useful in the ablation of this arrhythmia.

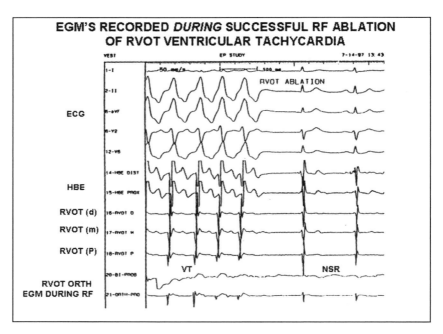

Figure 9. RVOT VT ABLATION: Recorded from top to bottom are surface ECG leads I, II, avF, V2 and V6. Below are intracardiac leads recorded from the bundle of His and three orthogonal electrograms recorded from the right ventricular outflow tract (RVOT) during the successful ablation of RVOT ventricular tachycardia. Although electrograms are not seen on the bipolar recording, the orthogonal electrogram (ORTH PRO) recorded during RF delivery demonstrates that the ablation site is the earliest recorded and that catheter position has remained stable.

In Figure 9, a multipolar orthogonal catheter is positioned in the RVOT. Its electrograms reflect local activation sequence.   The earliest signal from this catheter is then used as a reference for the ablation catheter which again 'maps' with orthogonal electrodes immediately behind the ablation tip prior to and *during* RF delivery. Again, catheter movement may be immediately detected by alteration in electrogram timing or characteristics.

8.   ORTHOGONAL ELECTRODES IN THE ABLATION OF ISCHEMIC VENTRICULAR TACHYCARDIA

The successful ablation of ventricular tachycardia associated with coronary artery disease and fibrotic tissue in the left ventricle is both difficult and hazardous.[12]   Orthogonal electrograms, here as elsewhere, may be useful in several regards. Localisation of sites of ventricular tachycardia in this setting is performed in several ways. Both during sinus rhythm and ventricular tachycardia, mid-diastolic potential may localise the reentrant pathway site. [13]   The near-field sensing ability of orthogonal electrodes amplifies these signals in comparison to more remote signals from 'distant' left ventricular sites.

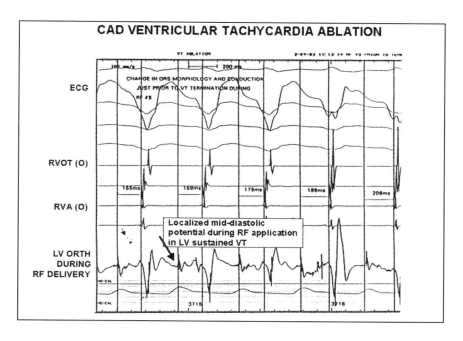

Figure 10. ORTHOGONAL EGM DURING LV VT ABLATION: During sustained monomorphic ventricular tachycardia associated with coronary artery disease, RF energy is applied to an area within the left ventricle where discrete diastolic potentials were recorded. On the electrograms recorded from the orthogonal sensors within the LV, the interval between the diastolic potential and the next tachycardia beat is seen to progressively prolong just prior to the termination of ventricular tachycardia. Orthogonal electrograms recorded from the right ventricular outflow tract (RVOT) and right ventricular apex (RVA) were used as reference electrodes for tachycardia mapping.

During pace and entrainment mapping, the ability of orthogonal sensors to record evoked responses and mid-diastolic potentials may be extremely important. Measurement of the interval between the last of a train of drive stimuli and the diastolic potential in ventricular tachycardia can be used to establish the catheter tip location relative to the entrance, isthmus or exit site of a sustained ventricular tachycardia.[14]

In addition, orthogonal electrograms recorded during RF application may shed light on the rhythm's mechanism as well as assist in determining successful sites and catheter movement. In Figure 10, RF energy is applied during an episode of sustained ventricular tachycardia of left ventricular origin. The mid-diastolic potential can be seen to occur with progressive delay in its time of onset as this tachycardia slows prior to successful ablation. Only with orthogonal electrograms is this type of recording possible.

SUMMARY

The key to successful ablation and cure of cardiac arrhythmias lies not so much in the energy source used to destroy localized areas of myocardium, as in the ability to localize the sites where ablation will be successful. Electrode catheter technology has progressed significantly over the past thirty year, however, the basic electrode design has remained unchanged. Recent studies employing small circumferentially placed electrodes have demonstrated that these orthogonal electrodes possess unique sensing capabilities. With powerful near-field sensing and virtually complete rejection of far-field signals, signal amplification may allow the recognition of localized intracardiac electrical activity previously unrecognised. The ability to record local evoked responses aids in the utility of entrainment mapping. Most importantly, however, the ability to record from orthogonal electrodes located immediately behind the tip of an ablation catheter *while* radiofrequency energy is being applied provides critical information. These recorded electrograms provide the unique ability not only to determine the precise location of the catheter tip but also whether failed applications are the result of site choice or catheter motion during RF.

REFERENCE:

1. Goldreyer B. Intracardiac electrocardiography in the analysis and understanding of cardiac arrhythmias. Ann Int Med. 1972; 77:117-136
2. DeCaprio V, Hurzeler P, Furman S. A comparison of unipolar and bipolar electgrograms for cardiac pacemaker sensing. Circ 1977; 56:750
3. Goldreyer B, Olive AL, Leslie J, Cannom DS, Wyman, MG. A new orthogonal lead for P synchronous pacing. PACE 1981; 4:638-644
4. Goldreyer B, Knudson M, Cannom D, Wyman M. Orthogonal electrogram sensing. PACE 1983; 6:464-469
5. Aubert A, Goldreyer B, Wyman, M, Jacquemlyn E, Ector H, DeGeest H. Filter characteristics of the atrial sensing circuit of a rate responsive pacemaker. To see or not to see. PACE 1989; 12:525-536

6. Aubert A, Goldreyer B, Wyman M, Denys B, Ector H, DeGeest H. Simultaneous right atrial appendage sensing with a target tip, a solid tip and J orthogonal electrodes. Am J Cardiol 1987; 59:610-614

7. Jackman W, Friday K, Yeung-Lai-Wah J, Fitzgerald D, Beck B, Bowman A, Stelzer P, Harrison L, Lazzara R. New catheter technique for recording left free-wall accessory atrioventricular pathway activation. Identification of pathway fiber orientation. Circ 1988:78,3: 598-610

8. Haissaguerre M, Gaita F, Fisher B, Commenges D, Montserrat P d'Ivernois C, Lemetayer P, Warin J. Elimination of atrioventricular nodal reentrant tachycardia using discrete slow potentials to guide application of radiofrequency energy. Circ 1992: 85,6: 2162-2175

9. Jentzer J, Goyal R, Williamson B, Man D, Niebauer M, Daoud E, Strickberger A, Hummel J, Morady F. Analysis of junctional ectopy during radiofrequency ablation of the slow pathway in patients with atrioventricular nodal reentrant tachycardia. Circ 1994; 90,6: 2820-2826

10. Schwartzman D, Callans D, Gottlieb C, Dillon S, Movsowitz C, Marchlinski F. Conduction block in the interior vena caval-tricuspid valve isthmus: association with outcome of radiofrequency ablation of type I atrial flutter. JACC 1996; 28,6: 1519-1531

11. Movsowitz C, Schwartzman D, Callans D, Preminger M, Zado E, Gottlieb C, Marchlinski F. Idiopathic right ventricular outflow tract tachycardia: narrowing the anatomic location for successful ablation. Am Heart J 1996; 131,5: 930-936

12. Stevenson W, Friedman P, Kocovic D, Sager P, Saxon L, Pavri B. Radiofrequency catheter ablation of ventricular tachycardia after myocardial infarction. Circ 1998; 98: 308-314

13. Bogun F, Bahu M, Knight B, Weiss R, Goyal R, Daoud E, Ching Man K, Strickberger A, Morady F. Response to pacing at sites of isolated diastolic potentials during ventricular tachycardia in patients with previous myocardial infarction. JACC 1997; 30:505-513

14. Stevenson W, Khan H, Sager P, Saxon L, Middlekauff H, Natterson P, Wiener I. Identification of reentry circuit sites during catheter mapping and radiofrequency ablation of ventricular tachycardia late after myocardial infarction. Circ 1993; 88:1647-1670

Chapter 7

MAPPING TECHNIQUES IN PATIENTS WITH PAROXYSMAL ATRIAL FIBRILLATION ORIGINATING FROM THE PULMONARY VEIN

Shih-Ann Chen, Ching-Tai Tai, Chin-Feng Tsai, Ming-Hsiung Hsieh, Yu-An Ding, Mau-Song Chang
Division of Cardiology, National Yang-Ming University School of Medicine and Taipei Veterans General Hospital, Taipei, Taiwan

INTRODUCTION

The so-called paroxysmal atrial fibrillation (AF) could be initiated by ectopic beats originating from the superior vena cava, cristal terminalis, ostium of coronary sinus, interatrial septum, atrial free wall, or ligament of Marshall; but most of the ectopic beats originate from the orifices of pulmonary veins (PVs) or from the myocardial sleeves inside the PVs.[1-9] Several laboratories have demonstrated that RF catheter ablation could effectively eliminate this type of AF, and suggest that AF is initiated by ectopic beats from a critical focus.[1-9] This article will discuss several critical issues regarding the mapping technique and interpretation of intracardiac electrograms in AF initiated by PV ectopic beats.

Supported in part by grants from the National Science Council (NSC 88-2314-B-010-094, 88-2314-B-010-093) and Tzou's Medical Foundation (VGHYM 87-S4-24, S3-17; VGH-23, 47, 61, 65, 254, 301), Taipei, Taiwan, R.O.C.

L. Bing Liem and E. Downar (eds.), Progress in Catheter Ablation, 79-92.

1.   MAPPING TECHNIQUE

1.1   Left atrium and PV angiography

As we described previously, left atrial and PV angiography is very important before we begin the mapping and ablation procedures. [10-11] From the left atrial angiography, the left atrial border can be visualized clearly; furthermore, location of the left atrial appendage can be confirmed to avoid inadevertant mechanical perforation caused by uncareful manipulation of mapping/ablation catheters outside the orifice of left PVs. Direct visualization of PVs by using different fluoroscopic views are very important to see the details of PV main trunk and branches; the oblique view (both the right anterior oblique 30 degree, left anterior oblique 60 degree), with or without cranial angulation 20 degree together with the anterior-posterior and lateral view are useful (Figure 1).

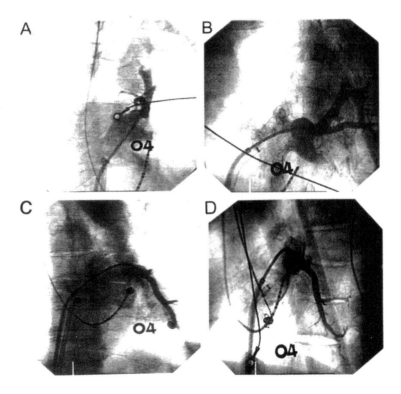

Figure 1. Panel A (RAO 30 degree) and B (LAO 60 degree) show the left superior PV and its branches; Panel C (AP view) and D (Lateral view) show the left inferior PV.

The anatomical variations of the PVs, especially their junction with the left atrium, and their branching patterns are quite common.[12-17] Several studies also demonstrated dilatation of PV ostium in patients with atrial arrhythmias originating from PVs; however, dilatation of PV ostium is not specifically related to the ectopic foci.[18-20]

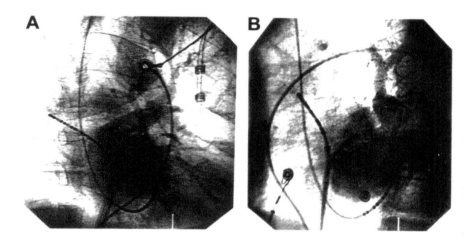

LSPV with vertical direction

Figure 2. The junction between LSPV and left atrium shows a nearly 90 degree angle in the LAO 60° fluoroscopic view.

The left PVs (superior and inferior PVs) are often (around 20-30%) known to have a common opening into the left atrium.[12-17] Our laboratory also shows the similar finding.[21] Some patients had a nearly vertical angle between left superior PV and left atrium, and makes the cannulation procedure very difficult (Figure 2). Trifurcation of the PVs (where the right middle lobe vein and the left lingual lobe vein open separately into the left atrium rather than join the upper PVs) is not rare. It is easy to mistaken the right middle lobe vein for the right inferior PV especially when the right middle lobe vein has a separate ostium or opens very proximally into the right superior PV, as the catheter points inferiorly in both these veins. The same mistake could be made for left lingual lobe vein and left inferior PV (Figure 3). Selective angiography in the lateral view can resolve this issue.[10,11] The right middle lobe vein and left lingual lobe vein are often small caliber veins and join with the right superior PV and left superior PV, respectively. They are noted to course downward, anterior to the spine, while the inferior PVs are noted to course posteriorly and overlap the shadow of the spine.[10-11]

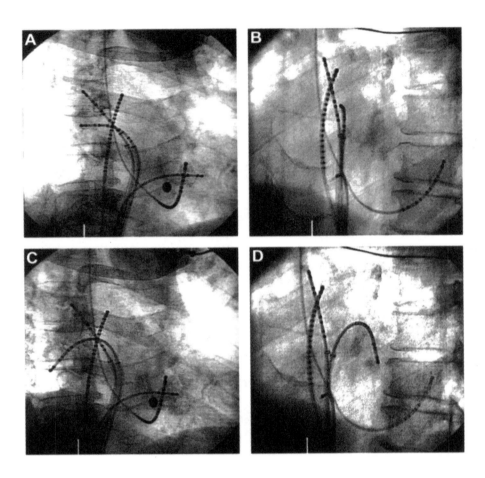

Figure 3. Panels A and B show the right anterior oblique 30 degrees and left anterior oblique 60 degrees, respectively; the same as Panel C and D. Arrow heads in Panel A and B denote mapping catheter in the right middle PV; whereas Panel C and D denote mapping catheter in the right inferior PV. Comparisons between Panel B and D show the anterior deviation of right middle PV, and posterior deviation of right inferior PV.

Using the CT or MRI for the 3-D reconstruction of the left atrium and PVs could be useful to delineate the anatomy of PVs, PV ostium junction between PV and left atrium before the invasive procedure. Intracardiac echocardiography is a promising tool for identifying the puncture site on the interatrial septum, and visualizing the PV ostia and branches.

1.2   Catheter Positions

The use of multiple mapping catheters in the PVs needs further discussion. Because two or more foci of trigger beats identified preceding AF, and simultaneous activation of trigger points from both PVs were not infrequent. Even in the same PV, ectopic beats arising from different branches may occur. Furthermore, during radiofrequency ablation, we needed one mapping catheter for guidance of ablation site. [6-11] Thus simultaneous mapping of two or multiple PVs using the regular size of double multielectrode catheters or multiple microcatheters would get the accurate activation pattern of ectopic beats which initiate AF, provide a good guide to select the optimal ablation site, and decrease the procedure and fluoroscopic times. Although the change of CS activation sequence or the relative activation sequence of His and CS would predict the presumed ectopic beats from the right or left PV (superior or inferior), some cases with simultaneous depolarization of two or more PVs, or simultaneous depolarization of SVC, upper cristal terminalis and right superior PV need more catheters to accurately locate the sites of ectopic beats.

This current multiple electrode catheters mapping technique may have safety and advantages when used for atrial fibrillation from the pulmonary veins, since the disadvantage of a single mapping catheter with few electrodes will be avoided. However, further studies will be required to establish an optimal mapping and ablation technique.

2.   INTERPRETATION OF PV ELECTROGRAM

2.1   Local PV Electrograms During Sinus Rhythm

During the sinus rhythm, PV potentials (with a sharp upstroke, narrow duration < 50msec, and an amplitude larger than 0.05 mV) in the right superior PV were usually preceded by a far field atrial potential with a slow slope (depolarization rate $dV/dt < 0.5$ mV/sec). However, PV potentials in the right superior PV may be preceded by a sharp potential if some portion of the right superior PV is very close to or contacts with the upper portion of the right atrial posterior wall, or superior vena cava; furthermore, SVC recordings can also get the near field potential of right superior PV (Figure 4). PV potentials are usually obscured by the left atrial potentials in the left side PVs. In patients with AF originating from PVs, the mean numbers of electrode pairs showing PV potentials and length of myocardial sleeve showing PV potentials were significantly less in the right side PVs than those in the left side PVs. The number of electrode pairs showing PV potentials and myocardial sleeve length were significantly less in the inferior PVs than those in both superior PVs;

furthermore, the amplitude of PV potential is usually higher in the proximal portion of PV than it in the distal portion of PV.[8,10,11,22]

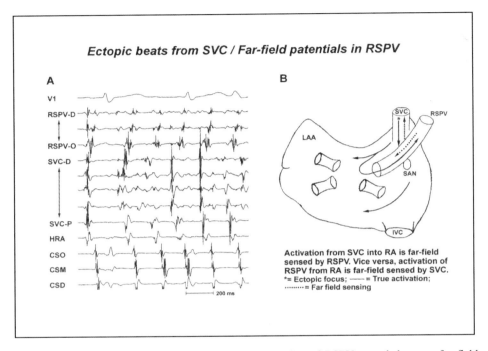

Figure 4. Panel A: during the sinus beat, the distal portion of RSPV record the near far field potentials of SVC potentials. During the initiation of AF, the first ectopic depolarization originated from SVC middle portion, and conducted to the right atrium, left atrium, proximal and distal parts of RSPV sequentially.

2.2   Local PV Electrogram During Ectopic Beats and Initiation of AF

2.2.1   Unusual Electrogram Morphologies of PV Ectopic Beats

The characteristics of typical PV potential include a very sharp and short duration electrogram. However, the morphologies of PV potentials during ectopic beats also depend on the anatomic sites of ectopic beats, and local property of myocardial sleeve inside the PVs. A fusion potential including PV potential and atrial potential from the PV ostium and surrounding atrial tissues, a wide, bizarre or fragmented electrogram from the PV ostium or inside the PV is possible (Figures 5, 6 and 7).

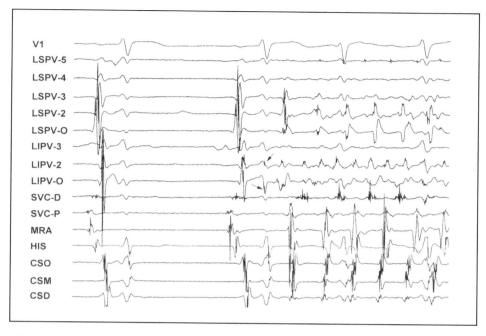

Figure 5. A sharp PV potential (arrows), inscribed on the terminal portion of V wave, was found nearly simultaneous on the left inferior PV ostium and the second electrode pair (2-5-2-5 mm spacing). After the ectopic beat, AF followed.

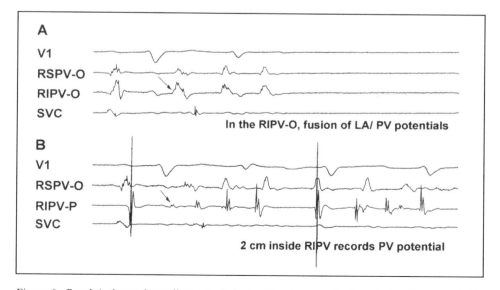

Figure 6. Panel A shows the earliest ectopic beat with a low amplitude wide duration potential in the right inferior PV ostium. However, when the mapping catheter was advanced 2 cm deep into the RIPV, the PV potentials with burst of depolarizations were demonstrated (confirmed by successful ablation).

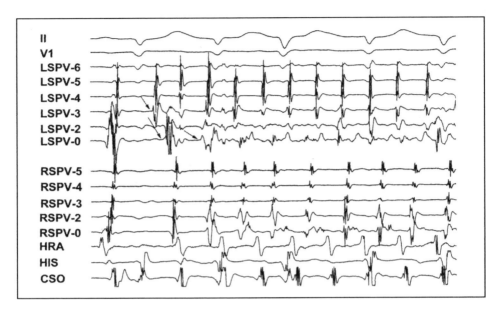

Figure 7. An atrial –like potential was recorded inside the LSPV (first arrow), and it conducted to the ostium (fusion potential with PV and atrial potential, with fibrillatory waves in the proximal portion of LSPV); however, the distal portions of LSPV (-4 to –6) and RSPV (-3 to –5) show organized activation.

2.2.2   Unusual Conduction Patterns of PV Ectopic Beats

During ectopic beats, PV potentials precede the far field right atrial or left atrial potentials. PV activity could conduct along the myocardial sleeve of PVs; however, unidirection or bidirection conduction block within the PVs (intra-PV conduction delay or block) with the phenomenon of concealed PV discharges is not rare. Intra-atrial conduction block (between different PVs) or interatrial conduction block (between PV and right atrium) is found occasionally (Figures 8 and 9). The role of some embryologic connection between PVs, superior vena cava, and CS must be considered, because the remanent myocardial tissues inside these venous vessels would change the activation sequences between PVs and other recording sites.

2.2.3   Double Potentials

The nature of double PV potentials, and the relation between first and second PV potential is not clear. The first PV depolarization may conduct very slowly, like the intra-atrial or intra-Hisian conduction delay, and the second PV potential is widely split from the first one. The second possibility is that the nearby myocardial tissue depolarizes spontaneously, and not related to the first PV potential (Figure 10).

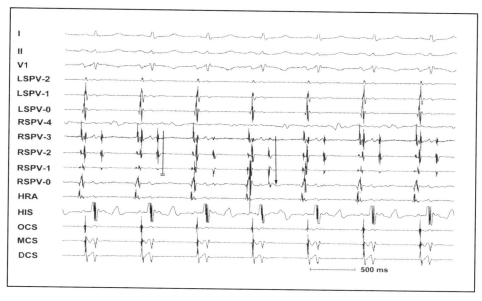

Figure 8. Eectopic depolarization originated from RSPV-3 with conduction block between RSPV-1 and RSPV-O, or between RSPV-O and left atrium.

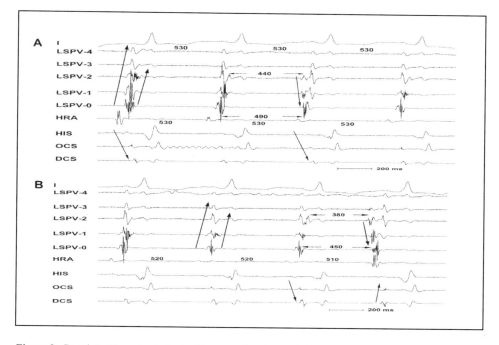

Figure 9. Panel A: The ectopic beat with a coupling interval 440 msec on LSPV-2 conducted to the LSPV-O, and collided with the impulse from sinus node, thus the AA intervals on HRA remain the same. Panel B: the ectopic beat with a shorter coupling interval (380 msec) on LSPV-2/3 conducted to the right atrium earlier than the regular sinus rate, and the AA interval on HRA was shortened.

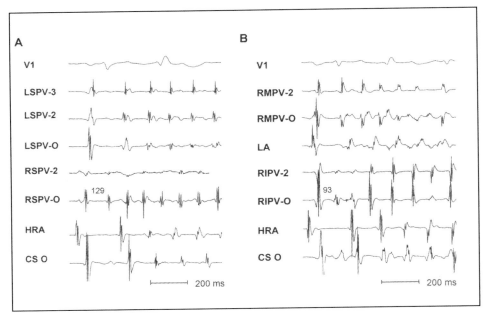

Figure 10.   Panel A showed the first episode of AF was from RSPV (Panel A), and the second episode of AF was from RMPV (Panel B), respectively.

2.2.4   Multiple Ectopic Foci with Independent, Simultaneous or Alternate Depolarization

Simultaneous or nearly simultaneous depolarization of two or more PVs, or simultaneous depolarization of PV and left atrial tissues is not common. However, the possibility of fusion beat, ectopic beats from PV ostium or from the area surrounded by the four PVs (posterior free wall or ligament of Marshall) should be considered. Alternate depolarization at different sites could occur within one PV, two PVs or different anatomic sites. For example, ectopic beats alternately arise from the proximal and distal ends of one PV, or ectopic beats alternately arise from different PVs or atrial tissues (Figures 10 and 11).

2.2.5   Proximal to distal conduction pattern

Especially in the ostial lesion, it is necessary to map the superior and inferior PVs simultaneously to avoid to the near far field recording or the bystander activation from the other branch (Figure 12).

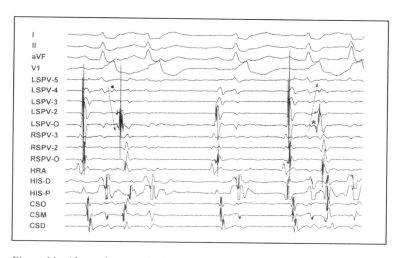

Figure 11. Alternating ectopic foci on LSPV distal and ostial areas.

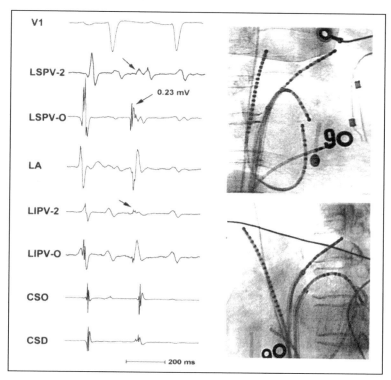

Figure 12. The ectopic beat from LSPV-ostium shows a fusion potential (PV potential with atrial potential). LSPV-2 shows low amplitude PV potential (arrow) and far-field left atrial potential. LIPV-O shows the small PV potential (passive depolarization of the LIPV myocardial sleeve) with left atrial potential. LIPV-2, as the LSPV-2, shows the low amplitude PV potential (arrow) and far-field left atrial potential. The right panels show the close distance between the proximal portion of left superior and inferior PVs.

2.2.6   Others

Detection of the fifth PV, anatomic route of Marshall vein, and the insertion site between Marshall vein and the left atrium may be necessary to find the "unknown" foci and improve the success rate.

3.   FUTURE DEVELOPMENT

The use of Ring catheter or Lasso catheter with multiple electrodes around or inside the PV ostium can identify the anatomic distribution of PV myocardial sleeves. Disconnection between these PV sleeves and left atrial tissue would block the conduction of ectopic beats to the atria and prevent occurrence of atrial fibrillation (Figure 13).

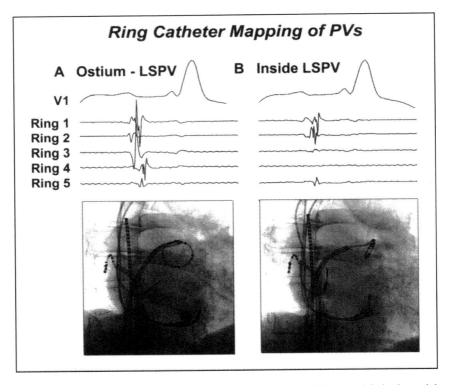

Figure 13. Panels A and B show the different distributions of PV potentials in the ostial and proximal area of left superior pulmonary vein (LSPV). In the ostial area, more bipolar recordings show PV potentials than those inside the PV (Ring-3 and Ring-4 do not record the PV potentials). From demonstration in New Delhi Batra Heart Center.

CONCLUSION

Mapping and interpretation of electrograms in the PVs becomes very important when we try to find the initiation mechanism of AF. More information about the basic knowledge of PV, advancement of mapping technique and development of new device is required for a detailed mapping and successful ablation of paroxysmal AF.

REFERENCES

1. Jais P, Haissaguerre M, Shah DC, Chouairi S, Gencel L, Hocini M, Clementy J. A focal source of atrial fibrillation treated by discrete radiofrequency ablation. Circulation 1997;95: 572-576.
2. Haissaguerre M, Jais P, Shah DC, Takahashi A, Hocini M, Quiniou G, Garrigue S, Mouroux AL, Metayer PL, Clementy J. Spontaneous initiation of atrial fibrillation by ectopic beats originating in the pulmonary veins. New Engl J Med 1998;339: 659-666.
3. Lau CP, Tse HF, Ayers GM. Defibrillation guided mapping and radiofrequency ablation of focal atrial fibrillation. J Am Coll Cardiol 1998;31: 61-A (abstract).
4. Wharton JM, Vergara I, Shander G, Sorrentino RA, Greenfield RA. Identification and ablation of focal mechanisms of atrial fibrillation. Circulation 1998;98: I-18 (abstract).
5. Natale A, Behiery S, Richey M, Pisano E, Sofferenza CS, Giovanni R; Fanelli R, Rajkovich K, Wides B, Martinez K, Tomassoni G, Leonelli F. Pulmonary vein ablation versus large dose of intravenous amiodarone for treatment of immediate recurrence of atrial fibrillation following electrical cardioversion. Circulation 1998;98: I-181 (abstract).
6. Hsieh MH, Chen SA, Tai CT, Tsai CF, V.S.Prakash, Yu WC, Liu CC, Ding YA, Chang MS. Double multielectrode mapping catheters facilitate radiofrequency catheter ablation of focal atrial fibrillation originating from pulmonary veins. J. Cardiovasc Electrophysiology 1999;10: 136-144..
7. Chen SA, Tai CT, Yu WC, Chen YJ, Tsai CF, Hsieh MH, Chen CC, Prakash VS, Ding YA, Chang MS. Right atrial focal atrial fibrillation - electrophysiologic characteristics and radiofrequency catheter ablation. J Cardiovasc Electrophysiol 1999;10: 328-335.
8. Chen SA, Hsieh MH, Tai CT, Tsai CF, Prakash VS, Yu WC, Hsu TL, Ding YA, Chang MS. Initiation of atrial fibrillation by ectopic beats originating from the pulmonary veins electrophysiological characteristics, pharmacological responses, and effects of radiofrequency ablation. Circulation 1999;100: 1879-1886.
9. Prakash VS, Hsieh MH, Tsai CF, Tai CT, Ding YA, Chang MS, Chen SA. Selective pulmonary vein angiography improves accuracy of catheterization and mapping in patients with paroxysmal focal atrial fibrillation. J Am Coll Cardiol 1999,33 (abstract).
10. Chen SA, Tai CT, Tsai CF, Hsieh MH, Ding YA, Chang MS. Radiofrequency catheter ablation of atrial fibrillation initiated by pulmonary vein ectopic beats. J Cardiovasc Electrophysiol 2000;11:218-227.
11. Chen SA, Tai CT, Hsieh MH, Tsai CF, Ding YA, Chang MS. Radiofrequency catheter ablation of atrial fibrillaiton initiated by spontaneous ectopic beats. Europace 2000;2:99-105.
12. Michelson E, Salik JO. The vascular pattern of the lung as seen on routine and tomographic studies. Radiology 1959;73:511-526.

13. Cory RAS, Valentine EJ. Varying patterns of the lobar branches of the pulmonary artery. Thorax 1959;14:267-280.
14. Hislop A, Reid L. Fetal and childhood development of the intrapulmonary veins in man-branching pattern and structure. Thorax 1973;28:313-319.
15. Rosse C, Caddum-Rosse P. The Lungs. In: Rosse C, ed. Hollinshead's Textbook of Anatomy. Philadelphia, PA: Lippincott-Raven Publications, 1997; 441-462.
16. Johnson CT, Zhong GW, Kall JG, Kopp DE et al. Morphometry and relationships of human left atrial anatomic structures. PACE 1998;21:816 (abstract).
17. Tsai CF, Tai CT, Hsieh MH , Yu WC, Lin WS, Ueng KC, Ding YA, Chang MS, Chen SA. Initiation of atrial fibrillation by ectopic beats originating from the superior vena cava-electrophysiologic characteristics and results of radiofrequency ablation. Circulation 2000;102:67-74.
18. Sivaram CA, Asirvatham S, Sebastian C, Patel A, Chandrashekaran S, Jackman W. Transesophageal echo abnormalities of pulmonary veins in atrial tachycardia originating from pulmonary veins. PACE 1998;21:888. (abstract).
19. Chiba N, Nakagawa H, Yoshioka K, Naiai K, Hotta K, Terui K, Hata Y, Yagi Y, Ito M, Hiramori K. Dilatation of the pulmonary veins in patients with idiopathic atrial fibrillation. Circulation 1998,17, I-702 (abstract).
20. Prakash VS, Hsieh MH, Tsai CF, Tai CT, Ding YA, Chang MS. Dilated pulmonary veins and focal atrial fibrillation originating from pulmonary veins. J Am Coll Cardiol 1999;33 (abstract).
21. Lin WS, Prakash VS, Tai CT, Hsieh MH, Tsai CF, Yu WC, Lin YK, Ding YA, Chang MS, Chen SA. Pulmonary vein morphology in patients with paroxysmal atrial fibrillation initiated by ectopic beats originating from the pulmonary veins implications for catheter ablation. Circulation 2000;101:1274-1281.
22. Hsieh MH, Tai CT, Tsai CF, Yu WC, Lee SH, Lin YK, Ding YA, Chang MS, Chen SA. Pulmonary vein electrogram characteristics in patients with focal sources of paroxysmal atrial fibrillation. J Cardiovasc Electrophysiol 2000;11:953-959.

Chapter 8

PULMONARY VENOUS ANGIOGRAPHY

Angelo A.V. De Paola, Roberto L. Farias, Almino C. Rocha Neto
Clinical Cardiac Electrophysiology, Paulista School of Medicine, Federal University of São Paulo, SãoPaulo, Brazil

INTRODUCTION

Successful radiofrequency catheter ablation of ectopic beats originating from the pulmonary veins can eliminate paroxysmal atrial fibrillation (AF),[1-4] but the complex anatomy of this region may limit mapping of AF. Information about the structure of the pulmonary veins and left atrial junction is poorly reported, especially in the adult population.

1. PULMONARY VENOUS, VENOATRIAL MORPHOLOGY AND VARIANTS

The four pulmonary veins (right superior, left superior, right inferior, and left inferior) originate in the hilum from the confluence of the pulmonary segmental vessels. In general, two pulmonary veins enter the left atrium on each side. Their course is longer on the right side than on the left.[5] Numerous variations and anomalies of the pulmonary veins have been identified. Doerr estimates their occurrence at 10%.[6]

The right superior pulmonary vein is in the hilum of the lung below and in front of the pulmonary artery. The right inferior pulmonary vein can be found below the principal bronchus. It collects the blood from the inferior lobe. Both veins run into the left atrium behind the superior vena cava. They enters separately into the atrium, the superior vein somewhat higher and more anteriorly than the inferior.

L. Bing Liem and E. Downar (eds.), Progress in Catheter Ablation, 93-104.

The left veins come together and return to the left atrium at 25% as a unique ostium. The superior vein enters the atrium at the top and the inferior vein enters in the left posterior corner of the left atrium.[5,7]

The diameter of the pulmonary vein ostium measures around 14 to 16 mm, with large variations in these measurements.[6,8-10] Ho and coworkers[11] reviewing the gross structure of the left atrium of 26 heart specimens, had some difficulty in determining the exact location of the venoatrial junction. The pulmonary vein ostia ranged from 2 to 17 mm. The shrinkage of the specimens due to fixation must have accounted for the low estimation of some of these measurements. Another cause for variation was the possibility that, instead of four, a different number of veins opened into the left atrium. On the right side, the number of the veins ranges from 2 to 6, and on the left side a common trunk may be formed within or outside of the pericardium (Figure 1).[12]

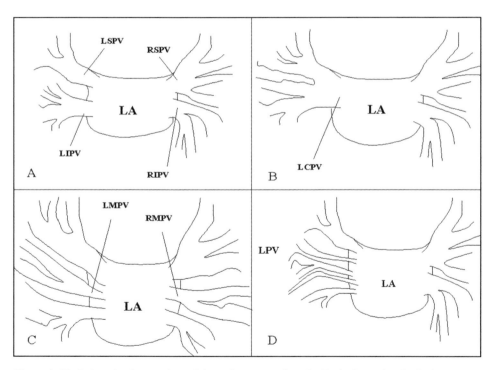

Figure 1. Variations in the opening of the pulmonary veins. A- Typical opening B: Left common trunk (LCPV) C- Separate opening of right and left middle veins D- Multiple.

In the absence of a total anomalous pulmonary vein connection,[13-15] morphologic variances do not have any clinical relevance. A partial anomalous connection (up to 50% in the left atrium) may not produce symptoms. Romada et al[16] found such anomalies in 10% of their autopsy studies.

The rapid development of endocardial mapping and radiofrequency ablation for drug-resistant AF has drawn attention to the left atrium and pulmonary vein structures. Precise mapping of the electrical activities along the pulmonary veins requires proper delineation of the pulmonary veins structures. Furthermore, the design of new devices, such as the ablation balloon for circumferential isolation of the pulmonary veins, requires careful evaluation of proximal pulmonary vein structures and diameters.[17]

2. EFFECTS OF RADIOFREQUENNCY ENERGY IN THE PULMONARY VEINS

The long-term complications of catheter ablation within pulmonary veins are unknown. The development of pulmonary vein stenosis has recently been described after catheter ablation to treat either chronic or paroxysmal AF.[18,19] Stenosis is an undesirable and potentially life-threatening complication, and the risk of this complication is greater in small vessels.

Unlike congenital narrowing of the pulmonary vein,[20,21] balloon dilatation of stenosis due to radiofrequency catheter ablation is feasible,[18] but the long-term prognosis is unknown. The early recognition of stenosis is important for the management of this complication.

3. PULMONARY VEIN MORPHOLOGY EVALUATION

Determining the optimal location for ablation catheters has challenged electrophysiologists' skills and yielded a worldwide search for new technologies. Vascular pulmonary circulation can also be assessed by a number of alternative imaging modalities, such as nuclear magnetic resonance, ultrafast computerized tomography, transesophageal echocardiography, intravascular ultrasound, and selective angiography. Nuclear magnetic resonance and ultrafast computerized tomography are very useful noninvasive tools for diagnosis of congenital heart diseases and may be used for the evaluation of pulmonary vein stenosis.[22-24] The main limitation of these techniques is the impossibility of performing them during the ablation procedure.

Transesophageal echocardiography is very accurate for defining the upper pulmonary vein anatomy. Doppler techniques can assess minimal alterations in blood flow in these vessels. However, assessment of inferior pulmonary veins and distal segments of pulmonary veins is difficult. Intravascular ultrasound provides intraluminal real-time, two-dimensional and cross-sectional images of the vessel wall and enables accurate measurement of the size of the lumen and vessel wall with minimal inter-observer variability. However, its use during fast comparative assessment of interventional results may be time-consuming in inexperienced hands. In addition, complete anatomical details of pulmonary veins and their branches cannot be obtained with this technique.

Despite some limitations, selective pulmonary vein angiography is the best tool for evaluating the anatomy of pulmonary veins. The most important factor for electing angiography is its immediate resolution capability in the fast decision-making process for assessment of vascular anatomy during interventional electrophysiological procedures. Stenosis, spasm, and thrombosis of pulmonary veins require prompt diagnosis to avoid additional radiofrequency applications and for planning effective treatment strategies (Figure 2). Moreover, a high-quality digital X-ray system, the well-tolerated nonionic dye agents and, finally, widespread use of well-standardized angiographic techniques recommend pulmonary venous angiography as a very good anatomical support for interventions in the pulmonary vein system.

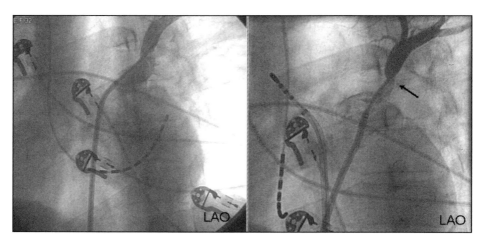

Figure 2: Left superior pulmonary venous angiography. A (left): before radiofrequency application. B (right): after ablation depicting vascular stenosis (arrow).

4.   SELECTIVE PULMONARY VEIN ANGIOGRAPHY

Robida[25] studied the diameters of pulmonary veins at the junction of individual pulmonary veins with the left atrium on the levophase of pulmonary trunk angiograms in children, but the view of the ostium of some of the left pulmonary veins was obscured by other structures. More recently, during mapping and ablation of AF, selective pulmonary vein angiography provided better visualization of this region than the conventional pulmonary trunk angiogram.

5. PULMONARY VEIN ANGIOGRAPHY AS SUPPORT DURING RADIOFREQUENCY CATHETER ABLATION OF ATRIAL FIBRILLATION

In performing pulmonary vein angiography, we introduce two 8.5 Fr sheaths (SL1 Daig, Minneapolis, MN, USA) into the left atrium. After making a standard transeptal puncture, we position the first sheath, which serves as a guide for the second puncture and sheath placement. The patient receives an initial intravenous bolus of 5000 IU of heparin to maintain an activated clotting time of > 300 seconds. We then introduce a deflectable soft-tip angiographic catheter (Naviport™, Cardima, Fremont, CA, USA) through the sheath, which is very helpful for selective cannulation of upper and inferior pulmonary veins. In our experience, deflectable soft-tip catheters are more appropriate than regular catheters for selective angiography of pulmonary veins. Their use aids in overcoming frequent difficulties such as repeated catheterization of the left atrium appendix during approaches for left superior pulmonary vein catheterization with regular NIH or multipurpose angiographic catheters. These catheters are also very useful not only in this situation but also for selective catheterization of inferior pulmonary veins.

Two or three injections of 5-cc dye using preferentially the left anterior oblique projections offer excellent angiographic definition of the ostium and proximal branches of each pulmonary vein. Modern catheterization laboratories have advanced digital display capabilities. The catheterization procedure can be shown on a video display unit. This visualization method is of the utmost importance for anatomical angiographic definition, and it offers instant replay, and postprocessing including measurements, subtraction capabilities, and contrast sensitivity during the procedures into these vessels.

When the angiographic study is completed, we keep the Naviport catheter in the left atrium for angiographic support during placement of electrophysiologic catheters for mapping and ablation of the AF. Because of the not uncommon frequency of multiple locations of pulmonary vein foci, we advocate simultaneous mapping of the four vessels and angiography to avoid misplacing the microelectrode catheters into secondary branches of the same main pulmonary vein. This approach is also very helpful in patients with scanty ectopy or recurrent onsets of AF during the procedure.

At this point, angiographic information of pulmonary vein anatomy has already been obtained, and the second sheath is placed in the same position as the first, in the ostium of the left pulmonary veins. Small injections of dye through the angiographic catheter assure the ˙correct longitudinal positioning of microelectrode catheters (3.3 Fr, Revelation™, Cardima, Fremont, CA, USA), which are inserted through the second sheath, with distal electrodes reaching the main branches of the pulmonary veins, and the proximal electrodes are placed into the ostium. Usually the left superior pulmonary vein is the first vessel cannulated followed by the left inferior pulmonary vein (Figures 3A and 3B)

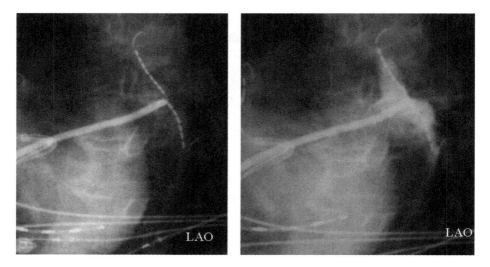

Figure 3. A (left panel): Microelectrode catheter placement in the left pulmonary veins. B (right panel): Catheter positioning was checked by angiography in this patient.

After placing microcatheters into the left pulmonary veins, pulling and giving a clockwise torque to the second sheath is enough to cannulate the right superior pulmonary vein. After checking correct positioning, we withdraw the angiographic catheter from the sheath and insert 2 microelectrode catheters into the right upper and inferior pulmonary veins. The right inferior pulmonary vein may be difficult to access. In this situation, we use the deflectable capability of the angiographic catheter positioning the sheath deeply into this vessel facilitating microcatheter placement. After this maneuver, we pull back the sheath to the ostium, directing the placement of the second right microelectrode catheter into the right superior pulmonary vein (Figure 4).

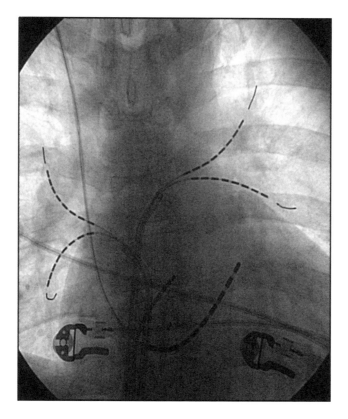

Figure 4: Selective catheterization of the 4 pulmonary veins with microelectrode catheters.

6.   VENOUS-ATRIUM JUNCTION DEFINITION

The pulmonary venous ostium is the junction of the pulmonary vein with the left atrium. It transmits ectopic electrical impulses from the pulmonary veins to the left atrium, and is a critical area for mapping and ablation of AF. Electrophysiologists have been using traditional fluoroscopic landmarks to define the ostium. These landmarks include the segment of the ablation catheter leaving the cardiac silhouette or, during the pullback maneuver, the entrance downward of the catheter tip into the left atrium chamber. However, this definition is not enough for interventional procedures, and a clear definition of the ostium may be reproducibly obtained with selective angiography (Figure 5).

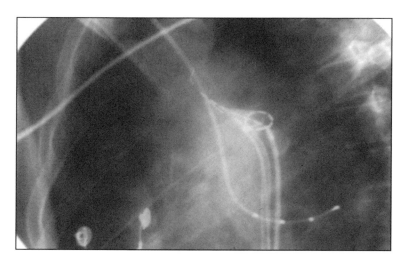

Figure 5: Circular shaping of microelectrode mapping catheter in the right superior pulmonary venous ostium (LAO projection)

7.   ANGIOGRAPHIC MEASUREMENTS

Knowing the diameter of the ostium is important for defining the mapping area, because the diameter provides anatomical information for strategies when electrical pulmonary vein-left atrium disconnection is contemplated (Figure 6).

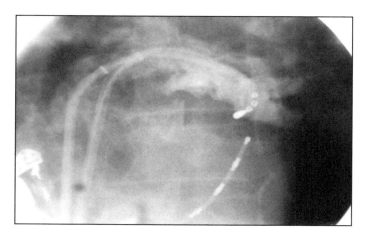

Figure 6: Pulmonary venous angiography (LAO projection): Ablation catheter positioned in the floor of the left inferior pulmonary vein during radiofrequency delivery for pulmonary vein-left atrium disconnection.

We performed pulmonary venous angiography during mapping and ablation of AF in 20 patients with the technique previously described. See Table 1 for a list of the ostium diameters of pulmonary veins, expressed in mean (mm) and ± standard deviation (SD) values. Electrophysiological mapping techniques are more effective in small areas or when landmarks are well defined. When the foci of AF are inside a small pulmonary vein, immediate angiography can provide the diameter of the targeted vessel and the risk of stenotic complications. Mapping proximal sites of pulmonary veins involves larger areas that are dependent on the dimensions of the ostium and the distance of branching of the main pulmonary vein.

	PVO (mm)	OB (mm)	AO (mm2)	MA (mm2)	OA/MA (%)
RSPV	14.7±5.7†	13.5±5.1*	185.3±72.0	836.0±608.9*	25.3±7.0*
LSPV	13.0±2.4	7.9±2.1*	164.1±30.3	497.6±148.6*	34.1±8.2*
RIPV	10.2±5.1†	13.2±6.0	127.3±63.7	608.8±486.2	25.6±10.7
LIPV	10.7±2.3	8.0±6.6	135.5±29.1	408.2±307.2	39.2±13.8

Table. 1: PV ostium diameter (PVO), distance from ostium to venous branching initiation (OB), the main ostium area (AO), the main mapping area (MA) and AO/MA ratio (values in percentage), right superior pulmonary vein (RSPV), left superior pulmonary vein (LSPV), right inferior pulmonary vein (RIPV), left inferior pulmonary vein (LIPV). Values in millimeters and standard deviation (SD). † * $p<0.05$, * Comparison of right and left side PV, † Comparisons of superior and inferior PV.

We studied the following characteristics of these "AF-related ablation areas", hypothesizing that the pulmonary vein acts as a cylinder: the pulmonary vein ostium, the distance from the ostium to the initiation of venous branching, the ostium area, the main pulmonary venous mapping area, and the ostium area to mapping area ratio (Figures 7A and 7B). We defined the main pulmonary venous mapping area as the area situated between the ostium area and proximal branching initiation.

The main right superior pulmonary vein mapping area was greater than the main left superior mapping area ($p=0.03$). Branching of the main left superior pulmonary vein was more proximal when compared with branching of the right superior pulmonary vein ($p<0.003$). These data were compared with mapping and ablation of foci located in the left posterior vein closer to the ostium ($p=0.01$) (Table 1). Diameters of the inferior pulmonary vein were smaller than diameters of the superior pulmonary vein, especially on the right side ($p=0.04$).

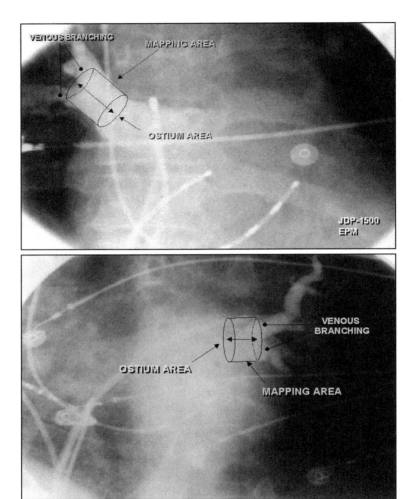

Figure 7: Schematic representation of the mapping area of the pulmonary veins, situated between the ostium and proximal branching. A: Right superior pulmonary vein B: Left superior.

Recently, pulmonary vein morphology has been associated with the presence or absence of ectopic beats that causes AF.[26]   Lin and coworkers[26] studied pulmonary vein morphology in patients with paroxysmal AF and found nonspecific dilatation of the ostia and the proximal portion of the superior pulmonary veins in patients with paroxysmal AF initiated by ectopic beats.

In conclusion, selective pulmonary vein angiography may be a useful tool during mapping and ablation of AF. Defining the pulmonary venous anatomy before and during catheter ablation of AF may show important variations in the caliber of the pulmonary veins. Checking the position of the ablation catheter and the caliber of the targeted vein may minimize complications and improve ablation results.

REFERENCES

1. Haissaguerre M, Jais P, Shah DC, Gencel L, Pradeau V, Guappigues S, Chouairi S, Hocini M, Metayer PLE, Clementy J. Right and left atrial radiofrequency catheter ablation therapy of paroxysmal atrial fibrillation. J Cardiovasc Electrophysiol. 1996;7:1132-1144.
2. Jais P, Haissaguerre M, Shah DC, Chouairi S, Gencel L, Hocini M, Clementy J. A focal source of atrial fibrillation treated by discrete radiofrequency ablation. Circulation. 1997;95:572-576.
3. Haissaguerre M, Jais P, Shah DC, Takahashi A, Hocini M, Quiniou G, Garrigue S, Mouroux AL, Metayer PLE, Clementy J. Spontaneous initiation of atrial fibrilation by ectopis beats originating in the pulmonary veins. N Engl J Med. 1998;339:659-666.
4. Chen AS, Tai CT, Yu WC, Chen YJ, Tsai CF, Hsieh MH, Chen CC, Prakash VS, Ding YA, Chang MS. Right atrial focal atrial fibrillation: electrophysiologic characteristics and radiofrequency catheter ablation. J Cardiovasc Electrophysiol. 1999;10:328-335.
5. Luzsa G: In: Blood vessels of the thorax. X-Ray Anatomy of the vascular system. Philadelphya and Toronto; J.B. Lippincott; 1974:19-119.
6. Doerr W. (1955) Die MiBbildungen des Herzens und dergroBen GefäBe (in: Lehrbuch der speziellen pathologischen anatomie. Ed. By Kaufmann, E. and Staemmler, M) W. de Gruyter, Berlin. (cit. by Luzsa G. 1974).
7. Michelson E, Salik JO. The vascular pattern of the lung as seen on routine and tomographic studies. Radiology. 1959;73:511-526.
8. Paturet G. In: Traité d'anatomie humane, volume 2-3, Masson; Paris; 1958.
9. Clemente CD. In: The veins. Gray's anatomy. Anatomy of the human body. 30th edition; Philadelphia; Lea & Febiger;1985:788-865.
10. Gardner H, Gray DJ, O'rahilly R. Em: Pleura e Pulmões. Anatomia. Estudo regional do corpo humano. 4° edição. Rio de Janeiro; Editora Guanabara Koogan; 1988:336-355.
11. Ho SY, Sanchez-Quintana D, Cabrera JA, Anderson RH. Anatomy of left atrium: Implications for radiofrequency ablation of atrial fibrillation. J Cardiovasc Electrophysiol 1999;10:1525-33.
12. Brantigan OC. Anomalies of the pulmonary veins: their surgical significance. Dis Chest 1952;21:174-178.
13. Amplatz K, Moller JH. In: Partial anomalous pulmonary venous connection. Radiology of congenital heart disease. St. Louis; Mosby Year Book; 1993:345-355.
14. Freedom RM, Culhan JAG, Moes CAF. In: Anomalies of pulmonary venous connections and obstruction to pulmonary venous flow. Angiocardiography of congenital heart disease. New York; Macmillan Publishing Company; 1984:274-302.
15. Culham JAG. In: Physical principles of image formation and projections in angiocardiography. Congenital heart disease. Textbook of angiocardiography. By: Freedom RM, Mawson JB, Benson LN. Volume I. Armonk, NY; Futura Publishing Company Inc., 1987:39-93
16. Romoda T, Istvánffy M, Záborasky B. A v. pulmonalis transpositio diagnosticus nehézségeiröl(About the diagnostic difficulties in case of transposition of the pulmonary vein). Orv. Hetil. 49, 2325.
17. Lesh MD, Guerra PG, Goseki Y, Sparks PB. An anatomic approach to prevention of atrial fibrillation: pulmonary vein isolation with through-the-balloon ultrasound ablation (TTB-

USA). Thorac Cardiovasc Surg;47 Suppl 3:347-51. Romoda T, Istvánffy M, Záborasky B. A v. pulmonalis transpositio diagnosticus nehézségeiröl (About the diagnostic difficulties in case of transposition of the pulmonary vein). Orv. Hetil. 49, 2325.

18. Robbins IM, Colvin EV, Doyle TP, Kemp WE, Loyd JE, McMohon WS, Kay NG. Pulmonary vein stenosis after catheter ablation of atrial fibrillation. Circulation 1998;98:1769-1775.
19. Sohn RH, Schiller NB. Left upper pulmonary vein stenosis 2 months after radiofrequency catheter ablation of atrial fibrillation. Circulation 2000;101:e154-e155.
20. Discroll DJ, Hesslein PS, Mullins CE. Congenital stenosis of individual pulmonary veins: Clinical spectrum and unsuccessful treatment by transvenous balloon dilation. Am J Cardiol 1982;49:1767-1772.
21. Lock JE, Bass JL, Castaneda-Zuninga W, Fuhrman BP, Rashkind WJ, Luca Jr. RV. Dilation angioplasty of congenital or operative narrowing of venous channels. Circulation 1984;70:457-464.
22. Chomka EV, Brundage BH. Cardiovascular ultrafast computed tomographic angiography. Am J Card Imaging 1993;7(3):252-264.
23. Hartnell GG, Meier RA. MR angiography of congenital heart disease in adults. Radiographics. 1995;15:781-794.
24. Hartnell GG, Hughes LA, Finn JP, Longmaid III HE. Magnetic resonance angiography of the chest veins. A new gold standard? Chest. 1995;107:1053-1057.
25. Robida A Diameters of pulmonary veins in normal children - an angiography study. Cardiovasc Intervent Radiol 1990;12:307-309.
26. Lin WS, Prakash VS, Tai CT, Hsieh MH, Tsai CF, Yu WC, Lin YK, Ding YA, Chang MS, Chen AS. Pulmonary vein morphology in patients with paroxysmal atrial fibrillation initiated by ectopic beats originating from the pulmonary veins. Implications for catheter ablation. Circulation 2000;101:1274-1281.

Chapter 9

ULTRASONIC GUIDANCE FOR RADIOFREQUENCY ABLATION

John D. Hummel
Riverside Methodist Hospital, Columbus, Ohio, USA

INTRODUCTION

Similar to transthoracic echocardiography, intracardiac echocardiography images cardiac structures with ultrasound waves. These sonic waves are emitted from an ultrasound crystal mounted onto the distal aspect of an intravascular catheter. The initial cardiac application was to evaluate intracoronary atherosclerotic lesions. Since tissue resolution varies inversely with the wavelength, and depth of penetration varies directly with wavelength, ideal imaging of the coronary endothelial surface requires high frequencies on the order of 30 mHz. For catheter ablation procedures, these ultrasound catheters were occasionally used to verify catheter tip-myocardial tissue contact.[1] Modification of the intracoronary ultrasound catheters to deliver lower frequencies (9 mHz) provided greater depth of penetration and not only allowed verification of tissue contact, but also facilitated identification of specific cardiac structures important in the ablation of arrhythmias and ablation location.[2-5] There are two commercially available ultrsound catheters. The first is a rotary driven transducer that images tangentially through a fluid filled catheter providing a 360° view around the catheter shaft that is angled at 15° consistent with the angle of the transducer (Figure 1). The second is a phased array system that mounts several transducers in an array on the shaft of a catheter, thus the image observed is pie shaped (Figure 2). In this chapter we will discuss the current and future role of intracardiac echocardiograpy (ICE) as an adjunctive imaging modality for electrophysiologic procedures.

L. Bing Liem and E. Downar (eds.), Progress in Catheter Ablation, 105-123.
© 2001 *Kluwer Academic Publishers. Printed in the Netherlands.*

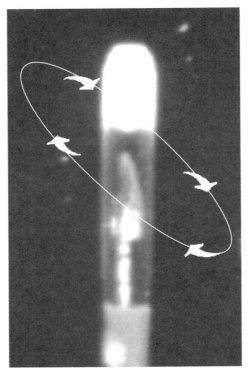

Figure 1. Diagram of a rotary driven intracardiac ultrasound catheter with a 360°field of imaging angled at 15°.

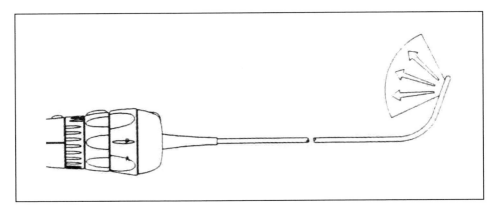

Figure 2. Diagram of a phased array ultrsound catheter. The handle allows the tip to be either turned in a circumferential manner or angled superior/inferior.

1.   TRANSSEPTAL PUNCTURE

Transseptal puncture for access to the left atrium and ventricle was pioneered by E.C. Brockenbrough, M.D. in the 1950's and 1960's. With the development of the retrograde aortic approach to left heart catheterization, it has become an infrequently used technique in the catheterization laboratory and, in fact, is more commonly used in the electrophysiology laboratory for left sided radiofrequency ablation procedures. Unfortunately, this technique is associated with a complication rate of 2-5%. Direct visualization of the right atrium, fossa ovalis, aorta, and left atrium by intracardiac echocardiography may minimize transseptal procedure duration and risk.[6]

1.1   Standard Transseptal Procedure

Detailed familiarity of the anatomy involved in this procedure is critical to its safety, particularly when only flouroscopy is used. A typical approach for transseptal puncture is described below. A transseptal sheath/dilator combination is advanced over a guidewire to the superior vena cava and a Brockenbrough needle is then advanced under fluoroscopy to just beneath the dilator tip. The needle hub is then connected to a pressure manifold. An arterial puncture is performed and a pigtail catheter is advanced to the aortic root to mark its position. At this point, the superior vena cava pressure is recorded and the needle and dilator are held in a constant relationship to each other as both are withdrawn as a unit from the superior vena cava to the right atrium under constant fluoroscopic guidance. As the unit is withdrawn it initially moves medially underneath the bulge of the ascending aorta and, subsequently, jumps medially into the fossa ovalis (Figure 3). At this point, slight advancement of the dilator/needle/sheath combination push it through a patent foramen ovale (which is present in approximately 10% of patients) or cause it to be halted by the rim of tissue that forms the superior edge of the fossa ovalis (the limbus). If satisfied with the position the operator will smoothly and forcefully advance the Brockenbrough needle tip so that it perforates the fossa ovalis (Figure 4). Successful entry into the left atrium is confirmed by documentation of left atrial pressure recordings from the hub of the needle, analysis of blood oxygenation from the tip of the needle, or injection of contrast media into the left atrium. If puncture of the fossa ovalis is unsuccessful, the needle is withdrawn, a guidewire is placed back into the superior vena cava and the entire procedure is repeated as there is no direct visualization of the needle position. In his textbook, William Grossman, M.D. refers to this standard procedure in the following way; " the infrequency with which the procedure is needed currently, has made it difficult for most laboratories to maintain operator expertise and to train cardiovascular fellows in transseptal puncture and has given the procedure an aura of danger and intrigue". The availability of intracardiac echo has helped to eliminate this aura of danger and allows one to abbreviate the previously delineated approach to transseptal puncture.

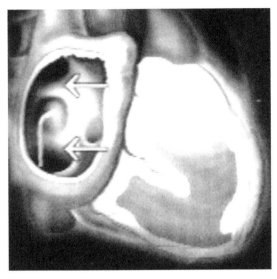

Figure 3. Illustration of right atrial anatomy demonstrating the position of the transseptal sheath in the fossa ovalis after withdrawl of the sheath from the superior vena cava.

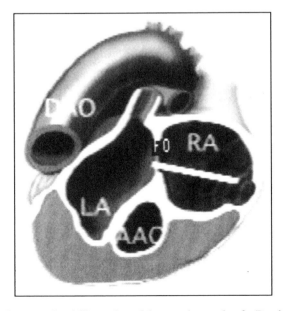

Figure 4. Cross sectional illustration of the crossing angle of a Brockenbrough needle through the fossa ovalis (FO). DAO indicates descending aorta; AAO, ascending aorta; LA, left atrium; RA, right atrium.

1.2   Intracardiac Echocardiographic Approach to Transseptal Catheterization

ICE simplifies transseptal puncture by allowing direct visualization of critical cardiac and extracardiac structrures in the following way. Under fluoroscopic guidance the ICE catheter is advanced through a 9 French sheath into the superior vena cava and slowly withdrawn into the right atrium. From superior to inferior the crista terminalis, aorta, aortic valve, interatrial muscular septum, fossa ovalis, left atrium and pulmonary veins, the coronary sinus, tricuspid and mitral valves and the right ventricle are inspected. The ICE probe is then positioned to continuously view the fossa ovalis. At this point, the operator can assess the length of the fossa ovalis, it's approximation to the left atrial wall and the presence or absence of a possible left atrial thrombus (Figure 5).

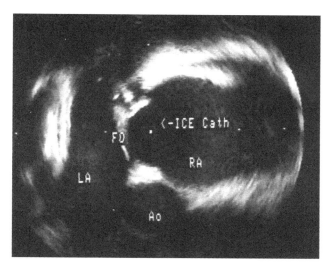

Figure 5. Typical image of the fossa ovalis (FO) obtained from a rotary driven ultrasound catheter positioned in the right atrium. LA indicates left atrium; RA right atrium; Ao, aorta.

The Brockenbrough needle, transseptal dilator and transseptal sheath are then withdrawn from the superior vena cava to the right atrium as previously described, however, the tip of the ultrasound probe is able to be used as a fluoroscopic marker for the location of the fossa ovalis. With septal displacement of the needle/dilator/sheath unit the unit is presumed to be in the region of the fossa ovalis. Ultrasound imaging, however, provides the operator detailed anatomic information for minute but critical adjustments in positioning of the dilator, safe transseptal puncture and avoidance of injury to important structures. Prior to advancing the needle through the fossa ovalis, tenting of the fossa ovalis is noted on intracardiac echo. At this point in the procedure the operator can appreciate the location of the aorta, the crossing angle of the Brockenbrough needle, and the proximity of the left atrial wall to the needle/dilator unit to avoid impingement upon this structure (Figure 6). After examination of the anterior/posterior and lateral/medial axes the intracardiac echo probe can be advanced superiorly and withdrawn inferiorly. This maneuver ascertains that the tip of the needle is neither positioned too far superior in the region of the limbus (with aorta above), nor that it is positioned too far inferior in the region of the coronary sinus (Figure 7). Once the needle trajectory and position is confirmed the needle is advanced through the fossa ovalis and the tenting of the fossa ovalis collapses. Upon collapse of the fossa ovalis a 0.014 high torque floppy guidewire is often advanced through the tip of the needle into the left atrium and often into the pulmonary veins to confirm that left atrial access has been achieved. There is no need for pressure monitoring at the hub of the Brockenbrough needle, checking oxygen saturation of blood withdrawn from the Brockenbrough needle, injection of contrast, or positioning of a pigtail catheter at the aortic root. With the completion of successful transseptal catheterization, ultrasound imaging provides additional information regarding possible complications.

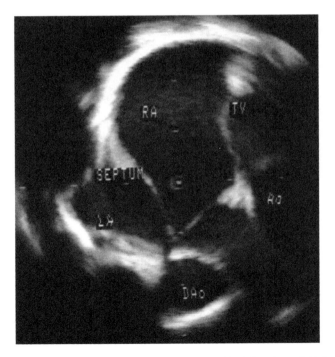

Figure 6.   Image of the fossa ovalis tented into the left atrium (LA) by the transseptal sheath and dilator. RA indicates right atrium; TV, tricuspid valve; Septum, interatrial septum; DAo, descending aorta; Ao, ascending aorta.

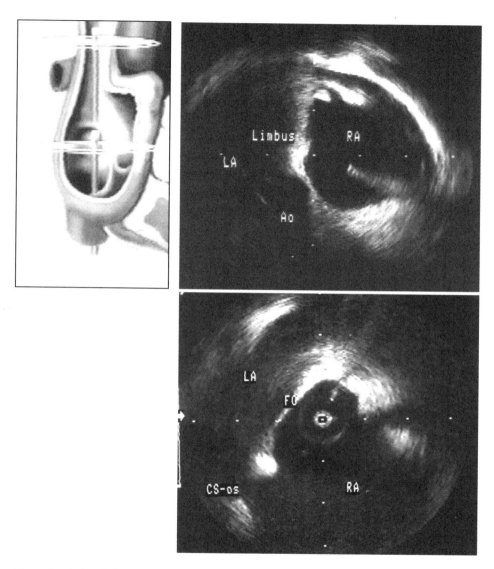

Figure 7. A (top left) Illustration of the movement of the ICE catheter from a superior to an inferior position in the right atrium with the cooresponding planes of imaging. B (top right) Image from the right atrium (RA) above the fossa ovalis, demonstrating the appearance of the ridge of tissue (limbus) lying immediately superior to the fossa ovalis. LA indicates left atrium; Ao, aorta. C (bottom) Image from the right atrium below the fossa ovalis demonstrating the relative position of the ostium of the coronary sinus (CSOS). FO indicates fossa ovalis.

2.   COMPLICATION MONITORING

Continuous ICE imaging during radiofrequency ablation procedures allows one to monitor for the development of complications.   The incidence of thromboembolic complications for ablation procedures performed in the left heart approaches 2% in some series.[7] Continuous intracardiac echocardiography during the procedure may potentially allow one to identify the early formation of coagulum at the tip of the radiofrequency ablation catheter during applications of RF energy and the presence or absence of any air entrapment into the left atrium from transseptal sheaths (Figure 8).   Furthermore, the use of ICE may potentially allow one to exclude the presence of left atrial thrombus prior to the placement of catheters in the chamber (Figure 9).   If there is ever a question of perforation during the transseptal or electrophysiology procedure, ICE affords visualization of the pericardial space to evaluate for this possibility. During ablation of inappropriate sinus tachycardia ICE monitoring of the diameter of the right atrial-superior vena cava junction allows one to identify developing stenosis of the junction during the ablation procedure. Other incidental findings such as vegetations, valvular abnormalities, and stenotic pulmonary veins may be helpful in avoiding complications at the time of the procedure (Figure 10).

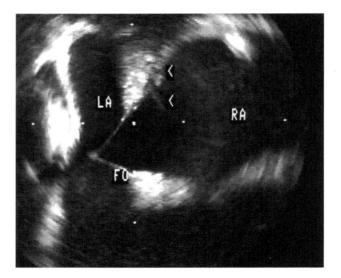

Figure 8.   ICE image of the right atrium (RA) with the fossa ovalis (FO) tented by the transseptal needle. A mural thrombus is noted (arrows) at the site of a previous radiofrequency energy application and transseptal puncture is aborted.

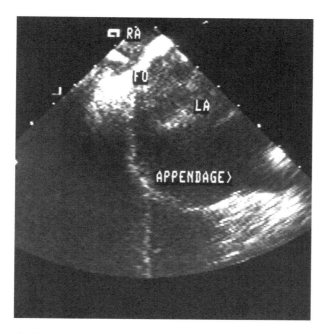

Figure 9: Image of the left atrium (LA) from the right atrium (RA) using a phase array ultrasound probe which affords clear views of the left atrial appendage (appendage). FO indicates fossa ovalis.

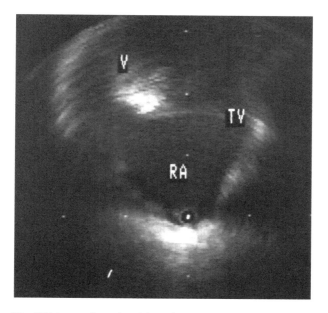

Figure 10. ICE image from the right atrium (RA). A large vegetation (V) is noted on the leaflet of the tricuspid valve (TV).

3.   ABLATION OF INAPPROPRIATE SINUS TACHYCARDIA

Inappropriate sinus tachycardia is characterized by an elevated resting heart rate and an inappropriate increase in heart rate with minor exertion. After secondary causes have been excluded, curative radiofrequency ablation can be employed. The sinus node arises from an area delineated on the right atrial endocardial surface by the crista terminalis. The crista terminalis originates at the junction of the superior vena cava and the right atrial appendage and travels inferiorly along the right atrial free wall toward the inferior vena cava (Figure 11).[8]

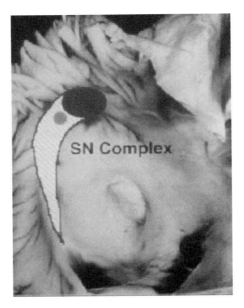

Figure 11. Gross pathologic specimen depicting the course of the sinus node complex. The sinus node complex is housed within the crista terminalis coursing superior to inferior along the lateral wall of the right atrium, separating the trabeculated muscular right atrial wall anteriorly from the smooth posterior right atrial wall.

Sinus node impulse origin and propagation within and out of the crista terminalis is dynamic and influenced by sympathetic and parasympathetic input.[8] Given this variability of electrophysiologic activation and propagation, the crista terminalis serves as an important anatomic target for modification of sinus node function by radiofrequency ablation. Successful ablation sites are typically along the superior-medial aspect of the crista terminalis and ICE provides imaging of this area as well as imaging of the position of the catheter tip relative to the crista terminalis (Figure 12). This technique assures ablation of the most rapid sinus node foci and minimizes excessive radiofrequency energy applications and the risk of permanent sinus bradycardia. Animal and clinical studies confirm the utility of ICE guided radiofrequency modification of the sinoatrial node and denote a reduction in fluoroscopy time with this approach.[4,9] Extensive, repeated ablation of the uppermost portions of the sinus node can sometimes be required for control of this arrhythmia. Such extensive applications can cause narrowing and stenosis of the superior vena cava-right atrium junction which can be monitored using ICE.[10]

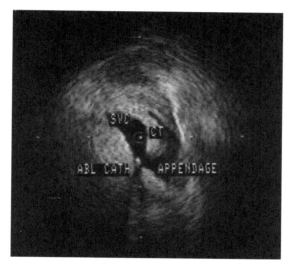

Figure 12. Fan shaped artifact generated by the 4mm tip of an ablation catheter (Abl Cath) as it positioned near the uppermost portion of the crista terminalis (CT) separating the right atrial appendage (appenadage) from the superior vena cava (SVC).

4.   ATRIAL TACHYARRHYTHMIAS

Atrial tachycardias often arise from well recognized anatomic sites including the crista terminalis, the coronary sinus ostium, the left or right atrial appendage, and the pulmonary vein ostia.[11-19] Ultrasound visualization facilitates positioning of either a roving ablation catheter or a multipolar mapping catheter along the crista terminalis, which helps assess the origin of the atrial tachycardia (Figure 13).[20,21] Furthermore, discriminating a right atrial tachycardia located in the superior aspect of the right atrium from a left atrial tachycardia originating from the right upper pulmonary vein is challenging with fluoroscopy alone. ICE visualization of anatomic electrode position and cooresponding electrophysiolgic activation patterns helps differentiate between these two anatomic locations (Figure 14).[5]

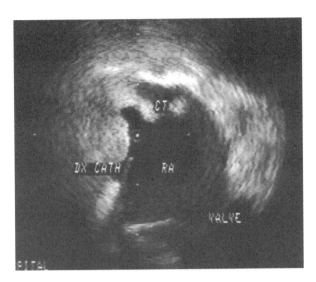

Figure 13. Image of the right atrium with the crista terminalis (CT) clearly visualized to serve as a target for intracardiac mapping. The shaft of a diagnostic catheter is seen along the septum (Dx Cath) medial to the tricuspid valve (Valve).

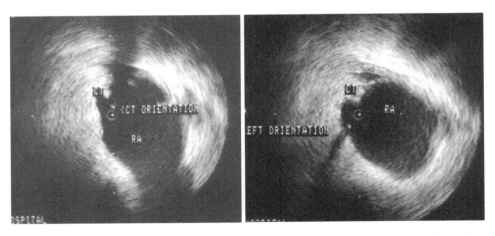

Figure 14. A (left): Image of the catheter in the right atrium (RA) with fan shaped artifact of the ablation catheter tip (CT orientation) directed toward the crista terminalis (CT). B (right): Image of the catheter in the right atrium (RA) with the small fan shaped artifact of the diagnostic catheter tip directed toward the left atrium (left orientation). RA indicates right atrium.

It is now well recognized that in some patients atrial fibrillation is initiated by atrial ectopy originating from the pulmonary veins and that ablation of these foci may eliminate atrial fibrillation.[22-24] However, one concerning complication of ablation in the pulmonary veins is pulmonic vein stenosis. ICE can be used to continuously monitor the pulmonary vein for early detection of stenosis (Figure 15).

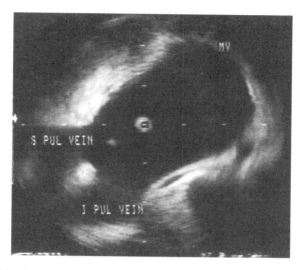

Figure 15: Image from an ICE catheter in the left atrium. The mitral valve (MV) lies anteriorly while the pulmonary veins lie posterior with clear appreciation of pulmonary vein ostial dimensions. S Pul Vein indicates superior pulmonary vein; I Pul Vein, inferior pulmonary vein.

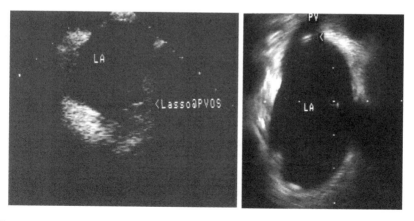

Figure 16: A. Image of the circular lasso catheter (Lasso @ PVOS) located in the ostium of the pulmonary vein. The phased arrary ICE probe is located in the right atrium. LA indicates left atrium. B. ICE image from the left atrium (LA). A 14mm ablation electrode from an investigational catheter (arrow) bridges the ostium of the pulmonary vein (PV).

The ablative approach to managing atrial fibrillation is appealing and numerous technologies are under investigation to simplify this procedure. ICE is helpful to position these newer ablation systems in the heart relative to important left atrial anatomy (pulmonary veins, mitral valve annulus, left atrial appendage) and to confirm appropriate endocardial contact to assure adequate lesion formation (Figure 16).[25]

Typical atrial flutter is dependent upon conduction through the right atrial isthmus tissue bordered by the inferior vena cava, coronary sinus ostium and tricuspid valve annulus.[26,27] The goal of atrial flutter ablation is to complete a line of radiofrequency lesions between the tricuspid valve annulus and the inferior vena cava. However, because of variable endocardial contour, this complex region can be difficult to ablate. In animal models, ICE provides confirmation of contiguous radiofrequency lesions and helps identify gaps in the line of block between these structures.[28] In humans the atrial flutter isthmus can be easily visualized using ICE and; therefore, ICE may provide a similar benefit (Figure 17).

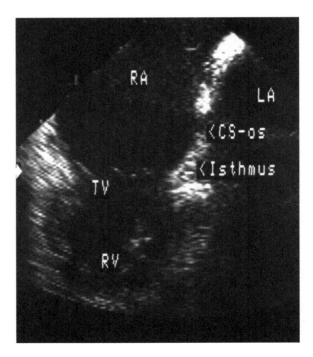

Figure 17. Image of from the right atrium (RA) with the phased array catheter oriented toward the right ventricle (RV). Isthmus indicates the atrial flutter isthmus; CSOS, coronary sinus ostium, LA, left atrium; TV, tricuspid valve.

5.　ATRIOVENTRICULAR NODAL REENTRANT TACHYCARDIA

The most common form of reentrant supraventricular tachycardia is atrioventricular nodal reentrant tachycardia. This tachycardia is easily ablated targeting the posterior slow pathway.[29] The risk of the procedure includes a small but real risk of heart block and at times localizing the slow pathway and stabilizing the catheter can be challenging. Fisher et. al. deployed ICE through a curved sheath into the right ventricle to provide visualization of the triangle of Koch.[30] The junction of the membranous interventricular septum and muscular interventricular septum identified the location the compact atrioventricular node while the insertion of the septal leaflet of the tricuspid valve into the muscular interventricular septum identified the location of the slow pathway (Figure 18). Use of ICE allowed reduction in the number of radiofrequency energy applications and a trend toward decreased use of flouroscopy.

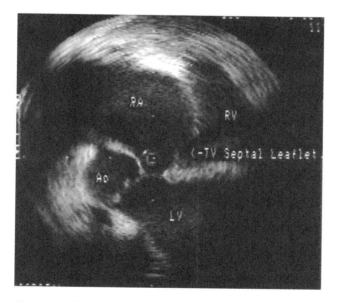

Figure 18. Image from an ICE catheter resting across the tricuspid valve just inside the right ventricle (RV). Immediately distal to the junction of the thin membranous interventricular septum and the thick muscular interventricular septum is the site of insertion of the septal tricuspid valve leaflet (TV septal leaflet) targeted for slow pathway ablation. RA indicates right atrium; Ao, aortic valve; LV, left ventricle.

6.   VENTRICULAR TACHYCARDIA

Ventricular tachycardias caused by a focus of triggered activity are commonly associated with an anatomic substrate. Most triggered ventricular tachycardias arise from the right ventricular outflow tract. This region is readily imaged using ICE which can help achieve contigous radiofrequency lesions at sites with early endocardial activation times and excellant pace maps (Figure 19).

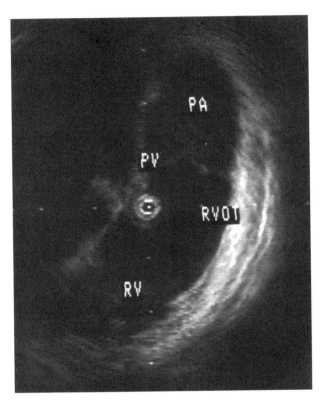

Figure 19. Image of the right ventricular outflow tract (RVOT) via an ICE catheter placed across the tricuspid valve into the right ventricle (RV). PV indicates pulmonic valve; PA, initial portion of the pulmonary artery.

The reentrant circuit of ischemic ventricular tachycardia often uses the border zone of scar tissue as the critical zone of slow conduction. Furthermore, these sites are located in areas of ventricular akinesis or dyskinesis which may serve as sites of thrombus formation. ICE has been shown to verify the presence of infarcted myocardial tissue suspected from low amplitude, fractionated electrograms.[31]   The potential utility of ICE is to exclude the presence of thrombus and to help identify the border zone of scar tissue to expedite mapping (Figure 20). Ablation of left ventricular tachycardia in the setting of ischemic heart disease may significantly benefit from the ICE identification of border zones of myocardial scarring, exclusion of the presence of left ventricular thrombus, and real time electroanatomical activation. This type of visualization has been successfully employed in animal models and is starting to be employed in humans.[32]

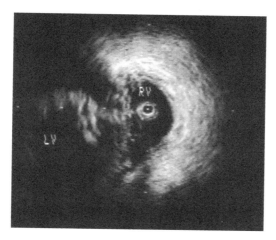

Figure 20. Image of the right ventricle (RV) and left ventricle (LV) via an ICE catheter placed in the right ventricular apex.

7. FUTURE USES

One of the most promising uses of ICE is to further define the role of anatomic structures as the substrate for arrhythmias (33). Another use for ICE is to monitor and guide placement of more complicated ablation systems and to evaluate ablation lesions. ICE guided placement of new ablation platforms (such as microwave antennae) in human and animal research have become increasingly common to help achieve ablation of the intended target, to create contiguous lesions and to perform the procedure safely.[34,35] Furthermore, the orientation of ablation catheter tip in relation to the endocardium greatly influences the diameter and depth of the lesion created. The use of ICE is therefore important when comparing ablation lesions from different ablation systems.[36] Three-dimensional models of cardiac chambers are now feasible using complete reconstruction of ICE images. This new imaging offers advantages not only for catheter ablation, but also potential insight regarding optimal placement of pacing electrodes for improving ventricular resynchronization.

REFERENCES

1. Haines DE. Determinants of lesion size during radiofrequency catheter ablation: The role of electrode-tissue contact pressure and duration of energy delivery. J Cardiovasc Electrophysiol 1991; 2:509-515.
2. Chy E, Kalman JM, Kwasman MA, et al. Intracardiac echocardiography during radiofrequency catheter ablation of cardiac arrhythmias in man. J Am Coll Cardiol 1994; 24:1351-1357.
3. Chu E, Fitzpatrick AP, Chin MC, et al. Radiofrequency catheter ablation guided by intracardiac echocardiography. Circulation 1994; 89:1301-1305.
4. Kalman JM, Lee RJ, Fisher WG, et al. Radiofrequency catheter modification of sinus pacemaker function guided by intracardiac echocardiography. Circulation 1995; 93:3070-3081
5. Kalman JM, Olgin JE, Karch MR, and Lesh MD. Use of intracardiac Echocardiography in Interventional Electrophysiology. Pace 1997; 20(Pt. 1):2248-2262.
6. Daoud EG, Kalbfleisch SJ, and Hummel JD. Intracardiac Echocardiography to Guide Transseptal Left Heart Catheterization for Radiofrequency Catheter Ablation. J Cardiovasc Electrophysiol 1999; 10:358-363.
7. Zhou L, Keane D, Reed G, Ruskin J. Thromboembolic complications of cardiac radiofrequency catheter ablation: a review of the reported incidence, pathogenesis and current research directions. J Cardiovasc Electrophysiol 1999; 10(5):680-691
8. Boineau JP, Schuessler RB, Hackel DB, et al. Widespread distribution and rate differentiation of the atrial pacemaker complex. Am J Physiol 1980; 239:H406-H415.
9. Lee RJ, Kalman JM, Fitzpatrick AP, et al. Radiofrequency catheter modification of the sinus node for inappropriate sinus tachycardia. Circulation 1995; 93:2918-2919.
10. Callans DJ, Ren JF, Schwartzman D, Gottlieb CD, Chaudhry FA, and Marchlinski FE. Narrowing of the superior vena cava-right atrium junction during radiofrequency catheter ablation for inappropriate sinus tachycardia: Analysis with intracaradiac echocardiography. J Am Coll Cardiol 1999; 6:1667-1670.
11. Boineau JP, Schuessler RB, Roeske WR, et al. Quantitative relation between sites of atrial impulse origin and cycle length. Am J Physiol 1983; 245:H781-H789.
12. Haines DE, DiMarco JP. Sustained intraatrial reentrant tachycardia: Clinical, electrocardiographic and electrophysiologic characteristics and long-term follow-up. J Am Coll Cardiol 1990; 15:1345-1354.
13. Chen SA, Chiang CE, Yang CJ, et al. Sustained atrial tachycardia in adult patients. Electrophysiological characteristics, pharmalogical response, possible mechanisms and effects of radiofrequency ablation. Circulation 1994; 90:1262-1278.
14. Lesh MD, Van Hare GF, Epstein LM, et al. Radiofrequency catheter ablation of atrial arrhythmias-Results and mechanisms. Circulation 1994; 89:1074-1089.
15. Tracy CM, Swartz JF, Fletcher RD. Radiofrequency catheter ablation of ectopic atrial tachycardia using paced activation sequence mapping. J Am Coll Cardiol 1993; 21:910-917.
16. Kay GN, Chong F, Epstein AE, et al. Radiofrequency ablation for treatment of primary atrial tachycardias. J Am Coll Cardiol 1993; 21:901-909.
17. Walsh EP, Saul JP, Hulse JE. Transcatheter ablation of ectopic atrial tachycardia in young patients using radio frequency current. Circulation 1992; 86:1138-1146.
18. Poty H, Saoudi N, Haissagguerre M, et al. Radiofrequency catheter ablation of atrial tachycardias. Am Heart J 1996; 131:481-489.
19. Shenasa H, Merrill JJ, Hamer ME, et al. Distribution of ectopic atrial tachycardias along the crista terminalis: An atrial ring of fire? (abstract) Circulation 1993; 88:I-29.
20. Weiss C, Hatala R, Carpinteiro L, et al. Topographic anatomy and in vitro fluoroscopic imaging of the crista terminalis: An attempt to more precisely localize the origin of ectopic atrial tachycardia. (abstract) Circulation 1994; I-595.
21. Tang CW, Scheinman MM, Van Hare GF, et al. P-wave morphology during automatic atrial tachycardia in man. J Am Coll Cardiol 1995; 26:1315-1324.

22. Haissaguerre M, Jais P, Shah DC, et al. Spontaneous initiation of atrial fibrillation by ectopic beats originating in the pulmonary veins. N Engl J Med 1998; 339:659-666.
23. Chen SA, Hsieh MH, Tai CT, et al. Initiation of atrial fibrillation by ectopic beats originating from the pulmonary veins. Circulation 1999; 100:1879-1886.
24. Jais P, Shah DC, Hocini M, Yamane T, Haissaguerre M, Clementy J. Radiofrequency Catheter Ablation for Atrial Fibrillation. J. Cardiovasc Electrophysiol, 2000; 11: 758-761
25. Roithinger FX, Steiner PR, Goseki Y, et al. Low-power radiofrequency application and intracardiac echocardiography for creation of continuous left atrial linear lesions. J Cardiovasc Electrophysiol 1999; 10(5): 680-691.
26. Feld GK, Fleck RP, Chen PS, et al. Radiofrequency catheter ablation for the treatment of human type 1 atrial flutter. Identification of a critical zone in the reentrant circuit by endocardial mapping techniques. Circulation 1992; 86:1233-1240.
27. Cosio FG, Goicolea A, Lopez-Gil M, et al. Catheter ablation of atrial flutter circuits. PACE 1993; 16:637-642.
28. Epstein LM, Mitchell MA, Smith TW, Haines DE. Comparative study of fluoroscopy and intracardiac echocardiographic guidance for the creation of linear atrial lesions. Circulation 1998; 17:1796-1801.
29. Kay GN, Epstein AE, Dailey SM, et al. Selective radiofrequency ablation of the slow pathway for the treatment of atrioventricular nodal reentrant tachycardia. Evidence for involvement of perinodal myocardium within the reentrant circuit. Circulation 1992; 85:1675-1688.
30. Fisher WG, Pelini MA, Bacon ME. Adjunctive Intracardiac Echocardiography to Guide Slow Pathway Ablation in Human Atrioventricular Nodal Reentrant Tachycardia: Anatomic Insights. Circulation 1997; 96:3021-3029.
31. Callans DJ, Ren JF, Michele J, Marchlinski FE, Dillon SM. Electroanatomic left ventricular mapping in the porcine model of healed anterior myocardial infarction. Correlation with intracardiac echocardiography and pathological analysis. Circulation 1999; 100(16):1744-1750.
32. Allan JJ, Smith RS, DeJong SC, McKay CR, Kerber RE. Intracardiac echocardiographic imaging of the left ventricle from the right ventricle: quantitative experimental evaluation. J Am Soc Echocardiogr 1998; 11(10):921-928.
33. Schumacher B, Jung W., Schmidt H, Fischenbeck C, et al. Transverse conduction capabilities of the crista terminalis in patients with atrial flutter and atrial fibrillation. J Am Coll Cardiol 1999; 34(2):363-373.
34. Tardif JC, Groeneveld PW, Wang PJ, Haugh CJ, et al. Intracardiac echocardiographic guidance during microwave catheter ablation. J Am Soc Echocardiogr 1999; 12(1):41-47.
35. Keane DK, Houghtaling C, Qin H, Aretz T, Ruskin JN. Linear Cryo Ablation of the Cavo Tricuspid Isthmus Under Guidance by Phased Array Intracardiac Echocardiography. (Abstract) Journal of the American College of Cardiology 2000; 35(2); 126A
36. Chugh SS, Chan RC, Johnson SB, Packer DL. Catheter tip orientation affects radiofrequency ablation lesion size in the canine left ventricle. Pacing Clin Electrophysiol 1999; 22(3):413-420.

Chapter 10

MAPPING USING THE LOCALISA SYSTEM

Fred H.M. Wittkampf
The Heart Lung Institute, Department of Cardiology, University Medical Center, Utrecht, the Netherlands

INTRODUCTION

Catheter ablation procedures have evolved from the relatively simple elimination of single arrhythmogenic structures to more complex procedures in which specific lesion patterns are created, e.g. a line of block in patients with atrial flutter or a lesion area in patients with ventricular tachycardia and relatively large arrhythmogenic substrates.[1-5] Uni- and even biplane fluoroscopy as a means to determine successive catheter positions then becomes inadequate.

We recently developed the LocaLisa system for real-time 3-dimensional (3D) localization of intracardiac catheter electrodes.[6] The system uses small transthoracic currents, applied via standard skin electrodes, to create an electrical field within the patient's thorax. Regular catheter electrodes are used as sensors, allowing determination of their position within the heart.

1. LOCALIZATION TECHNIQUE

The LocaLisa system is a battery operated device, approximately the size of an RF generator, which transmits three 1 mA, 30 kHz currents through the patient's chest using standard skin electrodes and detects the resulting electrical signals from standard catheter electrodes. These signals are used to calculate and display the real time catheter position on a standard Macintosh computer.

The skin electrodes are placed such that three approximately orthogonal fields are created. (Figure 1) The most critical electrode pair, nearest to the heart, is

L. Bing Liem and E. Downar (eds.), Progress in Catheter Ablation, 125-135.

relatively large to improve the homogeneity of the electrical field: a disposable Valleylab E7506 adhesive gel electrode (9 cm x 16 cm) at approximately the V2 position and a similar size conductive rubber pad on the back. Both are fluoroscopically positioned directly over the presumed area of interest. The second electrode pair consists of two standard ECG electrodes, which are placed laterally at both sides of the thorax, in line with the center of the first pair. For the axial direction, one standard ECG electrode is placed at the patient's neck and the other on the left leg.

Figure 1

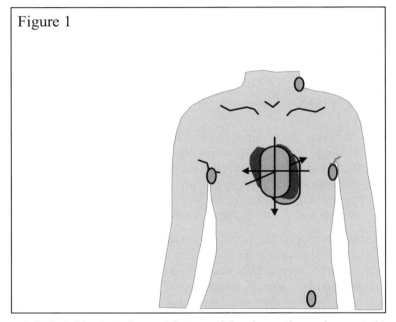

Figure 1. Patient skin electrodes used for transmitting three orthogonal currents through the thorax. Standard ECG electrodes are placed at the right and left mid-axillary line at the fourth intercostal space (V2) level, and at the left leg and left shoulder. Two 10 x 15 cm skin patches, one posterior under the heart on the back, and the other anterior above the heart, at the V2 position, are used to create the third field.

Three electrodes are used as location sensors: one reference electrode, and two electrodes on the mapping catheter. Preferably, the reference electrode is a catheter electrode at a stable position in one of the heart chambers. Respiratory excursions are then minimalized because both the reference electrode and the mapping catheter electrodes are similarly affected. Stability of the reference electrode is crucially important; dislocation invalidates all previously recorded positions. In critical cases, we therefore use the 6416 (Medtronic Inc, Minneapolis) screw-in tempory pacing wire. Alternatively, a skin electrode can be used, but then respiratory movements are approximately a factor 2 larger. [6]

1.1   Calibration and Accuracy

During mapping, LocaLisa measures the localization signals from two mapping catheter electrodes; the tip and the last ring electrode. Translation of a change in signal amplitudes into a shift in electrode position, however, requires knowledge about the magnitude of the three applied orthogonal electrical fields (in Volts per centimeter). The LocaLisa software automatically performs this 'calibration' by using the known interelectrode distance of the two mapping catheter electrodes as a caliper for the electrical field. This field is, however, never perfectly homogeneous. A stronger field will cause a larger potential difference between these two electrodes and thus a seemingly larger interelectrode distance and vice versa. Measured distances between various electrode positions are subject to local inhomogeneities. The magnitude of these variations can be estimated by measuring the variation in calculated distances between the two mapping catheter electrodes for all catheter positions. This variation or standard deviation can then be expressed as a percentage of the true interelectrode distance; a standard deviation of e.g. 10 % then implies that a true distance between two electrode positions of 5 cm will be measured by the LocaLisa system as 5 cm ± 5 mm.

1.2   Interaction with other equipment.

LocaLisa uses regular catheter electrodes to detect the 30 kHz localization potentials. All electrograms remain unaffected. An RF generator, however, may cause a current leak from electrode to ground pad and affect electrode localization. The calibration method is then also affectedbecause the current leak will also affect the potential difference between the two mapping catheter electrodes. Moreover, the high frequency RF current itself may also disturb detection of the localization signal. Consequently, various electronic measures are required to ensure correct operation of the LocaLisa system during RF ablation. Interference by the RF current itself is the biggest challenge, but also the most important one to ensure safety, e.g. with ablation near the atrioventricular (AV) node and His bundle and to facilitate the creation of drag lesions.

2.   COMPARISON WITH OTHER SYSTEMS

At present there are two comparable systems for three dimensional catheter localization; the Biosense-Webster Carto™ system which is commercially available and the LocaLisa system that will soon start clinical evaluation. Both Carto and LocaLisa display the position of the mapping catheter 3-dimensionally and in real time. There are, however, two main differences between both methods. Carto requires the use of a specially designed catheter with a magnetic sensor. With LocaLisa, the standard electrodes are used as sensors and the user can use any commercially available catheter by selecting the catheter type in one of the menus. Also during a procedure, the catheter can be exchanged. This allows for the choice of specific catheter characteristics, e.g. different curves or other tip electrode configurations, for difficult procedures.

The second difference is the absence of activation time information on LocaLisa. Colored activation maps are not generated. This may be regarded as an important limitation. Activation maps may create beautiful images of reentry patterns in various arrhythmias. In practice, however, these maps are often of very limited value. In the Wolff-Parkinson-White (WPW) syndrome, His bundle ablations, atrioventricular nodal reentrant tachycardia (AVNRT), atrial flutter, idiopathic ventricular tachycardia (VT) from the right ventricular outflow tract or left ventricular septum, and in patients with frequently firing arrhythmogenic atrial foci, the success rate is very high since the ablation target site or area is either known anatomically or relatively easily identifiable by activation mapping. Activation maps are very rarely required.

There may be three types of arrhythmia where treatment may benefit from 3-dimensional activation maps: Post-infarct and right ventriclular dysplasia related VT, and post incisional atrial reentrant tachycardia. In VT patients, activation maps can only be created by sequential mapping if the patient has inducible, hemodynamically tolerable, monomorphic VT's. These, however, are the relatively easy cases and activation maps are typically only useful to identify the exit site, but not the ablation target site. More important is the identification or reentry circuit sites which requires more detailed analysis of local electrograms plus entrainment analysis. In patients in whom sequential catheter mapping can not be applied, only systems which are capable of creating activation maps within a single or a few cycles, like the EnSite™ system (Endocardial Solutions Inc) or basket catheters may be useful to guide catheter positioning to the area of interest. In post incisional atrial reentrant tachycardias, activation maps have been constructed and successfully used to identify ablation target sites.[7] Activation maps beautifully demonstrated isolated channels between surgical scars. These detailed maps may limit the number of RF applications. The maps,however, confirmed that most if not all patients can be cured by interconnection of the surgical scars, or by connecting scars with anatomical barriers.

3.   MAPPING AND ABLATION STRATEGIES WITH LOCALISA

So far, LocaLisa has been used in more than 500 catheter ablation procedures. Besides LocaLisa, we use a second specially designed tool during these procedures: a custom designed large screen triggered monitor on which the 8 most important electrograms are continuously displayed (Figure 2). Triggering on a stable reference electrogram results in a real time image showing the precise timing of local mapping catheter electrograms. The monitor is positioned next to the LocaLisa screen and both monitors are slaved to the catheterizing physician.

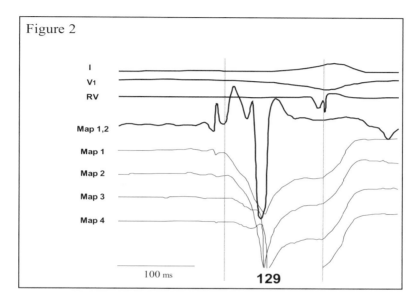

Figure 2. Copy of the image of the 8 channel triggered monitor, specially developed for catheter ablation procedures. The monitor enables quick assessment of local activation times. This example shows two surface electrocardiograms, lead I and V1, an electrogram from a stable right ventricular (RV) catheter, and 5 electrograms from the mapping catheter: one bipolar electrogram from the distal electrode pair (Map 1,2) and 4 unipolar recordings (Map 1 to 4). The RV electrogram is used for triggering which results in a stationary position of the surface and RV electro(cardio)grams whereas the mapping catheter electrograms change in position and morphology with different catheter positions. The two cursors lines are manually regulated and used for measurement of local activation time relative to one of the stable recordings, in this case the RV electrogram.

The mapping and ablation strategies which we were able to develop due to the availability of the LocaLisa system are described below.

3.1 WPW syndrome

Catheter ablation is guided mainly by electrophysiological measurements: earliest activation of the preexcited chamber with a unipolar, initially steep, negative deflection and preferably a Kent potential. In the vast majority of cases, fluoroscopic exposure times are relatively short and 3D catheter localization is not required. The importance of accurate catheter localization increases, however, with the complexity of the case. Collected late and early sites near the bypass serve as road signs for obtaining a more optimal catheter position. The LocaLisa image may show areas near early sites which have not (yet) been mapped and applications near the His bundle may be carried out with greater precision and safety. If the perfect electrode position can not be reached, multiple pulses may be delivered closely around early sites to achieve permanent success. Repetitive ablations at previously unsuccessful sites can be avoided and extra pulses may be delivered at and around sites with late interruption of the bypass or with unstable contact.

3.2   AVNRT

With the anatomical approach, accurate catheter localization is extremely useful. Using the femoral approach, a regular quadripolar ablation catheter is first advanced a few cm into the coronary sinus (CS). The catheter is then slowly withdrawn, while marking successive catheter tip positions, until it drops into the right atrium. The catheter is subsequently advanced to the His bundle area and again slowly withdrawn to the most proximal His bundle recording site while marking positions with His bundle potentials on the distal unipolar electrogram. If necessary, a few additional and different catheter orientations are collected to calibrate the LocaLisa system.

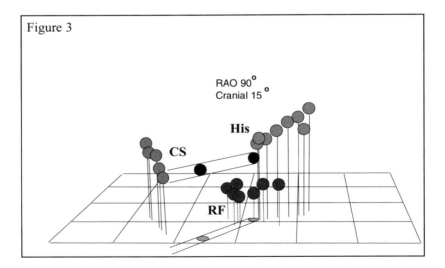

Figure 3

Figure 3. Copy of LocaLisa image during catheter ablation of the slow atrioventricular nodal pathway. The view angle is right anterior oblique 90 °. The moving catheter is continuously displayed with its shadow on the ground plane to create a three dimensional image. Marking of previous catheter positions inside the coronary sinus (CS) and against the His bundle created a road map for positioning the ablation catheter in the area of interest. Radiofrequency (RF) pulses are then applied approximately 1 cm below the most proximal His bundle recording site until the arrhythmia is no longer inducible.

The distance between the ablation electrode and that site remains continuously displayed on the LocaLisa screen from that moment on. With a 90° right anterior oblique LocaLisa view, approximately perpendicular to the area of interest, successive RF pulses are then applied 0.8 to 1.2 cm below the most proximal His bundle recording site. During RF application, the right atrium is paced to allow continuous monitoring of antegrade conduction. Frequent junctional activity, which may impair the monitoring of antegrade conduction is suppressed by increasing the stimulation frequency. All ablation sites are marked with LocaLisa. (Figure 3) Sites with accelerated junctional activity during RF delivery are specially labelled and used as target areas for next ablations until the arrhythmia is no longer inducible. Using this approach, our success rate is above 98% without a single case of inadvertent permanent AV block; only transient first-degree AV block has been observed in a few cases.

3.3   Atrial Flutter

As in the case of AVNRT, the predominantly anatomical approach makes a 3D mapping system like LocaLisa an indispensable tool for the creation of a line of block in the isthmus. The positions of the CS and His bundle are marked and calibration is performed as described above. Then, the position of the Eustachian ridge is marked on the basis of double potentials inferior to the CS ostium during CS pacing. Either the tricuspid to Eustachian ridge or tricuspid to inferior vena cava line is then drawn, depending on catheter maneuverability in the isthmus.[3,4] Initially, a drag lesion is created while marking ablation electrode positions every few mm. Special care is taken to create a narrow ablation line. In our experience, the localization of leaks is complicated by patchy ablation patterns and the presumable zig-zag pathways. The presence of bidirectional conduction block is analyzed while using the LocaLisa system to position the catheter tip on and at both sides of the ablation line. Holes in the line are closed with extra pulses.

3.4   Idiopathic VT

In patients with VT originating from the right ventricular outflow tract, the ablation target site is characterized by the earliest negative deflection in the unipolar tip electrogram. In case of too infrequent ventricular ectopy, the ablation target site is identified by pacemapping. At and around that target site 5 to 10 RF applications are then delivered within a distance of approximately 5 to 10 mm from the target to create an homogeneous lesion area. One or more of these applications often induce rapid ventricular ectopy with the clinical morphology; that site is then used as the new central target for area ablation.

In patients with idiopathic verapamil sensitive left ventricular tachycardia, the left ventricular septum is mapped to identify the site with earliest ventricular activation. Sites with Purkinje potentials are also collected to mark the course of the posterior fascicle (Figure 4). After identification of the ablation target site, a few RF pulses are applied at and around that site to create a relatively small lesion area. In two patients in whom the optimal catheter position could not be reached, we achieved permanent success by ablation of the distal posterior fascicle, very close to the ventricular exit.

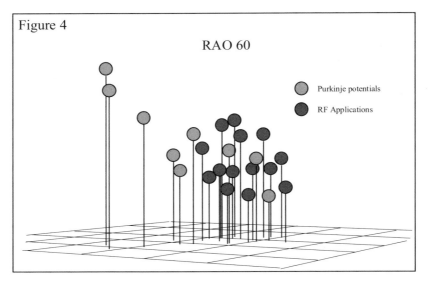

Figure 4. Copy of the LocaLisa screen after successful catheter ablation in a patient with idiopathic verapamil sensitive left ventricular tachycardia. Sites with Purkinje potentials that were detected during catheter mapping were marked on the LocaLisa image and multiple adjacent radiofrequency (RF) pulses were delivered to create a relatively small lesion area at and around the site with earliest ventricular activation.

3.5   VT Post Myocardial Infarction

In patients amendable to catheter mapping, scar tissue and early sites are identified and marked on LocaLisa. Sites isolated early and/or fractionated potentials near the endocardial exit are also marked and mapping continues to identify sites at which the detected potentials have their maximum amplitude. Pacing is then performed via the distal mapping electrode pair to identify sites with entrainment and concealed fusion and post-pacing intervals which are less than 30 ms longer than the VT cycle length following the criteria of Stevenson.[8] This mapping part of the procedure thus does not differ from the classical approach except that color marking of different sites on LocaLisa facilitates a more structured approach. RF energy is then delivered at the identified target site. Multiple pulses are then delivered within an approximately 1 to 1.5 cm radius around that target site. An RF ablation site that terminates the tachycardia is used as new central target for expanding the lesion area. Using this area ablation strategy, we have been able to achieve a very high success rate in this patient population.[5]

3.6   Arrhytmogenic Atrial Foci

In these patients, LocaLisa is used to mark early sites and nearby anatomical structures as road signs to identify the earliest site. There, we routinely apply a few pulses to create a small lesion area a few mm around the target site.

3.7   Post Incisional Atrial Reentry Tachycardia

After exclusion of typical atrial flutter, the location of the right lateral surgical scars are recognized by demonstrations of split potentials and markedly disparate activation times on contiguous electrode pairs and marked on the LocaLisa image. Activation and entrainment mapping is then performed between scars, and between scars and anatomical barriers, to understand the course of the reentrant wave front. In case of confirmation of a critical isthmus at those sites or if electrophysiological analysis remains inconclusive, a few lesions are then delivered in the isthmus between the surgical scars or between scars and the nearest anatomical barrier, superior or inferior vena cava or the tricuspid annulus. So far we have only treated 6 patients which were all successfully cured using this strategy.

4.   REDUCTION IN X-RAY EXPOSURE

Multiple reports about skin erosion in patients who underwent a lengthy catheterization procedure illustrate that patient radiation levels may reach critical levels.[9-13]   Total yearly operator exposure levels may also be significant.[14] LocaLisa enables precise catheter positioning without fluoroscopy, but the insertion of catheters through veins and arteries, passage of the aortic valve and catheter manipulation to the general area of interest still requires fluoroscopy. To measure the true reduction in fluoroscopy exposure, patients should be randomized to catheter ablation with and without LocaLisa. After our learning curve, however, the advantages of LocaLisa were so obvious that it would be unethical not to use the system in catheter ablation procedures. The exact reduction in fluoroscopy time can therefore not be specified. Since the introduction of the system in our center, we have, however, experienced a considerable reduction in fluoroscopy exposure with a factor 2 as our best estimate.[15]

SUMMARY

The clinical experience with the LocaLisa system is limited to our own center where the system has been developed. The availability of precise and reproducible location information facilitated more structured mapping and ablation and improved our success rate, especially in the more complex procedures. We strongly believe that the system offers substantial benefits to the user at amazingly low 'costs'; the only efforts required are the placement of the six skin electrodes and a few mouse clicks.

REFERENCES

1. Borggrefe M, Budde T, Podczeck A, Breithardt G. High frequency alternating current ablation of an accessory pathway in humans. J Am Coll Cardiol. 1987;10:576-582.
2. Jackman WM, Wang X, Friday KJ, Roman CA, Moulton KP, Beckman KJ, McClelland JH, Twiidale N, Hazlitt HA, Prior MI, Margolis PD, Calame JD, Overholt ED, Lazzara R. Catheter ablation of accessory atrioventricular pathways (Wolff-Parkinson-White syndrome) by radiofrequency current. N Eng J Med. 1991;324:1605-1611.
3. Cosio FG, Lopèz-Gil M, Goicolea A, Arribas F, Barroso JL. Radiofrequency ablation of the inferior vena cava-tricuspid valve isthmus in common atrial flutter. Am J Cardiol. 1993; 71:705-709.
4. Nakagawa H, Lazzara R, Khastgir T, Beckman KJ, McClelland JH, Imai S, Pitha JV, Becker AE, Arruda M, Gonzales MD, Widman LE, Rome M, Neuhauser J, Wang X, Calame JD, Goudeau MD, Jackman WM. Role of the tricuspid annulus and the eustachian valve/ridge in atrial flutter. Circulation. 1996;94:407-424.
5. Elvan A, Wittkampf FHM, Wever EFD, Ramanna H, Derksen R, Magnin I, Hauer RNW, Robles de Medina EO: Radiofrequency catheter ablation of ventricular tachycardia using a new non-fluoroscopic localization technique (LocaLisa). Circulation 1998;98,17-I:p566 (abstract)
6. Wittkampf FHM, PhD, Wever EFD, MD, Derksen R, Wilde AAM, Ramanna H, Hauer RNW, Robles de Medina EO. LocaLisa: New technique for real-time 3D localization of regular intracardiac electrodes. Circulation 1999;99:1312-1317
7. Nakagawa H, Asirvatham S, Shah N, Beckman K, Gonzalez M, Arruda M, Calame J, Imai S, Otomo K, Lazzara R, Jackman W: Improved catheter mapping of macroreentrant right atrial tachycardia associated with scar frequently allows focal (as opposed to linear) ablation. Pacing and Cardiac Electrophysiology 1998;12:p832 (abstract)
8. Stevensen WG: Catheter mapping of ventricular tachycardia. In Zipe DP and Jalife J (eds): Cardiac Electrophysiology From Cell to Bedside. 2nd ed. Philadelphia, P, WB Saunders Company, 1995, pp1193-1112.
9. Park TH, Eichling JO, Schechtman KB, Bromberg BI, Smith JM, Lindsay BD. Risk of radiation induced skin injuries from arrhythmia ablation procedures. Pacing Clin Electrophysiol. 1996;19:1363-9.
10. Nahass GT. Acute radiodermatitis after radiofrequency catheter ablation. J Am Acad Dermatol. 1997;36:881-4.
11. Rosenthal LS, Beck TJ, Williams J, et al. Acute radiation dermatitis following radiofrequency catheter ablation of atrioventricular nodal reentrant tachycardia. Pacing Clin Electrophysiol. 1997;20:1834-9
12. E. Vañó, L. Arranz, J.M. Sastre, et al. Dosimetric and radiation protection considerations based on some cases of patient skin injuries in interventional cardiology. British J Radiol. 1998;71:510-6.

13. Kovoor P, Ricciardello M, Collins L, Uther JB, Ross DL. Risk to patients from radiation associated with radiofrequency ablation for supraventricular tachycardia. Circulation. 1998; 98:1534-40.

14. Calkins H, Niklason L, Sousa J, El-Atassi R, Langberg J, Morady F. Radiation exposure during radiofrequency catheter ablation of accessory atrioventricular connections. Circulation. 1991;84:2376-82.

15. Wittkampf FHM, Vos C, vanderTol J, Wever EFD, Hauer RNW, Robles de Medina EO. Reduction of Radiation Exposure in the Cardiac Electrophysiology laboratory. Circulation 1998;98,17-I: p567 (abstract)

Chapter 11

ELECTROANATOMICAL MAPPING USING THE CARTO® SYSTEM
Technical Concept, Validation and Basic Application

L. Bing Liem
Cardiac Arrhythmia and Electrophysiology, Stanford University, Stanford, California, USA

INTRODUCTION

Mapping during catheter ablation is an essential component of the procedure in several aspects. In terms of "localization", in addition to the mere fact that it is necessary for identification of the region of the heart that is the "focus" of the arrhythmia, mapping should also provide some insight into the mechanism of the arrhythmia. Furthermore, to facilitate the ablation process, mapping should also provide some information about the anatomy and geometry of that particular portion of the heart. Finally, if the ablation process involves more than a single point ablation, mapping should also provide guidance in terms of navigation.

The CARTO® mapping system is intended to provide the clinician with electroanatomical data. The system, which uses magnetic technology to locate and recall the location of the roving endocardial mapping catheter, provides three-dimensional reconstruction of the cardiac chambers involved superimposed on the electrophysiological information obtained using conventional endocardial electrogram recording. Without using fluoroscopy, the system provides the operator with navigation of the mapping catheter.

In this chapter, the technology of the CARTO® system, its validation and application for a variety of arrhythmias will be discussed.

1. TECHNOLOGY

The magnetic-base system comprises an ultralow magnetic field emitter in the form of an external pad, a miniature passive field sensor within the locatable catheter, and a processing unit. The locatable catheter is typically an 8F

L. Bing Liem and E. Downar (eds.), Progress in Catheter Ablation, 137-148.

deflectable/steerable catheter similar to conventional mapping/ablation catheter and is equipped with radiofrequency (RF) delivery capability for ablation. The sensor is imbedded just behind the distal electrode tip (Figure 1). The external locator pad is intended to be placed beneath the procedure table. It generates ultralow magnetic fields (5×10^{-6} to 5×10^{-5} T). It comprises of three coils that generates a magnetic field that would enable the sensor to determine its distance from each coil (Figure 1).

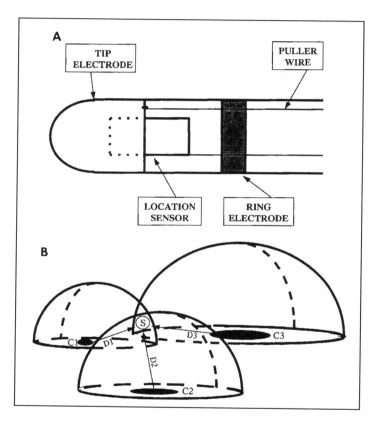

Figure 1. A = catheter. B = the process of location. The three coils (C1, C2, C3) generate a magnetic field that decays as a function of distance from the coil which enable the sensor to determine its distance from each coil (D1, D2, D3). Reproduced with permission from reference 1.

The system uses two locatable catheters. The first is a reference catheter to be placed in the coronary sinus (CS) or right ventricular (RV) apex. The second is the mapping catheter. The location of the mapping catheter is gated to a particular point (such as the ventricular or atrial electrogram) in the cardiac cycle and recorded relative to the location of the fixed reference catheter to compensate for cardiac motion. The location of the mapping catheter and is determined by the system in three-dimensional planes (on the x, y, and z axes) and is presented to the operator to assist in navigating without using fluoroscopy. The system also displays the tip configuration and motion ("roll, pitch, and yaw") to assist the operator in determining its directionality. As the mapping catheter is positioned at various points, local activation time (LAT) is calculated from the selected reference point. The LAT is color coded to identify its relative prematurity to the fixed reference time, with red being the earliest and purple the latest (please see Chapter 12 and Color Plate section). Thus, reconstruction of the mapped sites would depend on the LAT and the number of sites obtained (Figure 2).

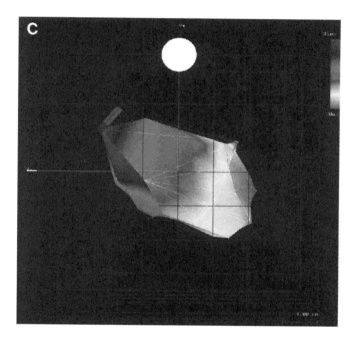

Figure 2. Shown above is the three-dimensional reconstruction of a pig left ventricle during RV pacing, obtained after collecting 52 sites. The head-and-eyes icon (white circle) is facing away from the picture, indicating that this is a posteroanterior view projection. The mapping catheter tip is represented by its icon, showing its angulation and direction towards to lateral wall. Reproduced from reference 1 with permission.

2. VALIDATION

2.1 Validation of Positioning and Distance Accuracy

Validation of the system was described in its early publication.[1] In-vitro validation was performed using a custom-made test jig with seven holes with known location and distances. One assessment was the accuracy of measurement calculated by the system after 25 positioning at each site with five different catheter rolls were obtained and presented as standard deviation (SD) and range of each "local cloud." The dispersion of repeated static location measurement showed an average SD measurement error of 0.16 ± 0.02 mm with 0.55 ± 0.07 mm range. Another comparison was of the system's calculation of distances between the seven sites against the known distances, which showed a mean measurement error of 0.42 ± 0.05 mm.[1]

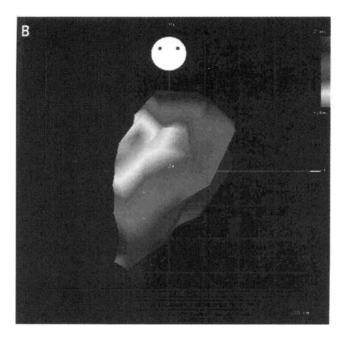

Figure 3. Activation map of the left ventricle during sinus rhythm. The earliest activation was noted to be arising from the high septum.

In-vivo validation was performed in animals using three protocols; repeated measurement at stationary sites, comparison of the system's distance calculation against a known distance, and acquisition of activation maps in the cardiac chambers (left ventricle, right atrium, and right ventricle). The SD of the "local cloud" of static measurement during 20 consecutive location determination inside the beating heart was 0.74 ± 0.13 mm. The comparison of the system's measurement of distances against known distance (based on marking on the catheters) showed an overall mean error of 0.73 ± 0.03 mm after 333 measurements using six different catheters. The results of the activation map were described in more qualitative terms. The investigators reported that the geometry of the respective chambers was similar in all cases and that the earliest activation coincided with the known source of activation (either sinus rhythm or pacing). Thus, for example, activation map of the left ventricle during sinus rhythm showed earliest activation at the high septum. (Figure 3). The authors also reported that after obtaining three sites within a chamber, the remaining sites could be collected without the use of fluoroscopy.[1]

2.2 Validation of Voltage Mapping

Voltage mapping, which potentially provides data for differentiating healthy from scarred tissue, was validated using echocardiographic and histology findings. Callans et al[2] performed comparison of voltage mapping to intracardiac echocardiogram (ICE) measurement and pathology in normal and infarcted pigs. Compared to areas remote from infarcted sites, akinetic areas were found to correlate with areas defined as having smaller (1.2±0.5 versus 5.1±2.1 mV) and more fractionated electrograms (74.2±26.3 versus 36.3±6.4 ms). Infarct size by pathology was found to correlate with area defined by contiguous electrograms with amplitude ≤ 1 mV. The clinical utility of such voltage mapping is described below.

3. CLINICAL UTILITY

The advantages of the system are several. One is its ability to combine electrical and spatial endocardial information, offering some insight into the role of anatomy in the mechanism of the arrhythmia and guidance to the operator in targeting ablation. It is also the first mapping method offering some navigation tool, which could be helpful in performing complex ablations, especially those requiring multiple applications.

3.1 Utility of Voltage Mapping

Roithinger et al[3] reported the utility of the mapping system in delineating trasseptal atrial conduction in humans. The mapping system was able to identify breakthrough points in the right atrium during left atrial pacing. Three distinct sites of intra-atrial conduction paths were noted; near the coronary sinus os in 9 of 18 patients, near the Bachmann bundle in 5 and near the fossa ovalis in 4. We performed mapping of the slow pathway of the atrioventricular node and found the retrograde breakthrough points to correlate with previous data. Such mapping data may become useful in targeting ablation. Electroanatomic voltage mapping can also be useful for identifying appropriate sites for permanent pacing, especially in complex congenital anomalies.[4] Another utility of voltage mapping is also described below under ablation for ventricular tachycardia (VT).

3.2   Utility in Focal Ablation

In its initial application, the mapping system was used for focal ablation both as a tool for navigation without fluoroscopy and as a tool for tracking previously ablated sites.[5-7] The advantage of the system in reducing fluoroscopy was evaluated in 79 patients undergoing ablation for atrioventricular (AV) nodal reentrant tachycardia (AVNRT), atrial tachycardia and flutter, VT and AV accessory pathways.[7] Significant fluoroscopic usage was found in all types of ablation; 10±7 versus 27±15 minutes for AVNRT, 18±17 versus 44±23 minutes for atrial tachycardia and flutter, 15±12 versus 34±31 minutes for VT, and 21±14 versus 53±32 minutes for accessory AV pathway. Total procedure time was also significantly shorter with the CARTO system for accessory AV pathway ablation.

3.3   Utility in Linear Ablation

Electroanatomical mapping is also intended to be used as a guide to linear ablation procedure. In one publication,[8] the authors reported the utility of the system in performing simple and linear ablation.

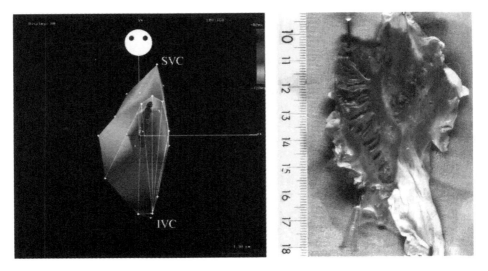

Figure 4. Right atrial linear ablation shown with CARTO® as contiguous dots and its histology. Reproduced from reference 2 with permission.

For performing single-point ablation, the system was used to navigate the tip of the ablation catheter to the same site for repeated application. Three ablations were performed in each of 9 pig's right atrium. Gross histological examination revealed the centers of the ablations to be at 2.3 ± 0.5 mm. The system was also tested for its ability in navigating the catheter tip for creating linear lesion and in estimating the lesion dimension (Figure 4). The system estimated accurately the linear ablation length with 0.96 correlation coefficient.

Utility for linear ablation is also evident in the case of isthmus ablation for atrial flutter. Complete conduction block can be better assessed with CARTO, eliminating the possibility of conduction leak in "apparent" bidirectional block. In addition, fluoroscopy time can also be significantly reduced. A prospective study comparing the addition of the mapping system to conventional fluoroscopy in atrial flutter ablation in 50 patients showed a significant reduction of fluoroscopy time from 22.0 ± 6.3 to 3.9 ± 1.5 minutes.[9]

3.4   Inappropriate Sinus Tachycardia

The utility of the CARTO® system for sinus node modification was described by Leonelli et al. in a case report of two patients undergoing the procedure.[10] The electroanatomical mapping was considered useful in several ways. First it showed that earliest atrial activation shifted cranially with the use of isoproterenol as the heart rate increased from a baseline range between 98 and 109 beats/min to a rate exceeding 170 beats/min (Figure 5). This is consistent with previous reports using other techniques for sinus node modification.

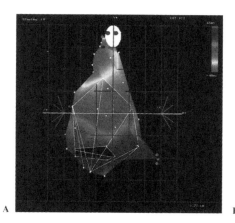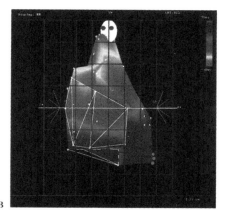

Figure 5. Shown above is the cranial shift of earliest atrial activation in a patient with inappropriate sinus tachycardia after infusion of isoproterenol. Reproduced from reference 10 with permission.

Second, the system facilitated a more precise targeting for ablation, resulting in only a few applications. The investigators reported that a marked effect (as evidenced by a marked decrease in heart rate) was accomplished after the first application. In addition, after delivery of RF ablation that resulted in reduction of sinus rate, a caudal and posterior shift of earliest atrial activation was noted (Figure 6). The investigators reported also that the fluoroscopy time in both procedures was less than 10 minutes.

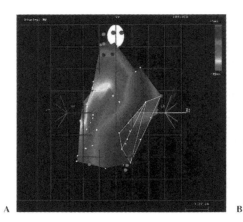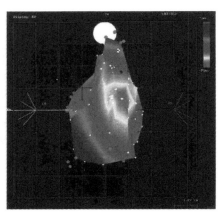

A   B

Figure 6. Shown above are the two views of earliest atrial activation after sinus node modification, identifying the site as being more caudal and posterior than at baseline. Reproduced from reference 10 with permission.

The authors concluded that the CARTO® system facilitated ablation of inappropriate sinus tachycardia. The accuracy of mapping of earliest activation was believed to be the reason for the limited number of RF applications necessary to achieve satisfactory result. The system's electroanatomical display was believed to have facilitated catheter positioning and reduced usage of fluoroscopy.

3.5   Paroxysmal Atrial Fibrillation

Pappone et al.[11] reported their work using the CARTO® system in creating linear lesions for the treatment of paroxysmal atrial fibrillation. Compartmentalization of both right (RA) and left atria (LA) was performed using RF ablation guided by CARTO® navigation method. Right and left atrial chamber mapping was performed during CS pacing at 100 bpm and chamber geometry was constructed after acquisition of an average of 81 ± 14 points (range 50 to 110 points). Compartmentalization of the RA was performed using three lines; intercaval, isthmic, and anteroseptal. The LA was compartmentalized using a single linear lesion encompassing all pulmonary veins. The CARTO® system was used to navigate the ablation catheter tip to create contiguous ablation sites. After the completion of linear ablation the CARTO® system was used in both atria to compare post-ablation activation sequence to pre-ablation (Figures 7 and 8). The procedure was performed in 27 patients. Biatrial approach was used in 14 patients, isolated LA in 5 and isolated RA in 8. The LA compartmentalization required an average of 98 ± 21 pulses while RA procedure required 61 ± 15 pulses. Completeness of linear ablation, which was confirmed by activation sequence, was noted in 21 patients.

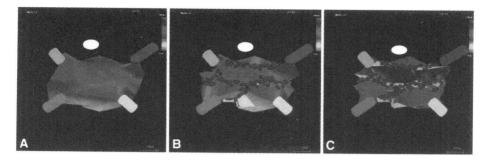

Figure 7. The reconstruction of LA is shown in panel A, viewed posteriorly. Protruding tubes represents pulmonary veins. The points corresponding to RF application are shown in panels B and C as dark spheres. A change in activation sequence is noted in panel C. Reproduced from reference 11 with permission.

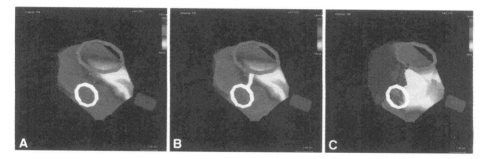

Figure 8. Shown above is the map of RA before (A) and after ablation (B and C). Dark ring represents tricuspid annulus, light ring inferior vena cava and dark tube CS. In panel C, after completion of ablation, activation map is changed.

The investigators concluded that the CARTO® system facilitated the selection of appropriate sites for ablation and the creation of linear ablation, assuring its completeness although in six patients, the lines were incomplete. The investigators were able to avoid using fluoroscopy during navigation, relying only on the mapping system. Fluoroscopy was only utilized for initial catheter placement and transseptal procedure, totalling 107 ± 44 minutes.

Ernst et al. reported their work in isolating pulmonary veins using the CARTO® system in a patient with prior failed attempt at LA and RA compartmentalization.[12] The investigators used the mapping system to create the electroanatomical map of the LA with 185 sites. They believed that the mapping system was helpful in identifying ablation gaps near the mitral annulus and on the roof of the LA. Completion of the lines resulted in complete conduction block and no inducible atrial tachyarrhythmia despite aggressive pacing. The fluoroscopy time was remarkably short, 21 minutes, despite a long procedure time of 10.6 hours.

Using the mapping system, the investigators were able to confirm completeness of ablation line from the change in activation pattern. Thus, macroreentrant atrial tachycardia along the mitral annulus that was noted after the failed first ablation was successfully prevented by completing the linear ablation. Such gaps is suspected to be the cause of recurrence of typical atrial flutter and therefore, this mapping system is also believed to be useful in identifying incomplete ablation lines.

3.6   Ventricular Tachycardia

The mapping system was also instrumental in the creation of complex linear ablation for the treatment of VT. Recently, several investigators have reported their use of a new method for controlling VT by creating conduction block to contain the site of tachycardia. Such method is potentially useful in patients with tachycardias that are difficult to map.

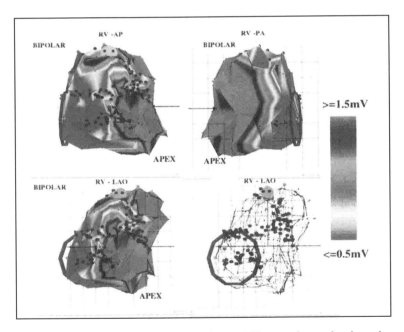

Figure 9. This figure shows the utility of CARTO's mapping and color scheme in displaying low voltage area (red zones) in a patient with right ventricular cardiomyopathy. Voltage mapping was then used to guide linear lesions (dotted lines) connecting dense scar to normal endocardium. Solid circle denotes the location of tricuspid valve. Reproduced with permission from reference 13.

Linear lesions along the border of abnormal myocardium are created by connecting dense scar to some anatomical boundary. The area of interest can also be estimated based on the morphology of VT on 12-lead ECG recording. For such procedures, the CARTO system was found to be quite useful.

Marchlinski et al[13] reported the result of such procedure in 16 patients with drug refractory, unmappable VT. These patients, with underlying ischemic and nonischemic cardiomyopathy and treated with antiarrhythmic drugs and implantable cardioverter defibrillator, had experienced frequent shocks from the device, ranging from 6 to 55 during the month prior to their procedures. Voltage mapping was performed using the system in 13 of 16 patients. Using the color scheme with the same spectrum as that used in activation pattern, the voltage of ventricular myocardium can be clearly displayed and areas with low voltage can be identified (Figure 9). In those patients, areas of abnormal endocardium ranged from 25 to 127 cm^2 (average 60±36 cm^2). The mapping system was also found to be useful in "tagging" ablated sites and in assessing completeness of the linear lesions, which ranged from 1.4 to 7.6 cm (average of 3.9 cm). For such cases, both total procedure and fluoroscopy time were noted to be high; at 8.8±1.9 hours and 121±38 minutes, respectively because of the complexity of the procedure. However, the voltage mapping and tracking ability of the system were believed to be useful for achieving the relatively high success rate of controlling the VT episodes.

SUMMARY

The CARTO mapping system is a novel system in that it provides useful adjunctive data for mapping. It provides anatomical correlate to the electrogram mapping and a tagging system to assist the creation of linear lesion. Activation mapping can be particularly useful for confirming conduction block created by the ablation while voltage mapping can be useful in identifying arrhythmogenic areas. The system dependence on the reference catheters is one disadvantage. Movement or dislodgement of the reference system may affect acquisition of mapping data significantly. However, overall, the system has proven to be useful in assisting complex ablation.

REFERENCES

1.   Gepstein L, Hayam G, Ben-Haim SA. A novel method for nonfluoroscopic catheter-based electroanatomical mapping of the heart. In vitro and in vivo accuracy results. Circulation 1997;95:1611-1622.
2.   Callans DJ, Ren J-F, Michele J, Marchlinski FE, Dillon SM. Electroanatomic left ventricular mapping in the porcine model of healed anterior myocardial infarction. Correlation with intracardiac echocardiography and pathological analysis. Circulation 1999;100:1744-1750.
3.   Roithinger FX, Cheng J, Sippens-Groenewegen A, Lee RJ, Saxon LA, Scheinmann MM, Lesh MD. Use of electroanatomic mapping to delineate transseptal atrial conduction in humans. Circulation 1999;100:1791-1797.

4.   Kloosterman EM, Yamamura K, Alba J, Mitrani RD, Myerburg RJ, Interian A, Jr. An innovative application of anatomic electromagnetic voltage mapping in a patient with Ebstein's anamoly undergoing permanent pacemaker implantation.   J Cardiovasc Electrophysiol 2000;11:99-101.
5.   Nademanee K Kosar EM. A nonfluoroscopic catheter-based mapping technique to ablate focal ventricular tachycardia. PACE 1998;21:1442-1447.
6.   Varanasi S, Dhala A, Blanck Z, Deshpande S, Akhtar M, Sra J. Electroanatomic mapping for radiofrequency ablation of cardiac arrhythmias.   J Cardiovasc Electrophysiol 1999;10:538-544.
7.   Khongphatthanayothin A, Kosar E, Nadamanee K.   Nonfluoroscopic three-dimensional mapping for arrhythmia ablation: tool or toy?. J Cardiovasc Electrophysiol2000;11:239-243.
8.   Shpun S, Gepstein L, Hayam G, Ben-Haim SA.   Guidance of radiofrequency endocardial ablation with real-time three-dimensional magnetic navigation system.   Circulation 1997;96:2016-2021.
9.   Kottkamp H, Hügl B, Krauss B, Wetzel U, Fleck A, Schuler G, Hindrikcks G. Electroanatomic versus fluoroscopic mapping of the inferior isthmus for ablation of typical atrial flutter. A prospective randomized study. Circulation 2000;102:2082-2086.
10.   Leonelli F, Richey M, Beheiry S, Rajkovich K, Natale A. Tridimensional mapping: Guided modification of the sinus node. J Cardiovasc Electrophysiol 1998;9:1214-1217.
11.   Papponne C, Oreto G, Lamberti F, Vicedomini G, Loricchio ML, Shpun S, Rillo M, Calabro MP, Conversano A, Ben-Haim SA, Cappato R, Chierchia S. Catheter ablation of paroxysmal atrial fibrillation using a 3D mapping system. Circulation 1999;100:1203-1208.
12.   Ernst S, Ouyang F, Schneider B, Kuck K-H. Prevention of atrial fibrillation by complete compartmentalization of the left atrium using a catheter technique.   J Cardiovasc Electrophysiol 2000;11:686-690.
13.   Marchlinski FE, Callans DJ, Gottlieb CD, Zado E. Linear ablation lesions for control of unmappable ventricular tachycardia in patients with ischemic and nonischemic cardiomyopathy. Circulation 2000;101:1288-1296.

Chapter 12

THREE DIMENSIONAL RECONSTRUCTION (CARTO®) IN PATIENTS WITH CONGENITAL HEART DISEASE

Joachim Hebe
Department of Cardiology, St. Georg Hospital, Hamburg, Germany

INTRODUCTION

Improvements in diagnostics, post operative care and surgery for congenital heart defects within the last two decades resulted in a higher survival rate and a significant prolongation of survival time, for more than 80% of these patients into far adulthood. As a side effect of this, the chance for the development of acquired tachycardias on the atrial or ventricular level is increased as additionally by the performance of a more complex cardiac surgery and the existence of residual volume or pressure overload of the ventricular chambers.[7,8,10]

As the hemodynamic tolerance of such tachycardias is often low due to hemodynamic or functional failure related to the underlying congenital heart defect, treatment is required more frequently than in patients with structurally normal hearts. Amongst the therapeutic options, antiarrhythmic medication, still as the most frequent chosen one, wears the disadvantage of an increased risk for potential side effects, like aggravation of preexisting cardiac failure or impairment of impulse generation and conduction.[2] Reliability for prevention of recurrences is low, at least on the long term course. Cardiac surgery in terms of a re-do surgery is rarely indicated at a time when tachycardias occur and primary antiarrhythmic surgery is not well accepted from the patient side due to its high invasive character. So, finally radiofrequency current ablation is increasingly asked for treatment of tachycardias after surgery for congenital heart defects, as it wears the potential for a substrate related and definitive treatment, at least for regular monomorphic tachycardias based on circumscribed substrates.

Early after stimulation techniques for the identification of essential areas for the maintenance of reentrant tachycardias were introduced in patients without

149

L. Bing Liem and E. Downar (eds.), Progress in Catheter Ablation, 149-186.
© 2001 *Kluwer Academic Publishers. Printed in the Netherlands.*

cardiac anomaly and ablation techniques consisting of linear lesions were established, like for the treatment of common type atrial flutter.[3,11-14,20-23]

While results in patients with more „simple" congenital heart defects and after more „ simple" surgical attempts for correction were promising, like e.g. in patients after closure of an atrial septum defect, success rates are still significantly lower and recurrence rates higher than compared to patients with e.g. common type atrial flutter and structurally normal hearts. The highly variable expression of the cardiac anomalies together with non-uniform surgical procedures resulting in unpredictable myocardial scars, are judged for being mainly responsible for the limited understanding of the individual anatomic situations, of the topography of barriers of electrical conduction and of the complete courses of reentry tachycardias. As these points are essential for the design of proper individual ablation strategies, the introduction of a 3-dimensional reconstruction and navigation system (CARTO) promised to open a new chapter in the treatment of such complex tachycardias.

The following article is aimed to show the application of the CARTO 3-D electro-anatomical reconstruction system in patients with tachycardias after surgery for congenital heart disease.

1. TACHYCARDIAS IN PATIENTS WITH POSTOPERATIVE CONGENITAL HEART DISEASE

Post-surgically acquired tachycardias are in the vast majority based on macro-reentrant circuits on the atrial or ventricular level. Residual myocardial scars possess a high potential to play a significant role in the process of arrhythmogenesis. Barriers of electrical conduction, like e.g. AV-rings, insertion of veins, myocardial scars or implants (patches) located in close topographical proximity to each other and separated by vital myocardium of potentially delayed conduction properties, may create critical zones for the perpetuation of a reentry circuit tachycardia. The best understood model for this type of tachycardia, so far, is the „common type atrial flutter", which can be observed similarly in patients with structural normal hearts and those with congenital defects. Here, the tachycardia takes its course along the tricuspid annulus, as a naturally given barrier of electrical conduction, through a narrow isthmus between the inferior aspect of the AV-ring and the orifice of the inferior caval vein.[3,17] After operation for congenital heart defects, there is an increased potential of developing macro-reentrant circuits due to the addition of surgery related barriers and in conjunction with global alterations of the surrounding myocardial tissue, named „incisional tachycardias". The stability and cycle length of the tachycardia is determined by the dimension of the circuit, the conduction properties of the myocardium involved and the degree of conduction delay within the critical zone. Global myocardial alterations, like dilatation, hypertrophy and fibrosis, together with the dimension of cardiac chambers are very likely to be important, but yet not sufficient explored cofactors for the development of such tachycardias. A rare number of post operatively acquired tachycardias is based on enhanced focal automaticity, mainly originating in tight topographical relationship to scars resulting from cardiac surgery.

2.   CONVENTIONAL TECHNOLOGY

2.1   Mapping (Conventional Maneuver for Understanding of Complex Tachycardias)

Detailed knowledge of the type of surgery and the individual expression of the cardiac anomaly are essential pre-requisites for the understanding of potential sites for the origin of ectopic automatic foci or sites of barriers of electrical conduction potentially involved in the creation of isthmic zones responsible for the maintenance of macro-reentry tachycardias.

In general, the techniques for identification of the underlying mechanism of the tachycardia as well as the identification and localization of the arrhythmogenic substrate are similar to those used in patients without cardiac anomalies.[13]

Due to the high variability of the postoperative cardiac situs, each chamber involved in the tachycardia circuit needs to be explored extensively by mapping of the localization and extension of myocardial scars, their topographical relation towards all naturally given barriers of electrical conduction and the position of implants. Like e.g. patches. Loss of local electrical activity or recordings of doubled local signals divided by an isoelectric line are reliable markers for an area of scar tissue or a bilateral activation of the myocardium surrounding a barrier.[16] Splitting or fractionation of local electrograms are signs for delayed conduction properties, often found in the neighborhood of scars. Such type of cartography can be performed during sinusrhythm, intracardiac pacing or during tachycardia, using multipolar electrode catheters in order to provide segmental recordings of the intraatrial activation sequence. Subsequently, the course of an already present and/or each inducible tachycardia along these barriers can be estimated. In order to achieve a maximum of local electrogram recordings from areas involved in the reentry circuit, corrections of the catheter positions are required according to the results of entrainment pacing.

2.2   Ablation Strategy

To our current understanding, the concept for the interventional treatment of macro-reentry is based on linear, continuous and transmural lesions consisting of multiple singular radiofrequency current applications. Combining laterally enclosing barriers, such linear lesions aim to electrically dissect a zone of myocardial tissue identified for being critical for the maintenance of the reentry circuit. The design of the ablation strategy needs to be individualized according to the variety of anatomical findings including the course of the physiologic conduction tissue.[1,4,6,19]

In patients after surgery for congenital heart disease, one of the challenging parts is to determine the precise anatomic location and extension of the confining barriers using exclusively fluoroscopy. Just with the help of catheter positions as intracardiac location markers and a „semi 3 dimensional" memory of the topographical relationship restricted to the investigators imagination, the ablation strategy can be planned and subsequently carried out.

2.3   Validation of Success

Validation of completeness of the ablation line is crucial for the acute success rate as well as to keep the recurrence rate low. Concepts developed and established for the treatment of common type atrial flutter[17] are partially transferred to postsurgical tachycardias. Due to the enormous variety of barriers confining targeted myocardial areas such procedure needs to be individualized with respect to the site of pacing, e.g. close to the entrance of an isthmic zone, and with respect to site of electrogram recording at sites close to its exit and representative surrounding myocardial areas. In case of a significant change in activation spread through an targeted zone, compared before and after ablative dissection, local electrograms recorded close to the ablation line are likely to show doubled activation signals, separated by an isoelectric line.[16] Additionally, multipolar electrograms recorded from surrounding myocardium, opposite to the pacing site, will show exclusive activation directed towards the electrically dissected area. Objectivation of such significant change in local activation while producing a linear lesion allows speculation about achievement of a complete block of activation through a targeted myocardial zone but requires proper catheter placement in relation to highly variable borders and interposed protected myocardial zones.

3.   3-D ELECTRO-ANATOMICAL RECONSTRUCTION

In order to overcome some of the limitations related to conventional mapping and ablation technology, modern technologies are increasingly introduced, like multi-electrode basket-catheter (Boston-Scientific¨) or 3-dimensional reconstruction systems, like e.g. the „non-contact-mapping" system (Endocardial Solutions Inc.¨) or the CARTO mapping system (Biosense¨). Such newer technologies aim to provide a more global recording of the intracardiac electrical propagation .[6,9]

The 3-dimensional electro-anatomical reconstruction system CARTO, which is described in this article, allows visualize the individual shape of selected cardiac chambers, the position and extension of electrical barriers and their topographical relationship. Furthermore, in addition to sinus rhythm or pacing, the course of monomorphic and regular tachycardias can be visualized along the barriers of electrical conduction within these reconstructed cardiac chambers. Combined with results from conventional pacing techniques, like entrainment maneuvers, such information allows to design a proper individual ablation strategy. If ablation fails due to inefficient lesion generation at sites of extensive scarring and myocardial at the targeted site, alternative ablation routes may be chosen, as the remaining tachycardias course is visualized.

In both ways conventional and 3-D reconstruction, specially developed stimulation techniques are used for the identification of the zone of critical conduction, its dimension, its entrance and its exit.[13,15,16]

Using the CARTO system, results of such maneuvers or any type of information can be marked within the reconstruction, as like zones of electrical block , slowed conduction or spots of electrically silence. Summarizing the results of the above mentioned maneuvers, an individual concept consisting of linear ablation lesions can be designed. These lines can be applied to the best and easiest accessible myocardial site with respect to catheter handling and/or to the potentially narrowest isthmic zone.

For validation of the ablations success, in terms of completion of the designated ablation line, the spread of electrical conduction across the targeted area can be visualized in relationship to the surrounding tissue, before, during and after ablation. Analogous to conventional technology, The dissection of an initially singular local activation signal into two components, separated by an isoelectric line will indicate sufficient lesion generation, at least for the single application. But detection of a complete blockade of conduction through the designated myocardium can be visualized by displaying latest local activation adjacent to the ablation line, opposite to the pacing site. Exclusive wave propagation towards this area within the targeted chamber after ablation has been performed, will be demonstrated by a complete repeat reconstruction.

As the site of physiologic impulse generation, sinus node or escape rhythm focus, and conduction (AV-node, His-bundle) might vary mainly according to the type of underlying cardiac anomaly and intraatrial or intraventricular conduction might be altered by surgery, identification of such structures and their implementation into the linear ablation concept is crucial for the success of such procedure.

3.1   3 D Procedure, Practical Issues

3.1.1   Technical Aspects

Production of a magnetic field around the chest of the patient and special designed catheters with magnetic sensors allow a point by point reconstruction of cardiac chambers. Each acquired point in space consists next to exact x,y,z coordinates of an information of the timing of the local electrical signal compared to a stable reference signal, gained from the surface ECG or intracardial. Adding such points subsequently acquired at the inner surface of a cardiac chamber, a virtual reconstruction of its shape as well as the spread of activation of the mapped rhythm within that reconstruction can be appreciated (see previous chapter about more details).

3.1.2   Selection of Chamber for Mapping

Study of the surgeons report about access to intracardiac structures and the type of attempted repair will allow suggestions about the cardiac chamber, which is critically involved in the maintenance of the targeted tachycardia, rather more than often unreliable analysis of the tachycardias surface ECG patterns. So, most of the patients after repair for an atrial septal defect, will present with an right-sided macro reentrant circuit, based on a scar resulting from the atriotomy at the lateral free wall or from a scar resulting from an indirect trans-myocardial cannulation of the systemic venous return or utilizing the tricuspid annulus. The same is true for most of the cardiac anomalies, which have undergone surgery via a trans-right-atrial approach, even if performed on the ventricular level. Analogous, ventricular tachycardias after cardiac repairs including a right sided ventriculotomy are most likely generated within the right ventricular chamber. In more complex types of surgery involving both atriums or both ventricles or those involving septal structures, generally tachycardias might be associated to each of the chambers or even utilize both sides on the atrial or on the ventricular level for their maintenance.

As from a technical point of view access to chambers connected to the systemic venous return is easier compared to those draining the pulmonary venous one, reconstruction should be started on the right atrial, or in case of ventricular tachycardia, on the right ventricular level, if surgical reports do not indicate exclusive surgery to the opposite chambers. Conventional mapping and entrainment maneuvers can help to identify myocardial zones, where „mid-diastolic" local electrograms can be recorded or critical zones may be detected by pacing maneuvers, both indicative for the crucial involvement of the mapped chamber in the perpetuation of the reentry tachycardia. If such criteria can not be identified quickly, a look to the spread of local electrograms of the 3-D reconstruction is very helpful answering this question. While the timing of the local electrograms recorded within a selected chamber should spread homogeneously over the cycle length of the reentry tachycardia, in terms of representation of the whole reentry circuit (Figure 1), a critical involvement of such chamber can be almost excluded, if significant gaps within the circuit cannot be filled, even with more intensive mapping of the whole entire chamber (Figure 2). In such cases, additional mapping and reconstruction of the opposite chamber at the atrial or ventricular level will allow identification of the searched reentry circuit.

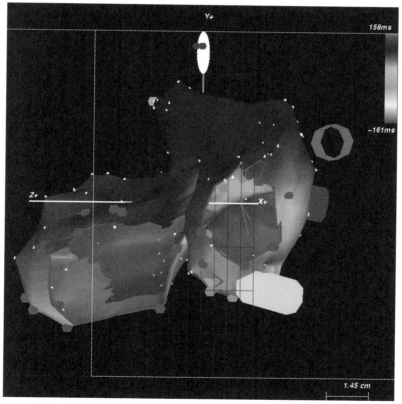

Figure 1 (see also Color Plate 3). Reconstruction of both atrial levels in a patient after a double switch procedure in order to correct a congenitally corrected transposition of the great arteries and an atrial tachycardia. On the trial level, a Senning type surgery was performed, displaying the pulmonary venous atrium on the pictures left side. Here, course of the tachycardia around the "right sided" mitral annulus can be suspected from the activation map, as a homogeneous display of the complete time span of the window of interest (equivalent to complete color range) is distributed around the mitral annulus, and relatively latest activation (purple) meets relatively earliest activation (red), termed "head meets tail".

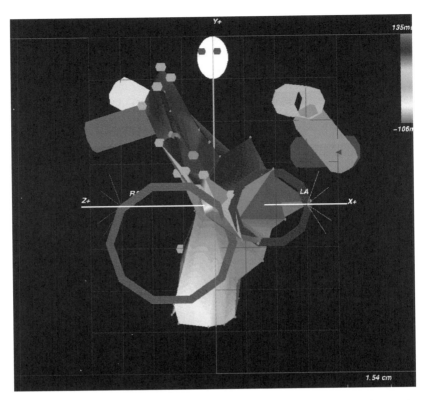

Figure 2 (see also Color Plate 4). Reconstruction of the systemic venous atrium in a patient after Senning type atrial switch procedure due to d-transposition of the great arteries. In case of a macro-reentry tachycardia, an incomplete display of the full color range (blue, light blue and green are missing) gives evidence for an incomplete reconstruction of the tachycardias circuit within that chamber. Differential interpretations are: 1. Chamber just as bystander of the tachycardia, 2. Chamber just as part of the circuit, compete in conjunction with the opposite chamber.

3.1.3   Selection of Rhythm for Mapping

In general, 3 D reconstruction can be performed during any type of constant rhythm, like sinus rhythm or constant escape rhythm, utilizing a permanent implanted or a transient „procedural" pacer or any monomorphic and regular sustained tachycardia. How to start the individual procedure will be mainly determined by the rhythm, present at the start of the procedure, as in case of the presence of a sustained tachycardia, it seems advisable to take the opportunity due to its often difficult or even impossible re-induction.

An initial basic mapping of the targeted chamber (see above) is concentrated on a complete reconstruction of its individual anatomical shape including the topography of electrical barriers, like e.g. insertion of systemic or pulmonary veins, atrioventricular rings, surgically created scars, areas of degenerated myocardium or implants. Additionally the site and course of the physiologic impulse generation (sinus node area) and atrioventricular conduction (His bundle) as like the position of the reference catheters electrode pair or, if present, the site of a transient or permanent pacing lead are marked in the entire map.

Starting the reconstruction during sinus rhythm allows the implementation of information about the sinus node localization as well as its the preferred course towards the AV node into the final ablation concept, all of which can extremely vary according to the underlying heart defect and the type of surgery that has been performed. After such basic reconstruction has been completed each inducible tachycardia involving such chamber can be mapped using this anatomic and topographic information, allowing visualization of its course along previously defined barriers of electrical conduction. Suspected critical zones for the maintenance of these reentry circuits can be proven by conventional pacing maneuvers, like e.g. concealed entrainment.

Information gained from above described maneuvers will determine the design of an individual ablation concept consisting of linear and continuous lesions aimed to combine electrical barriers confining zones of critical conduction. Furthermore, alternative ablation routes ca be selected, if radiofrequency current application fails in terms of sufficient lesion generation due to scarred, fibrotic or hypertrophic myocardium at the targeted site.

As a third step, electrical conduction through the area selected for ablation is electro-anatomically reconstructed utilizing a rhythm, originating in close proximity to this zone. For this, a stable sinus rhythm or pacing through the reference catheter can be used each, if properly located. Alternatively an additional transient screw electrode can be placed selectively close to the targeted area and utilized for pacing during the procedure. A proper reconstruction of the conduction properties before ablation will allow validation of the completeness of the attempted ablation line during and at the end of radiofrequency current application.

3.1.4   Selection of Electrogram Reference, Site of Pacing

The signal for the reference channel typically is chosen from the endocardial level rather more than from the surface electrocardiogram as the latter wears the disadvantage, that the QRS-morphology is likely to change during the procedure, e.g. due to the occurrence of a bundle branch block pattern or any type of intracardiac conduction delay related to the speed of the tachycardia. Additionally, if tachycardias on the atrial level are to be reconstructed, the QRS complex might have variant relation to atrial signals due to variable atrioventricular conduction properties provided by the physiologic conduction system.

3.1.4.1   Atrial tachycardias

In most of the cases the coronary sinus is chosen for the placement of the reference catheter around the mitral valve annulus, as such anatomic structure offers the highest probability for a stable catheter position throughout the procedure. Despite its selective representation of left atrial activation patterns, both left and right sided tachycardias can be reconstructed electro-anatomically sufficient. In contrast to this, for validation purposes (see below), pacing from the coronary sinus is very likely not to be appropriate case of attempted linear ablations at the right atrium, especially at the lateral free wall. For this, the additional use of a transient screw electrode is advisable. Alternatively, in case of an abnormal or undetected drainage of the coronary sinus, the atrial appendages can be used as a relatively stable place for positioning of non screwed electrodes.

3.1.4.2   Ventricular Tachycardias

If the QRS morphology during sinus rhythm or tachycardia is unchanged throughout the mapping procedure, a surface QRS complex can be used as an electrical reference signal. Alternatively an intracardiac signal can be used, ideally gained from the opposite chamber to the targeted one, as it prevents unintentional manipulation of the reference catheter while mapping.

3.1.5   Setting „Window of Interest"

Selective acquisition of electrical information from the chamber of interest or exclusion of pacing artifacts can be provided by a free adjustable „window of interest", defined by a timing filter related to a reference signal during sinus rhythm, pacing or any type of sustained regular tachycardia. Within the postoperative course of congenital heart defects, tachycardias are based in the vast majority on macro-reentry circuits, where the proper adjustment of the „window of interest" is crucial for the final understanding of its complete course. In contrast to a focally originating rhythm, like sinus rhythm or constant pacing, we expect in a macro reentry to record local signals representing homogeneously the complete duration of the tachycardias cycle length by mapping those anatomical sites critically involved in the perpetuation of the circuit. The relatively earliest recordings within the „window of interest" are color coded in red, the relatively latest in deep purple, which meet directly as zones coded in red at some area within the circuit, as we are dealing with a continuous loop. Such „head meets tail" zone, used as a modern identification criterion for the identification of a macro reentry circuit, can be placed at any site if the reconstructed circuit, as its position is determined by the setting of the borders of the „window of interest" and its relation to the timing of the signal gained from the reference catheter. Typically the duration of the „window of interest" is set to 90% of the tachycardias cycle length, in case of significant variations, to 90% of the shortest measured A-A or R-R intervals. By this, recording and annotation of signals of two sequential circuits within a singular tachycardia beat can be excluded.

3.1.6   Start of Mapping

Guided by conventional criteria for the decision which cardiac chamber needs to be mapped at the beginning of the procedure (see above), the basic reconstruction initially concentrates on the identification of representative landmarks like the insertion of veins into the atrial chambers (superior and inferior caval vein, pulmonary veins, coronary sinus), site and course of the specific conduction system and the atrioventricular rings, latter are equivalent important in case of ventricular mapping in addition to the insertion of the great arteries. Furthermore, for the sake of a better understanding of the final reconstruction, identification of the localization of the reference catheters electrode pair and if existing, the position of a permanent or transitional pacing electrode is advisable. Such initial landmarks are mapped with the help of a conventional fluoroscopic view to the catheter manipulations, especially with respect to the high variety of native and postsurgical anatomy in patients with congenital heart defects. Depending on the investigators experience, the use of fluoroscopy can be dramatically reduced, after the rough dimension and orientation of the targeted chamber is stored and above mentioned landmarks are visualized on such initial reconstruction.

As a second step of this initial map, the complete endocardial surface of the chamber needs to be explored and reconstructed by a fair number of mapping points, which should for this step not count less than 1 mapping point per square centimeter. Such performance provides basic information about the rough shape of the chamber, allowing now to concentrate on the detection of splitted and doubled signals or such significantly reduced in amplitude as the third step of the reconstruction. Additionally, at this step, the mapped chamber can be proven to be critical for the tachycardia, as a homogeneous distribution of the local electrograms timing filling the tachycardia cycle length is expected.

Requirements to a higher density of acquired points are related to the exact identification of areas of conduction functional or anatomical block, on transition zones from vital towards diseased and relatively slower conducting myocardium or towards fibrotic tissue, like e.g. insertion of vessels, atrioventricular rings, scars or implants (patch). The careful reconstruction of such zones serves as a crucial requisite for the planning and performance of the individual ablation strategy.

3.1.7   Annotation of Local Electrograms

The CARTO software provides algorithms for automated annotation of local electrograms, which basically offer annotation targeting the maximum amplitude of or the maximum slope within an electrogram. As many electrophysiologists prefer to record bipolar electrograms for reconstruction of macro-reentry tachycardias, automated annotation targeting the maximum amplitude is chosen mostly, at least for gaining a quick orientation about the course of a tachycardia or about the spread of activation across an area of interest while a certain rhythm. But as the maximum amplitude component of a bipolar signal is placed more accidentally within the duration of the whole local electrogram recorded at the endocardial myocardium and often additionally shows beat to beat variations at unchanged catheter positions, such automated annotation does not allow a more precise reconstruction of an electro-anatomical situation, e.g. with a focal origin. If requested, such automated annotation can be manually corrected according to any algorithm, that is believed to be the most reproducible and correct one. In our experience, manual re-annotation targeting the initial main deflection of the local bipolar signal is preferred, defined as a deviation of a signal with a steepnes of more than 45° in relation to the isoelectric line and an amplitude exceeding the noise level by more than 50%.

Areas, where instead of sufficient wall contact a reduction of the local signal amplitude below noise level is objected, are suspicious to represent myocardial scars resulting from surgical procedures, like e.g. incisions or implants, or from disease related ischemia and cyanosis. So far the only available way to prove sufficiency of electrode contact to the mapped endocardial surface is gained from the additional use of fluoroscopy showing simultaneous movement of myocardium and catheter tip.

In case of small or narrow scars resulting in blockade of electrical conduction, doubling of the local electrogram can be detected if electrical activation occurs with a difference in timing on opposite sites of the scar and if additionally signals from these sites can be detected with the same electrode pair in place. Annotation of such double potentials is guided by the signal with the higher amplitude as it typically represents of direct recording of local activation at one site of the conduction block. The smaller amplitude signal is believed to be due to a far field recording of the activation of the opposite site of the block.

The degree of separation of the two components is determined by the length of the area of blocked conduction next to other factors like e.g. local conduction velocity.

3.1.8   Markers

In addition to the automated color coded display of the electroanatomical map, each single point can additionally be marked by differently colored dots in order to introduce a third level of information to the map. Thus, on top to the coordinates for the position in space and the relative timing towards the reference signal for each acquired point of the map, manually any type of information can be coded with markers in different colors, as like e.g. the occurrence of fractionated, splitted or double electrograms, the identification of the atrioventricular rings or the specific conduction system, the transition from myocardium towards veins or arteries a.s.o. (Figure 3). Furthermore, results from conventional pacing maneuvers, like identification of critical zones for the tachycardia, proven by concealed entrainment or the identification of bystander areas as well as spots outside the reentry circuit can be added to the electro-anatomical information of such points. Finally, spots, where radiofrequency current is applied, can be marked selectively and thereby help to control the ablation course along the designated ablation line.

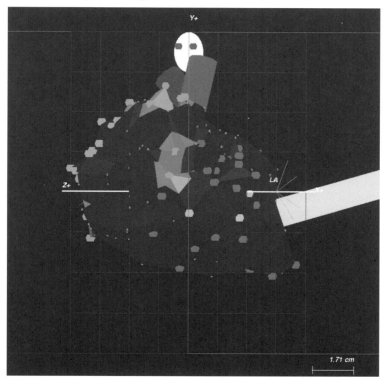

Figure 3 (see also Color Plate 5). 3-D electroanatomical reconstruction of the right atrium of a patient after Fontan surgery (LAO projection, propagation map mode). Yellow tube shows rough course of the coronary sinus, gray and brown tubes show transition to and course of the pulmonary trunk. Blue dots mark areas with doubled potentials (line of electrical block), gray dots mark areas with loss of electrical signals (scars), brown dots mark occurrence of A and V signals (area of the right sided atrioventricular junction at atretic tricuspid annulus), yellow dots where solely V signals were detected.

3.2   Ablation Strategy

After all necessary and available information about the individual anatomy, the position of components of the specific conduction system, the topography of barriers and the complete course of the tachycardia or those of multiple tachycardias have been summarized in the 3-D electroanatomical reconstruction, an individual concept for the ablation procedure can be developed. As mentioned earlier, in most of the post operative congenital heart patients such interventional concept will consist of linear ablation lesions, aiming to continuously combine electrical barriers confining a myocardial zone, identified to be critical for the maintenance of the tachycardia due to a macro reentry circuit as underlying mechanism for the majority of tachycardias.

The decision where to create an ablation line, will be influenced on the atrial level by the position of the sinus node, the preferential course of its impulse towards the AV-node, the position of the His bundle and on the ventricular level by its continuation into the bundle branches. The avoidance of a direct damage of components of the conduction system is a crucial part in the process of designing the ablation strategy as like the preservation of its preferential tracts for impulse propagation via myocardial tissue.

The efficacy of the translation of the decided ablation strategy towards the myocardium is depending on the length of the designated ablation line, the accessibility of the targeted area by catheter maneuvers and the degree of hypertrophy, fibrosis or scarring the local myocardium. In case of failed ablation with respect to effective lesion generation along the primary elected area, with the use of the 3-D visualization of the complete tachycardia course, an alternative ablation route can be chosen involving better accessible or less altered myocardium offering an improved chance for sufficient lesion generation.

Especially in patients after surgery for congenital heart disease, the likelihood for the induction of multiple reentry tachycardias is high due to the number of myocardial scar resulting from disease related degeneration and surgery at the involved chambers. Therefore, after having identified the course and critical zones of the clinically relevant tachycardia, more than one thought must be spent to the possibility of further tachycardias based on the reconstructed anatomy and additionally their potential creation by an ablation line. Following this, the ablation concept should implement proven data about critical zones for reconstructed tachycardias and speculative thoughts about potential new ones after the ablation session has been stopped.

If two or multiple tachycardias are inducible involving the same cardiac chamber, the 3-D animated visualization allows the identification of common utilized myocardial zones representing an appropriate ablation target.

3.3   Validation

As the termination of the tachycardia by radiofrequency current application is inducing the investigators enthusiasm rather more than ensure the completeness of the ablation line with respect to its continuity and possibly its transmurality, a concept for validation of the conduction block needs to be introduced into the ablation strategy. Such validation concept basically consists of the 3-D reconstruction and visualization of the electrical propagation through a myocardial zone, which carries the targeted ablation line, including the propagation along the alternative routes via the surrounding myocardium, before and after radiofrequency current has been applied (Figure 4).

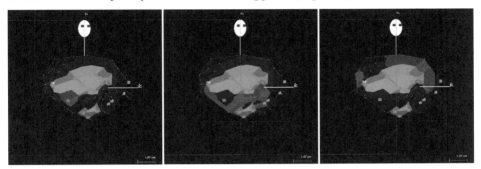

Figure 4 (see Color Plate 6). Partial reconstruction in a patient after Fontan procedure (RAO projection) showing two scars (gray fields) at the lateral atrial wall confining an area of vital myocardium, identified before for being critical for the maintenance of a reentry tachycardia. In preparation of an ablation line, aiming to combine both scars, propagation through this area was visualized by pacing in its close proximity (yellow marker: position of transient screw electrode). Figures a (left) – c (right) display electrical conduction trough the designated area before ablation was started.

For such validation concept a proper selection of the site of impulse generation is mandatory, providing a homogeneous electrical propagation through the targeted myocardial zone resulting in a collision of the wave-fronts generated by alternative routes along the remaining myocardium. Such collision zone, ideally identical with the area activated latest within the selected chamber, should be far distant from the pacing site and the area, where ablation is attempted. Following such strategy, after completion of the linear ablation, a block of electrical conduction can be visualized by a new reconstruction, displaying now a shift of the latest activation in closest proximity to the ablation line, on the opposite site of the impulse generation (Figure 5).

If the position of the sinus node accidentally appears not to be proper serving as impulse generator for validation of the decided ablation site, any other place can be selected following the above mentioned advice using a standard pacing catheter or a transient screw electrode.

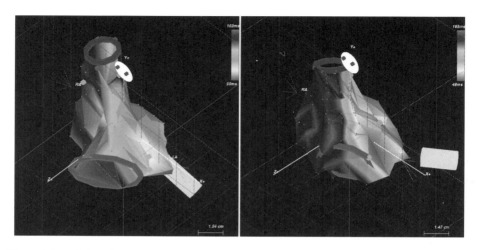

Figure 5 (see Color Plate 7). LAO-anterior view the right atrium in a patient, where an ablation line was incompletely carried out, attempting a complete block between the insertion of the superior caval vein (green ring) and the anterior aspect of the tricuspid annulus (brown ring). Pacing was carried out close to the ostium of the coronary sinus displaying a homogeneous propagation from the pacing site towards the attempted ablation line. Note the difference between site of latest activation before the ablation line was completed, purple color located at the lateral free atrial wall (a) and after successful block of the targeted area, purple color located adjacent to the ablation line, opposite to the pacing site (b).

4.   CASE PRESENTATIONS

4.1   Atrial Reentry Tachycardia in A Patient After Fontan Procedure (Figure 6 and Color Plate 8)

Reconstruction of right atrium in a patient after Fontan procedure due to an imperforate tricuspid valve type tricuspid atresia (LAO projection). As tachycardias circuit was identified to cruise around the atretic tricuspid annulus, utilizing the posterior isthmic region as a critical zone, ablation was attempted to combine the center of the tricuspid annulus, where from the atrial level solely local ventricular signals were recorded (yellow markers), and the insertion of the tricuspid annulus. Red Markers show sites of radiofrequency current applications along the designated ablation line. Note the difference of site of latest activation while pacing at the coronary sinus ostium (yellow tube) before ablation (a) and after completion of ablation line (b). Pictures c to f show propagation of the activation before ablation, homogeneously from the pacing site through the posterior isthmic region and along the anterior right atrial wall towards, colliding at the lateral free atrial wall. Pictures i to h show exclusive propagation along the anterior right atrial wall, with latest activation adjacent to the ablation line, opposite to the pacing site after block in the posterior isthmus was achieved.

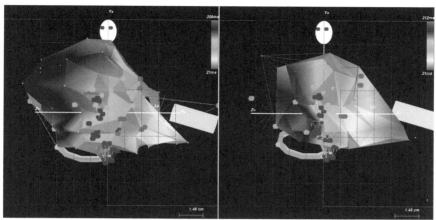

Figure 6 a

Figure 6 b

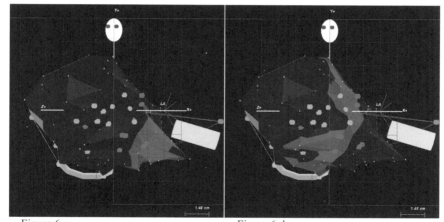

Figure 6 c

Figure 6 d

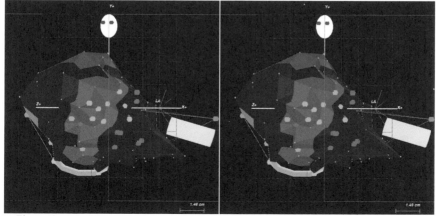

Figure 6 e

Figure 6 f

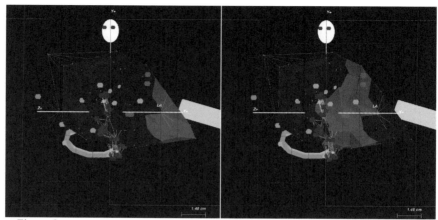

Figure 6 g

Figure 6 h

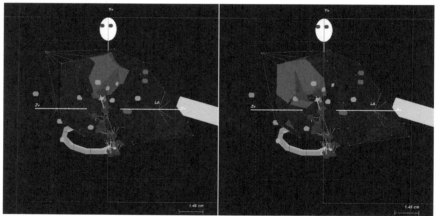

Figure 6 i

Figure 6 j

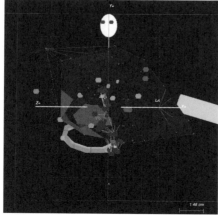

Figure 6 k

4.2 Atrial Reentry Tachycardias in a Patient After Surgical Closure of an Atrial Septal Defect (Figure 7 and Color Plate 9)

Reconstruction of 2 different atrial reentry tachycardias in an adult patient 2 years after surgical closure of an atrial septum defect (secundum type) via a conventional lateral atriotomy.

7a (RAO view) and 7 b (right lateral view) show an activation map of the initial tachycardia, which was permanently present in this patient for > 6 months, previously a failed attempt to block the posterior isthmus has been done in the referring institution. Gray ring depicts the insertion of the inferior caval vein, green ring the insertion of the superior caval vein, brown ring the tricuspid annulus, gray tube represents the coronary sinus, gray fields represent areas of myocardium with loss of local activation. Superior-anterior scar presumably resulting from the atriotomy, inferior-dorsal one from cannulation of the systemic veins via the myocardium, scar on the posterior isthmus as a result of incomplete block of that region.

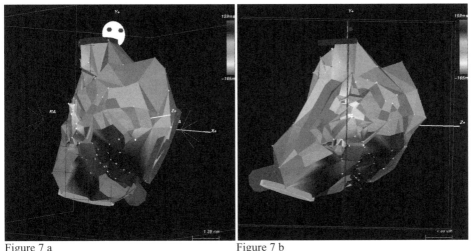

Figure 7 a   Figure 7 b

7 c Pink dots mark areas with concealed entrainment of the reentry tachycardia.

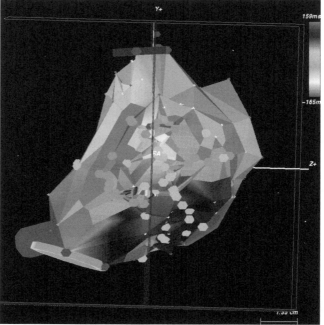

Figure 7 c

7 d – j   Propagation map of the tachycardia shows a course of the circuit through both surgically created scars in caudo-cranial direction and a reentry via the anterior and posterior right atrial free wall.

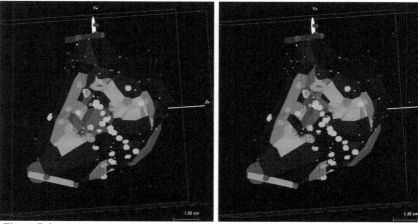

Figure 7 d   Figure 7 e

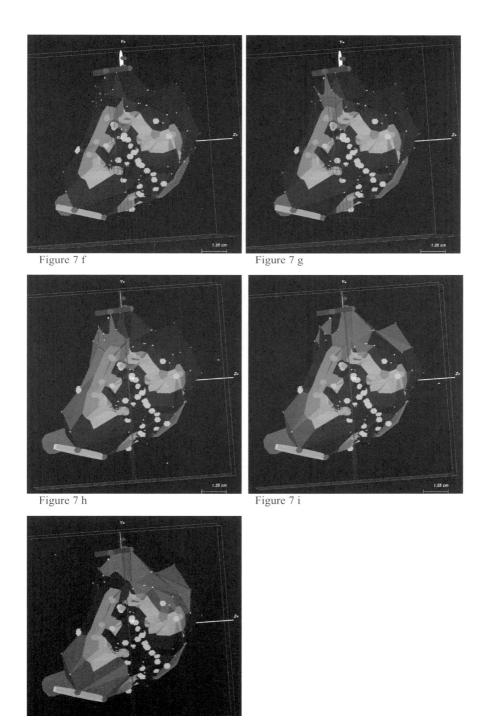

Figure 7 f

Figure 7 g

Figure 7 h

Figure 7 i

Figure 7 j

7 k (RAO view) Activation map of second tachycardia following successful ablation of the first tachycardia by combining both scars with radiofrequency current ablation (note additional gray area between superior and inferior scar)

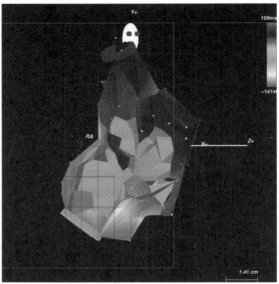

Figure 7 k

7 l Pink dots mark areas with concealed entrainment of the reentry tachycardia.

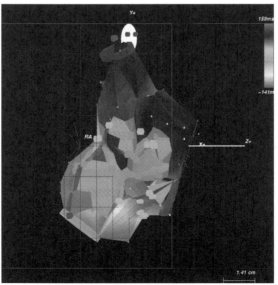

Figure 7 l

7 m – t   Propagation map of the second atrial tachycardia with a caudo-cranial course along the dorsal right atrial wall around both surgically created scars and a cranio-caudal course along the anterior wall between the lateral tricuspid annulus and the anterior border of the atriotomy scar. Radiofrequency current applications combining these barriers were successful in blocking the second tachycardia permanently.

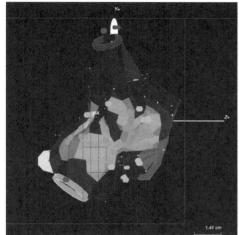

Figure 7 m

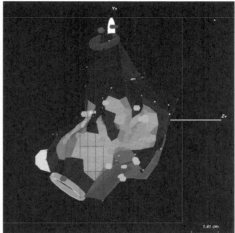

Figure 7 n

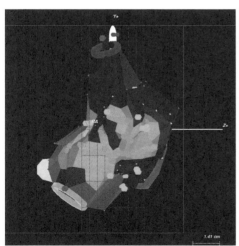

Figure 7 o

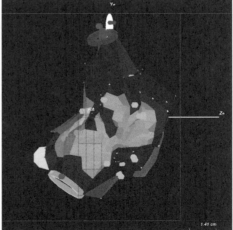

Figure 7 p

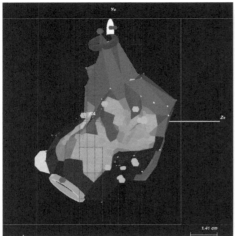

Figure 7 q

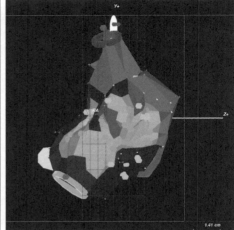

Figure 7 r

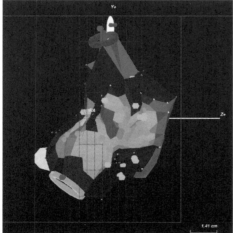

Figure 7 s

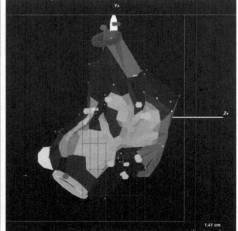

Figure 7 t

7 u surface ECG of incessant and initial atrial tachycardia, cycle length at atrial level of 310 msec., 2:1 atrioventricular conduction, positive p wave polarity in inferior leads II, III, aVf.

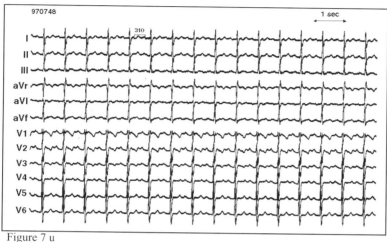

Figure 7 u

7 v surface ECG of second atrial tachycardia, cycle length 360 msec, inverted p wave polarity in inferior leads.

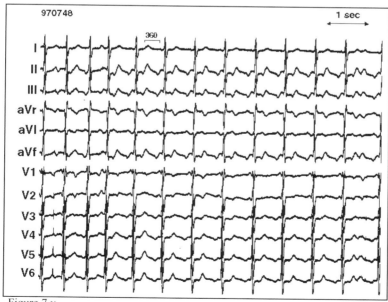

Figure 7 v

7 w schematic view to the postoperative right atrial situs of the patient, showing 2 separate scars at the lateral free wall and depicted in red, the course of the ablation line for tachycardia N° 1.

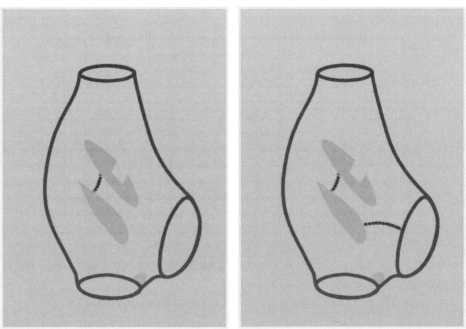

Figure 7 w   Figure 7 x

7 x display of both ablation lines (grey dots), combining both lateral surgery related scars and the lateral tricuspid annulus, for tachycardia N° 1 + 2.

4.3   Atrial Reentry Tachycardia in a Patient After Atrial Switch Procedure of the Mustard Type Due to d-Transposition of the Great Arteries (Figure 8 and Color Plate 10)

8 a (left lateral view) 8 b (posterior-anterior view) show reconstruction of both the pulmonary venous atrium (right side on picture 8 a) and the systemic venous atrium (left side on picture 8 a) in the activation map mode while reentry tachycardia. Tricuspid annulus is depicted by the brown ring, the mitral annulus by the red ring, tube display entrance of pulmonary veins into the pulmonary venous atrium. Grey areas on systemic venous atrium depict connection to superior and inferior caval vein, on pulmonary venous atrium scar resulting from lateral atriotomy.

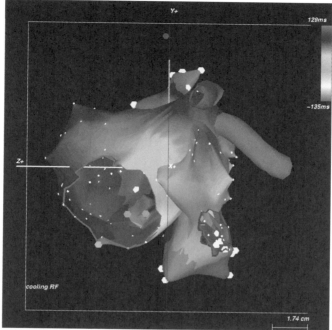

Figure 8 a

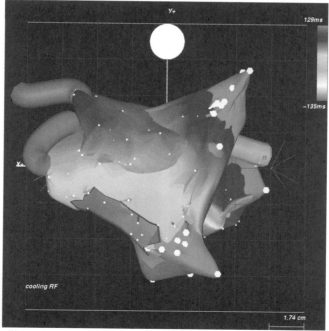

Figure 8 b

8 c – m   (left lateral view) propagation map of the tachycardia circling around the tricuspid annulus in a counter-clock wise manner, comparable to common type atrial flutter in patients with structural normal hearts. Ablation concept consisted in production of a continuous linear lesion combining the posterior tricuspid annulus and the atriotomy scar, visible through the tricuspid annulus (gray area).

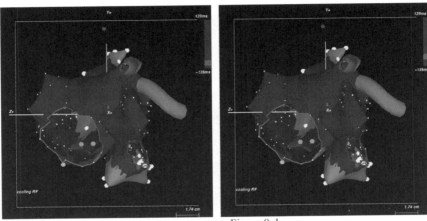

Figure 8 c   Figure 8 d

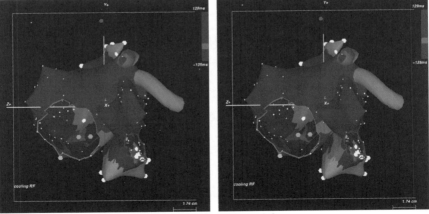

Figure 8 e   Figure 8 f

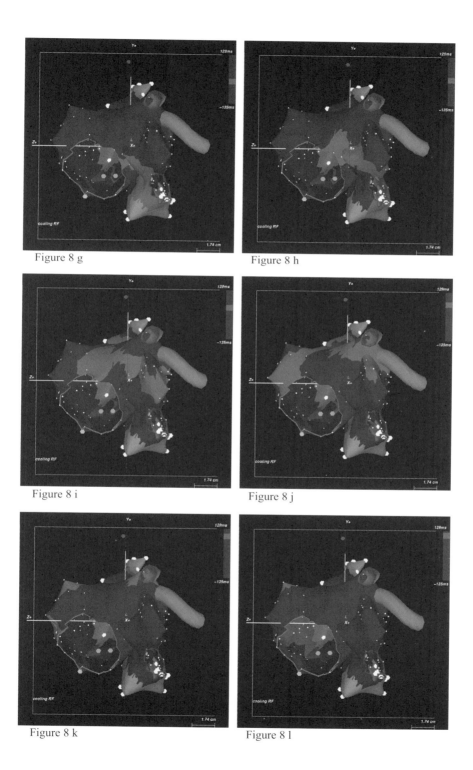

Figure 8 g

Figure 8 h

Figure 8 i

Figure 8 j

Figure 8 k

Figure 8 l

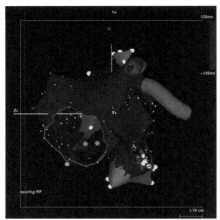

Figure 8 m

8 n surface ECG during tachycardia with a stable 2:1 atrioventricular conduction, next to surface leads, an intraatrial signal from the proximal electrode pair of the mapping catheter is depicted (Map prox 3-4).

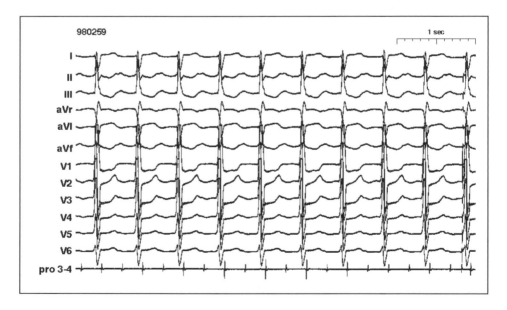

Figure 8 n

4.4 Atrial Reentry Tachycardia in a Patient After Atrial Switch Procedure of the Senning Type Due to d-Transposition of the Great Arteries (Figure 9 and Color Plate 11)

9 a (LAO view) 9 b (posterior anterior view) show reconstruction of the systemic venous atrium in the activation map mode during atrial reentry tachycardia. Red ring depicts mitral annulus, gray ring the tricuspid annulus. Tube display course of pulmonary veins close to the pulmonary venous atrium (not to be seen on this pictures). Blue dots mark areas with splitted local electrograms, orange dot at site of His bundle recording, yellow dots at site of fractionated local electrograms.

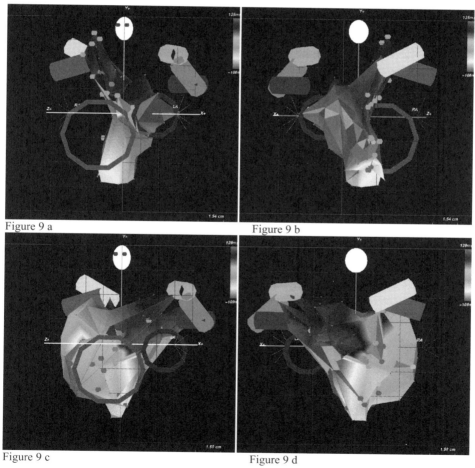

Figure 9 a

Figure 9 b

Figure 9 c

Figure 9 d

9 c (LAO view) 9 d (posterior anterior view) show the pulmonary venous atrium during tachycardia, brown dots mark areas with doubled local signals.

9 e (LAO view) 9 f (posterior anterior view) display both reconstructed atriums while tachycardia. Course of the reentry circuit was similar to the Mustard case (see above), as like the ablation strategy that has been carried out successfully.

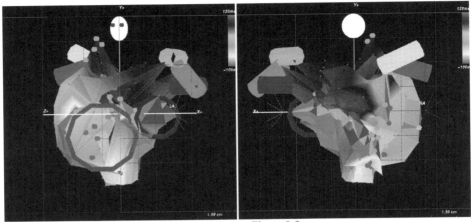

Figure 9 e   Figure 9 f

4.5   Atrial Reentry Tachycardia in a Patient After Fontan Surgery Due to an Atresia of the Tricuspid Annulus (Figure 10)

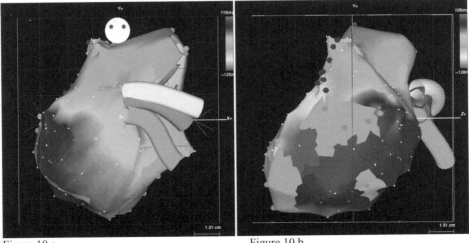

Figure 10 a   Figure 10 b

10 a (AP view) 10 b (right lateral view) show reconstruction of the tachycardia circling around a scar at the lateral free atrial wall utilizing a critical zone additionally confined by a second scar close to the insertion of the inferior caval vein and another zone, confined by the central scar and a third one close to

the connection towards the pulmonary trunk. Green frame depicts connection to the pulmonary trunk, tubes display course of an enormous dilated coronary sinus. Orange dot marks site of reference electrode (transient screw electrode). Dark dots depict the ablation line combining scar area close to pulmonary trunk and central scar area, where successful block of the tachycardia was achieved.

10 c – p (right lateral view, slight dorsal rotation) Propagation map of the tachycardia displaying its course around the central scar at the free lateral wall in a clockwise manner.

For prevention of accidentally cutting off the preferential course of the sinus nodal impulse towards the AV-node, the superior ablation line was chosen, as the position of the sinus node was identified close to the inferior border of the central scar area.

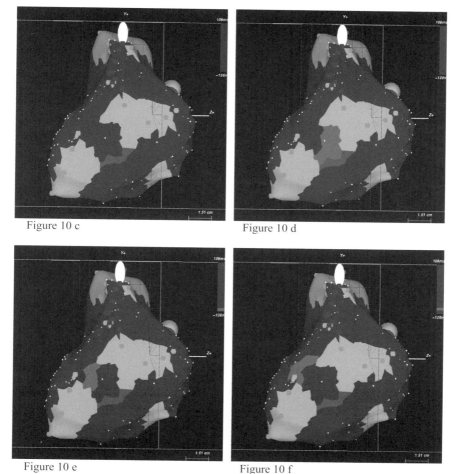

Figure 10 c

Figure 10 d

Figure 10 e

Figure 10 f

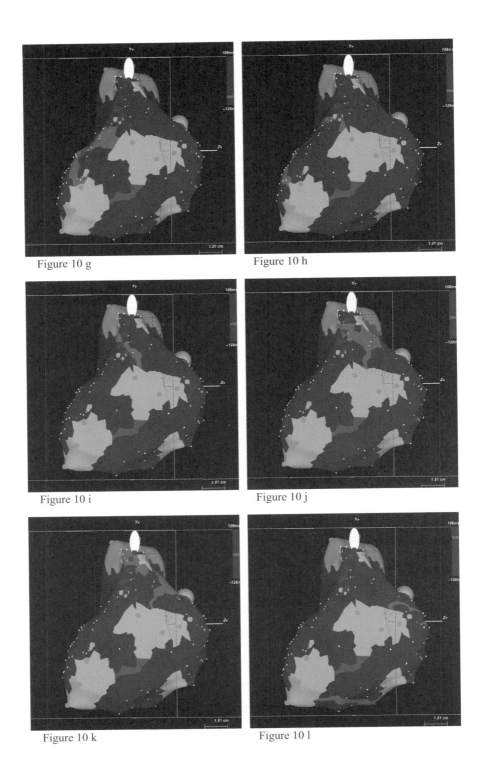

Figure 10 g

Figure 10 h

Figure 10 i

Figure 10 j

Figure 10 k

Figure 10 l

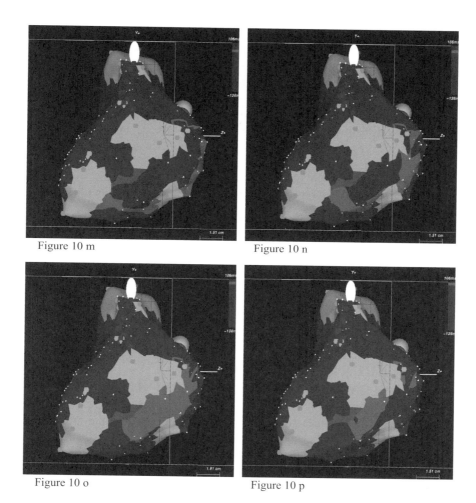

Figure 10 m

Figure 10 n

Figure 10 o

Figure 10 p

5. ADVANTAGES 3-D ELECTROANATOMICAL MAPPING IN PATIENTS WITH POSTOPERATIVE CONGENITAL HEART DISEASE

Since introduction in the field, 3-D electroanatomical reconstruction using CARTO has given us a new insight into the highly variant individual expression of congenital cardiac anomalies, their postoperative anatomy and into their often complex tachycardias. The system provides in a so far unique way visualization of "true" anatomical point by point information, as well as the course of electrical propagation of any regular rhythm, like sinus rhythm, pacing or any stable sustained tachycardia. The implementation of conventional mapping criteria and pacing maneuvers for the identification of potentially vulnerable zones is possible and still crucially required. The topographical relation of such data within the 3-D reconstruction is very helpful in understanding the tachycardias course, its critical zones and potentially successful sites for intervention by radiofrequency current application. The visualization of the complete tachycardia course provides the chance for alternative ablation strategies, if the originally targeted zone carries the risk for damage of essential cardiac structures or if at this zone radiofrequency current application is inefficient due to local difficulties in catheter manipulation or due to tissue related failure in lesion generation. Furthermore the application of such system offers the chance to reduce the procedural fluoroscopy time significantly, but provides a permanent online control of the catheters tip position throughout the procedure, which can be extremely important, if we e.g. think about mapping in patients with mechanical valve replacements.

By the use of such technology, validation concepts can be developed and sufficiently carried out, even for complex ablation strategies in even more complex postoperative cardiac situations. This together with a better understanding of the individual situs provides a high potential for an improvement of the acute success rates and a reduction of a still relatively high recurrence rate reported in this patient cohort.

6. CURRENT LIMITATIONS 3-D ELECTROANATOMICAL MAPPING

Due to the point by point acquisition of the reconstruction and the need for a manual re-annotation of the local electrograms, such procedure can even be in experienced hands time consuming, possibly extending procedure duration up to 8 hours and more for complex hearts or tachycardias. This limitation is even more significant, as by the time, tachycardia cycle length may change and thereby eventually confuses the process in understanding its course.

If the cycle length of the tachycardia is shorter than compared to the maximum activation time of the complete mapped cardiac chamber, activation fronts resulting from the same circuit may appear twice within the window of interest. Such situation might occur in any patients with significant enlargements or conduction delay of the mapped chamber, like e.g. in patients after Fontan surgery. Interpretation of reconstruction under such circumstances is very likely to fail, as no pacing maneuver for clarification can be added at this stage of mapping.

REFERENCES

1. Anderson RH, Becker AE, Arnold R, et al. (1974) The conducting tissues in congenitally corrected transposition. Circulation 50:911-923.
2. Balaji S, Johnson TB, Sade RM, Case RL, Gillette PC, Management of atrial flutter after the Fontan procedure. J Am Coll Cardiol, 1994 Apr, 23:5:1209-1215.
3. Cosio FG, Arribas F, Lopez-Gil M, et al. Radiofrequency ablation of atrial flutter. J Cardiovasc Electrophysiol 1996;760-770.
4. Davies MJ, Anderson RH (1983) The conduction system of the heart. In Davies MJ, Anderson RH (eds): Conduction system in congenital heart disease. London, Butterworths 95-166.
5. Dickinson DF, Wilkinson JL, Smith A, et. al. (1982) Variations in the morphology of the ventricular septal defect and disposition of the atrioventricular conduction tissues in tetralogy of Fallot. Thorac Cardiovasc Surg 30:243-249.
6. Dorostokar PC, Cheng J, Scheinman MM, Electroanatomical mapping and ablation of the substrate supporting intraatrial reentrant tachycardia after surgery for complex congenital heart disease. Pacing Clin Electrophysiol, 1998 Sep, 21:9, 1810-1819.
7. Garson A Jr, Bink-Boelkens M, Heslein PS, et al. (1985) Atrial flutter in the young: a collaborative study of 380 cases. J Am Coll Cardiol 6: 871-878.
8. Gelatt M, Hamilton RM, McCrindle BW, Gow RM, Williams WG, Trusler GA, Freedom RM (1994)Risk factors for atrial tachyarrhythmias after the Fontan operation. J Am Coll Cardiol, 24;7:1735-1741.
9. Gepstein L, Evans SJ: electroanatomical mapping of the heart: basic concepts and implications for the treatment of cardiac arrhythmias. Pacing Clin. Electrophysiol., 1998 June, 21;6:1268-1278.
10. Flinn CJ, Wolff GS, Dick M (1984) Cardiac rhythm after the Mustard operation for complete transposition of the great arteries. N Engl J Med 310:1635-1642.
11. Hebe J. Radiofrequency catheter ablation of tachycardia in patients with congenital heart disease, Ped. Cardiol.
12. Hebe J. Antz M. et al, Radiofrequency current ablation of supraventricular tachycardias in congenital heart disease. Herz 1998;23:231-250
13. Kalman JM, VanHare GF, Olgin JE, Saxon LA, Stark SI, Lesh MD (1996) Ablation of „incisional" reentrant atrial tachycardia complicating surgery for congenital heart disease. Use of entrainment to define a critical isthmus of conduction. Circulation, 93;53:502-512.
14. Kanter R.J., Papagiannis J, Carbory M.P., et al, Radiofrequency catheter ablation of supraventrucular tachycardia substrates after mustard and senning operations for d-transposition of the great arteries. J Am Coll Cardiol 2000 (Feb); 35;2):428-441.
15. Lesh, M.D., Kalman J.M. (1996) To fumble flutter or tackle „tach"? Toward updated classifiers for atrial tachyarrhythmias. J Cardiovasc Electrophysiol, Vol 7, pp 460 - 466, May 1996
16. Lesh MD, Spear JF, Simson M. (1988) A computer model of the electrogram: what causes fractionation? J Electrocardiogr 1988 (suppl): S69-73
17. Nakagawa H, Lazarra H, Khastgir T, et al., Role of the tricuspid annulus and the eustachian valve/ridge on atrial flutter. Relevance to catheter ablation of the septal isthmus and a new technique for rapid identification of ablation success. Circulation 1996;94:407-424.
18. Saul JP, Triedman JK. Radiofrequency ablation of intraatrial reentrant tachycardia after surgery for congenital heart disease. Pacing Clin Electrophysiol, 1997 Aug, 20 (8 Pt 2) 2112-2117.
19. Thiene G, Wenink AC, Frescura C, et. al. (1981) Surgical anatomy and pathology of the conduction tissues in atrioventricular defects. J Thorac Cardiovasc Surg 82: 928-937.
20. Triedman JK, Saul JP, Weindling SN, Walsh EP (1995) Radiofrequency ablation of intra-atrial reentrant tachycardia after surgical palliation of congenital heart disease. Circulation, 91; 3:707-714.

21. Triedman JK, Bergau DM, Saul JP, Epstein MR, Walsh EP. Efficacy of radiofrequency ablation for control of intraatrial reentrant tachycardias in patients with congenital heart disease. J Am Coll Cardiol, 1997 Oct, 30;4:1032-1038.
22. Triedmann JK, Jenkins KJ, Colan SD, Saul JP, Walsh EP (1997) Intra-atrial reentrant tachycardia after palliation of congenital heart disease: characterization of multiple macroreentrant circuits using fluoroscopically based three-dimensional endocardial mapping. J Cardiovasc Electrophysiol, 8; 3: 259-270.
23. Van Hare GF, Lesh MD, Stanger P (1993) Radiofrequency catheter ablation of supraventricular arrhythmias in patients with congenital heart disease: results and technical considerations. J Am Coll Cardiol, 22;3:883-890.

Chapter 13

ENDOCARDIAL MAPPING USING REAL TIME THREE DIMENSIONAL ULTRASOUND-RANGING TRACKING SYSTEM
Results of In-Vitro, In-Vivo, and Clinical Studies

L. Bing Liem, N. Parker Willis
Cardiac Arrhythmia and Electrophysiology, Stanford University, Stanford, CA and Cardiac Pathways Corporation, Sunnyvale, CA, USA

INTRODUCTION

Mapping during a catheter ablation procedure is needed for a variety of reasons. The main objective is the visualization of catheter position at a particular time. Such a static identification of catheter location can be achieved with standard fluoroscopy coupled with the information obtained from the intracardiac electrical signal. In the performance of a more complex ablation, such as the creation of a large or linear lesion, additional information would be needed. To facilitate the formation of contiguous ablations and to minimize overlapping of lesions, the mapping procedure would have to include identification of previous catheter tip locations. Furthermore, to guide the direction of the proposed lesion, the mapping data should ideally provide other cardiac landmarks. Also of great importance, the data should be available almost instantly because catheter positioning is frequently not stable.

Various new mapping techniques were recently made available. Some, such as the basket recording system offers simultaneous multiple recordings but still relies on fluoroscopy for its placement.[1] Others utilize electromagnetic field to assist localization or computer-assisted acquisition without contact with the endocardium.[2-7] The system, discussed in this chapter, offers a combination of features that are intended to assist catheter positioning, and navigation to previous sites in three-dimensions with minimal usage of fluoroscopy. The utility of this system has been assessed in pre-clinical, animal experiments as well as clinical studies. Data from these studies will be reviewed.

L. Bing Liem and E. Downar (eds.), Progress in Catheter Ablation, 187-202.

1.   TECHNICAL COMPONENTS

The ultrasound-ranging tracking system, Realtime Position Management (RPM®, Cardiac Pathways Corporation, Sunnyvale, CA) is a multi-component system that integrates ultrasound-based catheter position data with electrocardiograms from intracardiac and body-surface recordings.

The system consists of two modules, the position acquisition module (PAM) and signal acquisition module (SAM) that are integrated with a workstation computer equipped with graphical monitors (Figure 1).

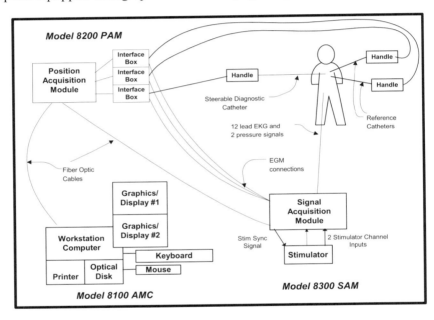

Figure 1. The above diagram illustrates the method of data acquisition and integration of the RPM whereby electrogram signals and position data are processed by the respective modules (SAM and PAM) and stored into the workstation computer for display and recall. The signal acquisition module can interface with a stimulator.

The PAM acquires data used to compute catheter positions, utilizing ultrasound-ranging to measure the distance between transducers mounted on specialized electrophysiologic (EP) catheters. The distance data is transferred to the workstation computer and processed to determine the three-dimensional position of the catheters.

The SAM acquires electrocardiogram data, including a 12-lead surface ECG, up to 48 catheter signals, and a pressure signal. In addition a stimulator can be integrated with the SAM to route pacing to catheter electrodes.

Thus, electrogram signals and ultrasound ranging data from specialized EP catheters are processed simultaneously but separately at the Signal Acquisition Module (SAM) and Position Acquisition Module (PAM) respectively. All data are synchronized and then processed through a workstation computer and displayed on graphical monitors.

Two specialized EP catheters form a stationary reference frame. These catheters are placed within the coronary sinus (CS) and at the right ventricular (RV) apex. These catheters are then used to track the position of other specialized EP catheters used for mapping or ablation.

Each of the reference catheters is 7F in size with a curved 6F tip, incorporating four ultrasound transducers in addition to conventional ring electrodes. The ultrasound transducers on the CS reference catheter are positioned to encompass the standard span of a decapolar electrode configuration. The transducers on the RV reference catheter are positioned to cover the distance from the mid right atrium to the RV apex (Figure 2).

The ablation catheter is a 7F catheter equipped with three ultrasonic transducers, three electrodes, a 4-mm tip, temperature sensing, and lumens for the delivery of cooled radiofrequency energy (Chilli®, Cardiac Pathways Corporation, Sunnyvale, CA). Two of the transducers are positioned on the distal tip providing the position of recording electrodes and the ablation tip. The third transducer is proximal to the catheter curve (Figure 3).

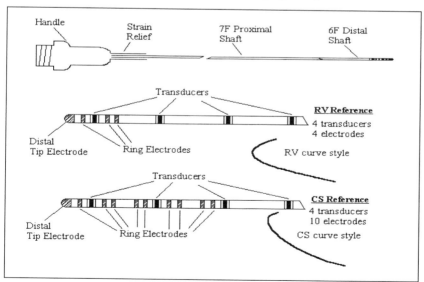

Figure 2. This diagram illustrates the relative positions of the standard ring electrodes and ultrasonic transducers in the right ventricular (RV, top) and coronary sinus (CS, bottom) reference catheters

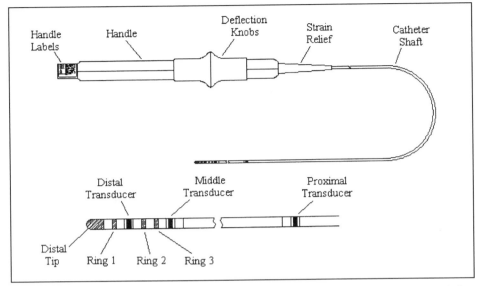

Figure 3. This diagram illustrates the typical ablation catheter with standard 4-mm tip and ring electrodes as well as ultrasonic transducers placed to provide positions of the distal electrodes and catheter curve.

The position acquisition module (PAM) transmits and receives ultrasound pulses between catheter transducers, measuring the time delays between the transmit and receive pulses. The time delays are directly proportional[1] to the distances between the transmitter and receiver (Figure 4).

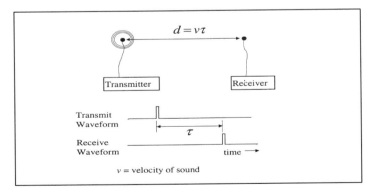

Figure 4. Distance (d) is estimated based on the above simple formula

---

[1] This is only true for medium with a constant velocity of sound. The relevant velocities for this application are blood = 1.57mm/usec and cardiac tissue = 1.58mm/usec.

A continuous cycle of transmit pulses is sent in a round-robin fashion to each of the reference catheter transducers, resulting in a matrix of distance data. The computer uses these data to triangulate the three-dimensional coordinates of the transducers. The transducer coordinates are then used to reconstruct a three-dimensional graphical representation of catheter positions and orientation (Figure 5).

Catheter position graphics are gated to the electrocardiography (ECG) or intracardiac electrogram to filter heart movement artifacts. One of the catheters in the graphical display can be selected for displaying a real time tip. This utilizes a graphical circle with a disappearing tail to indicate tip movement, providing motion information to assess wall contact and feedback during catheter navigation.

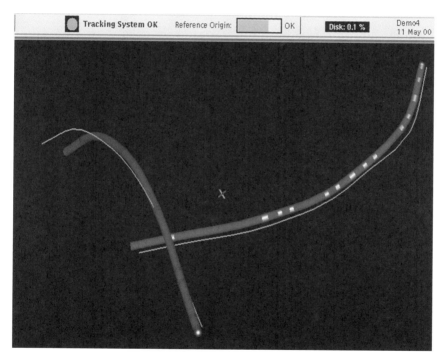

Figure 5. The computerized display of the two reference catheters (the right ventricular and coronary sinus catheters) are shown above in an orientation that is similar to the left anterior oblique view. The ultrasound transducers are widely separated while the recording electrodes are positioned in the standard configuration. The green lines indicate the original position of the reference catheters (see also Figure 14).

The system also continuously monitors the position of the reference catheters relative to their initial placement, providing a warning mechanism and feedback for repositioning if the reference catheters shift. In Figure 5, the initial reference catheter placement is indicated by the green lines and the reference origin gauge at the top of the figure measures how closely this reference position matches the initial position.

Adjustment of the three-dimensional graphic can be done to provide standard right and left anterior oblique (RAO and LAO) views as well as cranial or caudal orientations.

Text can also be added to the display at the location of any catheter tip or recording electrode, providing a method for labelling anatomical locations, and mapping and ablation sites. Electrocardiogram and position data are synchronised and stored together, allowing recall of catheter positions from recorded signal data. This provides a convenient mechanism for returning to previously mapped sites.

2.   IN VITRO DATA

The accuracy of the system was tested in-vitro using a test jig with six holes arranged in a rectangular grid. The catheter tip was positioned in each of six holes of the test jig while the RPM® system marked the position of the catheter. This cycle was repeated 5 times. The 30 data points, consisting of 6 clusters with 5 points each (Figure 6), were analyzed for accuracy and precision of targeting the catheters. This test showed a mean error, defined by the average radius of each cluster, of 0.47 mm.

A relative distance error was defined as the difference between two points reported by the system and the exact distance between the corresponding holes of the test jig. The test showed that the system has a precision of 0.8 mm and an accuracy of 1.0 mm.

3.   IN VIVO DATA

Three methods of in-vivo testing were performed. The first, simple method was comparing the actual distance between distal transducers on ablation catheter with distance reported by RPM system. This test showed a mean error of 0.47 mm.

The second test was performed by computation of equivalent radius of point cluster created by recording the ablation catheter tip position for at least 20 cardiac cycles (Figure 7). The result showed an average radius of 1.5 mm.

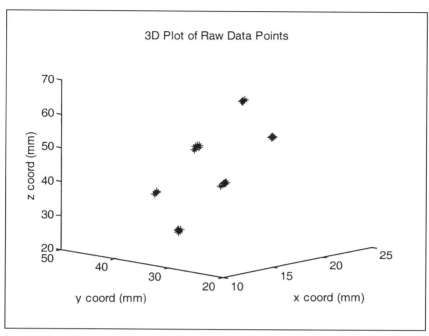

Figure 6. This figure shows clusters of position data produced by repositioning the catheter tip in a six-hole test jig.

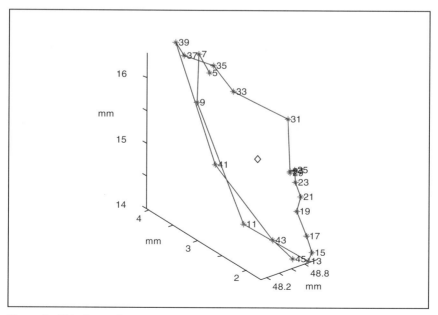

Figure 7. This figure shows an example of the computation of radius of the point cluster of an ablation catheter tip recorded for several cardiac cycles.

The utility of the RPM system was tested against histology data in animals. The study was performed to test the accuracy of the system in identifying predetermined sites and its ability to guide the operator to position and reposition the ablation catheter to those sites without using fluoroscopy.

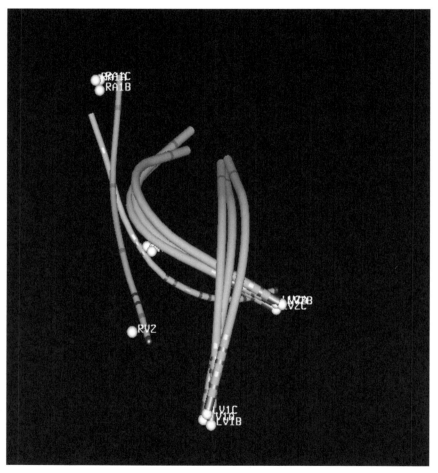

Figure 8. This figure shows the final positions of the catheter tip as a result of the three attempts at repositioning at the two pre-determined left ventricular sites (LV1 and LV2, respectively). The position display is in the LAO view.

The animals (four pigs) were instrumented in the standard fashion for catheterization. The reference catheters were positioned to the right ventricular apex and coronary sinus, respectively using fluoroscopy. The ablation catheter (equipped with ultrasound transducers) was advanced to the selected sites also using fluoroscopy at first. The ablation catheter was positioned to two right atrial and two left ventricular sites, respectively, and the positions of these sites were recorded and stored. Afterwards, using only the RPM system, the ablation catheter was repositioned to those pre-identified sites three times and ablation applied using radiofrequency energy. The operator was to attempt to reposition the ablation catheter as closely as possible to the pre-determined sites (Figure 8). Ablations were then applied at the best positions. The final positions were then stored and compared with histological data after the animals were sacrificed.

The ablation catheter could be maneuvered within the cardiac chamber, without fluoroscopy, to the ablation sites without difficulty. As shown in Figure 8, the tip, electrodes and curvature of the reference catheters and the ablation catheter could be visualized such that the approach to the desired sites can be replicated. The display of catheter curvature also facilitated catheter manipulation in and out the cardiac chambers.

In the event of reference catheter displacement, the ability to recall its original position allows for repositioning. This feature may prove to be useful during mapping. In the case of electroanatomical mapping with the CARTO system, displacement of reference catheter may result in inability to complete mapping and necessity in repeating the procedure after repositioning.

In most cases, superimposed positioning recorded by the RPM data was confirmed histology, showing single lesions both by gross examination and sectional views (Table 1, Figures 9 and 10). In some instances, coalescing lesions were found on histology (Figure 11).

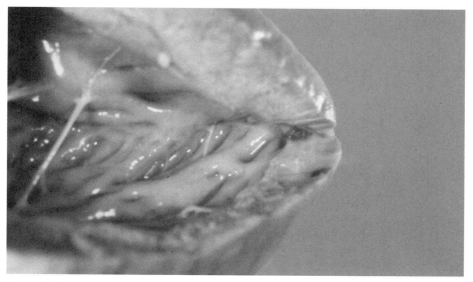

Figure 9. Shown above is the single lesion in the LV apex resulting from three superimposed ablations performed by repositioning the Clili® catheter using the RPM system.

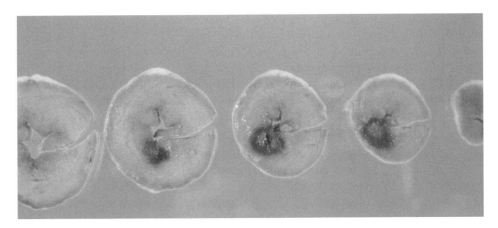

Figure 10. Cross sections of the lesion shown in Figure 9

In the event that the catheter could not be repositioned to the previously marked site, a coalescing lesion would result, as shown in Figure 11 below. In the in-vivo experiment, the inability to reposition the catheter tip to the desired position was caused by mechanical issues unrelated to the mapping system performance. Indeed we believe that such circumstances may occur in clinical setting, such as at a location at or near trabeculated endocardium.

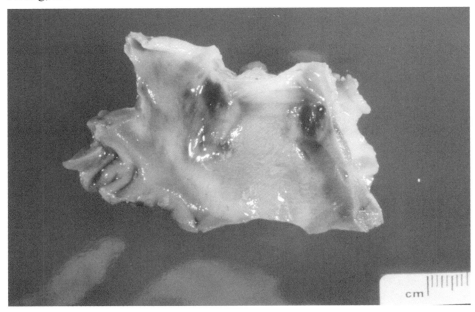

Figure 11. In this experiment (study #1), the series of ablations in the right atrium (RA1 and RA2) resulted in coalescing but separate lesions at the RA1 site and contiguous lesions at RA2 site. These non-superimposed lesions, however, were predicted by positioning data from the RPM (Figure 12).

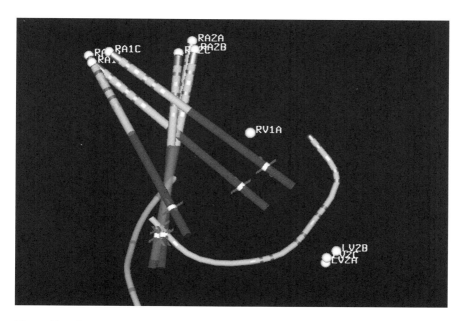

Figure 12. The RPM positioning data of study #1, where the ablations resulted in separate lesions (Figure 13).

The RPM positioning data were derived from measurement during acquisition. Repositioned sites that were more than 0.5 cm apart from the prior site were considered to be "separate" while those that were closer than 0.5 cm from each other were regarded as "superimposed." Similarly, identification of "separate" ablation sites was made if there were distinct lesions, usually with separation of the nidi by more than 1 cm apart. Those with no distinct healthy myocardium in between were labelled "coalescing", usually with nidi separation of 0.5 to 1.0 cm. Those with nidi separation of less than 0.5 cm apart were considered as "overlapping" lesions (Figure 13). Those with only single nidus were annotated as "single lesion."

The results listed in Table 1 showed that the estimate made based on the RPM closely predicted the histology except for the second LV site of study # 4, which produced two distinct lesions separated by 1.3 cm distance. Of note, the overall lesion dimensions were large, with a diameter of 1.0 cm on the average with single lesion and 1.5 cm for overlapping lesions. However, although most lesions were transmural, there was no cardiac perforation noted. It thus appears that multiple lesion generation can create lesions with broader dimension without risking over penetration.

Table 1

Study	Site	RPM Data	Histology Data	Lesion Dimension
Study 1	RA1	2 separate sites	3 coalescing lesions (separated by 0.7-0.9 cm)	1.7 x 1.6 cm (total)
	RA2	2 separate sites	overlapping lesions	0.9 x 0.8 cm
	LV1	separate sites	2 overlapping lesions	1.5 x 1.1 cm
	LV2	superimposed	1 large lesion	1.2 x 0.8 cm
Study 2	RA1	superimposed	2 overlapping lesion	1.9 x 1.0 cm
	RA2	superimposed	1 lesion	0.7 x 0.5 cm
	LV1	superimposed	1 lesion	0.9 x 0.7 cm
	LV 2	superimposed	1 lesion	0.9 x 0.7 cm
Study 3	RA1	superimposed	coalescing lesions (separated by 0.5 – 0.8 cm)	1.5 x 1.1 cm
	RA2	superimposed	1 lesion	1.0 x 0.5 cm
	LV1	superimposed	2 overlapping lesions	0.5 x 1.6 cm
	LV2	superimposed	2 separate lesions (separated by 1.3 cm)	1.0 x 0.8 cm 1.0 x 0.3 cm
Study 4	RA1	superimposed	3 overlapping lesions	1.0 x 0.5 cm
	RA2	superimposed	1 lesion	1.0 x 0.8 cm
	LV1	superimposed	1 lesion	1.2 x 1.1 cm
	LV2	superimposed	1 lesion	1.4 x 0.9 cm

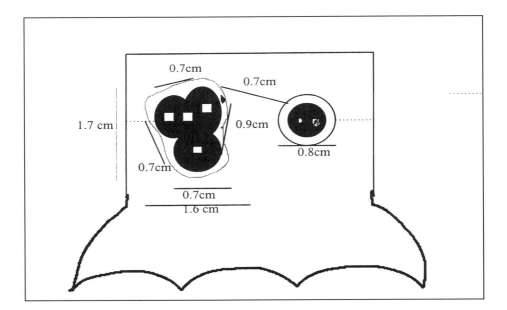

Figure 13. The above figure illustrates the two types of lesions in the first experiment within the right atrium. The nidi of lesions on RA1 could be identified separately but the total area of the lesions coalesced with one another with nidi separation of 0.7 – 0.9 cm. Lesions at RA2 also have separate nidi but the lesions overlap each other.

4. CLINICAL DATA

Recently, de Groot et al.[8] reported the utility of the system in patients. The system was utilized in 30 patients undergoing catheter ablative therapy for atrial flutter (10 patients), ventricular tachycardia (VT, 15 patients) or accessory pathway (AP) arrhythmia (5 patients). One reference catheter was positioned at either the right atrium or CS while the second at the RV apex. In general, the study assessed the utility of the system in facilitating mapping and ablation and in reducing fluoroscopy exposure. In particular, the study assessed the relative stability of the reference catheters and the possibility of navigating to a previously marked site.

The investigators found that the reference catheters did not hinder positioning of other catheter and that although there were some ultrasonic transducer failures, mapping was completed in all cases. The fluoroscopy time was 10 ± 3 minutes for atrial flutter, 17 ± 8 for VT, and 8 ± 3 for AP cases. The mean displacement distances for the RV reference catheter ranged from 2.1 ± 1.6 mm for AP ablation to 6.1 ± 4.1 mm for VT (Figure 14). The RA reference catheter was displaced by as little as 1.2 ± 0.6 mm during AP ablation to as much as 6.0 ± 1.5 mm during flutter ablation.

The ability to recall original catheter positions, which would allow such a comparison, is also an advantage of this mapping system. If displaced, the reference catheter can be repositioned to the original configuration (Figures 5 & 14) and hence, acquisition of mapping sites does not need to be repeated.

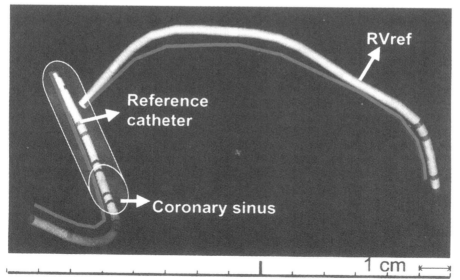

Figure 14. Reference catheter positions, current and original (green line) are displayed, allowing repositioning, if necessary.

The investigators also assessed the utility of navigation to a previously marked site. Such a feature is particularly useful for identifying an optimal point in a complex ablation procedure such as for postmyocardial infarction VT. The investigators showed several examples of the utility of such a feature in this case. Thus, for example, sites with mid diastolic potentials can be identified and simultaneously displayed, allowing for identification of the region for an encircling ablation (Figure 15). Ablation for VT was successful in 9 of 12 of postmyocardial infarction VT and in 3 of 3 of VT in patients with right ventricular dysplasia. Although there was no mention of comparison with their usual success rate and whether or not the navigation system was instrumental in their ability to ablate such complex VT, these results are very promising.

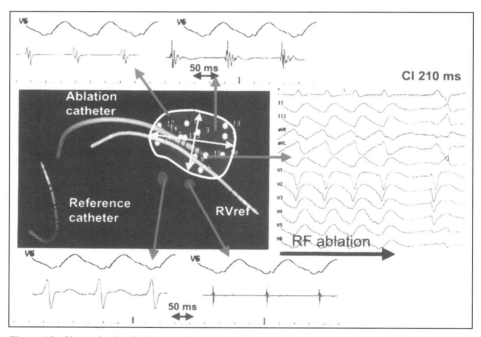

Figure 15. Shown in the display are the positions of reference catheters and sites with mid diastolic potentials. Ablation was performed around these sites.

The investigators concluded that while the accuracy of mapping still depends on stability of reference catheters, which can be displaced or dislodged, especially after DC cardioversion, the ability to recall original position(s) facilitates completion of mapping, unlike the case with other systems. In terms of the usefulness of the system for navigation, the investigators found that they were able to navigate back to previously marked sites with an accuracy of ± 2 mm, which, in their opinion, is comparable to the results obtained with CARTO and LocaLisa systems.[2-4,9] The investigators also believe that the use of the

RPM® will result in reduction of fluoroscopy, as shown in the short fluoroscopy usage in the clinical application of the system.

SUMMARY

The RPM system enables catheter positioning to a predetermined site without the use of fluoroscopy with good accuracy. The in-vivo experiment, which was designed to assess the practicality of the system and its accuracy in predicting lesion position, resulted, at times, in overlapping lesions because the catheter could not be repositioned exactly to the original location. However, such imprecision was confirmed by histology in most cases. Thus, the accuracy of the system is, in general, quite good. Incidentally, we learned that in the case of overlapping lesions, a large ablation surface was created, while in the case of single, superimposed lesions, the total depth of ablation appeared to be safe.

This form of mapping with tracking capability can be used to create large lesions if desired. With the availability of catheter curvature display, catheter maneuvering is likely to be intuitive and similar to that using fluoroscopy. Similarly, visual display of reference catheter positions would facilitate repositioning in the event of reference catheter movement. Finally, the availability of cardiac contour that could be generated by this system may further aid catheter positioning as it would assist the operator with the estimate distance between the mapping catheter and the wall of the cardiac chambers.

The disadvantage of this system is similar to the Biosense mapping system in that mapping of tachycardia requires positioning of the catheter to multiple locations and can therefore only be performed during a sustained form of tachyarrhythmia. Another disadvantage is the dependence of the reference catheters to provide a stable reference frame for position information. The system, however, alerts the operator of such an event and provides a method for repositioning the reference catheters to their initial position.

REFERENCES

1. Downar E, Parson ID, Yao L, Cameron DA, and Waxman MB: Endocardial catheter mapping of unstable and pleomorphic ventricular tachycardias. Circulation 1984;70(suppl II):1488.
2. Ben-Haim S, Gepstein L, Hayam G, Ben-David J, Josephson M. A new electro-anatomical mapping system. Pacing Clin Electrophysiol 1996;19(Pt 2)4:709-711.
3. Gepstein L, Hayam G, Ben-Haim SA. A novel method for nonfluoroscopic catheter-based electroanatomical mapping of the heart: In vitro and in vivo accuracy results. Circulation 1997;95:1611-1622.
4. Shpun S, Gepstein L, Hayam G, Ben-Haim SA. Guidance of radiofrequency endocardial ablation with real-time three-dimensional magnetic navigation system. Circulation 1997;96:2016-2021.

5. Marchlinski FE, Callans DJ, Gottlieb CD, Zado E. Linear ablation lesions for control of unmappable ventricular tachycardia in patients with ischemic and nonischemic cardiomyopathy. Circulation 2000;101:1288-1296.
6. Schilling RJ, Peters NS, Davies WD. Simultaneous endocardial mapping in the human left ventricle using a noncontact catheter comparison of contact and reconstructed electrograms during sinus rhythm. Circulation 1998;98:887-898.
7. Gornick CC, Adler SW, Pederson B, Hauck J, Budd J, Schweitzer J. Validation of a new noncontact catheter system for electroanatomical mapping of left ventricular endocardium. Circulation 1999;99:829-835.
8. De Groot NMS, Bootsma M, Van Der Velde ET, Schalij MJ. Three-dimensional catheter positioning during radiofrequency ablation in patients: First application of a real-time position management system. J Cardiovasc Electophysiol 2000;11:1183-1192.
9. Wittkampf FHM, Wever EFD, Derksen R, Wilde AM, Ramanna H, Hauer RNW, Robles de Medina EO. LocaLisa: New technique for real-time three-dimensional localization of regular intracardiac electrodes. Circulation 1999;99:1312-1317.

Chapter 14

ENDOCARDIAL CONTACT MAPPING USING MULTIPOLAR BASKET ELECTRODE CATHETERS

Eugene Downar, Stéphane Massé, Elias Sevaptsidis, Mei-Hao Shi, Menashe B. Waxman.

Toronto General Hospital, University Health Network Toronto, Ontario, Canada

INTRODUCTION

The most commonly used method for cardiac mapping has changed little in principle from that developed by early pioneers almost a century ago. A single exploring electrode collects temporal data over an imaginary spatial grid projected onto a surface of the heart. Local activation times, referenced to the surface ECG are then collected sequentially over a time period that may measure ten minutes or more. A further ten to fifteen minutes may be required to collate the temporal data so as to produce a stereotypical isochronal map of activation. This process is predicated on the sequence of activation being precisely reproduced with each heart beat throughout the mapping procedure. When this process is applied to ventricular tachycardias, a major limitation is that the tachycardia must be sustained, without change or hemodynamic compromise for the duration of the mapping period. In practice this means that tachy-arrhythmias that fluctuate in morphology or cycle length and those that are unstable hemodynamically, can not be adequately mapped by a roving catheter.

One approach to try and overcome these limitations has been to develop multi-electrode arrays that allow recordings of a large number of local electrograms to be made simultaneously. Endocardial activation maps can then be obtained for each cardiac cycle on a beat-by-beat basis. With appropriate computer processing it is even possible to provide an on-line display of activation in real time. Such mapping systems were initially developed for the intraoperative environment and were used with great success for guiding surgical ablation. Multi-electrode arrays were mounted on a pre-shaped balloon that upon inflation would mold and adapt fairly accurately to the shape of the endocardial

203

L. Bing Liem and E. Downar (eds.), Progress in Catheter Ablation, 203-223.
© 2001 *Kluwer Academic Publishers. Printed in the Netherlands.*

chamber being mapped. Such balloon arrays obliterate the cardiac chamber and can only be used during cardiopulmonary bypass. They can not be used as a percutaneous technique without circulatory assist.

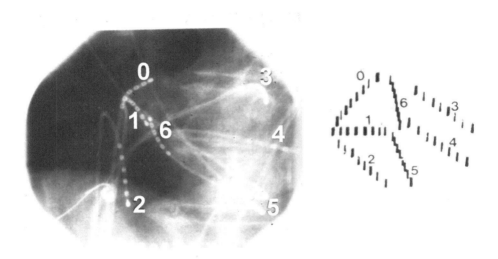

Figure 1. An early attempt at on-line multipolar catheter mapping. Left panel shows a fluoroscopic image of seven separate hexapolar catheters. These were positioned to conform with the standardized configuration shown on the right and displayed as a video image. Activation at each electrode was determined by an algorithm which lit up the appropriate electrode on the video display.

In an early attempt[1] to achieve online beat-by-beat catheter mapping of biventricular endocardial activation, we utilized an array of seven separate octapolar (or hexapolar) catheters deployed in a standardized fashion (Figure 1). Three catheters were positioned in the right ventricle to monitor the basal inflow, mid ventricular septum to apex and the right ventricular outflow tract regions. Two catheters were introduced by transeptal sheaths to monitor the left ventricular inflow and lateral regions. Finally, another two catheters were passed retrogradely to monitor the left ventricle septal and apical regions. This approach provided some measure of success. Maintaining each catheter in its designated position, however, especially throughout the transition of rhythm from sinus to ventricular tachycardia and cardioversion back to sinus proved to be challenging. One solution to maintaining several catheters in a stable array was to tether their distal and proximal ends into a fixed geometry reminiscent of an eggbeater. The resulting basket catheter had the advantages of a reliable spatially fixed multi-electrode array that could be deployed through a single percutanous portal. Although the first prototype of a basket catheter[2] was first tried in the early 80's, clinically acceptable versions did not appear until a decade later.

At the present time three versions are available for clinical use. All three are similar in principle in that the basket comprises up to eight longitudinal struts each carrying up to eight electrodes for a maximum of 64 electrodes. The electrodes can be distributed as four bipolar pairs or at even intervals along the strut for unipolar recordings. Our own observations have been primarily with the EPT Constellation™ 64 electrode catheter with electrodes evenly spaced (Figure 2).

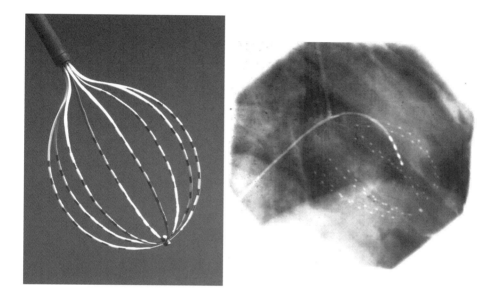

Figure 2. Left panel shows the 64 electrode basket catheter. Right panel is a fluoroscopic image of the catheter positioned in the left ventricle in 30° RAO.

TABLE 1. Advantages of Electrode Array Mapping vs. Roving Electrode

Electrode Array	Single Electrode
- Simultaneous recordings	- Sequential recordings
- No need for collation	- Collation
- Self-referencing spatial grid	- Reference grid difficult to establish
- Whole grid is covered if basket is fully deployed	- Difficult to access whole grid
- Beat by beat mapping:	- Beat by beat mapping impossible therefore:
1) Does not require stability in activation therefore can map polymorphic tachycardias	1) Requires stability in activation sequence
2) Can map hemodynamically unstable arrhythmias	2) Requires hemodynamic stability
3) Multiple morphologies can be mapped expeditiously	3) Time consuming especially with multiple morphologies
- Provides spatial reference for roving/ablation catheter	

With such a basket catheter our experience has been that the theoretical advantages of mapping with a multipolar array over a roving catheter are easy to realize in practice. Table 1 itemizes these advantages.

The success of the basket array, however, does not mark the demise of traditional catheter mapping which is still the technique of choice for mapping many common arrhythmias such as those of the preexcitation syndromes and AV nodal reentrant tachycardia. Furthermore there are also very real technical limitations which pose restrictions to the applicability of basket mapping. These are itemized in Table 2 and should be carefully considered before using the catheter. The diagnostic category of an arrhythmia is also something that should be taken into consideration. In general arrhythmias that are best suited for basket mapping are those with large diffuse macro entrant substrates or those that are more focal in origin but occur in diffuse disease processes such as the cardiomyopathies.

TABLE 2. Limitations of Basket Catheter Mapping

- Fixed Geometry not ideal for all anatomic chambers.
- Needs proper sizing
       Too large a basket causes collapse or distortion.
       Too small causes minimal electrode contact.
- Limited to single chamber
       Does not provide global mapping.
       Difficult to move from chamber to chamber.
- As with all endocardial mapping cannot identify deep intramural or epicardial targets.
- Electrode distribution/spatial resolution fixed.
       Electrode wastage on passive region of little interest.
       Need for asymmetrical electrode arrays.
- Difficult to identify specific electrodes fluoroscopically.
- Potential for snaring/catheter entanglement
- Potential for thrombus formation.
- Potential for mural thrombus dislodgment.
- Need for full anticoagulation.
- Requires 11F - 12F introducing sheath - therefore potentially traumatic for diseased arteries.
- Left ventricular mapping requires two retrograde catheters +/- transseptal catheters (one for mapping and one for ablation).
- Need for computer assisted interpretation / activation display.
- Expense.

Suitable arrhythmias are indicated in Table 3 and include those of atrial as well as ventricular origins. Indications for basket mapping arrhythmias with a recognized anatomic substrate such as bundle branch reentry and fascicular ventricular tachy-arrhythmias are less clear.

TABLE 3. Arrhythmias Suitable for Basket Mapping

- Ventricular Tachycardias in the setting of:
        Chronic ischemic heart disease
        Dilated Cardiomyopathy
        Right Ventricular Dysplasia
        Idiopathic Right Ventricular Arrhythmias
        Tetralogy of Fallot Repair
        VSD Repair
- Supraventricular Tachycardias:
        Refractory Typical Atrial Flutter
        Atypical Atrial Flutter
        Incisional Atrial Reentry
        ? Ectopic Focal Atrial Tachycardia
        ? Atrial Fibrillation

1.   TECHNIQUE

After determining that a tachycardia is suitable for basket mapping the next stage is to determine which cardiac chamber is the most likely to enclose the ablation target. The ECG morphology of the tachycardia, history and location of previous cardiac surgery or myocardial infarction and specific disease processes such as right ventricular dysplasia may all be useful in this determination. In instances where ECG morphology is absent or suggests a ventricular septal origin, a preliminary EP study may be necessary for a "scout" mapping with a conventional exploring catheter to identify the appropriate cardiac chamber. Such a study also serves to establish that the arrhythmia is indeed inducible and determine the required stimulation protocol for its induction.

Once the appropriate cardiac chamber has been identified it is important to select the right size of basket catheter for that chamber. Too large a basket fails to unfold correctly and may even torque into a complex cross-over of struts that defy identification of electrode position, thwarting any attempt at mapping. Too small a basket will greatly reduce the number of electrodes making endocardial contact as well as being unstable in position. Both factors defeat the purpose of multi-electrode array mapping. An echocardiogram is essential to obtain accurate measurements of the chamber to be mapped. The basket nearest in size is then selected from a choice of five options ranging from 38-94 mm. In general it is better to select a basket slightly smaller than one too large.

A choice also has to be made regarding electrode spacing. As mentioned earlier each strut has eight electrodes that can be evenly spaced or arranged in four bipolar pairs. The latter disposition generates a total of 32 bipolar signals, which in our estimation provides an inadequate spatial resolution. We have always used the evenly spaced configuration from which we record 64 unipolar electrograms as well 56 bipolar electrograms derived in a sequential chain from electrodes 1-2, 2-3, 3-4, etc. In this way we are able to improve the spatial resolution while maintaining the advantage of recording high gain bipolar electrodes down to a 50-100 μV range for enhanced detection of diastolic potentials. By simultaneously recording 64 unipolar signals through a separate bank of amplifiers we tried to ensure that useful timing data can be obtained even from electrodes that do not maintain contact with the endocardial surface.

Introduction of a basket catheter into any chamber of the heart can only be achieved through a guiding sheath since the basket is not itself steerable. These sheaths are precurved to angles varying from 15-120 degrees to facilitate entry of a basket into the target chamber. Correct positioning of the tip of the guiding sheath is extremely important. Because the basket is too floppy to be advanced when fully unsheathed and because the tip of the basket is rigidly stiff and thus potentially injurious when protruded from the sheath, the basket is deployed by withdrawal of the sheath back from over the collapsed struts. In practice this requires that the tip of the sheath first has to be maneuvered (over a guide wire and guiding catheter) to where the distal end of the basket is to be delivered. Whereas in right atrial mapping this is relatively straightforward, in left ventricular mapping it may be more challenging. At present the latter procedure is usually achieved by a retrograde approach in which it is essential to ensure the sheath has crossed the aortic valve and sits close to the left ventricular apex before delivering the basket. To ensure smooth entry of the guiding sheath it is passed into the femoral artery through a 12 French short introducing sheath.

Care must also be taken to avoid air and thrombus embolization. The basket catheter is introduced into the diaphragm of the guiding sheath while immersed in a kidney dish of saline, after thoroughly wetting the struts of the basket and ensuring that no air bubbles are entrapped in the collapsed struts. The guiding sheath is slowly perfused with heparinized saline. Although the basket has a heparin coat, once it has been satisfactorily positioned additional heparin is given to maintain the Activated Clothing Time (ACT) above 300 seconds throughout the procedure. Generally the duration of basket mapping is restricted to two hours. Repositioning of the basket catheter is performed by first advancing the sheath to cover the struts, redirecting the sheath, then uncovering the basket by sheath withdrawal.

At the end of the mapping the sheath is again advanced over the basket and only then is the basket withdrawn. This sequence also serves to minimize the likelihood of entrapment of other catheters or chordae tendinae.

Once the basket is in position the quality of local electrogram recordings is checked and gains optimized. Provided that sufficient care is taken in sizing and positioning of the basket, good quality electrograms can be obtained consistently from 85% - 95% of the electrodes.[3-4] After these signals have been optimized the tachycardia can be induced and the endocardial mapping begins. Identification of the earliest electrograms is simple in unifocal tachycardias and can be done by scanning each spline as though it were a discreet octapolar catheter. Unless a 64 channel recording system is available, it may be necessary to make two or more separate recordings during the tachycardia and collate these through a common reference signal. This of course may to some extent diminish the value of basket mapping. Having obtained all 64 electrograms, directly or by collation, a further problem may be interpretation of complex activation sequences. This may be especially true in macro-reentrant circuits. Interpretation is greatly enhanced by an automatic computer mapping system, which unfortunately up till now has only been available in centers with custom-built systems. Potential targets for ablation are identified by conventional criteria including earliest site of activation, a coherent activation map exhibiting sequential spatial-temporal excitation, pace-mapping and functional tests for concealed reentry. All of this can be achieved with the basket electrodes alone.

Identification of target electrode is facilitated by specific markers on the different struts that can be identified by fluoroscoping in multiple obliquities. Since the basket catheter electrodes can not deliver RF energy, a conventional steerable ablation catheter also has to be advanced into the chamber being mapped. In the case of the left ventricle the ablation catheter is usually passed retrogradely from the contralateral femoral artery.

This ablation catheter is also used to further explore the electrograms between the basket struts. Although the possibility exits of interference and entanglement between the two catheters provided care is exercised as discussed earlier, this has not proved to be a practical problem. Delivery of RF energy with the basket in place is also not restricted. In patients with severe arterial and aortic disease it is usually easier to pass the guiding sheath retrogradely into the left ventricle then it is to pass the ablation catheter, which can not be passed over a guide wire. In these cases the ablation catheter may be passed through a transseptal sheath. Alternatively after mapping with the basket has identified an anatomic site, the basket can be removed and its guiding sheath used to introduce the catheter into the left ventricle.

2.   CASE STUDIES

2.1   PATIENT #1

A 75 year-old-man had a history of a remote anteroseptal infarct. He presented with recurrent monoform ventricular tachycardia which initially responded to amiodarone but after two years the patient had clinical recurrences and underwent electrophysiological study with basket mapping of the left ventricle.

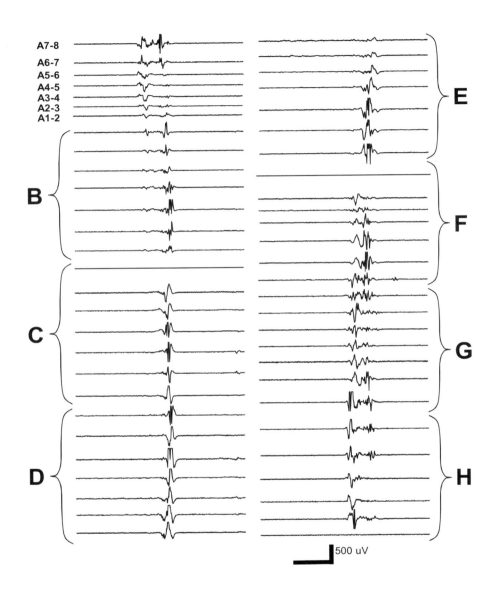

Figure 3. Local bipolar electrograms from the left ventricular endocardium of patient #1 during sinus rhythm. See text.

Figure 3 shows local bipolar electrograms from the entire basket array during sinus rhythm. Each of the eight splines is identified alphabetically from the index spline A through to H. Seven bipolar electrograms were recorded off each spline by chaining the electrodes in sequence starting on A spline distally with A 1-2, A 2-3, through to 7-8, at the proximal end. Note that with the exception of two channels, which malfunctioned due to amplifier failure in the recording system, good quality bipolar electrograms with low noise were recorded from the entire basket array. Also note the complex fractionated electrograms that were recorded from virtually all electrodes except splines C and D. This reflects the marked extent of left ventricular endocardial scarring and was often seen at intraoperative mapping of patients with chronic ischemic heart disease.[5]

Figure 4 shows a continuous ECG strip of surface lead III of the same patient throughout one attempt at induction of ventricular tachycardia. The first five beats are sinus followed by eight beats of a basic drive and a single extra stimulus. This initiates a nonsustained run of fast polymorphic tachycardia of which the last nine beats stabilize into one morphology before abruptly terminating.

Figure 5 shows termination of the same salvo on seven of the twelve surface ECG leads recorded. The morphology of these beats was identical to the morphology of the clinical ventricular tachycardia. In the weeks prior to the study the patient's dose of amiodarone had been increased while he waited for his study. This must have inhibited the induction and maintenance of his ventricular tachycardia since sustained runs of ventricular tachycardia could not be initiated. Previous to this dose increase, two extra stimuli reproducibly induced sustained tachycardia of the same morphology.

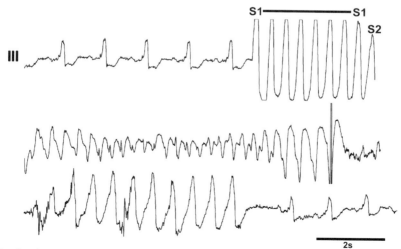

Figure 4. Continuous recording of ECG lead III of previous patient showing programmed pacing inducing non-sustained run of ventricular tachycardia. See text.

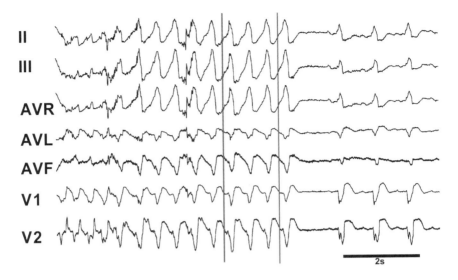

Figure 5. Termination of ventricular tachycardia shown in figure 4 as seen on seven surface ECG channels. The last nine beats were identical in morphology to the patient's clinical tachycardia. See text.

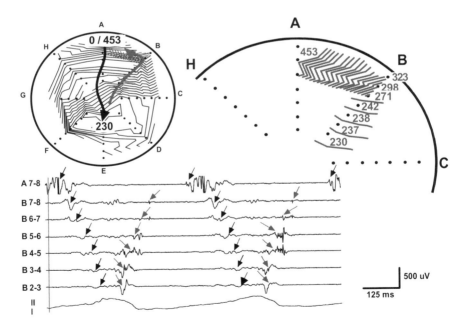

Figure 6. Top left panel shows left ventricular endocardial activation in 10 ms isochrones of one of the terminal beats of ventricular tachycardia seen in figure 5. Top right panel shows diastolic activation of return pathway. Lower panel shows selected bipolar electrograms of the same terminal beats. Grey arrows show diastolic activation. See text for discussion.

Figure 6 shows in the top left panel a 10 ms isochrone map of activation of one of the terminal beats of the tachycardia shown on figure 5. The left ventricular endocardium is depicted in a polar projection on the basket array with the apex in the center and the base on the periphery. Electrode rows A through to H represent the corresponding struts with electrodes A 1-2 at the apex and A 7-8 at the base. The lower panel shows surface ECG lead III as well as selected bipolar electrograms from two sequential cycles of the nine beat runs shown in figure 5. The top right panel shows isochronal details of the electrograms depicted in red in the lower panel. As can be seen in the top left isochrone map, each beat starts at the base of row A (electrodes A 7-8) indicated by time 0. Systolic activation then spreads down like a descending curtain, towards the apex ending at 230 ms on the apical portion of row E. This activation is summarized with a black arrow. The activation pattern on row B initially follows this same sequence as that on A but after reaching the apex it reverses and proceeds back to the base reaching B 7-8, at 323 ms then across to its close neighbor A 7-8, by 453 ms thus starting the next VT cycle. This diastolic activation is summarized by the red arrow in the top left panel. Although the distance between B 7-8, and A 7-8, is depicted as being great this is in fact a distortion of the polar projection used since all the rows/splines are united at the base just as they are shown to be at the apex. The diastolic electrograms forming the return path along row B are indicated by the red arrowheads.

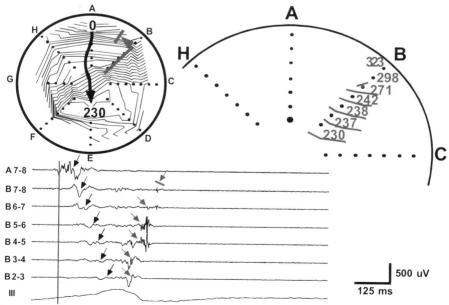

Figure 7. Activation maps and selected electrograms of last beat of the tachycardia seen in figure 5. The panels are arranged as in figure 6. Tachycardia terminates spontaneously because of block in the pre-exit portion of the return path. See text.

This macro-reentrant circuit was seen in each of the nine beats. Variations in morphology but not in relative timing occurred from one beat to the next. These may represent minor movements of the basket array with cardiac contraction and relaxation. Figure 7 shows the end of the ninth beat, where diastolic potentials can be traced back along row B as far as B 7-8 but fail to conduct across to A 7-8 resulting in termination of the VT run. This is an example of block of conduction in the pre-exit portion of the return path. Similar examples have been reported from intraoperative mapping studies.[6]

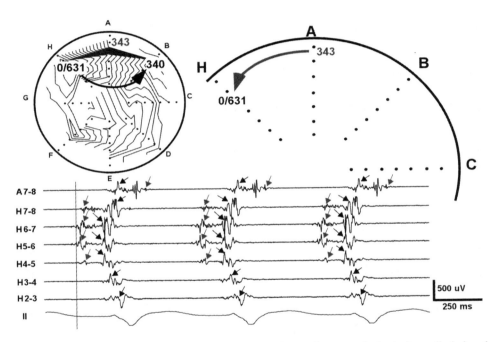

Figure 8. Activation maps of a second morphology of monoform ventricular tachycardia induced in patient #1. The panel arrangement is similar to that seen in the previous figures. See text.

In the same patient a second morphology of ventricular tachycardia could be induced with burst ventricular pacing. Basket mapping of this tachycardia revealed the earliest origin of each beat on H 6-7, and H 5-6. Figure 8 shows the isochrone map of activation of this VT as well as selected key bipolar electrograms in surface lead II. Each beat is initiated by complex protracted electrograms starting in mid diastole and persisting locally for 240 ms. The latest activation is seen in A 7-8, 340 ms later. This is closely adjacent to H 6-7, where the next beat starts at 631 ms. There is a temporal gap with electrical silence lasting 248 ms most likely due to a portion of the return path lying deep in the subendocardium of the septum, beyond the recording capabilities of the basket array.

The anatomic locations of the basal electrodes of rows H, A, and B were all closely adjacent on the crest of the septum. This region was ablated with RF energy and no recurrences of ventricular tachycardia have occurred in three years despite the discontinuation of amiodarone.

2.2   PATIENT #2

This 79-year-old man also had a history of an anterior infarct but remained free of symptoms until he presented with ventricular tachycardia at rate of 130 per minute. The tachycardia proved not only to be completely refractory to all antiarrhythmic drugs, but also failed to respond to antitachycardia pacing and repeated cardioversion attempts (shown in figure 9). After eighteen days of incessant ventricular tachycardia he was referred for catheter mapping and ablation. Figure 10 shows an isochrone map of left ventricular endocardial activation and selected bipolar electrograms plus surface lead V1 and V6 recorded during tachycardia. Each beat of the tachycardia started in the left ventricular apex at electrodes E 1-2, as indicated by the asterix. Activation then proceeds in a figure 8 manner around a functional arc of block to end at closely adjacent electrodes A 1-2. Exploration of these sites with an ablation catheter confirmed the early pre-potential around E 1-2, and is shown in the tracing labeled "exit". Furthermore, the electrogram labeled "entrance" was recorded within 1 cm of E 1-2, close to A 1-2 and shows an early diastolic potential indicated by the arrowhead.

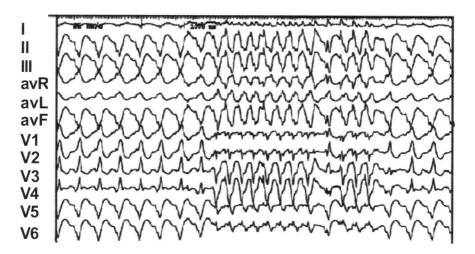

Figure 9.   Twelve lead ECG recording of an incessant ventricular tachycardia seen in patient #2. The figure shows an unsuccessful attempt of pace-termination. See text.

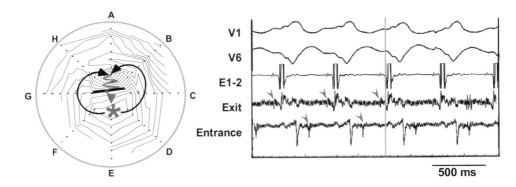

Figure 10.   Left panel shows isochronal map of left ventricular endocardial activation of tachycardia shown in figure 9.   Right panel shows surface ECG leads V1 and V6, one bipolar electrogram from site of earliest activation with a small pre-systolic potential (E 1-2).   Bottom two tracings are of bipolar electrograms from the ablation catheter at the entrance and exit sites of the figure 8 reentry sequence.   Red arrow heads indicate early diastolic and adjacent pre-systolic potentials.   RF ablation was performed at the site with early diastolic potentials presumed to be at the entrance to the return path.   See text.

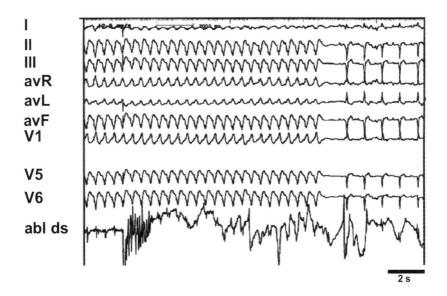

Figure 11. Result of RF energy delivered at site shown in figure 10.   The incessant ventricular tachycardia was terminated within 10 seconds for the first time in 18 days.

    The presence of such an early diastolic potential suggested the possibility of this truly being the site of entrance of the return path across the functional arc of block to the exit site at E 1-2. As shown on figure 11 radio-frequency energy was applied to this entrance site and within ten seconds resulted in termination of the tachycardia for first time in eighteen days! The ablation lesion was enlarged and programmed stimulation failed to induce any further arrhythmias.

2.3   PATIENT #3

A 66-year-old man with an idiopathic dilated cardiomyopathy presented with syncope. Investigations revealed runs of nonsustained ventricular tachycardia. He received an implantable defibrillator and was treated empirically with amiodarone. He remained well for four years then presented in an electrical storm with repeated episodes of ventricular tachycardia refractory to antiarrhythmic agents thus resulting in multiple discharges of his defibrillator. Because the ventricular tachycardia episodes were all monoform and suggested a left ventricular origin, basket catheter mapping was undertaken.

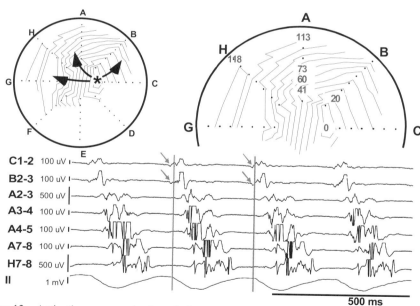

Figure 12. Activation maps and selected electrograms from left ventricular endocardium during ventricular tachycardia in patient #3. Panels are arranged as in the previous figures except both upper panels show systolic activation (right panel magnified depiction of the left panel). The lower panel shows selected bipolar electrograms from the array. Each beat of the tachycardia started at C1-2 and B2-3 at 0 ms and spread radially. At these sites there were small pre-systolic potentials - 20 ms relative to earliest surface ECG. See text.

Figure 12 shows the isochrone map of the ventricular tachycardia with selected bipolar electrograms. As shown by the asterix the map indicates a monofocal origin of each beat in the left ventricular apex at C 1-2. The bipolar electrogram from these electrodes showed just a small presystolic potential preceding the surface ECG signals by merely 20 ms. The subsequent spread of activation from the earliest site was then radial with no indication of a macro-reentrant return path. The underlying mechanism of the tachycardia was either micro-entrant or abnormal automaticity. Exploration with an ablation catheter confirmed that presence of a small pre-potential. Radiofrequency ablation of that site resulted in the inability to reinduce the ventricular tachycardia. No clinical recurrences or discharges of the patient's defibrillator have occurred in three years of follow-up.

2.4   PATIENT #4

This 50-year-old woman had a surgical repair of an atrial septal defect at the age of 12. Postoperatively the patient remained asymptomatic until age 26 when she began to complain of increasingly frequent episodes of sudden onset irregular palpitations lasting hours or days. During these attacks the ventricular rate was 130/min. Amiodarone and sotalol produced unacceptable side effects. ECG documentation revealed an atrial flutter of atypical morphology. On the presumption that the patient may have had an incisional atrial reentrant tachycardia caused by either repair of her ASD or around the site of her atrial cannulation, basket catheter mapping of the right atrium was performed.

Figure 13 shows the fluoroscopic image of the basket catheter in position in the right atrium in a 30° right anterior oblique projection.

Figure 14 shows an isochronal map of her right atrial activation in the upper panel. Key local bipolar atrial electrograms are shown in the lower panel. During the atrial tachycardia earliest atrial activation occurred at the base of spline D at D7-8. Activation then progressed counterclockwise around the base of the right atrium and upwards along D to reach its tip at D 1-2 by 60 ms. From there activation crossed over to the tip of the closely neighboring electrode E 1-2 and down strut E reaching its base at E 7-8 by 100 ms. The electrograms from D and E clearly show this in their sequential activation seen in the lower panel. This activation sequence is consistent with a conduction block between struts D and E, which anatomically corresponded to the lateral free wall of the right atrium. At the base of E at E 7-8, there are double potentials, the diminished second component of which (indicated by arrowheads) gives rise to a fully developed electrogram on closely neighboring D 7-8, setting off the next cycle (D 7-8 is shown at the top and bottom of the electrogram panel to facilitate orientation). In the entire circuit of activation, the greatest delay of conduction (95 ms) occurs at a single location on E 7-8, suggesting this was the critical portion of the return path. Although functional tests for concealed entrainment were not performed, application of RF energy at this site resulted in termination of the atrial tachycardia within five seconds. The patient has remained free of clinical recurrences over the follow-up period of one year.

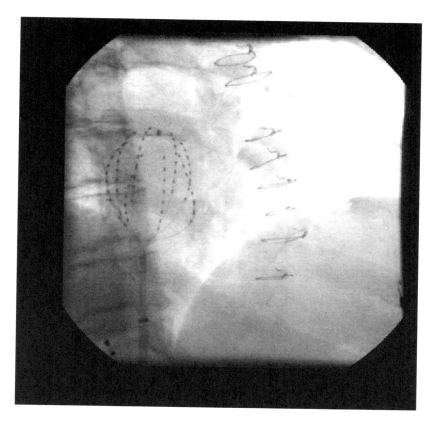

Figure 13. Fluoroscopic image of basket catheter in the right atrium in a 30° right anterior oblique projection of patient #4. See text.

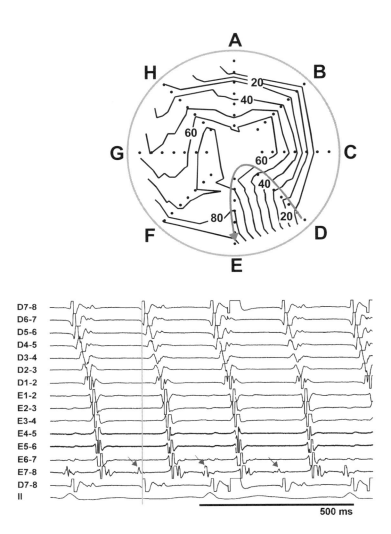

Figure 14. Upper panel: Right atrial activation during the atrial tachycardia of patient #4 shown in lower panel. Lower panel shows selected bipolar atrial electrograms and surface lead II during atrial tachycardia. Red arrowheads indicate second component of double potentials seen on E7-8. These immediately preceeded start of next atrial cycle which started on D7-8. See text.

3.   RESULTS

The cases presented in the foregoing are clearly not comprehensive but rather serve to illustrate the utility of basket mapping. The detail of underlying arrhythmia mechanisms can sometimes be revealed in astonishing detail, which may be critical to the successful outcome of an ablation attempt. As already discussed care has to be taken to ensure that the basket is appropriate in both size and its placement in the correct cardiac chamber. Before placement it is advisable to first check that the clinical arrhythmia is inducible. Our total experience includes 16 patients with ventricular tachycardia in which 11 underwent left ventricular mapping and 5 right ventricular mapping. The mapping contributed to a successful ablation in twelve patients. In four patients (two right ventricular and two left ventricular) ablation was unsuccessful. Failure was attributed to the target tissue being in deeply intramural or epicardial in 3 patients and to a broadly diffuse return path with multiple exits in one patient. Thirteen atrial arrhythmias were mapped with a basket catheter - eleven in the right atrium and two in the left atrium. Ablation of these arrhythmias was successful in eight of the right atrial cases. In the two patients with left atrial mapping the clinical atrial arrhythmia switched to a right atrial flutter which preempted evocation of the left atrial arrhythmia. Throughout the entire experience there were no complications attributable to the basket catheter. One patient had a cerebro-vascular accident from a left ventricular mural thrombus that was dislodged by manipulation of the ablation catheter. That patient had undergone an extensive left ventricular ablation one week earlier at the referring hospital and had not been covered by anticoagulants in the intervening week. After that experience, it has been our practice to try and avoid performing left ventricular ablation within a month of a previously failed ablation attempt.

CONCLUSION

Basket catheter mapping has proved to be effective in guiding and achieving successful catheter ablation in cases where conventional mapping has failed or is unlikely to succeed by virtue of the nature of the arrhythmia or its hemodynamic consequences. Refractory ventricular tachycardias and supraventricular arrhythmias, particularly atrial tachycardia resulting from prior atriotomies should be considered for basket mapping.

In comparing basket mapping with alternative new mapping techniques such as the non-contact method, both advantages and limitations are apparent and should be taken into consideration before deciding on one technique. These are itemized in Table 4. Electroanatomic mapping techniques are restricted in their applicability to arrhythmias that are electrically and hemodynamically stable because they depend on sequentially collected data.

These very different new techniques should not be viewed as competing alternatives but rather as different tools to be chosen from to best address the challenge of a particular arrhythmia. Future developments of the basket catheter are likely to include an asymmetric electrode distribution to improve spatial resolution in a region of interest. Combination of the basket with intracardiac echocardiography also promises high resolution true electrode-anatomic mapping on a beat-by-beat basis. Utilization of actual electrograms from the basket electrode to compute virtual electrograms in the intervening space, theoretically could also greatly enhance the electrical resolution of basket mapping.

TABLE 4. Comparison of Basket with Non-Contact Mapping Systems

Basket	Non-Contact
- Spatial resolution limited to 64 electrodes.	- Extremely high resolution > 3000 virtual electrograms.
- Contact or close proximity necessary.	- Contact unnecessary.
- Geometry of array restricted by basket.	- Geometric shell complies closely with anatomy.
- Electrograms are real and without distorsion.	- Virtual electrograms are computed - Despite good correlation with real electrograms some distorsions occur.
- Electrograms seen are at the anatomic position of the electrodes and are derived from electrically excitable myocardium at that site.	- Electrograms are projected onto endocardial surface and assigned to that specific site even if there is no electrically excitable myocardium there e.g. dacron patch. This may lead to misdirected ablation attempts.
- Movement of basket does not invalidate mapping since basket array is self-referencing.	- Movement of mapping balloon may invalidate spatial construct of mapping.
- Although interpretation may be complex, it is usually feasible using standard recording systems.	- Requires separate dedicated console for display and analysis which may be complex.
- Provided basket is sized appropriately even the largest cardiac chambers can be encompassed.	- Comparatively "near-sighted": beyond 3 cm may miss critically vital real electrograms.

REFERENCES

1.   Downar E, Parson ID, Yao L, Cameron DA and Waxman MB: Endocardial Catheter Mapping of Unstable and Pleomorphic Ventricular Tachycardias, Circulation 1984;70(Supp II):1488.

2.   Browne KF, Chilson DA, Waller BF and Zipes DP: Use of a Spatially Distributed Multielectrode Catheter to Activation Map the Left Ventricular Endocardium Simultaneously and Destroy Selected Areas, Circulation 1983;68(Supp III):84.

3.   Jenkins KJ, Walsh EP, Colan SD, Bergau DM, Saul JP and Lock JE: Multipolar Endocardial Mapping of the Right Atrium During Cardiac Catheterization: Description of a New Technique, J Am Coll cardiol 1993;22:1105.

4.   Eldar M, Fitzpatrick AP, Ohad D, Smith MF, Hsu S, Whayne JG, Vered Z, Rotstein Z, Kordis T, Swanson DK, Chin M, Scheinman MM, Lesh MD and Greenspon AJ: Percutaneous Multielectrode Endocardial Mapping During Ventricular Tachycardia in the Swine Model, Circulation 1996;94:1125.

5. Downar E, Kimber S, Harris L, Mickleborough L, Sevaptsidis E, Massé S, Chen TCK and Genga A: Endocardial Mapping of Ventricular Tachycardia in the Intact Human Heart II. Evidence for Multiuse Reentry in a Functional Sheet of Surviving Myocardium, J Am Coll Cardiol 1992;20:869.
6. Downar E, Saito J, Doig JC, Chen TCK, Sevaptsidis E, Massé S, Kimber S, Mickleborough L and Harris L: Endocardial Mapping of Ventricular Tachycardia in the Intact Human Ventricle III. Evidence of Multiuse Reentry With Spontaneous and Induced Block in Portions of Reentrant Path Complex, J Am Coll Cardiol 1995;25:1591.

Chapter 15

ENDOCARDIAL GLOBAL NONCONTACT MAPPING (ENSITE™)

Bradley P. Knight, Fred Morady
Department of Internal Medicine, Division of Cardiology, University of Michigan Medical center, Ann Arbor, Michigan, USA

INTRODUCTION

Multisite epicardial activation mapping has advanced our understanding of arrhythmia mechanisms and has served as a valuable tool during arrhythmia surgery. Conventional endocardial mapping during percutaneous radiofrequency ablation procedures generally is performed using 1-3 catheters, each with a limited number of electrodes. In fact, some arrhythmias, such as AV nodal reentrant tachycardia, can be diagnosed and cured with radiofrequency ablation using only two quadrapolar catheters. However, current catheter-based mapping techniques have significant limitations when attempts are made to ablate complex arrhythmias, such as ventricular tachycardia in patients with a history of myocardial infarction.

Noncontact mapping has been developed to permit high-resolution global activation mapping of the endocardium without the need for endocardial contact.[1,2] The technique is based on the ability to compute far-field endocardial electrograms from analysis of intracavitary potentials. This chapter reviews the commercially available Ensite 3000 noncontact mapping system developed by Endocardial Solutions, Inc. (St. Paul, MN) and describes its use during ablation of cardiac arrhythmias. Because the value of the mapping system is heavily dependent on the accuracy of the virtual electrograms and locator signal, a detailed review of published validation studies is also included.

L. Bing Liem and E. Downar (eds.), Progress in Catheter Ablation, 225-240.
© 2001 *Kluwer Academic Publishers. Printed in the Netherlands.*

1. DESCRIPTION OF ENSITE 3000™ NONCONTACT MAPPING SYSTEM

The Ensite 3000™ noncontact mapping system derives information from two sources - a multielectrode array (MEA) and a catheter locator signal. Data from these two sources are used to construct a high-resolution, three-dimensional graphical representation of endocardial activation using dynamic isochronal or isopotential color maps.

1.1 Multielectrode Array (MEA)

The MEA is designed to record cavitary potentials. The array is a mesh of 0.003-inch diameter polyimide-coated stainless steel wire that covers an inflatable 7.5-ml balloon (Figure 1). Sixty-four electrodes are created by removing a small amount of the insulation from the wires at specific locations. The MEA is mounted on a 9 -French lumenal pigtail catheter that can be advanced percutaneously into any cardiac chamber over a 0.035 guidewire. Ring electrodes are positioned on the catheter with one distal and three proximal to the balloon.

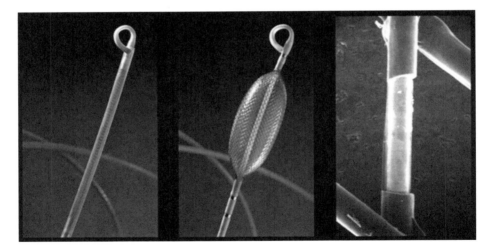

Figure 1. The multielectrode array catheter. The 9 French pigtail catheter is shown with the balloon deflated and the protective sheath that has been advanced near the end of the catheter (Left). The wire mesh of 0.0003-inch diameter polyimide-coated stainless steel is visible on the surface of the inflated balloon (Middle). A photomicrograph is shown of one of the electrodes that are created by removing the insulation with a laser (Right).

1.2 Locator Signal

The tip of any standard electrode catheter can be located relative to the MEA by use of the locator signal. A 5.68-kHz signal is emitted from the distal electrode and is detected by the electrodes on the MEA. The location of the mapping catheter is updated 100 times per second on the display. The locator signal is used to define the geometry of the endocardial border and to pinpoint the position of the mapping/ablation catheter.

1.3 Determination of Chamber Geometry

After the MEA and mapping catheters are positioned in the heart, the chamber geometry is determined. This permits construction of a three-dimensional model of the endocardium on which the activation maps are displayed. Accurate identification of the endocardial border as a reference is critical to the accuracy of the activation maps. The roving contact catheter is systematically moved within the cardiac chamber to identify as much of the endocardial border as possible. The endocardial display is continuously updated as more distant sites are reached to construct a multifaceted model. A smoothing process is applied to create a more realistic endocardial model (Figure 2). This process takes approximately 5 minutes to complete.

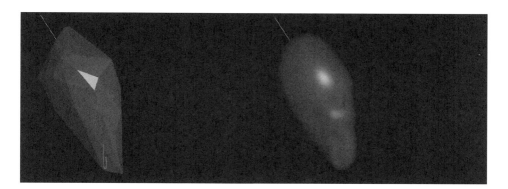

Figure 2. A three-dimensional model of the endocardium is constructed on which the activation maps are displayed. A multifaceted model is continuously updated during its creation, as more distant sites are reached with the roving catheter (Left). A smoothing process is applied to make a more realistic endocardial model (Right).

1.4 Generation and Display of Activation Maps

Low-amplitude, low-frequency, far-field cavitary signals are sampled at 1200 times per second from the 64 noncontact balloon electrodes. A custom-designed amplifier is used and the potentials are filtered with a programmable bandwidth between 0.1 and 300 Hz. The data is processed using a Silicon Graphics workstation with custom software. A boundary-element method based on an inverse solution to Laplace's equation is used to compute 3,360 unipolar endocardial electrograms from the cavitary potentials.[1] Sophisticated algorithms are also applied to the data to minimize noise.

Isopotential or isochronal activation maps are displayed on a computer screen (Figure 3). A color range is used to define the voltage or the timing of onset. The three-dimensional image of the heart chamber can be "cut away" and interactively rotated using a mouse, to allow visualization from different angles (Figure 4). The position of the tip of the roving catheter is continuously displayed on the virtual endocardial model. Local virtual electrograms can also be selected using a cursor and displayed as waveforms along with the contact catheter and surface electrograms (Figure 5).

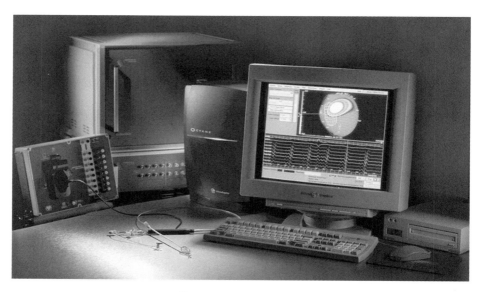

Figure 3. Shown is the Ensite 3000™ System and display with the multielectrode catheter in the foreground.

2.   ENSITE SYSTEM VALIDATION

2.1   Validation of the Locator Signal

A validation study of the locator signal was performed using a saline-filled tank to simulate intracardiac noncontact mapping.[2] Using this model, the precision of the locator signal was found to be 0.33±0.45 mm at distances of <50 mm from the MEA balloon and 0.75±1.13 mm at distances of >50 mm. The roving electrode could be guided to within 2.33±0.44 mm of the signal source as displayed on the isopotential map at distances of <50 mm from the MEA balloon and to within 7.50±1.13 mm at a distances of >50 mm. The major source of error was determined to be granularity, due to the finite number of grid vertices on which endocardial sites can be labelled, and was amplified at greater distances from the array catheter.

Accuracy of the locator signal was also studied in the right atrium of normal dogs. The mean absolute difference between computed and actual interelectrode distances was 0.96±0.77 mm^3.

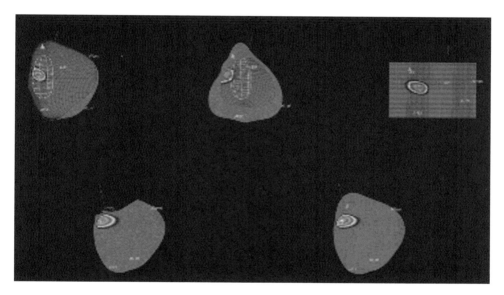

Figure 4. The three-dimensional image of the heart chamber can be "cut away" and interactively rotated using a mouse (left and middle images). Activation maps can also be displayed on a "flat" representation of the endocardium (right).

2.2   Validation of the Computed Waveforms

2.2.1   Animal Studies

Initial validation studies of the Ensite system were performed in dogs[2] (Table 1). Endocardial left ventricular pacing was performed in open-chest dogs with normal hearts using transmural plunge electrodes. The timing of the maximum -dV/dT and morphology of waveforms generated from the array catheter were compared to the timing and morphology of waveforms recorded from the contact catheter. In addition, radiofrequency lesions were created at sites determined to be the pacing site based on the computed isopotential maps.

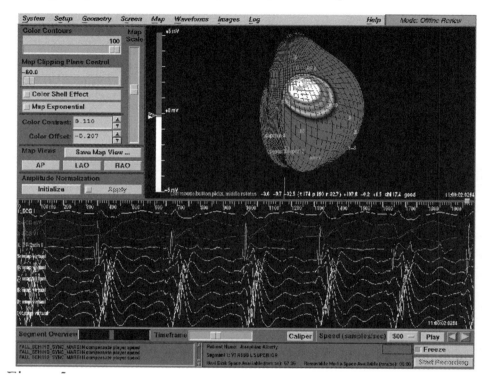

Figure 5. The monitor displays the endocardial reconstruction on which an isopotential map is superimposed (top). Local virtual electrograms can be selected using a cursor and displayed as waveforms along with the contact catheter electrograms and surface electrograms (bottom).

The timing difference between computed and contact electrograms was -0.64±2.48 msec. The mean waveform correlation was 0.966. The mean distance from the center of the radiofrequency lesion to the pacing site was 4 mm, although some lesions were as far away as 8 mm. It is important to note that these results were obtained in hearts that are significantly smaller than the hearts of most patients with ventricular tachycardia and that only every fourth beat was paced to minimized the hemodynamic changes that occur when the ventricle is activated from the free wall.

Kadish et al performed validation studies of the Ensite system in the right atrium in normal dogs.[3] The mean correlation coefficients during sinus rhythm, pacing-induced atrial flutter and pacing-induced atrial fibrillation were 0.80±0.12, 0.85±0.17, and 0.81±0.18 msec, respectively. The accuracy of electrogram reconstruction was found to be lowest at sites that were more than

4.0 cm from the center of the balloon and at sites with a high spatial complexity of activation.

2.2.2   Human Studies

Validation studies were performed using data obtained in the first 15 patients who underwent ablation of ventricular tachycardia using the Ensite system at the University of Michigan[4] (Table 1). After the MEA balloon was placed in the left ventricle, the steerable roving catheter was positioned at three different left ventricular endocardial sites.   Unipolar recordings were obtained from the noncontact mapping system and from the contact roving catheter at each site during sinus rhythm, right ventricular pacing, and ventricular tachycardia. Morphology coefficients and timing differences were used to compare electrograms. The results are summarized in Table 1. The overall accuracy of the computed electrograms was good. Accuracy was better during sinus rhythm compared to during ventricular tachycardia and at sites within 3.4 cm compared to sites greater than 3.4 cm from the center of the MEA balloon. Similar results were obtained during sinus rhythm from human validation studies performed by Schilling, et al at St. Mary's Hospital in London.[5]

Table 1. Results of Validation Studies Comparing Contact Waveforms to Computed Waveforms Using the Ensite Noncontact Mapping System

| Chamber | Subject | Rhythm | Study | Timing Difference (ms) | | | Morphology Correlation | | |
| | | | | (Median or Mean ± Standard Deviation) | | | | | |
				Overall	Close (<3.4cm)	Far (>3.4cm)	Overall	Close (<3.4cm)	Far (>3.4cm)
LV	Dogs	SR	Gornick[2]	-0.64±2.48	-	-	0.966	-	-
LV	Humans	SR	Strickberger[3]	1.8	1.7	2.8	0.86	0.88	0.81
LV	Humans	RVP	Strickberger[3]	4.0	3.0	7.4	0.82	0.85	0.78
LV	Humans	VT	Strickberger[3]	2.8	1.9	5.3	0.78	0.83	0.72
LV	Humans	SR	Schilling[4]	-	-1.94±7.12	-14.16±19.29	-	0.87	0.76
RA	Dogs	SR	Kadish[5]	-	-	-	0.80	-	-
RA	Dogs	AFL	Kadish[5]	-	-	-	0.85	-	-
RA	Dogs	AF	Kadish[5]	-	-	-	0.81	-	-

3.   USE OF NONCONTACT MAPPING FOR SPECIFIC ARRHYTHMIAS

Initial human studies in the United States were conducted under two different Investigational Device Exemptions (IDE). One IDE covered studies of left ventricular tachycardia and a second IDE covered studies of right atrial arrhythmias. This section reviews the experience at the University of Michigan using the Ensite system during mapping and ablation of left ventricular tachycardia and right atrial flutter.

Since approval of the Ensite system in Europe in 1998, several centers have used the Ensite system during mapping and ablation of a variety of arrhythmias including atrial fibrillation, atrial tachycardia, and tachycardias following corrective cardiac surgery. The experience with the Ensite system for these arrhythmias has not yet been published.

3.1   Ventricular tachycardia

The Ensite noncontact mapping system has been used during mapping and ablation of 25 patients with left ventricular tachycardia at the University of Michigan. The results from the first 15 patients are summarized.[4] Patients had recurrent monomorphic ventricular tachycardia and had previously undergone placement of an implantable cardioverter-defibrillator. The mean age of the patients was 70±6 years and 2 were women. Thirteen of the patients had a history of myocardial infarction, and 2 patients had a nonischemic dilated cardiomyopathy. Nine patients were being treated with amiodarone at the time of the procedure.

Programmed electrical stimulation was performed using a conventional 7 - French pacing catheter inserted into a femoral vein and positioned in the right ventricle. The inducibility of ventricular tachycardia was assessed with 4 extrastimuli using basic drive cycle lengths of 350, 400, and 600 msec.

After the clinical ventricular tachycardia was found to be reproducibly inducible, the Ensite noncontact MEA catheter was positioned. Intravenous heparin was administered to achieve and maintain an activated clotting time greater than 350 seconds. Using a retrograde aortic approach, the MEA catheter was advanced over a 0.035-inch guidewire through the left femoral artery into the left ventricle using fluoroscopic guidance. The pigtail tip of the catheter was placed at the apex in most patients. In patients who appeared to have ventricular tachycardia arising from the lateral wall of the left ventricle, the pigtail tip was positioned more laterally. The array was expanded using a plunger on the handle of the catheter and the balloon was inflated with a mixture of radiopaque contrast and saline. Fluoroscopy was used to confirm that the balloon was clearly below the aortic valve during inflation of the balloon. A conventional 7-French steerable electrode catheter was inserted into the right femoral artery and positioned in the left ventricle using a retrograde aortic approach. The roving catheter was used to construct a 3-dimensional model of the endocardium, as described above.

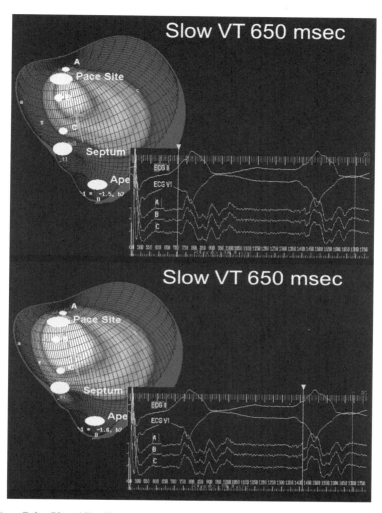

Figure 6 (see Color Plate 12). Shown is an example of concealed entrainment during a ventricular tachycardia that has a cycle length of 650 msec. The top panel shows the isopotential map at the time of the onset of the last entrained QRS complex, immediately following pacing (from the site marked Pace Site) which resulted in concealed entrainment. The pacing stimulus can be seen at the beginning of the electrograms. The bottom panel shows the isopotential map of the ventricular tachycardia at the onset of the QRS complex, which identifies the exit site of the ventricular tachycardia reentry circuit. Note that the exit site of the entrained ventricular beat has a similar exit site as that of the native ventricular tachycardia, as would be expected after concealed entrainment. The septum and apex are marked.

Ventricular tachycardia was induced by programmed stimulation and recorded using the Ensite system. Recordings of ventricular tachycardia were completed in less than 10 seconds and isopotential maps were displayed in less than 30 seconds. Adjusting the color controls at the time of QRS onset identified the exit site of the reentrant circuit that was generating the ventricular tachycardia (Figure 6). Presystolic activation was traced back as far as possible to identify sites critical to the ventricular tachycardia circuit (Figure 7). The entire diastolic component of the reentrant circuit could be identified in only one patient. The virtual electrograms were also sampled to identify regions of isolated diastolic potentials.

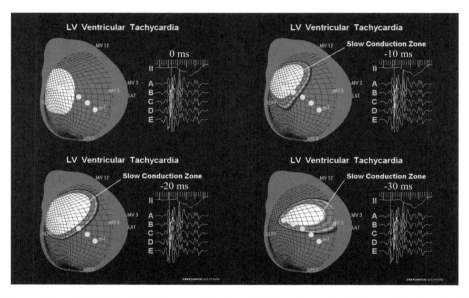

Figure 7 (see Color Plate 13). An example of ventricular tachycardia is shown. The isopotential map at the time of the onset of the QRS is shown in the upper left corner. Each of the next three panels show a presystolic isopotential map at progressively earlier times relative to the onset of the QRS complex during ventricular tachycardia: −10 msec (upper right corner), -20 msec (lower left corner), and −30 msec (lower right corner). Note progressive activation from the base to the apex of the left ventricle. Lat=lateral wall, MV3=3 o'clock on the mitral annulus in the lateral anterior oblique view, MV5=5 o'clock, and MV12=12 o'clock, sept=septal wall. The closed yellow circles represent the recording sites of the virtual electrograms A through E.

Mapping and ablation of 19 ventricular tachycardias was attempted in 14 patients. Ablation was not attempted in one patient who developed a severe hypotension after ventricular tachycardia was induced. The mean ventricular tachycardia cycle length was 383±111 msec. Ablation of 9 of the ventricular tachycardias was performed during sinus rhythm because the ventricular tachycardia was hemodynamically unstable. Using the locator signal and fluoroscopy, the roving catheter was moved to the site selected for ablation (Figure 8). Radiofrequency current was delivered to a target temperature of 60°C.

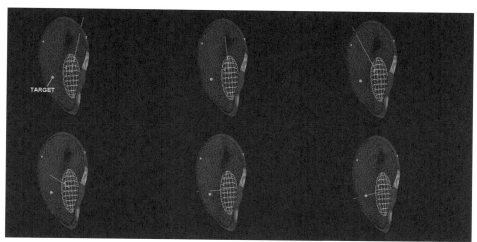

Figure 8 (see Color Plate 14). An example of the locator signal being used to guide the roving catheter to a target site. The green line originates from the center of the balloon (denoted by the yellow wire mesh) and meets the endocardial reconstruction to denote the position of the roving catheter at the endocardium. From left to right and top to bottom, the roving catheter is steered to the target site.

Successful ablation, defined as the inability to induce ventricular tachycardia, was achieved in 15 (78%) of the 19 ventricular tachycardias. Five of the 9 ventricular tachycardias that were hemodynamically unstable were successfully ablated. The mean procedure time was 125 minutes and the mean fluoroscopy time was 79 minutes. Three complications occurred and included tamponade, an embolic stroke, and transient electromechanical dissociation after transthoracic cardioversion. The latter patient died several days after the procedure from progressive hemodynamic deterioration.

Our initial experience using the Ensite noncontact mapping system for mapping and ablation of human ventricular tachycardia demonstrated that the virtual isopotential maps are sufficiently accurate to aid in ablation of human ventricular tachycardia. The system allows ablation of hemodynamically unstable ventricular tachycardia to be accomplished in some patients. Identification of endocardial exit sites and sites of presystolic and diastolic activity during ventricular tachycardia is facilitated by the system. In addition, the locator signal accurately guides movement of the ablation catheter during ventricular tachycardia without the use of fluoroscopy.

3.1.1   Additional Experience with the Ensite System during Ventricular Tachycardia

The initial experience at St. Mary's Hospital using the Ensite system during mapping and ablation of 81 ventricular tachycardias in 24 patients has been published.[6] An exit site was demonstrated in 99% of the ventricular tachycardias and the complete ventricular tachycardia circuit was demonstrated in 21% of the ventricular tachycardias. Ablation was more successful when radiofrequency was delivered at sites that were identified as part of the diastolic portion of the circuit compared to sites that were identified as exit sites using the Ensite system.

The same investigators from St. Mary's Hospital were unable to identify any endocardial waveform characteristics recorded during sinus rhythm that could predict successful ablation sites for ventricular tachycardia.[7] Other investigators have also concluded that the latest sites of endocardial activation during sinus rhythm correlate poorly with sites of ventricular tachycardia presystolic zones of slow conduction and exit sites.[8] However, sites displaying isolated diastolic potentials during ventricular tachycardia may share a similar activation pattern during sinus rhythm and during ventricular tachycardia, suggesting that areas critical for ventricular tachycardia potentially may be localized during sinus rhythm.[9]

3.2   Atrial Flutter

The Ensite noncontact mapping system has been used during mapping and ablation of 16 patients with atrial flutter at the University of Michigan.[10-11] The mean age of the patients was 53±15 years and 4 were women. Three patients were being treated for hypertension, 2 patients had undergone repair of an atrial septal defect, 2 patients had coronary artery disease, and 1 patient had cor pulmonale.

The Ensite noncontact MEA catheter was advanced over a 0.035-inch guidewire through a femoral vein into the right atrium using fluoroscopic guidance. The catheter was positioned and the balloon was inflated so that the equator of the balloon was adjacent to the low right-atrial isthmus region. Intravenous heparin was administered to achieve and maintain an activated clotting time greater than 350 seconds. A conventional 7 -French steerable electrode catheter was inserted into a femoral vein and positioned in the right atrium for ablation. A second steerable catheter was inserted into a femoral vein and positioned into the right atrium for atrial pacing. The roving catheter was used to construct a 3-dimensional model of the right atrial endocardium.

Atrial flutter was recorded using the noncontact mapping system. The mean cycle length was 231±22 msec. The color controls were adjusted to allow identification of as much of the flutter circuit as possible (Figure 9). Virtual electrograms from the right atrial isthmus were sampled and displayed for analysis. The rhythm was counterclockwise, isthmus-dependent atrial flutter in each case.

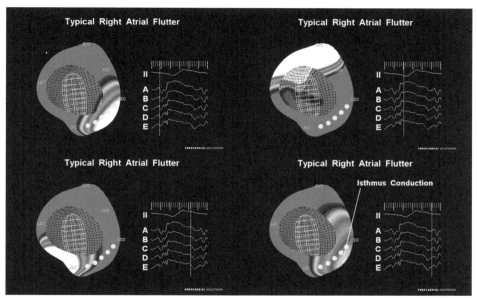

Figure 9 (see Color Plate 15). Isopotential maps are shown during the circuit typical counterclockwise atrial flutter. Each map denotes the endocardial activation at different times. The virtual electrograms are also displayed from the right atrial isthmus with the time of each activation map denoted by the vertical time line. The bottom right panel shows the endocardial activation during conduction through the low right atrial isthmus. The yellow wire mesh denotes the noncontact balloon. The closed yellow circles represent the recording sites of the virtual electrograms A through E.

Serial radiofrequency lesions were delivered from the tricuspid annulus to the inferior vena cava to create a line of conduction block through the low right-atrial isthmus region. Individual lesions were made by delivering 60-second applications of radiofrequency current through the distal 4-mm electrode of a standard ablation catheter. The target temperature was 60°C. The locator signal was used to catalog sites of radiofrequency delivery and to assure continuity of the lesions.

Successful ablation was defined as termination of the atrial flutter and creation of bi-directional isthmus conduction block as determined by the noncontact mapping system. The presence or absence of bi-directional conduction block was determined during coronary sinus pacing and posterolateral tricuspid annulus pacing at cycle lengths of 300 and 400 msec.

Isopotential maps were constructed during pacing and the isthmus region was inspected. Block was present when the isopotential map showed that conduction through the isthmus was absent during pacing. When isthmus conduction persisted after delivery of a complete ablation line, the isopotential map was used to identify the "gap" in the ablation line where further applications were required.

Successful ablation was achieved in each patient. The mean procedure time was 99 minutes and the mean fluoroscopy time was 64 minutes. No complications occurred. However, four patients experienced a recurrence of typical atrial flutter within 2 months after the procedure.

Our initial experience using the Ensite noncontact mapping system for mapping and ablation of human atrial flutter demonstrated that the isopotential maps allowed visualization of low right atrial isthmus portion of the endocardial circuit during typical counterclockwise atrial flutter. However, a significant amount of color gain adjustment was required to permit visualization of the flutter circuit. The locator signal was valuable for creating contiguous radiofrequency lesions and identified movement of the ablation catheter that was not appreciated fluoroscopically. The virtual isopotential maps helped achieve complete conduction block by identifying conduction gaps during atrial flutter or during atrial pacing. Our high recurrence rate of 25%, however, suggests that the isopotential maps may have suggested that isthmus block was present when it was not.

3.2.1   Additional Experience with the Ensite System during Atrial Flutter

Other centers have published preliminary data from their experience using the noncontact mapping system during ablation of human atrial flutter.[12-13] The Ensite system was used to guide successful ablation in 5 patients, 3 of whom had failed previous attempts at ablation using conventional techniques. The mapping system was able to identify the entire atrial flutter circuit in 3 of the 5 patients.

3.3   Atrial Fibrillation

There is little published on the use of the Ensite noncontact mapping system during atrial fibrillation. Kadish et al published preliminary data in their experience using the Ensite system in 2 patients with atrial fibrillation.[14] They found that the system could rapidly evaluate atrial activation and potentially localize sites of repetitive reentry.

4.   LIMITATIONS OF NONCONTACT MAPPING

The Ensite system displays an isopotential map of a tachycardia on a model of the endocardium that is derived during sinus rhythm. Theoretically this might result in inaccuracies from the geometric distortion that occurs during the tachycardia. However, validation studies of the virtual electrograms suggest that minimal accuracy is lost during tachycardia.

A limitation of the Ensite system is the heavy dependence on the operator for adjustments of the isopotential map color gains. Recent upgrades in the system software appear to be more automated and may minimize this problem. Another limitation is that the accuracy of the system depends on the stability of the noncontact multielectrode catheter. Although the balloon catheter is very stable in most cases, the catheter must be repositioned if it moves and endocardial reconstruction must be repeated.

Although the safety of the noncontact balloon catheter appears to be high, it must be remembered that more equipment is often associated with more complications. It will be important to identify which arrhythmias are best treated using a minimal approach and which arrhythmias require the use of an advanced mapping system. Cost-effectiveness of the system remains to be determined.

Practical considerations include taking time to carefully reconstruct the chamber geometry, becoming familiar with unconventional views of the cardiac chambers, and pacing with the least amount of current needed to allow recording during pacing.

CONCLUSIONS

The Ensite noncontact mapping system generates global endocardial activation maps that are sufficiently accurate to be used during mapping and ablation of human cardiac arrhythmias. A major advantage of noncontact mapping is the ability to map hemodynamically unstable and nonsustained arrhythmias. Perhaps its greatest potential is to permit ablation of hemodynamically unstable ventricular tachycardia. In addition to the isopotential maps, useful features of the system include the ability to rapidly sample and display a line or block of virtual electrograms from a region of interest, and a locator signal that facilitates accurate guidance of conventional ablation catheters without the use of fluoroscopy.

REFERENCES

1. Taccardi B, Arisi G, Macchi E, Barufi S, Spaggiari S. A new intracavitary probe for detecting the site of origin of ectopic ventricular beats during one cardiac cycle. Circulation 1987;75:272-281.
2. Gornick CC, Adler SW, Pederson B, Hauck J, Budd J, Schweitzer J. Validation of a new noncontact catheter system for electroanatomic mapping of left ventricular endocardium. Circulation 1999;99:829-835.
3. Strickberger SA, Knight BP, Man KC, Goyal RG, Pelosi F, Flemming M, Hasse C, Morady F. Mapping and ablation of ventricular tachycardia guided by virtual electrograms using a noncontact, computerized mapping system. J Am Coll Cardiol (In Press).
4. Schilling RJ, Peters NS, Davies DW. Simultaneous endocardial mapping in the left ventricle using a noncontact catheter. Comparison of contact and reconstructed electrograms during sinus rhythm. Circulation 1998;98:887-898.
5. Kadish A, Hauck J, Pederson B, Beatty G, Gornick. Mapping of atrial activation with a noncontact, multielectrode catheter in dogs. Circulation 1999;99:1906-1913.
6. Schilling RJ, Peters NS, Davies DW. Feasibility of a noncontact catheter for endocardial mapping of human ventricular tachycardia. Circulation 1999;99:2543-2552.
7. Schilling RJ, Davies DW, Peters NS. Characteristics of sinus rhythm electrograms at sites of ablation of ventricular tachycardia relative to all other sites: a noncontact mapping study of the entire left ventricle. J Cardiovasc Electrophysiol 1998;9:921-933.
8. Chung MK, Niebauer MA, Kidwell GA, Augostini R, Al-Khadra A, Beatty GE, Tchou PJ. The yield of endocardial mapping during sinus rhythm or pacing in localization of slow zone or exit sites during ventricular tachycardia (Abstract). J Am Coll Cardiol 1999;123A
9. Bogun F, Bender B, Li YG, Gronefeld G, Beatty G, Hohnloser S. Comparison of activation patterns during sinus rhythm and ventricular tachycardia in postinfarction patients using a non-contact mapping system (Abstract). J Am Coll Cardiol 1999;123A
10. Goyal R, Oral H, Tse HF, Kim M, Pelosi F, Flemming M, Michaud G, Knight BP, Strickberger SA, Morady F. Identification of a gap in linear radiofrequency lesions in humans using a noncontact mapping catheter (Abstract). J Am Coll Cardiol 1999; 124A.
11. Goyal R, Pelosi F, Flemming M, Souza J, Zivin A, Knight BP, Man KC, Strickberger SA, Morady F. Trans-isthmus conduction block in patients with atrial flutter assessed with a noncontact mapping catheter (Abstract). J Am Coll Cardiol 1999; I282.
12. Schilling RJ, Peters NS, Davies DW. Characterisation of functional and anatomical components of human atrial flutter using a non-contact mapping system (Abstract). J Am Coll Cardiol 1999;123A.
13. Schilling R, Peters N, Kadish A, Davies DW. Characterisation of human atrial flutter using a novel non-contact mapping system (Abstract). Pacing and Cardiac Electrophysiol 1997;20:1055.
14. Kadish A, Schilling R, Peters N, Hauck J, Davies DW. Endocardial mapping of human atrial fibrillation using a novel non-contact mapping system (Abstract). Pacing and Cardiac Electrophysiol 1997;20:1063.

Chapter 16

ENDOCARDIAL NON-CONTACT MAPPING IN PEDIATRIC AND GROWN UP CONGENITAL HEART ARRHYTHMIAS

Tim R. Betts, John M. Morgan
Wessex Cardiac Center, Southampton General Hospital, Southampton, United Kingdom

INTRODUCTION

Pediatric patients undergoing electrophysiology procedures are a heterogeneous group, ranging from small children with structurally normal hearts and WPW syndrome, to young adults with congenital heart disease who have undergone extensive palliative surgery and have multiple complex arrhythmias. For over a decade radiofrequency ablation has been an effective therapy for "simpler" arrhythmias such as atrioventricular reentry tachycardias, which account for 60- 82% of pediatric ablation procedures.[1-3] Conventional mapping and ablation techniques abolish accessory pathways with long term success rates of 83-98%.[2-7] Radiofrequency ablation of focal atrial tachycardias (a minority of patients) is less successful, with higher recurrence rates.[1-3] Pediatric patients with idiopathic ventricular tachycardia have also been successfully ablated.[8]

Most pediatric patients undergoing electrophysiology procedures have structurally normal hearts. Mapping and ablation presents more of a challenge in patients with coexisting structural heart disease. Approximately 10% of accessory pathways are associated with congenital heart disease.[1] The most common association is with Ebstein's anomaly. Multiple pathways may be present, and arrhythmia recurrence is more likely.[9] Up to 75% of pediatric patients with atrial flutter will have had previous palliative surgery for congenital heart defects.[10] As the long-term success of palliative surgery increases, many patients with complex congenital heart disease are surviving for longer. Ventricular, and in particular, atrial tachyarrhythmias are a significant long-term complication, with the incidence increasing with length of follow-up. After the Fontan procedure, atrial tachyarrhythmias occur in 20% of patients at 5 years and with long enough follow-up, may be ubiquitous.[11-13] Following the Mustard or

L. Bing Liem and E. Downar (eds.), Progress in Catheter Ablation, 241-270.
© 2001 *Kluwer Academic Publishers. Printed in the Netherlands.*

Senning procedure, 28% of patients may have spontaneous atrial flutter and 55% have inducible arrhythmias at electrophysiological study.[14] Surgical correction of tetralogy of Fallot (the most common cyanotic congenital defect with the most adult survivors) may be followed in the long-term by atrial arrhythmias in 33% of patients and ventricular arrhythmias in 6%.[15] These complex patients are particularly vulnerable to tachyarrhythmias, may suffer hemodynamic compromise, and may not tolerate medical therapy due to the presence of coexisting sinus node disease.

1.   THE CHALLENGE OF ARRHYTHMIA THERAPY POST-RECONSTRUCTIVE SURGERY

Mapping and ablation of arrhythmias in patients who have undergone palliative surgery presents particular challenges, including difficult access to the appropriate cardiac chamber, poorly tolerated arrhythmia due to impaired ventricular function and distorted anatomy such that conventional fluoroscopic views may not apply (Table 1).

Table 1. Mapping challenges in pediatric and grown-up congenital heart patients

Challenges to complex arrhythmia mapping in GUCH patients
Distorted anatomy
Poorly tolerated arrhythmia
Access to appropriate cardiac chambers
Complex anatomy
Surgical barriers
Multiple arrhythmia circuits

The arrhythmia substrate may include the original congenital defect, anatomical barriers, suture lines and incisions and artificial barriers to conduction such as baffles, patches and conduits (Table 2). There may also be changes induced by increased wall stress and volume overload, as well as changes in atrial refractoriness due to associated sinus node dysfunction and bradycardia. Under these circumstances the resulting arrhythmia mechanism is usually macroreentry, hence the nomenclature "incisional tachycardia" or "intra-atrial reentrant tachycardia". Multiple circuits may be present. In reported series (usually small groups containing a variety of congenital heart conditions), activation mapping, pace mapping and entrainment have all been used to locate sites critical to the arrhythmia circuit and suitable for radiofrequency ablation.[15-20] In these reports, identification of surgical boundaries relied heavily on operation records. Atriotomy incisions were identified by double potentials. Patches and baffles were presumed to occur at sites with no electrograms and where pacing stimuli failed to capture. Radiofrequency burns were applied as focal lesions or as lines across the narrowest gap between two critical barriers to conduction. Using these methods, initial success rates of 73-90% were achieved, although recurrence rates of up to 50% by 6 months follow-up were recorded. Patients with single reentrant circuits (those with surgical repair of atrial septal defects and tetralogy of Fallot) were more likely to have procedural success than those with complex chambers with multiple circuits (e.g. following the Fontan procedure).

Table 2. Arrhythmic substrate in the surgically altered cardiac chamber

Natural barriers	Artificial barriers	Hemodynamic and structural changes
Valve annuli	Suture lines	Raised pressures
Caval veins	Baffles	Increased wall stress
Coronary sinus	Patches	Chamber dilatation
Septal defects	Conduits	Myocardial fibrosis
Crista terminalis	Incisions	Myocardial hypertrophy

More complex arrhythmias require more detailed electrophysiological mapping (Table 3). A number of advances in mapping technology, including the basket catheter,[21] electroanatomical mapping[22,23] and non-contact mapping, have been developed to provide high-density activation maps of complex cardiac chambers (Table 4). In this chapter we will describe the use of non-contact mapping in the setting of pediatric arrhythmias, commenting on general techniques and considerations as well as our personal experience.

Table 3. Electrophysiological mapping techniques

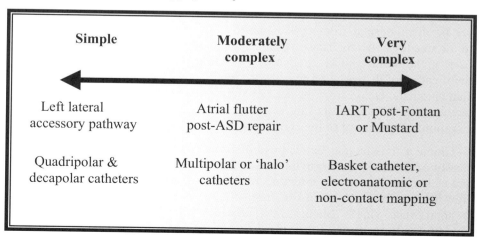

Simple	Moderately complex	Very complex
Left lateral accessory pathway	Atrial flutter post-ASD repair	IART post-Fontan or Mustard
Quadripolar & decapolar catheters	Multipolar or 'halo' catheters	Basket catheter, electroanatomic or non-contact mapping

Table 4. Advanced mapping technologies

Technology	Catheter locator signal	3 dimensional reconstruction	Non-sustained arrhythmia	Data points collected	Peak voltage map	Electrograms
Basket catheter	No	No	Yes	10's	No	Requires basket contact. Bipolar
Electroanatomic mapping	Yes	Yes (requires new geometry for each new arrhythmia)	No	10's – 100's	Yes	Requires catheter contact. Unipolar or bipolar
Non-contact mapping	Yes	Yes	Yes	>3,000	Yes	Non-contact. Unipolar. Accuracy reduced at sites >4cm from MEA center

2.   NON-CONTACT MAPPING

Non-contact mapping using the EnSite 3000 system (Endocardial Solutions Inc., St. Paul, MN) has been described in detail in the previous chapter and in other publications.[24-26] Although initially designed to guide ablation of ischemic ventricular tachycardia, it has subsequently been applied to a whole spectrum of arrhythmias involving every cardiac chamber. The system enables high density, multisite mapping of the entire endocardial surface of the cardiac chamber under examination. Reconstruction of chamber geometry produces a three-dimensional image that can be viewed from any angle, externally, internally or in an open view (where the whole surface is seen). The image can be manipulated to represent standard fluoroscopic views. Important cardiac structures are labeled on the geometry allowing their role in arrhythmia propagation to be determined. Isopotential color maps represent wave fronts of depolarisation that not only indicate when a point on the endocardial surface is activated, but also where the activation traveled from and where it subsequently goes. Thus, bystander circuits may be distinguished from critical diastolic pathways that are appropriate for radiofrequency ablation. Tracking an isopotential map back in time to before the onset of the surface ECG, gradually increasing the sensitivity, allows precise identification of the earliest site of endocardial activation. This may be the focus of an automatic tachycardia, or the exit site from a zone of slow conduction in a macroreentrant tachycardia. In some cases it is also possible to visualize activation within part of or the entire protected zone of slow conduction.[24,27]

Global activation may be recorded in a single beat. This is particularly useful in cases of non-sustained arrhythmia, such as idiopathic right ventricular outflow tract tachycardia, or poorly tolerated arrhythmias which may be terminated after a few beats before the patient becomes compromised. Theoretically, mapping of an appropriate single ectopic beat provides enough information to guide successful radiofrequency ablation of a tachyarrhythmia.

In contrast to electroanatomical mapping, if a new arrhythmia is induced it may be mapped without the need to recreate chamber geometry. This is based on the assumption that activation at the critical point in an arrhythmia circuit (the focus or exit site from a zone of slow conduction) occurs during late diastole, before the onset of the surface QRS or P wave. The chamber under examination will be at maximum distension i.e. with the endocardial surface at its greatest distance from the balloon array, and thus identical to the shape of the reconstructed geometry, regardless of the tachycardia origin. Therefore, isopotential recordings can be made during sinus rhythm, any induced arrhythmia or during pacing manoeuvres.

The non-contact nature of the EnSite system also has advantages over conventional mapping with multipolar catheters by avoiding the need for good electrode contact. This may be particularly important in large, dilated or distorted chambers, especially if they contain inert material such as patches or baffles. The ability to create reconstructed "virtual" unipolar electrograms at any site on the geometry facilitates the differentiation of true activation from repolarization artefact and adds further information to that gained from the isopotential maps when assessing activation patterns and timing.

In complex congenital heart disease, situs abnormalities may make orientation confusing, with standard fluoroscopy planes difficult to interpret. Non-contact mapping has the advantage of navigation via the geometry, once a few labels have been added to orientate the operator. Conduction tissue may be in an unusual location (e.g. a more posterior location near the CS os, as in ostium primum atrial septal defects), increasing the risk of heart block. Non-contact mapping can identify the site of His potentials and, providing retrograde conduction is via the atrioventricular node, locate the site of earliest atrial activation during ventricular pacing as the area containing the compact node.

One limitation of non-contact mapping is that only one chamber can be mapped using the system. However, any number of additional contact catheters may be used and their electrograms displayed alongside the EnSite data. Far-field activity from adjacent cardiac chambers may be detected, but this can be avoided by judicious use of adenosine (to provide transient atrioventricular block and avoid ventricular artefact when recording atrial arrhythmias) or by examining electrograms in the appropriate contact catheters.

Non-contact mapping calculates endocardial potentials and provides electrograms and isopotential maps of endocardial activity. Although this is appropriate for arrhythmias that are endocardial in origin, other arrhythmia circuits may have a critical epicardial or intramural component. It is not yet clear how deep into the myocardium non-contact mapping can record, although the amplitude of an electrical potential will obviously play a role in whether it is detected or not.

Another limitation is the need to recreate chamber geometry if the multielectrode array becomes displaced. Fortunately, this is a rare occurrence.

3.   SPECIAL CONSIDERATIONS FOR PEDIATRIC PATIENTS:

3.1   Chamber size

The dimensions of the multielectrode array when fully expanded are 4.5x1.8cm, with a volume of 7.5ml. It is conceivable that in small chambers it will obstruct blood flow, resulting in hemodynamic compromise. The smallest patient we have studied to date weighed 32 kilograms. However, it is the chamber dimensions that are the most important factor. The majority of pediatric patients undergoing non-contact mapping are likely to have complex arrhythmias in abnormal cardiac chambers that may have undergone surgical correction. These chambers are usually dilated and sometimes have reduced contractility, allowing multielectrode array deployment without compromise.   Chamber dimension should be carefully measured by echocardiography, angiography and if necessary, magnetic resonance imaging, to ensure that the multielectrode array has adequate room.

3.2   Catheter size and characteristics

The catheter shaft on which the multielectrode array (MEA) is mounted is 9-French in diameter. This has not caused difficulties with vascular access to date but may potentially prevent the MEA from being deployed across baffle leaks or fenestrations (see below). The rigidity of the shaft improves catheter stability, but may result in difficulties in MEA placement if acute angles need to be negotiated. Right atrial deployment via the superior or inferior caval veins, and left ventricular deployment retrogradely across the aortic valve, is easily attained. Right ventricular deployment, particularly when aiming for the apex via the inferior caval vein, can be difficult. We have found that the use of extra-stiff guide wires that may be bent into a desired shape can facilitate deployment. It is important, however, to be aware of the risk of myocardial perforation when manipulating the stiff catheter within pediatric cardiac chambers.

3.3   Accessibility

In structurally normal hearts, the right atrium and left ventricle are accessed without difficulty and the multielectrode array may be placed in a stable position. Access to the right ventricle, as previously mentioned, may require extra manipulation with the aid of stiff guide wires. The left atrium may be accessed via patent foramen ovale or trans-septal puncture. However, it should be noted that access for both the MEA and an ablation catheter is required. Prosthetic or stenosed aortic valves may prevent access to the left ventricle. As with any electrophysiology procedure in complex congenital heart disease, surgical interventions may result in limited or difficult access to the cardiac chamber that needs to be mapped. Baffles and patches (such as the lateral tunnel in the modified Fontan operation) may exclude the MEA from the dominant chamber responsible for the arrhythmia. Although it may be possible to cross baffles via fenestrations or eccentric leaks, it may be more appropriate to do so with small diameter, flexible or steerable multipolar catheter than with the stiff MEA. To access the venous return chamber, the MEA may be inserted via the inferior caval, subclavian or internal jugular veins. Previous surgery, such as a bi-directional Glen anastomosis, will mean that access is limited to the inferior caval vein route.

3.4   Patient preparation

Patient consent needs to include additional information of the use of anticoagulation to prevent thromboembolism. The use of heparin, combined with the 9-French catheter shaft, may result in an increased risk of bruising and hemorrhage at the site of vascular access. Otherwise, consent must include information on the risks of perforation, pneumothorax and heart block etc in common with other ablation procedures.

In our institution, pediatric patients have their procedures carried out under general anesthesia. We have extended this policy to include young adults with complex congenital heart disease who are undergoing non-contact mapping. As the majority will have complex arrhythmias, often with multiple circuits, procedure times are long. Patient comfort is increased by general anesthesia, which also minimizes the risk of MEA displacement.

3.5   Fluoroscopy and procedure times

One of the perceived advantages of 3-dimensional non-contact mapping is a reduction in fluoroscopy dosage. Although we have found this to be the case in some adult scenarios (such as ablation of ischaemic ventricular tachycardia or common atrial flutter), the fluoroscopy times in complex congenital heart disease are still high. Fluoroscopy is used during creation of chamber geometry to check on catheter tip position and ensure that only points from the chamber under examination are collected. Accurate geometry is vital, and in complex, distorted and surgically altered chambers, it can take up to 45 minutes to complete the process. If additional contact catheters are used, either in the same chamber or in other areas of the heart, their positioning and manipulation is still performed under fluoroscopic guidance.

3.6   Anatomical landmarks – identification and labeling

By attaching the locator signal to the steerable ablation catheter, its precise position can be plotted on the chamber geometry. Using fluoroscopy and ablation catheter tip electrograms, the position of cardiac valves, vessel orifices and anatomical landmarks can be labeled on the chamber geometry. In the right atrium, for example, it is conventional to label a number of points on the inferior and superior caval vein orifices, the coronary sinus os and at least 4 points around the tricuspid valve annulus. The septum, free wall and atrial appendage may also be marked. This allows accurate orientation around the chamber, reduces the need for fluoroscopy, and guides linear lesion placement, ensuring that the appropriate margins are reached.

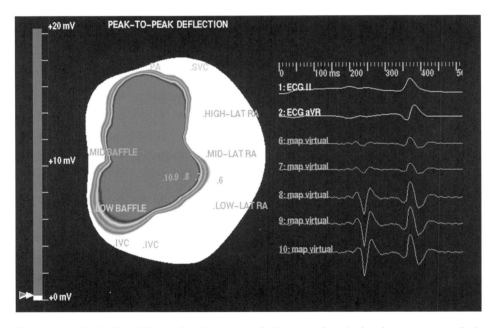

Figure 1 (see Color Plate 16). Peak voltage map of a Fontan atrium (atriopulmonary connection). Right atrial geometry is displayed in a right posterior oblique plane. Peak voltages are measured from >3000 sites on the endocardial surface during a single cycle (of sinus rhythm in this example). Areas with peak voltages >0.4mV are displayed in purple and areas <0.4mV are displayed in white. Virtual unipolar electrograms are displayed alongside, with the sites from which they are recorded indicated by the numbered position on the geometry. This example demonstrates that the majority of atrial mass in the chronic Fontan atrium consists of diseased, hypertrophied myocardium plus inert surgical material. Only a small area of the posterior wall displays electrical potentials of significant value. Electrograms recorded from the white area are small, fractionated or absent. During isopotential mapping activation was seen to spread over the purple area. The remainder of the atrium was electrically silent.

In cardiac chambers that are distorted through congenital malformation or have undergone surgical alteration, identification of anatomical landmarks is a more convoluted process. Fluoroscopy, angiography, electrogram characteristics, response to pacing stimuli, plus an in-depth review of all operation records are required for an accurate and detailed chamber reconstruction. Cardiac valves and vessel and conduit openings may be identified by fluoroscopy and angiography, together with changes in electrogram morphology (e.g. absence of contact electrograms from the catheter tip when touching vessel or conduit walls). Baffles and patches, which are electrically inert materials, can be identified by the loss of contact electrograms and the failure of pacing stimuli to capture at maximum output. The latest version of software also has a peak voltage map. The peak voltages reached on the endocardial surface between two designated points in time are displayed as a color map. Areas with peak voltages close to 0 mV represent electrically inert material or myocardium (figure 1).

Suture lines and incisions, such as atriotomy scars, may be identified by the presence of double potentials during tachycardia.[17] This will only be the case if the incision is acting as a line of block, with differing activation times on either side (figure 2). All these techniques rely on the use of contact catheters and electrograms, and have been applied in previous studies.[16-20] When applied to non-contact mapping, there is the additional advantage of being able to visualise the three dimensional position of the catheter tip and relate its position to chamber geometry and other anatomical landmarks. Reconstructed virtual electrograms may also be examined from selected points on the endocardial surface to look for similar changes in morphology that relate to underlying structures. Finally, isopotential maps recorded during tachycardia, sinus rhythm or pacing may add further information by demonstrating the site of barriers to conduction.

Review of operation notes will allow the operator to determine the likely chamber geometry, remembering that it may have been remodeled subsequently by pressure or volume overload. Also, hypertrophy, scarring and fibrosis induced by these changes, may cause areas to be electrically inactive or display small, fractionated electrograms. This is more likely in older patients with long follow up since initial surgery. Inert or abnormal areas may be mistaken for surgical material if not accurately located on the geometry. We have found this to be a particular feature of atriotomy scars in the Fontan atrium. Rather than displaying a discrete line of double potentials, these grossly abnormal atria often demonstrate a large area of low amplitude or absent electrograms in the lateral wall area where the atriotomy incision is presumed to be (Figure 1).

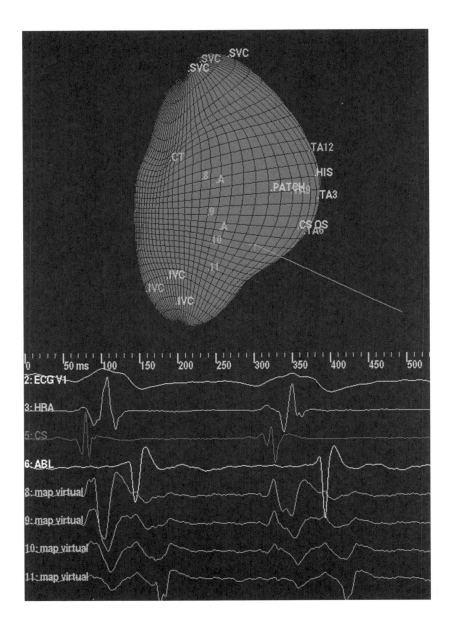

Figure 2 (see Color Plate 17). Double potentials around an atriotomy incision during atrial flutter: Right atrial geometry is viewed in a right anterior oblique plane. Virtual electrograms in channels 8-10 are recorded from the sites labeled on the map, along the presumed atriotomy incision on the lateral right atrial wall. The position of the ablation catheter tip is indicated by the locator signal (green line). Double potentials are seen in the virtual electrograms, indicating that the incision acts as a line of conduction block. Labels in green are on the near side of the geometry. Labels in yellow are on the far side and seen through the geometry. SVC, superior vena cava; IVC, inferior vena cava; CS OS, coronary sinus ostium; TA, tricuspid valve annulus; CT, crista terminalis.

3.7   Additional catheters and techniques

Non-contact mapping is best utilized as an adjunct rather than alternative to conventional mapping techniques. As previously mentioned, conventional catheters are still required for geometry creation and labeling, identification of anatomical landmarks and recording of activity in adjacent cardiac chambers. Small diameter multipolar catheters may be required for access across fenestrations or baffles.

Following identification of a target site for radiofrequency ablation and navigation of the ablation catheter to the proposed site, examination of the contact electrogram from the catheter tip will confirm electrogram timing. We routinely perform pace mapping or entrainment prior to ablation for further reassurance that the target site is within the arrhythmia circuit or is at the earliest site of activation. Although entrainment has been successfully used to guide ablation in complex congenital heart disease (such as Fontan[16] or Mustard[20] patients), we have found it on occasions to be an inconclusive technique. In large, diseased chambers containing significant amounts of inert surgical material, P wave morphology may be difficult to determine and may be predominantly derived from the adjacent, healthier atrial chamber. Pacing stimuli may only intermittently capture, either through poor catheter stability lack of capture in diseased myocardium. Non-contact mapping allows accurate determination of the arrhythmia circuit even when these other conventional techniques fail.

4.   WHO TO STUDY

Non-contact mapping is not required for the majority of pediatric patients. Results of radiofrequency ablation of accessory pathways, AV nodal reentry tachycardia and most cases of sustained idiopathic ventricular tachycardia have excellent success rates using conventional methods.[2-6,8] Automatic atrial tachycardias have a lower success rate. In the structurally normal heart, we therefore reserve non-contact mapping for pediatric patients who have either failed previous attempts at ablation (arrhythmia recurrence or no initial procedural success), have focal atrial tachycardias, or have non-sustained arrhythmias (such as right ventricular outflow tract tachycardia).

At our institution, pediatric patients who have congenital heart disease, particularly if they have undergone palliative surgery, undergo non-contact mapping unless there is a contraindication (such as chamber size or accessibility). Patients with complex cardiac conditions are more likely to suffer arrhythmia recurrence following conventional methods and often have multiple arrhythmia circuits. Use of non-contact mapping at the initial electrophysiology procedure may increase the likelihood of success (although in heavily diseased cardiac chambers emergence of a new arrhythmia may be inevitable) and reduce the need for subsequent therapies.

Table 5. Pediatric and GUCH patient non-contact mapping procedures performed at Southampton General Hospital

Patient (age)	Condition	NCM Chamber	Tachycardia mechanism	Critical area targeted for ablation	Procedure (fluoroscopy time) minutes	Outcome
ML (24)	ASD repair	RA	IART	Cavotricuspid isthmus	245 (60)	No recurrence after 4 months
LS (25)	ASD repair	RA	IART	Superior atriotomy-SVC os	345 (132)	No recurrence after 7 months
HC (63)	ASD repair	RA	IART	Cavotricuspid isthmus	235 (46)	No recurrence after 8 months
MD (10)	Normal heart	RA	Focal AT	Mid-lateral crista terminalis	220 (16)	No recurrence after 8 months
JV (17)	Normal heart	RA	Focal AT	Mid-lateral crista terminalis	150 (30)	No recurrence after 3 months
SF (16)	Tricuspid atresia	LA	Focal AT	Left inferior septum	420 (72)	New tachycardia at 11 months
NA (17)	Normal heart	RV	Mahaim	RV septum	210 (27)	No recurrence after 10 months
CC (36)	Fallots tetralogy	RV	Incisional VT (macroreentry)	Inferoapical septum between VSD patch and ventriculotomy	385 (99)	New tachycardia at 3 months
ZP (17)	Normal heart	RV	Focal	Septal RVOT	260 (38)	No recurrence after 6 months
CH (11)	Ebstein's	RA	AVRT	Posteroseptal space	170 (17)	Recurrence after 1 month. Repeat procedure successful
JBe (23)	Fontan (APC)	RA	IART	Atriotomy-TV patch	270 (45.2)	Unable to terminate tachycardia
JBu (15)	Fontan (APC)	RA	IART	Atriotomy-IVC	300 (59.5)	Recurrence at 3 weeks
DC (19)	Fontan (APC)	RA	IART	Atriotomy-IVC	405 (46)	No recurrence at 5 months
GS (21)	Fontan (APC)	RA	IART	Atriopulmonary connection-TV patch	320 (73)	Infrequent, asymptomatic episodes
KT (17)	Fontan (APC)	RA	IART	Atriotomy-IVC	420 (58)	Recurrent non-sustained attacks
KS (18)	Fontan (RA-RV conduit)	RA	IART	RA-RV conduit-CS os-IVC	45 (7)	No recurrence at 15 months
GH (23)	Fontan (lateral tunnel)	Lateral tunnel	IART (left sided)	Inferior lateral tunnel margin (on left and right sides)	350 (103)	Immediate recurrence

Pediatric and grown-up congenital heart patients who have undergone non-contact mapping studies at our institution are summarized in Table 5

5.   SPECIFIC EXAMPLES

5.1   Atrial arrhythmias

Non-contact mapping is ideally suited to the treatment of right atrial arrhythmias. The limiting factor is the size of the atrial chamber. Validation studies show that the relationship of virtual electrogram timing and reconstruction becomes less reliable when the centre of the MEA is greater than 4.0 cm from the endocardial surface, and this limit may be approached in the giant Fontan right atrium.[25,28] The right atrium is best approached via the inferior vena cava (Figure 3).

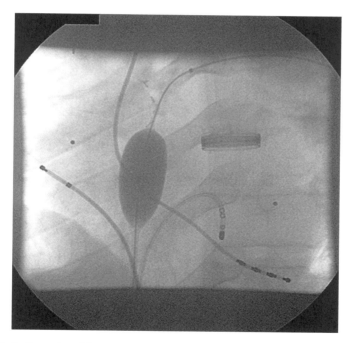

Figure 3. Left anterior oblique view. The contrast-filled MEA is seen in the middle of the right atrium. The guidewire extends from the distal catheter into the pulmonary artery through the anastomosis. A bipolar catheter is positioned against the anterolateral wall and a quadripolar catheter is positioned in the coronary sinus via a superior vena cava approach. The ablation catheter is positioned near the coronary sinus ostium. Note the wide dimensions of the chamber. The patient also has a prosthetic aortic valve.

If the superior vena cava is patent the catheter may be orientated with the guidewire extending up into the SVC to increase stability and position the balloon in the middle of the atrial chamber. If the SVC has been closed (e.g.

following a bi-directional Glen anastomosis and subsequent Fontan procedure) the catheter may be orientated towards the right atrial-pulmonary artery anastomosis with the guidewire extending into the pulmonary artery. Intravenous heparin is required to keep the ACT > 300. Intravenous adenosine injection may be used during recording of atrial activation to induce temporary complete heart block and allow atrial mapping without artefact from far-field sensing of ventricular activation.

5.1.1   Atrial flutter (post-atriotomy and atrial septal defect repairs)

Atrial flutter may occur following repair of atrial septal defects and other atrial surgical procedures. In addition to the substrate found in normal hearts (unidirectional block and slow conduction in the cavotricuspid isthmus plus functional block in the crista terminalis), the right atrial atriotomy incision and the septal patch may also act as barriers to conduction. The substrate is therefore more complex and an "incisional" flutter with atypical ECG morphology may arise. These flutters may not be amenable to anatomically based ablation of the cavotricuspid isthmus.

We have mapped and ablated 3 patients with atrial flutter after ASD closure. Non-contact mapping demonstrated the exit site from the zone of slow conduction in each case. Although all three patients had surgically altered atria, the critical point in the arrhythmia circuit was the cavotricuspid isthmus in 2 patients. Activation was seen to emerge from the isthmus 20-30 msec before global activation and climb the posterior septum and cross the posterior wall in a caudo-cranial direction. The ASD patch limited septal activation, with the wavefront rotating around the patch in a clockwise direction (when viewed from a right anterior oblique angle). In this situation, the atriotomy scar acted as a barrier between the posterior and anterolateral walls in a similar fashion to the crista terminalis (which is in close proximity). Although this circuit is similar to the common atrial flutter circuit, surface ECG morphology may be atypical as the ASD patch can influence the electrical mass of the septum and may affect left atrial activation patterns, changing electrical vectors.

The third patient had a flutter circuit that rotated around the lateral atriotomy scar. The cycle length was shorter with atypical P wave morphology on the surface ECG. Activation was seen to ascend the anterolateral wall between the tricuspid valve annulus and the atriotomy incision. The wavefront slowly turned around the superior margin of the atriotomy to descend across the posterior wall. A linear lesion from the superior aspect of the atriotomy incision to the superior vena cava terminated the tachycardia. Non-contact mapping allowed accurate localization of the upper margin of the atriotomy, represented by the pivot point for the wavefront on the isopotential map. The gap between this site and the SVC was 1.8 cm and was the narrowest point in the arrhythmia circuit. The catheter locator signal was able to determine the ablation catheter tip position to ensure linear lesion accuracy and continuity.

5.1.2   Intra-atrial reentrant tachycardia in the Fontan atrium

Patients who have undergone the Fontan procedure for tricuspid atresia or double inlet ventricle have a high incidence of late onset atrial arrhythmias. The substrate is complex, including the original congenital malformation, the (often multiple) surgical procedures resulting in incisions, baffles, patches and conduits, and the resultant hemodynamic and pathological changes that occur in the remaining atrial myocardium (Table 2). Within published series of ablation in pediatric patients, Fontan patients often have the lowest success rates. This is either due to the inability to locate a site suitable for ablation, or due to early arrhythmia recurrence. The complexity of arrhythmia circuits in a grossly dilated, diseased chamber makes mapping and ablation by conventional means a challenging procedure.

We have performed non-contact mapping on 6 patients with the classic atriopulmonary Fontan procedure. Each patient required a thorough work up with angiography, echocardiography and detailed review of the operation records to help identification of anatomical landmarks. The average time from last surgery was 6.5 years. The hemodynamic strain placed on the Fontan circuit can dramatically distort atrial architecture. Large areas of myocardium may gradually become hypertrophied, fibrosed and electrically inert, which may add to the substrate and be difficult to distinguish from prosthetic surgical material. Although large chamber size may limit the accuracy of non-contact mapping, we found that the balloon often sat in the middle of the chamber with most of the endocardial surface within 4 cm from the balloon center (Figure 3). Multipolar catheters were introduced to augment non-contact mapping information with bipolar contact electrograms. Very limited information was gathered from these multipolar catheters due to a combination of poor contact and the large amount of inert myocardium. Similarly, entrainment techniques were frustrated by intermittent capture of the pacing stimulus and non-distinct P wave morphology. The bulk of the surface P wave appeared to be derived from left atrial activation. The right atrium was largely inert and added very little to P wave appearance. Consequently, ablation was predominantly guided by isopotential mapping and virtual electrogram morphology.

Patients typically had multiple tachycardia circuits. One advantage of non-contact mapping was that the initial reconstructed geometry could be used for each arrhythmia. Arrhythmias with P wave morphologies and cycle lengths similar to those previously recorded on 12-lead ECGs were identified as clinical arrhythmias and were the principal targets for ablation. Arrhythmia circuits were macroreentrant, using surgical and anatomical structures as barriers to conduction. An example is shown in Figure 4. Ablation lesions were targeted at the narrowest gap between two barriers that appeared to be crucial to the arrhythmia circuit. The positions of radiofrequency lesions were labeled on the geometry using the locator signal. Linear lesions were attempted until the arrhythmia terminated and conduction block could be demonstrated during pacing. Non-contact mapping was used to record activation following pacing from the ablation catheter when placed adjacent to the linear lesion. This allowed identification of gaps within the lesion that could then be targeted by steering the ablation catheter to that site using the locator signal. In common with other reported studies we found that the atriotomy incision was the most commonly targeted barrier, necessitating a linear lesion from its inferior margin to the inferior vena cava os.

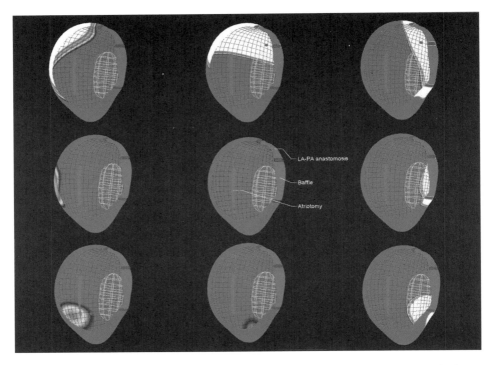

Figure 4 (see Color Plate 18). Fontan (atriopulmonary connection): Right atrial geometry is shown in a left lateral plane. The medial wall has been clipped away to allow an internal view of the structure. The left atrial roof to pulmonary artery anastomosis plus the pericardial baffle that helps direct flow from the IVC to the anastomosis have been drawn on the geometry. The lateral wall atriotomy scar is also depicted. The yellow frame depicts the position of the MEA. The colored areas represent negative endocardial potentials (depolarization) against the purple background. Macroreentry is visualised moving around the atrium in an anti-clockwise fashion. The atriotomy acts as a central barrier to conduction. As the activation wavefront descends anterior to the atriotomy is becomes low amplitude with reduced velocity. A radiofrequency linear lesion between the lower atriotomy and inferior vena cava terminated tachycardia.

Despite short-term success in 5/6 patients, the recurrence rate remains high with 4/5 patients having further arrhythmias by 6 months. One patient who underwent intraoperative non-contact mapping and cryoablation during conduit replacement has had no further arrhythmias. Four patients have subsequently undergone surgical conversion to total cavopulmonary connection with an extra-cardiac conduit and cryotherapy lesions. During their operations the right atrial endocardial surface was examined for evidence of radiofrequency lesions. The section of the lateral wall (including the atriotomy incision) that is removed during conversion surgery was examined histologically. There was no macroscopic evidence of scarring from radiofrequency energy in any of the hearts examined. The myocardium was over 1cm thick with significant fibrotic changes. We believe that non-contact mapping identified suitable sites for ablation (as radiofrequency energy transiently stopped the arrhythmia in the majority of cases) but the ablation technology used was not capable of providing transmural, continuous lesions. In addition to the fibrotic, hypertrophied myocardium, the low flow hemodynamics in the Fontan circuit result in excessive heat loss into the blood pool during RF application. Future ablation technologies may help to overcome these obstacles.

Patients who have undergone lateral tunnel surgery present a greater challenge. A significant proportion of the systemic venous return chamber (the tunnel) is made up of inert baffle material. The majority of atrial myocardium is on the left side (pulmonary venous return) and may be inaccessible. A fenestration may have been placed in the baffle, or a leak may be present, providing a communication between the two. Although conventional catheters may be placed across this communication to provide left atrial mapping, we have not positioned the EnSite catheter across. The large gauge and relative stiffness of the catheter shaft preclude this. As a consequence, mapping is more limited.

Providing it is large enough to accommodate the balloon, non-contact mapping of the tunnel will identify sites where activation breaks through across the baffle suture line from the left side into the tunnel myocardium. If a critical part of the arrhythmia circuit involves the tunnel, then ablation of these breakthrough sites may terminate the arrhythmia. If the tunnel is activated as a bystander circuit then ablation needs to be guided by conventional mapping in the left atrial chamber. Non-contact mapping may identify the exit site from the tunnel and aid positioning of mapping and ablation catheters on the left side.

5.1.3 Intra-atrial reentrant tachycardia after the Mustard / Senning procedure

Atrial arrhythmias are common following the Mustard or Senning procedure with an incidence of up to 43% by 5 years follow-up.[10,14] Following the onset of atrial flutter there is a 5-fold increase in sudden death, presumed to be due to 1:1 conduction.[29] Both procedures result in extensive surgical alteration of the atria with atriotomies and baffle material. They provide a particular challenge, as the pulmonary venous return chamber (containing the pulmonary veins, trabeculated right atrium and tricuspid valve) is inaccessible unless there is a baffle puncture or leak or a retrograde approach is undertaken. In a small series of 10 patients using activation timing and entrainment, successful sites were predominantly found in the posteroinferior systemic or pulmonary venous atrium, near or at the opening of the coronary sinus.[20] Success was more likely when the coronary sinus drained into the systemic venous atrium.

Non-contact mapping in these patients plays a similar role to that in patients whom have undergone the lateral tunnel variant of the Fontan procedure. The balloon catheter may only be positioned in the systemic venous return chamber. It cannot be maneuvered into the pulmonary venous return chamber via the retrograde approach. We would not recommend attempting to position the catheter across a baffle puncture or leak. Providing the critical component of the arrhythmia circuit is in the same chamber as the balloon catheter, non-contact mapping may readily identify the tachycardia circuit. This may be the case for patients in whom the coronary sinus drains into the systemic venous return chamber. Otherwise, non-contact mapping has little more to add over conventional contact catheter techniques.

5.1.4   Focal atrial tachycardias

Non-contact mapping is ideally suited to treatment of focal arrhythmias. Using isopotential maps, activation may be tracked back in time to the point of earliest endocardial activation. By increasing amplifier gain and color contrast and offset sensitivity, the earliest site can be pinpointed to a precise area a few millimeters in diameter. Using the cursor, virtual unipolar electrograms from this site can be displayed. The presence of a QS complex confirms that this site is likely to be the true tachycardia origin. Activation times may be referenced to the surface ECG and the ablation catheter may be steered to the precise area using the locator signal (see Figure 5).

Non-contact mapping has revealed that within a few msec of the onset of activation, depolarization can spread out from the focus into adjacent myocardium. Within 5 msec of onset an area of 1-2 cm^2 may have been activated. Identification of the precise site of earliest activation may be difficult using contact catheter bipolar electrogram timings. Pace mapping may confirm that the catheter tip is close the correct area but the pacing stimulus may capture a significant area of myocardium, again limiting precision. With non-contact mapping, identification of the exact site of onset enables tachycardia ablation with a single radiofrequency lesion. With high right atrial tachycardias, non-contact mapping during sinus rhythm allows identification of the sinus node complex, which may be labeled onto chamber geometry. This reduces the risk of damage to the sinus node and may be helpful for sinus node modification in those patients with inappropriate sinus tachycardia. Likewise, identification of His bundle and slow pathway potentials on chamber geometry will decrease the risk of damage to the AV junction.

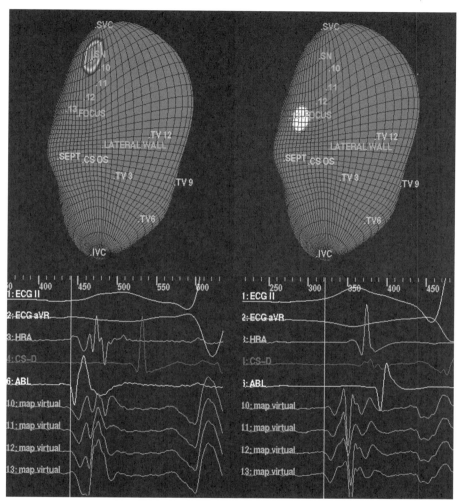

Figure 5 (see Color Plate 19). Focal atrial tachycardia. An external view of right atrial geometry in a right anterior oblique plane. Negative potentials (depolarization) are depicted as colors against a purple background. Contact and virtual electrograms are shown. Virtual unipolar electrograms (channels 10–13) are taken from the points on the geometry marked by the appropriate numbers. The yellow vertical line indicates the point in time that corresponds to the isopotential map. A) Sinus rhythm. The site of earliest activation is the high right atrium/SVC junction (i.e. the sinus node complex). This coincides with the onset of the surface P wave. The high right atrial catheter (HRA) and ablation catheter (ABL) are also positioned close to the sinus node. The virtual unipolar electrograms confirm that activation begins at number 10 and spreads in a caudal direction. The earliest electrogram has a QS configuration. B) Automatic atrial tachycardia. The site of earliest activation is on the mid lateral wall within the crista terminalis. Activation in the high right atrial and ablation catheters occurs later in the cycle. The earliest activation in the virtual electrograms is now in number 13, with activation spreading in a cranial direction. Labels in green are on the near side of the geometry. Labels in yellow are on the far side and seen through the geometry. SVC, superior vena cava; IVC, inferior vena cava; SEPT, atrial septum; CS OS, coronary sinus ostium; TV, tricuspid valve; SN, sinus node.

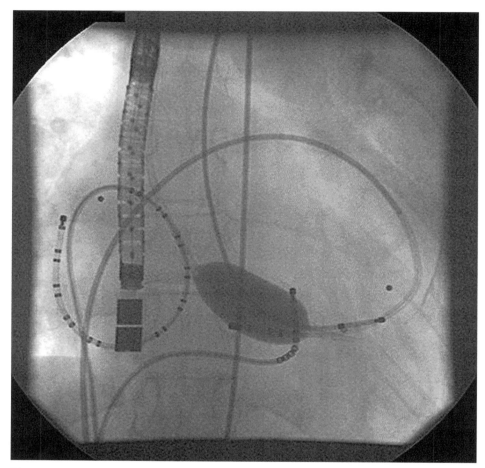

Figure 6. Anteroposterior view. The patient has uncorrected tricuspid atresia, a large atrial septal defect (ASD) and an automatic left atrial tachycardia. The MEA has been positioned across the ASD via a superior approach. A multipolar catheter is positioned in the right atrium. A coronary sinus catheter has been positioned via an inferior approach. A bipolar electrode has been positioned in the left ventricle via a retrograde approach. The ablation catheter has been positioned across the ASD and looped inside the left atrium to place the tip on the left side of the inferior septal remnant. A transoesophageal probe is in-situ.

We have employed non-contact mapping in pediatric patients with structurally normal hearts and focal atrial tachycardias in order to reduce fluoroscopy time and the number of radiofrequency lesions. We have also studied a patient with uncorrected tricuspid atresia with a focal tachycardia arising from the left side of the interatrial septum (Figure 6). A previous ablation attempt at this site had been abandoned due to the proximity of the His bundle. The balloon was passed across the atrial septal defect into the left atrial chamber with the tip of the catheter positioned in the left atrial appendage. Non-contact mapping confirmed the earliest site of activation to be on the inferior margin of the left atrial septum. The His bundle was identified using ablation catheter electrograms and labeled onto chamber geometry. The site of earliest activation was ablated and the tachycardia rendered non-inducible. At 10 months follow-up there had been no arrhythmia recurrence.

5.2   Accessory pathways

5.2.1   Accessory pathways and Ebstein's anomaly

Uncomplicated accessory pathway ablation can be treated with a high success rate using conventional catheter techniques. In certain circumstances where there may be unusual anatomy, multiple pathways and a greater risk of recurrence, non-contact mapping may be advantageous. The positioning of the MEA depends upon the size of the chambers involved and the direction of activation through the accessory pathway. In Ebstein's anomaly, the right atrium is usually large enough to accommodate the balloon, but the right ventricle may be small and distorted, particularly if the attachment of the septal leaflet of the tricuspid valve is towards the ventricular apex. Non-contact mapping will locate the earliest site of activation within that chamber. Consequently the balloon needs to be positioned in the chamber that receives the distal end of the accessory pathway conduction during tachycardia or pacing (i.e. the right atrium for orthodromic tachycardia with a right-sided pathway). Activation may be mapped during tachycardia or pacing from within the chamber at the proximal end of the accessory pathway. If multiple pathways are present within the same chamber, activation maps for each tachycardia can be recorded without the need for re-creation of chamber geometry. An example of a patient with an accessory pathway and Ebstein's anomaly is shown in Figure 7.

5.2.2   Mahaim tachycardias

We have also used non-contact mapping to guide radiofrequency ablation of Mahaim tachycardias in pediatric patients. Long atriofascicular or nodofascicular pathways may have distal arborization and a wide distal insertion of up to 2cm.[30] Non-contact mapping is used to locate the body of the Mahaim bundle or the distal insertion site during tachycardia or paced atrial extrastimuli. The right bundle branch may also be identified, reducing the risk of iatrogenic right bundle branch block. Retrograde conduction over the Mahaim pathways is unusual; ablation of the proximal atrial insertion site is usually not feasible with non-contact mapping and ventricular pacing.

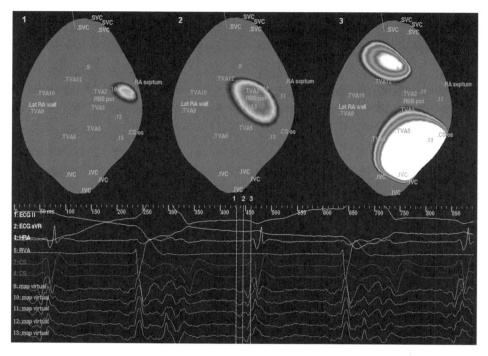

Figure 7 (see Color Plate 20). Accessory pathway and Ebstein's anomaly: 3 frames from a single cycle of tachycardia are shown. Right atrial geometry is depicted in a left anterior oblique view. Negative endocardial potentials (depolarization) are indicated by the colors on the isopotential map against a purple background. Contact and virtual electrograms are shown below. The virtual electrograms (channels 9-13) are taken from the corresponding sites labeled on the right atrial geometry. The vertical yellow lines correspond to the points in time that are displayed on the isopotential maps. 1) Earliest right atrial activation. A small, low amplitude area of depolarization is seen on the anteromedial septum. 2) Activation moves in an anterior direction towards the tricuspid valve annulus, still low amplitude. This is depicted as a small negative potential in the virtual electrograms. 3) Global activation begins and spreads around the tricuspid valve annulus and over the right atrial endocardial surface. This corresponds with a larger, steeper QS complex in the virtual electrograms. In this case, tracking activation back to the earliest site facilitated successful ablation without harm coming to the conduction system (note the presence of a right bundle branch potential within the activation route). Labels in green are on the near side of the geometry. Labels in yellow are on the far side and seen through the geometry. SVC, superior vena cava; IVC, inferior vena cava; CS os, coronary sinus ostium; TVA, tricuspid valve annulus; RBB pot, right bundle branch potential.

5.3 Ventricular Tachycardias

Non-contact mapping was originally developed as a tool for the mapping and ablation of ischemic left ventricular tachycardias. The technique may also be applied to other forms of ventricular tachycardia. Positioning of MEA in the left ventricle requires a retrograde transaortic approach that is prohibited by prosthetic aortic valve replacement or significant aortic stenosis. Once across the aortic valve, the tip of the catheter lies in the ventricular apex, providing a relatively stable and central MEA position.

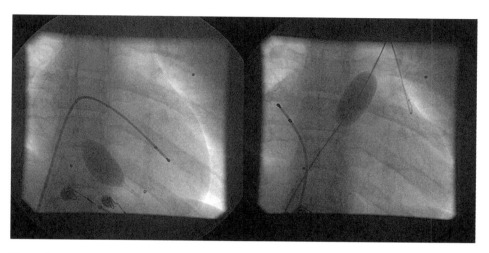

Figure 8. Anteroposterior views. When performing right atrial studies the MEA may be positioned towards the apex via a superior approach or towards the outflow tract via an inferior approach. The most appropriate position will depend upon the tachycardia mechanism.

Positioning the MEA in the right ventricle may be more complicated. The eccentric shape and trabeculated ventricular walls can impair positioning and stability. Particular attention must be paid to geometry creation, as it is easy to miss significant "pockets" within the chamber. This will limit the accuracy of non-contact mapping and necessitate recreation of chamber geometry when discovered, adding time to the procedure. Access to the right ventricle via the tricuspid valve may be obtained via the inferior or superior caval vein approach. The stiff catheter shaft prevents easy manipulation across the valve and extra-stiff guidewires, which can be bent into a desired shape, may be required to facilitate catheter positioning. Preoperative assessment of the likely source of the tachycardia will help to decide whether an apical or outflow tract position is most appropriate. Balloon insertion via the femoral vein is suitable for right ventricular outflow tachycardias, whereas insertion via the subclavian or internal jugular veins allows a more apical positioning (figure 8). We do not recommend the femoral route if an apical position is required. Not only is catheter manipulation towards the apex extremely difficult from this route, but also, excess torque may be placed on the catheter shaft and transmitted to the catheter tip. Continued friction and abrasion of the catheter tip against thin-walled right ventricular apex places the patient at risk of perforation and cardiac tamponade.

5.3.1   Ventricular tachycardia after repair of Tetralogy of Fallot

Up to 6% of patients who have undergone surgical correction of tetralogy of Fallot may have documented VT or sudden cardiac death.[15] Previous studies have demonstrated that macroreentry is the arrhythmia mechanism, either involving the ventricular septal defect (VSD) patch or the ventriculotomy scar. Other studies have shown that reentry may occur in fibrotic, disorganized myocardial tissue, distant from scars or patches. Large macroreentrant circuits may occur, with broad pathways between areas of anatomical or functional conduction block.[31]. Such circuits require ablation with linear lesions joining two barriers to conduction.

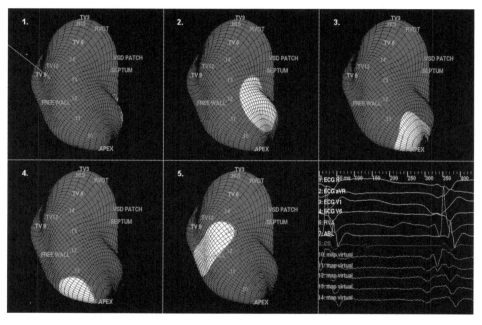

Figure 9 (see Color Plate 21). Fallots VT: Right ventricular geometry view from a cranially orientated left anterior oblique plane. Virtual electrograms (channels 10-14) are recorded from the anterosuperior free wall along the site of the presumed ventriculotomy incision. The appropriately numbered labels on the geometry indicate the recording sites. Frames 1 and 2 show activation spreading up the apical septum from inferior to superior. The VSD patch prevents activation heading towards the base of the septum. Frames 3 and 4 show how the ventriculotomy acts as a barrier, with the wavefront having to turn around the apical end of the incision. Frame 5 shows activation now able to depolarize the free wall from apex to base. This line of block is confirmed by the presence of double potentials in the virtual electrograms along the site of the ventriculotomy. The position of the ablation catheter (ABL) is indicated by the locator signal (green line) in frame 1. Labels in green are on the near side of the geometry. Labels in yellow are on the far side and seen through the geometry. TV, tricuspid valve annulus; RVOT, right ventricular outflow tract.

Ventricular arrhythmias are more likely to occur in older patients with larger ventricles. The MEA is usually positioned in the right ventricle without difficulty. The VSD patch and ventriculotomy may be identified by low amplitude contact or virtual electrograms plus the absence of color on isopotential mapping. The peak voltage map facility also allows identification of low amplitude or absent electrical activity consistent with prosthetic material or inert myocardium. During ventricular tachycardia the ventriculotomy scar may be identified by the presence of double potentials in virtual or contact electrograms (Figure 9). If the tachycardia is poorly tolerated it may be terminated after a few beats by pacing or cardioversion and the acquired data reviewed off-line. Only a few beats are required to provide global activation timings of the entire endocardial surface. Anatomical and surgical structures, including the entire length of the ventriculotomy scar, may then be labeled on the map using reconstructed virtual electrograms obtained by moving the cursor around the map of the endocardial surface.

In common with patients who have undergone extensive atrial surgery, multiple morphologies of tachycardia may be present. We have performed ablation on a patient with surgical correction of tetralogy of Fallot who had 4 different morphologies of ventricular tachycardia with cycle lengths varying between 285 and 335 msec. Despite their different morphologies, all 4 shared a common broad diastolic pathway between the VSD patch and the ventriculotomy. Three of the tachycardias proceeded through the diastolic pathway in a clockwise fashion whereas the 4th tachycardia used the same circuit but in reverse. A long lesion placed at the exit site and reaching to the VSD patch terminated all 4 tachycardias.

5.3.2   Idiopathic right ventricular outflow tract tachycardia

Ventricular tachycardia in the structurally normal heart most commonly arises from the right ventricular outflow tract. Although it is essentially a benign arrhythmia, symptoms may warrant treatment by radiofrequency ablation. It accounts for only a small fraction of procedures performed (<5%) with success rates of 60-90%.[3,4,8,32] The arrhythmia usually arises from an automatic focus in the right ventricular outflow tract. Conventional techniques such as activation mapping and pace mapping are employed. Often, tachycardia is difficult to induce and may be non-sustained, rendering identification of the earliest site of activation difficult, leading to procedural failure.

We have used non-contact mapping to guide ablation in pediatric patients who have non-sustained right ventricular outflow tract tachycardia. The MEA is inserted via a femoral vein, passed across the tricuspid valve and positioned in the right ventricular outflow tract with the guidewire extending into the left pulmonary artery. Activation mapping of the entire endocardium is performed during each beat and theoretically a single ectopic is all that is required to guide positioning of the ablation catheter at the exact site of earliest activation. We always perform activation and pace mapping at target sites prior to ablation. An example of non-contact mapping of idiopathic right ventricular outflow tract tachycardia is shown in Figure 10.

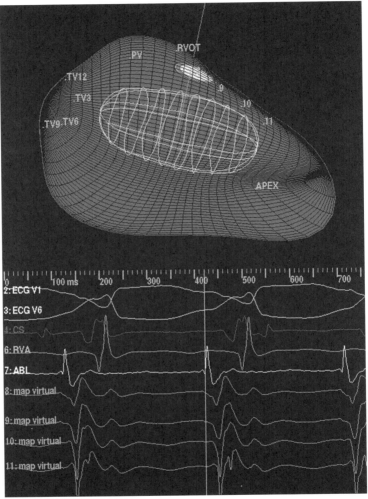

Figure 10 (see Color Plate 22). Right ventricular outflow tract tachycardia. Right ventricular geometry is displayed in a right anterior oblique view with the free wall clipped away to provide an internal view of the septum, medial outflow tract and inferior wall. The yellow frame indicates the MEA position. Contact and virtual electrograms are displayed below. The virtual electrograms (channels 8-11) are taken from the numbered sites on the geometry. The vertical yellow line indicates the point in time displayed on the isopotential map. Earliest systolic activation is shown occurring 20 msec before the onset of the surface QRS. The site is indicated by the white spot of color (negative potential) on the isopotential map. The virtual electrogram from this point (channel 8) shows the earliest activation and a QS morphology. The green line on the geometry represents the locator signal, which has guided the ablation catheter tip to this site. The bipolar contact electrogram is shown in channel 7.   TV, tricuspid valve; PV, pulmonary valve; RVOT, right ventricular outflow tract.

5.3.3   Idiopathic left ventricular tachycardia

Idiopathic left ventricular tachycardia (fascicular tachycardia, verapamil-sensitive ventricular tachycardia), arising from the posterior left ventricular septum, is also found in structurally normal hearts. It accounts for a small minority of pediatric ablations. Studies conducted in the adult population have determined that the most common form is reentrant in nature, yet opinion is still divided as to the exact mechanism of tachycardia and the most suitable technique to guide ablation. Activation and pace mapping has been successful in some series.[32,33] Other authors have reported the presence of a diastolic potential (Purkinje potential or late diastolic potential) found at the base of the septum that is a marker for successful ablation.[34-36] This potential may reflect activation of part of the specialized conducting system. The site of the earliest potential is the target for radiofrequency energy.

When tachycardia is difficult to induce or non-sustained, non-contact mapping may be the preferred technique for guiding radiofrequency ablation. We have found that it can accurately locate the site of earliest endocardial activation to a precise area, usually towards the inferoapical septum. Although non-contact mapping detects activation within the main body of the left bundle branch and the posterior fascicle, we have only detected discrete diastolic activity at the base of the septum in 1 out of 6 patients. This was also present on contact electrograms at this site. One other patient had a small diastolic potential at their successful ablation site seen only in the contact electrogram. Four other patients were successfully ablated at sites of earliest activation as demonstrated by isopotential mapping. In all 6 cases, 1-4 radiofrequency applications were required. No patient has suffered a recurrence of tachycardia. We have concluded that there is a protected zone of slow conduction within the septum with an entrance site deep within the base of the septum and an exit site towards the apex. The earliest diastolic potential represents the entrance whereas the earliest point of activation with a perfect pace map represents the exit. Although conduction along the zone of slow conduction is of too low amplitude to be detected by non-contact mapping, this technique readily identifies the precise exit site and can guide successful ablation.

CONCLUSION

There is a growing experience with non-contact mapping in pediatric patients. The combination of real-time global activation mapping of the entire endocardial surface superimposed on a three-dimensional model of chamber geometry, plus the reconstruction of unipolar electrograms at over 3,300 sites, allows precise mapping of tachyarrhythmias. The technique provides particular advantages with non-sustained or poorly tolerated arrhythmias, and in patients with complex congenital heart disease and surgically altered cardiac chambers in which conventional techniques have proved limited. Non-contact mapping has offered additional insights into arrhythmia mechanism in pediatric patients. Coupled with recent advances in ablation technology, more patients are treatable with electrophysiological techniques. The principle disadvantage is the size of the MEA, which prohibits the use of the catheter in cardiac chambers that have dimensions smaller than 4.5 by 2.0 cm or require access via baffle punctures.

REFERENCE

1. Kugler JD, Danford DA, Deal BJ, et al: Radiofrequency catheter ablation for tachyarrhythmias in children and adolescents. The Pediatric Electrophysiology Society. N Eng J Med 1994;330:1481-1487.
2. Hsieh IC, Yeh SJ, Wen MS, Wang CC, Lin FC, Wu D: Radiofrequency ablation for supraventricular and ventricular tachycardia in young patients. Int J Cardiol 1996;54:33-40.
3. Van Hare GF, Witherell CL, Lesh MD: Follow-up of radiofrequency catheter ablation in children: results in 100 consecutive patients. J Am Coll Cardiol 1994;23:1651-1659.
4. Tanel RE, Walsh EP, Triedman JK, Epstein MR, Bergau DM, Saul JP: Five-year experience with radiofrequency catheter ablation: implications for management of arrhythmias in pediatric and young adult patients. Journal of Paediatrics 1997;131:878-887.
5. Dorostkar PC, Dick M: The use of radiofrequency energy in pediatric cardiology. J Interv Cardiol 1995;8:557-568.
6. Kugler JD, Danford DA, Houston K, Felix G: Radiofrequency catheter ablation for paroxysmal supraventricular tachycardia in children and adolescents without structural heart disease. Pediatric EP Society, Radiofrequency Catheter Ablation Registry. Am J Cardiol 1997;80:1438-1443.
7. Danford DA, Kugler JD, Deal B, et al: The learning curve for radiofrequency ablation of tachyarrhythmias in pediatric patients. Participating members of the Pediatric Electrophysiology Society. Am J Cardiol 1995;75:587-590.
8. Smeets JL, Rodriguez LM, Timmermans C, Wellens HJ: Radiofrequency catheter ablation of idiopathic ventricular tachycardias in children. Pacing Clin Electrophysiol 1997;20:2068-2071.
9. Reich JD, Auld D, Hulse E, Sullivan K, Campbell R: The Pediatric Radiofrequency Ablation Registry's experience with Ebstein's anomaly. Pediatric Electrophysiology Society. J Cardiovasc Electrophysiol 1998;9:1370-1377.
10. Gow RM: Atrial fibrillation and flutter in children and in young adults with congenital heart disease. Can J Cardiol 1996;12:45A-48A.
11. Peters NS, Somerville J: Arrhythmias after the Fontan procedure. Br Heart J 1992;68:199-204.
12. Fishberger SB, Wernovsky G, Gentles TL, et al: Factors that influence the development of atrial flutter after the Fontan operation. J Thorac Cardiovasc Surg 1997;113:80-86.
13. Driscoll DJ, Offord KP, Feldt RH, Schaff HV, Puga FJ, Danielson GK: Five- to fifteen-year follow-up after Fontan operation. Circulation 1992;85:469-496.
14. Vetter VL, Tanner CS, Horowitz L: Inducible atrial flutter after the Mustard repair of complete transposition of the great arteries. Am J Cardiol 1988;61:-428
15. Saul JP, Alexander ME: Preventing sudden death after repair of tetralogy of Fallot: complex therapy for complex patients. J Cardiovasc Electrophysiol 1999;10:1271-1287.

16. Kalman JM, Van Hare GF, Olgin JE, Saxon LA, Stark SI, Lesh MD: Ablation of 'incisional' reentrant atrial tachycardia complicating surgery for congenital heart disease. Circulation 1996;93:502-512.

17. Baker BM, Lindsay BD, Bromberg BI, Frazier DW, Cain ME, Smith JM: Catheter ablation of clinical intraatrial reentrant tachycardias resulting from previous atrial surgery: localising and transecting the critical isthmus. J Am Coll Cardiol 1996;28:411-417.

18. Triedman JK, Bergau DM, Saul JP, Epstein MR, Walsh EP: Efficacy of radiofrquency ablation for control of intraatrial reentrant tachycardia in patients with congenital heart disease. J Am Coll Cardiol 1997;30:1032-1038.

19. Saul JP, Triedman JK: Radiofrequency ablation of intraatrial reentrant tachycardia after surgery for congenital heart disease. Pacing Clin Electrophysiol 1997;20:2112-2117.

20. Van Hare GF, Lesh MD, Ross BA, Perry JC, Dorostkar PC: Mapping and radiofrequency ablation of intraatrial reentrant tachycardia after the Senning or Mustard procedure for transposition of the great arteries. Am J Cardiol 1996;77:985-991.

21. Triedman JK, Jenkins KJ, Colan SD, Saul JP, Walsh EP: Intra-atrial reentrant tachycardia after palliation of congenital heart disease: characterisation of multiple macroreentrant circuits using fluoroscopically based three-dimensional endocardial mapping. J Cardiovasc Electrophysiol 1997;8:259-270.

22. Dorostkar PC, Cheng J, Scheinman MM: Electroanatomical mapping and ablation of the substrate supporting intraatrial reentrant tachycardia after palliation for complex congenital heart disease. Pacing Clin Electrophysiol 1998;21:1810-1819.

23. Gepstein L, Evans SJ: Electroanatomical mapping of the heart: Basic concepts and implications for the treatment of cardiac arrhythmias. Pacing Clin Electrophysiol 1998;21:1268-1278.

24. Kadish A, Hauck J, Pederson B, Beatty G, Gornick CC: Mapping of atrial activation with a non-contact, multielectrode catheter in dogs. Circulation 1999;99:1906-1913.

25. Schilling RJ, Peters NS, Davies DW: Simultaneous endocardial mapping in the human left ventricle using a non-contact catheter: Comparison of contact and reconstructed electrograms during sinus rhythm. Circulation 1998;98:887-898.

26. Schilling RJ, Peters NS, Davies DW: Mapping and ablation of ventricular tachycardia with the aid of a non-contact mapping system. Heart 1999;81:570-575.

27. Schilling RJ, Peters NS, Davies DW: Feasibility of a noncontact catheter for endocardial mapping of human ventricular tachycardia. Circulation 1999;99:2543-2552.

28. Gornick CC, Adler SW, Pederson B, Hauck J, Budd J, Schweitzer J: Validation of a new noncontact catheter system for electroanatomic mapping of left ventricular endocardium. Circulation 1999;99:829-835.

29. Gewillig M, Cullen S, Mertens B, Lesaffre E, Deanfield J: Risk factors for arrhythmia and death after Mustard operation for simple transposition of the great arteries. Circulation 1991;84:III-187-III-192

30. Haissaguerre M, Cauchemez B, Marcus F, et al: Characteristics of the ventricular insertion sites of accessory pathways with anterograde decremental conduction properties. Circulation 1995;91:1077-1085.

31. Stevenson WG, Delacretaz E, Friedman PL, Ellison KE: Identification and ablation of macroreentrant ventricular tachycardia with the CARTO electroanatomical mapping system. Pacing Clin Electrophysiol 1998;21:1448-1456.

32. Coggins DL, Lee RJ, Sweeney J, et al: Radiofrequency catheter ablation as a cure for idiopathic tachycardia of both left and right ventricular origin. J Am Coll Cardiol 1994;23:1333-1341.

33. Wellens HJJ, Smeets LRM: Idiopathic left ventricular tachycardia; cure by radiofrequency ablation. Circulation 1993;88:2978-2979.

34. Nakagawa H, Beckman KJ, McClelland JH, et al: Radiofrequency catheter ablation of idiopathic left ventricular tachycardia guided by a Purkinje potential. Circulation 1993;88:2607-2617.

35. Tsuchiya T, Okumura K, Honda T, et al: Significance of late diastolic potential preceding Purkinje potential in verapamil-sensitive idiopathic left ventricular tachycardia. Circulation 1999;99:2408-2413.
36. Zardini M, Thakur RK, Klein GJ, Yee R: Catheter ablation of idiopathic left ventricular tachycardia. Pacing Clin Electrophysiol 1995;18:1255-1265.

Part III

New Ablation Approaches and Modalities

Chapter 17

THE ADVANTAGES AND DISADVANTAGES OF CREATING LARGE RADIOFREQUENCY ABLATION LESIONS

Munther K. Homoud, Craig Swygman, Mark S. Link, Caroline B. Foote, N. A. Mark Estes, III, Paul J. Wang
New England Cardiac Arrhythmia Center,Division of Cardiology, New England Medical Center, Boston, Massachussets, USA

INTRODUCTION

Radiofrequency ablation has become a major therapeutic modality in the treatment of cardiac arrhythmias. Most forms of supraventricular tachycardia have been successfully treated with catheter-based techniques using focal ablative radiofrequency lesions. A large range of other arrhythmias, however, may be treated using longer, wider, and deeper lesions. A long linear lesion may be particularly important in the ablation of reentrant arrhythmias that have a critical zone 1-cm or more in length. Such a critical zone may exist between two or more anatomic structures, such as in atrial flutter, scar-related reentrant tachycardias, some atrial tachycardias, and some ventricular tachycardias (Figure 1). A series of linear lesions may also be effective in preventing perpetuation of reentrant wavefronts in such disorders as atrial fibrillation (Figure 2). A line of lesions may be placed circumferentially when it is not possible or desirable to ablate the arrhythmia focus itself (Figure 3). This approach may be useful in some ventricular tachycardias and in focal atrial fibrillation ablation in pulmonary veins. There are situations in which the reentrant circuit may be complex and it is not possible to ablate all the critical zones. It may be possible to transect the zone in such cases as ischemic-based ventricular tachycardia (Figure 4). Wide lesions may be necessary when the reentrant circuit spans a large surface area subendocardially (Figure 5). Deep lesions may have a particular utility when a reentrant circuit lies beneath the endocardium and within the myocardium, for example in ischemic ventricular tachycardia or epicardial accessory pathways (Figure 6).

L. Bing Liem and E. Downar (eds.), Progress in Catheter Ablation, 273-291.
© 2001 *Kluwer Academic Publishers. Printed in the Netherlands.*

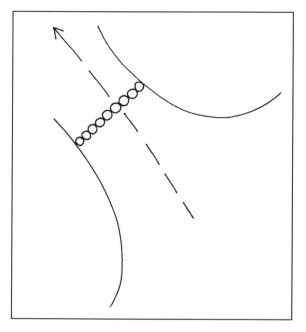

Figure 1. Schematic drawing of long linear lesions between two anatomic structures to prevent reentry within a critical zone.

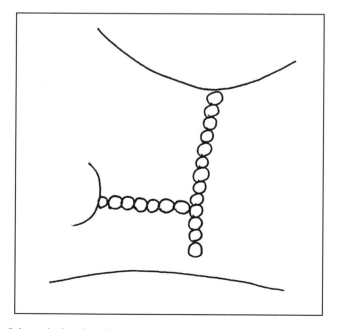

Figure 2. Schematic drawing of a series of linear lesions to prevent reentrant wavefronts.

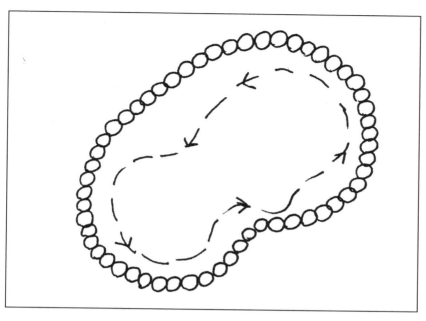

Figure 3. Schematic drawing of circumferential lesion

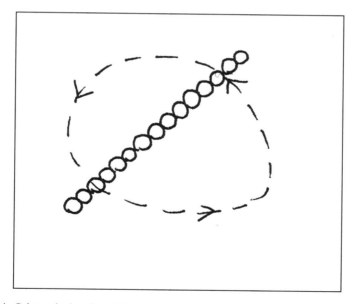

Figure 4. Schematic drawing of linear lesions that transect the reentrant circuit

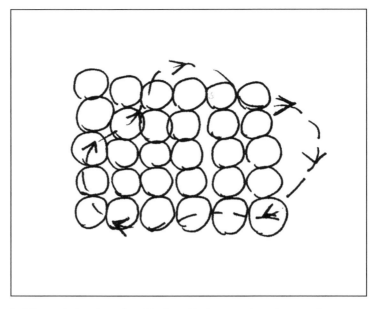

Figure 5. Schematic drawing of a wide, broad lesion covering a large surface area

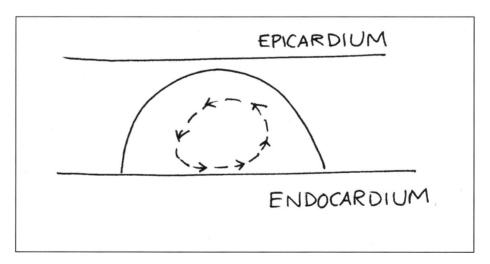

Figure 6. Schematic drawing of a deep lesion

1.   LINEAR LESIONS

1.1   Role of Linear Lesions between Anatomic Structures

Reentry requires one or more circular functional or anatomic paths.   Linear ablative lesions may be quite effective in interrupting these reentrant circuits by creating a line of block from one anatomic structure to another.   This strategy may be used to take advantage of existing anatomic structures such as the vena cavae, the mitral and tricuspid annuli, the crista terminalis, and surgical scars or patches.   A critical zone has been identified for atrial flutter that permits such an effective use of linear ablation.   Other reentrant rhythms may utilize a surgical scar as an important substrate.   Some forms of intra-atrial reentry and ventricular tachycardia may also use anatomic boundaries for reentry.

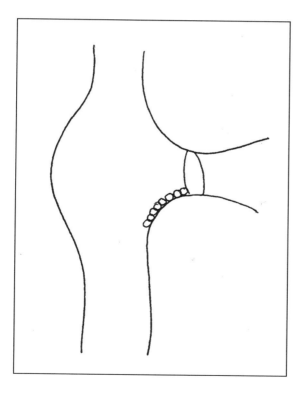

Figure 7. Linear ablative lesion between the inferior vena cava and the tricuspid valve annulus to prevent atrial flutter

1.1.1   Catheter Ablation for Atrial Flutter

Atrial flutter is the prototypical disorder for which a linear lesion is used to interrupt the reentrant circuit between two anatomic boundaries.[1] In so-called isthmus-dependent atrial flutter, the catheter ablation of the isthmus of tissue separating the annulus of the tricuspid valve from the eustachian ridge and the ostium of the inferior vena cava successfully eliminates the ability to sustain atrial flutter, Figure 7).[1-7] Both counterclockwise and clockwise atrial flutter demonstrate this dependence on the same area of the low right atrium. Ablation of this region prevents perpetuation of atrial flutter since the remaining tissue is unable to support a reentrant circuit. The anatomic approach of creating a linear ablation from the annulus of the tricuspid valve and to the inferior vena cava has become the standard approach to atrial flutter. Because recurrence of atrial flutter is related to the creation of incomplete lines of block, several techniques have been introduced to help determine the completeness of the line of block along the isthmus.[7,8] Wider and larger lesions may also be more effective in creating bi-directional block and larger tipped and irrigated tip ablation catheters have been used for this purpose.

1.1.2   Post-surgical Reentrant Tachycardias

Cardiac surgery may result in multiple regions of block or impaired conduction that may form the basis for reentrant arrhythmias. Atrial cannulation sites may serve as the basis for intra-atrial reentry. Patches used in closure of atrial or ventricular septal defects or in Tetralogy of Fallot surgery may also be substrate for reentry. Surgery for congenital heart disease such as the Fontan procedure or the Mustard or Senning repair for transposition of the great vessels may result in intra-atrial reentrant tachycardias.[9-13] Reentry is supported by the presence of these surgical scars and natural barriers such as the tricuspid valve annulus, os of the coronary sinus, superior and inferior vena cavae (Figure 8).[12,13] Entrainment with concealed fusion can be used to identify the areas of slow conduction and target them for radiofrequency ablation. These sites include the atriotomy site(s), margins of the atrioseptal patch, the atrial insertion of the Fontan conduit, and the zones adjacent to the Mustard and Senning baffles.[13] An important strategy to treat these arrhythmias is the creation of linear ablative lesions from the incision to an anatomic boundary such as the superior vena cava. Lesions created at these areas of slow conduction were successful in treating these arrhythmias in greater than 73% of cases.[12,13]

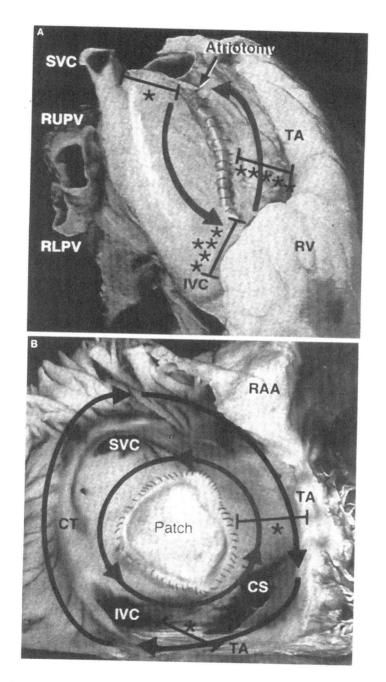

Figure 8. Linear ablative lesion between a surgical incision to an anatomic boundary

1.1.3 Ventricular Tachycardia due to Macroreentrant along Mitral Valve Annulus

In most ventricular tachycardias, the reentrant circuit is a complex macroreentrant circuit within the border zone of infarct and intact tissue. Simply connecting the border zone to an anatomic structure would not be likely to treat the ventricular tachycardia. However, a specific type of ventricular tachycardia complicating inferior myocardial infarction may be particularly amenable to treatment with linear ablation. Wilber et al have shown that a linear ablation from the mitral valve annulus to the infarct border[14] may successfully treat this form of ventricular tachycardia (Figure 9). It is quite possible that other anatomic substrates will be identified that will permit linear ablation for other ventricular tachycardias.

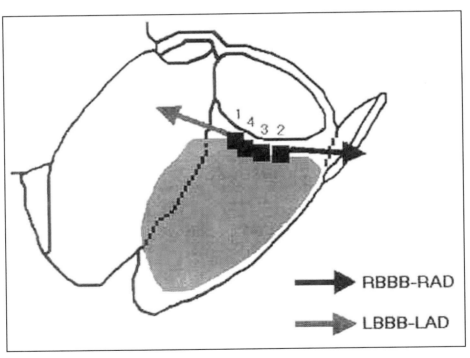

Figure 9. Linear ablation from infarcted border to mitral valve annulus to treat ventricular tachycardia

1.2 Linear Ablation for Transection of Reentrant Circuit

1.2.1 Catheter Ablation for Ventricular Tachycardia

The multiplicity of clinical and induced tachycardias and complexities of mapping have limited radiofrequency ablation of ventricular tachycardia. Ventricular tachycardia complicating healed myocardial infarction usually is the result of reentry at the edge of the scar. Catheter radiofrequency ablation is directed at the zone critical to the perpetuation of the reentrant tachycardia. Because of the complexity of the reentrant circuit, focal ablation of the critical zone may be difficult. As a result, a method of creating linear lesions to transect the critical zone has been attempted.

Recently, magnetic electroanatomic mapping and bipolar sinus rhythm mapping have been used to identify border zones separating scar from normal tissue (Figures 10A and B).[15] Linear lesions were drawn to cross the border zones while incorporating the site where pace mapping replicated the morphology of documented ventricular tachycardia. Seven of fifteen patients with inducible ventricular tachycardia became no longer inducible.[15] Clinically, only four patients had clinical ventricular tachycardia during a mean follow-up period of 8 months (range 3-36 months). Such an approach may dramatically decrease the time and extent of mapping and permitting the ablation of ventricular tachycardia to become partially anatomically based.

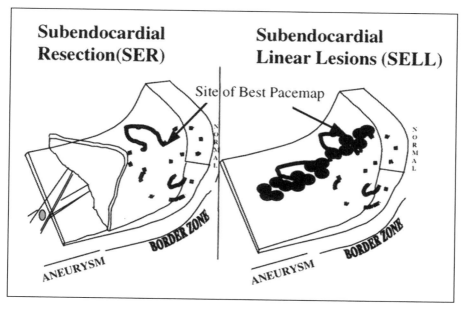

Figure 10A. A linear ablative lesion transects the critical reentrant zone

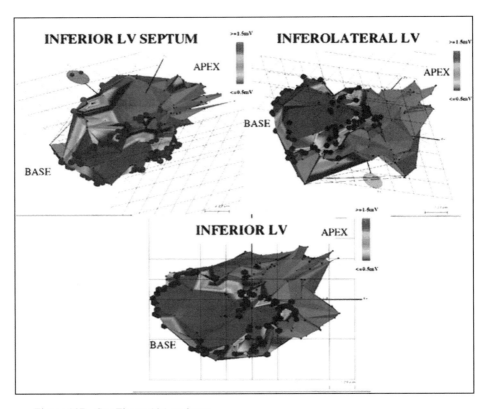

Figure 10B. See Figure 10A and text.

The development of widely applicable catheter ablation techniques for ventricular tachycardia may have an important impact on the quality of life of patients with sustained ventricular tachycardia. Although implantable defibrillators have improved the survival of patients with sustained ventricular arrhythmias, spontaneous tachycardias may occur. The high success rate and low complication rate associated with implanting antiarrhythmia devices have eclipsed the role arrhythmia surgery had on controlling ventricular tachycardia. Although prior surgical techniques such as subendocardial resection, cryoablation, encircling endocardial ventriculotomy, and laser ablation[16-20] have been successfully applied to the treatment of ventricular arrhythmias, because of surgical morbidity and mortality, they have been nearly completely abandoned in current therapy. Therefore, a simplified and effective catheter technique for the treatment of ventricular tachycardia would be extremely appealing.

1.3 Linear Ablation in the Presence of Functional Reentrant Wavefronts

1.3.1 Catheter Ablation for Atrial Fibrillation

The work of Moe and Allessie has shown that atrial fibrillation requires multiple reentrant atrial wavelets for its perpetuation.[21,22] Work by Cox et al. has demonstrated the successful treatment of atrial fibrillation by the creation of surgical incisions in the right and left atria.[23,24] These incision lines preclude the development of reentrant wavelets while maintaining propagation of sinus impulses to the atrioventricular node. Catheter techniques creating linear ablative lesions may potentially offer patients with atrial fibrillation an alternative to surgery.

A number of different arrangements of linear lesions have been proposed for the radiofrequency ablation treatment of atrial fibrillation. Most strategies are derived from the surgical work by Cox et al.[23,24] These involve a method of preventing reentry around the pulmonary veins and within the free walls of the right and left atria. Several studies have employed right atrial lesions from the superior vena cava to the inferior vena cava, circumferentially around the right atrium to the tricuspid annulus, from the superior vena cava to the tricuspid annulus, and septally through the fossa ovalis to the inferior vena cava. Left atrial lesions have largely consisted of lesions connecting the pulmonary veins with the mitral annulus and from the right superior pulmonary vein to the fossa ovalis (Figure 11).

The goal of creating transmural linear lesions within the atria has been difficult to achieve. The length of the lesions required to create lines in the right and left atria have been measured on cadaveric hearts by Jaïs et al and Jensen et al.[25,26] They vary from 15 to 177 mm, the thickest part of the atria, the trabeculated right atrium and the paramitral band were measured at 10 mm, whereas the thinnest, at 0.5 mm. The creation of such lesions may require energy sources that can easily penetrate these depths. Lavergne et al described their attempt at creating linear right and left atrial lesions in animals using 50W energy delivered via a 4 mm irrigated tip catheter.[27] The procedure was relatively safe with no hemopericardium and a 2% incidence of coagulum formation at trabeculated sites. Gaps in the lines were consistently seen if only one drag lesion was created.

Linear ablation for atrial fibrillation has been reported.[28-33] Results from the delivery of lesions limited to the right atrium have been disappointing with a high rate of recurrence.[29,32,34] Results were significantly better when lines were drawn in the left atrium.[28,29,33] Recurrences were predominantly left atrial flutter, the result of gaps in the line delivered.[28,29,33] The commonest site of gaps are at the junction of the right superior pulmonary vein-mitral annulus line with the mitral annulus, gaps in the roof line and the left superior pulmonary vein-mitral annulus line favoring left atrial flutter.[33]

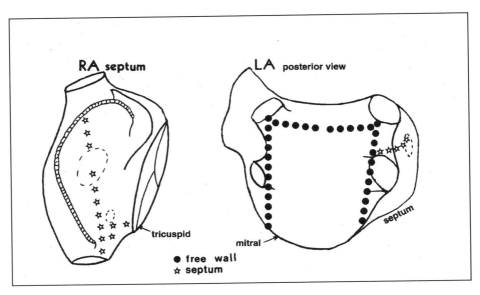

Figure 11. A series of linear ablative lesions are used to prevent multiple reentrant wavefronts in atrial fibrillation

The determinants of success were the ability to deliver at least one complete line of block without gaps, the ablation of focal atrial fibrillation and a smaller sized left atrium.[29,33] The development of catheters that would allow the creation of linear lesions would improve the outcome of this procedure and reduce the time required for a successful outcome. This would potentially reduce the amount of time catheters spend in the left atrium and reduce the risk of thromboembolism. The long-term consequences of the creation of these long linear lesions remain unclear. There is a theoretical risk of converting short term, infrequent bursts of paroxysmal atrial fibrillation to sustained atrial fibrillation.[28] There is also the risk of creating the substrate for new reentrant arrhythmias.[35] The success rate of biatrial linear ablation increased from 57% to 84% when previously ineffective antiarrhythmic agents were reintroduced.[33]

Enhanced and novel methods of mapping may also add importantly to the success of atrial fibrillation linear ablation. Three-dimensional non-fluoroscopic activation mapping has been used to confirm the continuity of linear lesions delivered in both atria in 27 patients with recurrent atrial fibrillation.[36]

Such techniques may make important advances in the treatment of a disorder that is present in over 2 million patients in the United States alone.[37] Atrial fibrillation accounts for one third of strokes in individuals over the age of 65.[38] In addition, atrial fibrillation causes symptoms of palpitations, increased fatigue, and dyspnea may require either medical therapy or the interruption of atrioventricular conduction, necessitating the concomitant implantation of a permanent pacemaker. Development of such techniques for atrial fibrillation may provide an important alternative to the existing pharmacologic and non-pharmacologic modes of therapy.

1.4   Circumferential Ablation

1.4.1   Role of Circumferential Ablation

An extension of a linear ablation is creation of a circumferential ablative lesion, completely isolating a focus or region. This strategy may prevent a focal tachycardia or reentrant circuit from depolarizing the rest of the heart. As such, it serves as a substitute for ablating the entire region of the critical focus. It may be particularly attractive when it is difficult to localize the critical region such as in ischemic ventricular tachycardia or when it is not desirable to ablate the tissue responsible for the focus such as in pulmonary vein focal tachycardia. Circumferential ablation has many of the same requirements as linear ablation: the ability to create transmural lesions, the need to demonstrate complete line of block, and the ability to identify the location of gaps.

2.   PULMONARY VEIN ISOLATION

In focal atrial tachycardias originating from a pulmonary vein, it may be difficult or not desirable to ablate the pulmonary vein directly. Pulmonary vein stenosis may result from ablation of the focus within the pulmonary vein. In an effort to avoid the development of pulmonary vein stenosis, circumferential ablation in the atrial tissue surrounding the pulmonary vein has been proposed. Once the pulmonary vein has been identified as the source of the atrial tachycardia focus, an anatomic circumferential lesion may be possible. This may further improve the speed of such procedures. The circumferential lesion might be made using a device with a circular array of electrodes or using a single electrode that is adjusted to trace a circular pattern. Pulmonary vein isolation may also be used in adjunct with linear ablation for atrial fibrillation. Lines may be used to connect these circumferential lesions to anatomic boundaries such as the mitral annulus. Circumferential lesions may be used to isolate two pulmonary veins, for example, the left superior and left inferior veins. Surgical isolation of all four pulmonary veins has been performed and with improved technology it may be possible to create a circumferential catheter ablative lesion in the future (Figure 12).

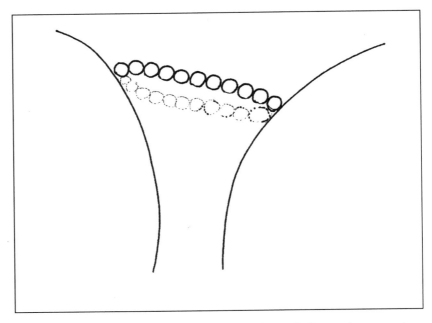

Figure 12. Schematic drawing of a circumferential lesion encircling a pulmonary vein

3. VENTRICULAR TACHYCARDIA ABLATION

Surgical procedures such as endocardial encircling ventriculotomy were designed to isolate electrically the region of the ventricular tachycardia. While effective in preventing ventricular tachycardia, endocardial encircling ventriculotomy was associated with a significant mortality. A catheter-based technique capable of encircling the reentrant circuit might be quite effective with a considerably lower mortality.

Although implantable cardioverter-defibrillators have proven benefit in patients with life-threatening ventricular arrhythmias,[39,40] frequent discharges from these defibrillators, are disturbing to the patients and reduce patient's tolerance to this form of therapy. Serious adverse effects and limitations of efficacy often limit antiarrhythmic drug therapy. Therefore, improvements in the catheter ablation of ventricular tachycardia may result in important advances in the treatment of this disorder.

4.   DISADVANTAGES AND LIMITATIONS OF LONG LESIONS

Long linear lesions may significantly increase the risk of complications of catheter ablation, particularly the risk of perforation and thromboembolism. Linear lesions may also create new reentrant tachycardias such as atrial tachycardias and ventricular tachycardias because of failure to complete a line of block to another line or anatomic structure (Figure 13).

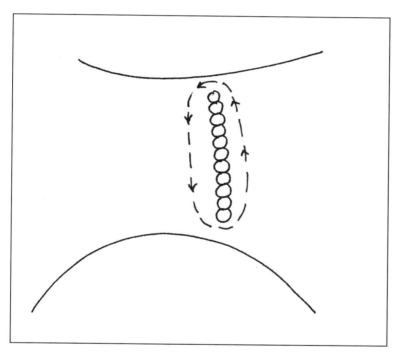

Figure 13. Schematic drawing of reentrant tachycardias created by a gap in a line of conduction block

Since some linear lesions have approximately the same width as depth, these linear lesions may have significant volume, potentially impairing myocardial contractility and distorting the heart chamber's geometry.   Creating linear lesions also takes significant periods of time, potentially increasing the total procedure time. Compared to using a single electrode to create a series of linear ablative lesions, using a multi-electrode catheter may decrease procedure time. However, use of a multielectrode catheter may not decrease procedure time as much as expected because of the time needed to determine the catheter location and to establish contact with the endocardium.

5.   WIDE LESIONS

There are several conditions in which lesions of greater surface area are desirable. In such conditions, the deeper lesions may not be needed but lesions of larger area may be needed.

5.1   Ventricular Tachycardia Originating from Myocardial Infarction

Ventricular tachycardia circuits originating from many myocardial infarctions lie subendocardially in the surviving tissue.   The surgical approach developed more than 2 decades ago consisted of the surgical resection of the scar tissue in the border zone region. In many surgical series, the resected region had a surface area of 4 to 9 cm^2 or more.[41]

Catheter ablation techniques have been employed to increase the surface area by creating a series of adjacent lesions. This may be achieved by moving a single electrode over a larger region,[42] guided by fluoroscopy or electroanatomic mapping. A single multielectrode catheter may be rotated about one of the mid electrodes to cover a large surface area.[43]   Novel catheters that may create a larger surface area have also been proposed. These may have a large surface area or be able to create a large surface area.[44,45]

5.2   Disadvantages

There may be important hemodynamic consequences of damaging a large region of endocardium, particularly extending into normal myocardial tissue. Because of the difficulty clinically to assess the depth of the arrhythmogenic focus, it is often incorrectly assumed that simply a deeper region must be ablated. Instead, an inadequate lesion leads to ablation failure.   The ability to create lesions with large surface area may result in careless application, resulting in damage to a large region of myocardium. Such techniques may often result in the operator's abandoning careful mapping, which is essential, to maximize safety.   Larger lesions may also result in pro-arrhythmia by creating new boundaries that may support reentry. Ablation over a greater surface area may increase the risk of thromboembolic events and increase the procedure time and associated complications.

6.   DEEP LESIONS

Conventional radiofrequency ablation techniques create lesions that have a limited volume. However, some arrhythmias may have critical zones or elements deep within the myocardium. There is significant evidence that the reentrant pathway in infarcted human tissue may follow a "zigzag" course, which at times may course subepicardially. Knowledge of this complex 3-dimensional reentrant circuit has come in great part due to the extensive work of de Bakker et al, examining ventricular tachycardia in Langendorff perfused human heart obtained at the time of heart transplantation. In many such patients superficial endocardial lesions may not be sufficient to terminate or prevent the tachycardia. For some ventricular tachycardias, epicardial ablation has been required, suggesting that transmural endocardial lesions would be necessary to treat such arrhythmias successfully. Littmann et al demonstrated the success of epicardial Nd:YAG laser ablation for this purpose. Some accessory pathways are more epicardial in extent and require ablation via the coronary sinus or deep from the endocardium under the mitral or tricuspid annuli. In such cases, saline-cooled radiofrequency ablation has been used to create deeper lesions.

CONCLUSIONS

Although many supraventricular arrhythmias may be treated with focal ablative lesions, any other arrhythmias may be ablated using longer and deeper lesions. Creating such lesions may require new catheter designs and ablative energies. Linear ablation may be suitable for arrhythmias having a particularly wide critical zone, often between two anatomic structures. Circumferential lesions also may be used to prevent spread of a depolarizing wavefront. Deeper lesions may be particularly well suited to treat foci located deep within the myocardium or subepicardium. New advances in catheter design will likely result in many more arrhythmias that can be successfully treated.

REFERENCES

1.　Olgin JE, Kalman JM, Lesh MD. Conduction barriers in human atrial flutter: correlation of electrophysiology and anatomy. Journal of Cardiovascular Electrophysiology. 1996;7:1112-1126.
2.　Olshansky B, Okumura K, Hess P, Waldo A. Demonstration of an area of slow conduction in human atrial flutter. Journal of the American College of Cardiology. 1990;16:1639-1648.
3.　Kalman JM, Olgin JE, Saxon LA, Fisher WG, Lee RJ, Lesh MD. Activation and entrainment mapping defines the tricuspid annulus as the anterior barrier in typical atrial flutter [see comments]. Circulation. 1996;94:398-406.
4.　Cosio G, M L-G, A G, F A, Barroso J. Radiofrequency ablation of the inferior vena cava-tricuspid valve isthmus in common atrial flutter. American Journal of Cardiology. 1993;71:705-709.
5.　Saoudi N, Atallah G, Kirkorian G, P T. Catheter ablation of the atrial myocardium in human Type I atrial flutter. Circulation. 1990;81:762-771.

6. Fischer B, Jais P, Shah D, Chouair iS, Haissaguerre M, Garrigues S, Poquet F, Gencel L, Clementy J, Marcus F. Radiofrequency catheter ablation of common atrial flutter in 200 patients. Journal of Cardiovascular Electrophysiology. 1996;7:1225-1233.

7. Johna R, Eckardt L, Fetsch T, Breithardt G, Borggrefe M. A new algorithm to determine complete isthmus conduction block after radiofrequency catheter ablation for typical atrial flutter. The American Journal of Cardiology. 1999;83:1666-1668.

8. Poty H, Saoudi N, Abdel A, Nair M, Letac B. Radiofrequency catheter ablation of type 1 atrial flutter. Prediction of late success by electrophysiological criteria. Circulation. 1995;92:1389-1392.

9. Flinn C, Wolff G, M. D. Cardiac rhythm after the Mustard operation for complete transposition of the great arteries. N Eng J Med. 1984;310:1635-1642.

10. Horvath K, Burke R, Collins JJ, LH. C. Surgical treatment of atrial septal defect: early and long-term results. J Am Coll Cardiol. 1992;20:1156-1159.

11. Driscoll D, Offord K, Feldt R, Schaff H, FJ P, Danielson G. Five and fifteen year follow-up after Fontan operation. Circulation. 1992;85:469-496.

12. Kalman J, VanHare G, Olgin J, Saxon L, Tark S, Lesh M. Ablation of 'incisional' reentrant atrial tachycardia complicating surgery for congenital heart disease. Use of entrainment to define a critical isthmus of conduction. Circulation. 1996;93:502-512.

13. Kanter R, Papajiannis J, Carboni M, Ungerleider R, Sanders W, Wharton J. Radiofrequency catheter ablation of supraventricular tachycardia substrates after Mustard and Senning operations for d-transposition of the great arteries. J Am Coll Cardiol. 2000;35:428-441.

14. Wilber D, Kopp D, Glascock D, Kinder C, Kall J. Catheter ablation of mitral isthma for ventricular tachycardia associated with inferior infarction. Circulation. 1995;3481-3489.

15. Marchlinski F, Callans D, Gotlieb C, E. Z. Linear ablation lesions for control of unmappable ventricular tachycardia in patients with ischemic and nonischemic cardiomyopathy. Circulation. 2000;101:1288-1296.

16. Manolis A, Rastegar H, Payne D, Cleveland R, Estes NAM III. Surgical therapy for drug-refractory ventricular tachycardia: results with mapping-guided subendocardial resection. J Am Coll Cardiol. 1989;14:199-208.

17. Rastegar H, Link M, Foote C, Wang P, Manolis A, Estes Nr. Perioperative and long-term results with mapping-guided subendocardial-resection and left ventricular endoaneurysmorrhaphy. Circulation. 1996;94:1041-1048.

18. Lee R, Mitchell J, Garan H, Ruskin J, McGovern B, Buckley M, Torchiana D, Vlahakes G. Operation for recurrent ventricular tachycardia. Predictors of short- and long-term efficacy. Journal of Thoracic and Cardiovascular Surgery. 1994;107:732-742.

19. Caceres J AM, Werner P, Jazayeri M, McKinnie J, Avitall B, Tchou P. Cryoablation of refractory sustained ventricular tachycardia due to coronary artery disease. Am J Cardiol. 1989;63:296-300.

20. Cox J, Gallagher J, Ungerleide R. Encircling endocardial ventriculotomy for refractory ischemic ventricular tachycardia.IV.Clinical indication, surgical technique, mechanism of action, and results. Journal of Thoracic and Cardiovascular Surgery. 1982;83:865-872.

21. Allessie M, Lammers W, Bonke F, al. e. Experimental evaluation of Moe's multiple wavelet hypothesis of atrial fibrillation. In: Zipes D, Jalife J, eds. Cardiac Electrophysiology and Arrhythmias. Orlando, FL: Grune and Stratton; 1985:265-276.

22. Moe G, WC R, Abildskov J. A computer model of atrial fibrillation. Am Heart J. 1964:200-220.

23. Cox J, Schuessler R, D'Agostino HJ, Stone C, Chang B, Cain M, Corr P, Boineau J. The surgical treatment of atrial fibrillation. III. Development of a definitive surgical procedure. J Thorac Cardiovasc Surg. 1996;101:569-583.

24. Cox J, Schuessler R, Lappas D, Boineau, JP. An 81/2-year clinical experience with surgery for atrial fibrillation. Ann Surg. 1996;224:267-275.

25. Jaïs P, Coste P, Shah D, et al. Biatrial dimensions relative to catheter ablation. Eur J CPE. 1996;6:87.

26. Jensen D, BK W, AG R. Human atrial dimensions relevant to intracardiac ablation "Maze" procedure for atrial fibrillation. Pacing Clin Electrophysiol. 1997;20:1146.

27. Lavergne T, Jaïs P, Haïssaguerre M, et al. Evaluation of a single passage RF ablation line in animal atria using an irrigated tip catheter. Circulation. 1997;96:259.
28. Haïssaguerre M, Jaïs P, Shah D, Clementy J. Catheter ablation for atrial fibrillation: clinical electrophysiology of linear lesions. In: Zipes D, Jalife J, eds. Cardiac Electrophysiology, From Cell to Bedside. Philadelphia, PA: W. B. Saunders Co.; 2000:994-1008.
29. Haïssaguerre M, Jaïs P, Shah Dea. Right and left atrial radiofrequency catheter therapy of paroxysmal atrial fibrillation. J Cardiovasc Electrophysiol. 1996;12:1132-1144.
30. Gaita F, R R, Lamberti F. Right atrium radiofrequency catheter ablation in idiopathic vagal atrial fibrillation. Eur Heart J. 1996;17:301.
31. Ching MK, Daoud E, Knight Bea. Right atrial radiofrequency catheter ablation of paroxysmal atrial fibrillation. J Am Coll Cardiol. 1996:188A.
32. Jaïs P, Shah D, Takahashi A, Hocini M, Haissaguerre M, Clementy J. Long-term follow-up after right atrial radiofrequency catheter treatment of paroxysmal atrial fibrillation. Pacing and Clinical Electrophysiology. 1998;21:2533-2538.
33. Jaïs P, Shah D, Haïssaguerre M, Takahashi A, T L, M H, S G, Barold SS, Le Metayer P, J. C. Efficacy and safety of septal and left-atrial linear ablation for atrial fibrillation. American Journal of Cardiology. 1999;84:139R-146R.
34. Calkins H, Hall J, Ellenbogen K, Walcott G, Sherman M, Bowe W, Simpson J, Castellano T, Kay G. A new system for catheter ablation of atrial fibrillation. Am J Cardiol. 1999;83:227D-236D.
35. Thomas S, Nunn G, Nicholson I, Rees A, Daly M, Chard R, Ross D. Mechanism, localization and cure of atrial arrhythmias occurring after a new intraoperative endocardial radiofrequency ablation procedure for atrial fibrillation. J Am Coll Cardiol. 2000;35:442-450.
36. Pappone C, Oreto G, Lamberti F, Vicedomini G, Loricchio M, Shpun S, Rillo M, Calabro M, A C, Ben-Haim S, Cappato R, Chierchia S. Catheter ablation of atrial fibrillation using 3D mapping system. Circulation. 1999;100:1203-1208.
37. Feinberg W, Blackshear J, Laupacis A, Kronmal R, J. H. Prevalence, age distribution and gender of patients with atrial fibrillation: analysis and implications. Arch Intern Med. 1995;155::469-473.
38. Wolf P, Abbott R, WB K. Atrial fibrillation: A major contributor to stroke in the elderly. The Framingham Study. Arch Intern Med. 1987;147:1561-1564.
39. Connolly S, Gent M, Roberts R, Dorian P, Roy D, Sheldon R, LB M, MS G, Klein G, O'Brien B. Canadian Implantable defibrillator study (CIDS). A randomized trial of the implantable cardioverter defibrillator against amiodarone. Circulation. 2000:1297-1302.
40. Investigators TAvIDA. A comparison of antiarrhythmic-drug therapy with implantable defibrillators in patients resuscitated from near-fatal ventricular arrhythmias. N Eng J Med. 1997;337:1576-1583.
41. Josephson M, Harken A, LN H. Long term results of endocardial resection for sustained ventricular tachycardia in coronary disease patients. American Heart Journal. 1982;104:51-57.
42. Stevenson W, Friedman P, Kocovic D, Sager P, Saxon L, Pavri B. Radiofrequency catheter ablation of ventricular tachycardia after myocardial infarction. Circulation. 1998;98:308-314.
43. Oeff M, Langberg J, Franklin J. Effects of multipolar electrode radiofrequency energy delivery on ventricular endocardium. Am Heart J. 1990;119:599-607.
44. Vanderbrink B, Gu Z, Rodriguez V, Link M, Homoud M, Estes NAM, 3rd, Rappaport C, Wang P. Microwave ablation using a spiral antenna design in a porcine thigh muscle preparation: in vivo assessment of temperature profile and lesion geometry. Journal of Cardiovascular Electrophysiology. 2000;11:193-198.
45. VanderBrink BA, Gilbride C, Aronovitz MJ, Lenihan T, Schorn G, Taylor K, Regan JF, Carr K, Schoen FJ, Link MS, Homoud MK, Estes NAM, III, Wang PJ. Safety and efficacy of a steerable temperature monitoring microwave catheter system for ventricular myocardial ablation. Journal of Cardiovascular Electrophysiology. 2000;11:305-10.

Chapter 18

NEW CONCEPTS IN RADIOFREQUENCY ENERGY DELIVERY AND COAGULUM REDUCTION DURING CATHETER ABLATION

Energy Delivery Management and a Quantitative Measure for Estimating the Probability of Coagulum Formation During Radiofrequency Ablation

Eric K.Y. Chan
CARDIMA, Inc, Fremont, California,, USA

1. RADIO FREQUENCY GENERATOR TECHNICAL FUNDAMENTALS

1.1 Operational Characteristics of Radio Frequency Generators and Waveforms

The primary functional building block of all radio frequency (RF) energy sources developed for tissue ablation is an electronic circuit called an oscillator which generates a sinusoidal waveform (sine wave) at a particular factory-preset operating frequency. This waveform is consequently amplified to deliver the required wattage required for tissue ablation. The operating frequency of this RF oscillator differs from one RF generator manufacturer to another; however, they all fall within the range from 470 to 510 kHz. A diagram of radio-frequency energy used in RF ablation in relation to the electromagnetic spectrum is shown in Figure 1.

L. Bing Liem and E. Downar (eds.), Progress in Catheter Ablation, 293-310.
© 2001 *Kluwer Academic Publishers. Printed in the Netherlands.*

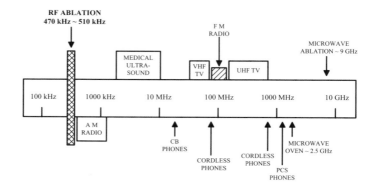

Figure 1. Radio and Microwave Frequency Spectrum

The quality of the oscillator and ancillary electronics design impinges on the stability of the resulting operating frequency. Hence, this operating frequency may "drift" slightly if the oscillator design is unstable. Typically, this frequency jitter has imperceptible influence on the resulting tissue lesion. However, a more serious problem is when a RF oscillator or its associated electronics system generate and deliver a skewed or distorted sine wave signal that has spurious noise spikes and/or harmonics riding on top of it. These undesirable noise artifacts may have the potential of promoting coagulum formation if they are present during the ablation process. Needless to say, it is desirable to use a RF source, which produces as pure and stable a sine wave as possible. Figure 2 shows an example of a desirable "clean" RF sinusoidal signal from a commercially available RF generator. With regards to patient safety, as well as meeting requirements for electromagnetic susceptibility and radiated emissions standards, the RF generator should be in compliance with international safety standards, such as the IEC 60601-2 set of standards, as well as the CE Mark standards.[1]

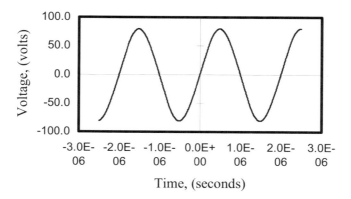

Figure 2. Typical RF generator sinusoidal output waveform

1.2   Catheter Ablation Systems Configuration

In catheter ablation, the amplified RF current is fed into biological tissue via electrodes arranged in various configurations at the distal end of a catheter. The RF current uses the ground pad as the return path to leave the body. This RF energy in turn heats the tissue by causing ionic and molecular friction within the tissue and fluid medium encompassed by the electric field.[2] The degree of tissue heating and resulting temperature rise is predominantly influenced by (i) tissue impedance, (ii) size and quality of electrode-tissue contact, and (iii) duration of RF application. When monitored, this temperature rise caused by the conversion of electrical to thermal energy can be used as a guide in RF catheter ablation. Its measurement is facilitated by the placement of thermal sensors, either thermocouples or thermistors, underneath or juxtaposed with the ablative electrodes. For example, a catheter that has been developed for right atrial linear MAZE ablation has eight electrodes with thermocouples located in between the electrodes rather than underneath the electrodes, to accurately sense localised tissue temperature at the ablation site.

Figure 3 shows a drawing of this catheter, the CARDIMA REVELATION™ Tx 3.7F microcatheter, which has eight 6 mm coil electrodes in a 2-2-2 spacing, and 8 thermocouples located proximal to each electrode in the inter-electrode spaces. Not only can the sensed temperature be used to ascertain the quality of electrode-tissue contact and predict lesion size, it can also be utilized by the RF generator as a feedback signal to automatically regulate the output power to arrive at or maintain a target temperature predetermined by the end-user. A 9F NAVIPORT™ steerable guiding catheter with either a 90 cm or 110 cm working length, also shown in Figure 3, is used in conjunction with this ablation catheter to aid in placement.

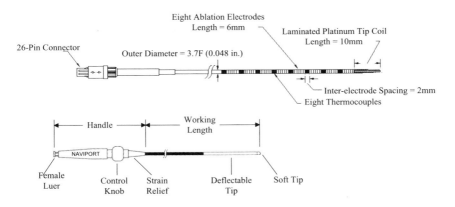

Figure 3. CARDIMA REVELATION Tx 3.7F Octapolar Microcatheter and NAVIPORT
Deflectable Tip Guiding Catheter (Drawings not to scale)

In order to switch between each of the multiple electrodes and their corresponding thermocouples or thermistors, manual switchboxes interfacing multi-electrode catheters with multiple thermocouples to single-channel RF generators have been developed. An example of such a switchbox is shown in Figure 4, the CARDIMA Tx-Select switchbox, which enables RF energy to be delivered to the ablation electrodes in a consecutive, sequential fashion. This switchbox interfaces the CARDIMA REVELATION Tx ablation catheter to a broad spectrum of commercially available RF generators simply by using different interchangeable connector cables. These RF generators include the Radionics RFG-3E, IBI-1500T4, Sulzer Osypka HAT300 Smart, Medtronic Atakr and Cordis EP-Shuttle Stockert.

There are also automatic-sequencing multi-channel RF energy generators that are now commercially available, such as the IBI 1500T4 RF generator. In addition, the IBI generator can also deliver RF energy *simultaneously* to four electrodes. By virtue of the higher energy requirements, this generator is capable of up to 150W power output in the simultaneous mode.

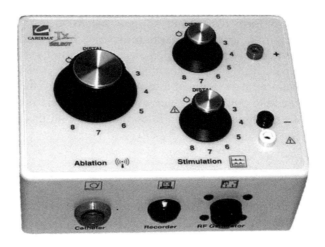

Figure 4. TX-SELECT Switchbox for interfacing a REVELATION Tx Octapolar Catheter (eight electrodes, eight thermocouples) to a Single Channel RF Generator. (Photo by Jason Franco).

Most RF generators have software modules, which run simultaneously on portable computers during RF energy delivery to record the ablation episode in real-time. The typical parameters logged are sensed impedance, power delivered, current and voltage, as well as tissue temperature sensed by either thermistors or thermocouples as described above. The software permits the end-user to select parameters that are displayed for post-procedural review. Figure 5 shows a typical screen display of the power, temperature and current logged during a 60-second ablation episode. These parameters were selected because they can be used in calculating a new measure for the probability of coagulum formation, to be discussed later in this chapter.

1.3   Delivery of RF Energy

All RF generators deliver RF energy in 2 phases: (i) the "ramp-up" phase in which a relatively high amount of power is delivered to the ablating electrode until a desired target temperature is sensed by the thermocouple or thermistor, and (ii) the "regulation" phase in which power is still being delivered but regulated at a lower level to maintain the desired target temperature. This target temperature is predetermined by the operator, and is generally set at 50^0 to 55^0 C in the linear ablation protocol using the REVELATION™ Tx catheter.

The challenge in RF ablation of cardiac tissue is to create deep lesions in the cardiac tissue while avoiding coagulum formation. It follows that RF energy has to be delivered *efficiently* into the tissue, and not delivered and lost into the blood medium. Hence, a primary objective in RF ablation is the achievement of *excellent electrode-tissue contact* to achieve deeper lesions, with the added benefit of reducing coagulum formation. The rest of this section explores this concept in greater depth.

An *in vitro* experiment was designed by Eick *et al* to test the hypothesis that increasing contact force at the electrode-tissue interface improves the flow of RF energy into tissue.[3] They found that contact force was indeed highly correlated, up to 97%, with temperature rise. Thus, when there is excellent electrode-tissue contact, there is a regular flow of RF energy transmitted into the tissue that is efficiently converted into heat energy. When this condition exists, the monitored tissue impedance and voltage is relatively constant.[4] In practice, the measured tissue impedance is another key parameter, because it is an indicator of electrode-tissue contact.

It follows that when tissue contact is good and stable, the impedance is relatively low and constant. As a result, less RF energy is required to reach the desired target temperature, with a shorter "ramp up" time and a lower wattage (less power) required to maintain the target temperature. The risk of coagulum formation is low because RF energy is effectively transmitted into the tissue, and heat is generated within the tissue rather than at the blood layer.

Conversely, when electrode-tissue contact is intermittent, the impedance value fluctuates and the power delivered also has to adapt rapidly in order to reach or maintain the target temperature. The rapid back and forth switching between high and low impedance causes the output power waveform to also fluctuate. If this fluctuating power waveform has high enough amplitude, it may be conducive for coagulum formation because it may undesirably approximate the coagulation waveform used by electrosurgical units.[5]

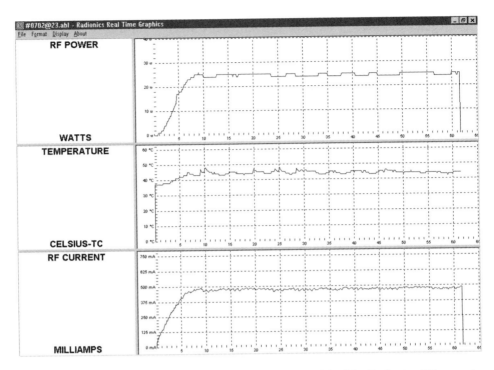

Figure 5. Screen capture of 60-second ablation episode as archived by Radionics RF generator software

When electrode-tissue contact is marginal or poor, impedance can rise rapidly, thereby requiring more RF energy to be delivered in a fast response to achieve the same target temperature. In this last scenario, because of poor electrode-tissue contact, there is a high probability that RF energy is lost into the blood layer surrounding the electrode, thus heating the blood rather than tissue and fostering coagulum formation. As coagulum forms on the electrode, it forms a resistive film between the tissue and electrode surface, and the RF generator has to emit more energy to reach or maintain target temperature. These conditions bring about a vicious cycle of climbing watts and escalation of thrombus formation. Hence, one has to terminate the power delivery immediately when there is a sudden impedance rise. The catheter should be withdrawn at this point to be inspected, and coagulum should be gently wiped off the electrodes if necessary.

1.4   Increasing Lesion Depth by Increasing Duration of RF Delivery

Assuming excellent electrode-tissue contact, *Hindricks et al* previously showed that lesion depth increases as a function of electrode size, for a given duration of RF energy application.[4] More importantly, for a given *electrode size*, their results indicated that one has to *triple* or *quadruple* the duration of RF application to *double* the resulting lesion depth. Their data for a 6F active tip electrode showed that it took approximately 22 seconds for the generated lesion depth to reach 2 mm. To double lesion depth to 4mm using the same electrode tip, it took about 70 seconds.[4]

One therefore has to be cognizant *that increasing RF application duration can increase lesion depth.* Therefore one must consider the differing myocardial thickness of anatomical regions of the heart, in determining the duration of RF application. For example, the duration of RF application at the isthmus region, which has an approximate average depth of 7 mm in the human heart,[6] can be increased to 90~120 seconds, in an attempt create a deeper lesion to achieve bi-directional conduction block.

In a series of *in vitro* experiments, *He et al* defined a quantitative *bio-battery* signal, which could be measured during RF energy delivery into tissue.[7] Their experiments showed that there was an optimal duration of RF energy delivery to develop deep lesions before the onset of rapid impedance rise. This duration coincided with a sudden change of slope in the *bio-battery* signal. Ablation durations beyond this sudden "bump" did not result in lesions that were much deeper than those created with RF energy terminated at the time of the "bump". While their initial data calls for further *in vivo* studies, their results parallel those of *Hindricks et al*, who showed that beyond certain duration of RF application, lesion depth and width tend to reach a steady-state condition and stop growing. One should also be cognizant from the work of *Hindricks et al* that the duration for RF energy application to arrive at a steady state for lesion diameter is much shorter than for lesion depth.[4] This is because there is no *deep, penetrative* heat transfer process involved in generating lesion width, especially in high bloodflow regions where convective heat transfer dynamics tend to whisk away heat from the tissue surface at the ablation site.

2. REDUCING COAGULUM FORMATION DURING RF ABLATION

While the above discussion has alluded to general insights on the interplay of electrode-tissue contact, temperature rise-time, sensed impedance and coagulum formation, we now discuss specific insights on how to reduce coagulum formation from the CARDIMA REVELATION Tx US Clinical Trials for right atrial MAZE ablation. The catheter MAZE procedure calls for the creation of linear barricades along anatomical trajectories within the right atrium, using RF ablation to compartmentalise the chamber and 'contain' pro-arrhythmic electrical propagation in a manner fashioned after the surgical MAZE procedure developed by Cox and others.[8]

2.1   Guidelines for Achieving Sufficient Electrode Tissue Contact in Linear Ablation

To underscore what has been discussed above, excellent electrode-tissue contact is paramount to achieving efficient tissue heating during RF ablation. In ideal situations, it is possible to achieve satisfactory tissue contact for all eight linear ablation catheter electrodes of the REVELATION Tx microcatheter. However, we have found that the procedural enhancement techniques listed here have provided successful ablation results in right atrial MAZE linear ablation procedures with the above mentioned octapolar microcatheter system, even when the anatomical or flow conditions prevent optimal *simultaneous* contact of all eight electrodes:

a. Aim for excellent tissue contact for as many linear array electrodes as possible.

b. A good measure of contact is low tissue impedance at 'baseline'; some RF generators permit this to be sensed and displayed prior to actual ablation by emitting a small RF current to interrogate tissue impedance at the ablation site.

c. Pacing threshold, if used as an indicator of contact, should be reasonable (1-2 mA); threshold values above 4-5 mA most likely indicate poor contact, and the catheter should be repositioned.

Flush the sheath periodically (say every 15 minutes) with a standard heparinized saline solution bolus. This improves contact by removing coagulum build-up on the electrodes and catheter shaft. If possible, the catheter should be pulled out of the NAVIPORT deflectable guiding sheath (see Figure 3) after each trajectory. The electrodes should be wiped clean if needed, before re-introducing the catheter into the NAVIPORT.

2.2   Power Delivery Management

In contrast to the excessive temperatures associated with the risk of char and coagulum as reported in earlier studies,[9] we have gained important insights on how to reduce coagulum formation by regulating the RF power settings:

a. It has been shown that the coiled electrodes of the 3.7F REVELATION Tx microcatheter permit high current densities that create transmural lesions as deep as a standard 8F ablation catheter. Importantly, these microcatheter lesions have less width and surface area than those created by a standard ablation catheter, thereby decreasing endocardial damage without sacrificing transmurality.[10] Furthermore, higher electrode current densities permit lower maximum RF generator power settings in the range of 30W to 35W, as opposed to 50W or higher.

b. Some generators may not provide the capability for manually setting the maximum power delivered. If so, the power delivered should be monitored continuously and the catheter should be repositioned as needed to maintain target temperature at a lower power level.

c. We have observed that coagulum formation is more evident when power required to maintain target temperature approaches 50W. Conversely, coagulum formation is minimized greatly when power required is less than 35W. This may be seen as a challenge when trying to reach target temperature. However, we have seen that *with excellent electrode-tissue contact*, the desired target temperature of 50°C to 55°C can be achieved with as low as 7W to 15W of power delivery. *In vivo* animal studies have verified deep, transmural lesions with these low power settings when there is sufficient electrode-tissue contact.

In addition to limiting the maximum output power setting, we have also discovered that the slope or gradient of the power curve plays an important role in minimizing coagulum formation. This is discussed in the next section.

3.   "COAGULUM INDEX" - A NEW ANALYTICAL MODEL FOR PREDICTING COAGULUM FORMATION

A working hypothesis has been developed for reducing the potential for coagulum formation. This has been based on RF ablation data from 398 independent ablation episodes from 15 patient cases in the REVELATION Tx U.S. clinical trials. The specific purpose for this research was to analyze the rate of RF power delivery from the REVELATION Tx catheter electrodes, with respect to target temperature set-points. The measurements made were the duration (t, seconds) for attaining a pre-determined target temperature, as well as the power (P, watts) and RF current (I, amperes) at that time. Each RF energy delivery episode corresponding to each electrode was thus analyzed. If the target temperature was not reached, the duration to reach the maximal recorded temperature closest to the target temperature was used instead.

After each linear ablation trajectory, the catheter was withdrawn from the steerable guiding sheath, and each electrode was visually inspected. The presence or absence of coagulum was duly noted on the clinical data sheets, thereby providing a record for future correlation analysis with other ablation parameters. Throughout the ablative process for each episode, ablation parameters such as power and current were logged automatically by software (see Figure 5). With these values, and the observation of coagulum as recorded in the clinical data sheets, it was possible to derive a mathematical model for data interpretation. From this model, a quantity called the *Coagulum Index* (C.I.) was defined:

> ***Coagulum Index, C.I.* = (P/t) / I^2**
>
> Power = P (watts)
> Current = I (amperes)
> Duration to reach Target Temperature = t (seconds)

It should be noted that the term on the right-hand-side of the equation, (P/t), is simply the slope or gradient of the power curve measured from the start of the ablation episode (baseline) to the time that the target temperature or maximum temperature is first reached in an ablation episode. It can be seen that as the slope defined by (P/t) increases on the right-hand-side of the equation above, the *Coagulum Index* (C.I.) also increases on the left-hand-side of the same equation. For the interested reader, the derivation of the *Coagulum Index* is included in Appendix A of this chapter.

3.1   Correlation of Coagulum Index with Presence of Coagulum

Upon further analysis of temperature and power curves from the CARDIMA U.S. Study series, a pattern emerged.   It was observed that there was a correspondence between C.I. and presence of post-ablation coagulum on the electrodes of the RF catheter.   The higher the calculated C.I., the higher the likelihood of coagulum being present.   Hence, whenever the slope (P/t) was large, a higher incidence of coagulum was recorded.

The lesson learnt from this analysis is that coagulum could be reduced if the slope (P/t) was gentle.   In practice, this amounts to gradually increasing the power delivered from the RF generator, as opposed to 'cranking up the watts' at the very start of an ablation episode.

Figure 6(a) and Figure 6(b) below are representative scatter-grams of C.I. values from two RF ablation patient cases.   It is evident that the derived C.I. value has pertinence and value in suggesting coagulum formation.   The series of ablation episodes depicted in Figure 6(b) illustrates an improvement from the ablation episodes depicted in Figure 6(a), where lower C.I. values correspond with an absence of coagulum.   This improvement stems from the fact that the power was gradually increased in the second study, in contrast to an immediate increase in power levels, demonstrated in the first study.   Furthermore, the maximum power setting was reduced from 50W to 30W.

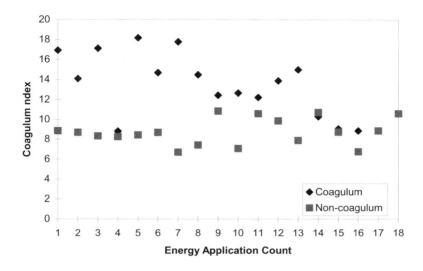

Figure 6(a). Typical data from a patient study when gradual power delivery was not applied. (Maximum power = 50W)

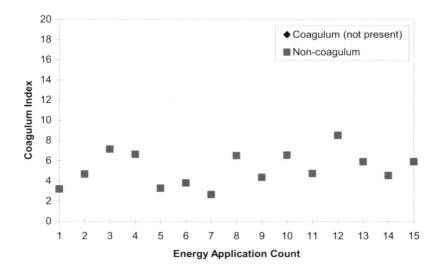

Figure 6(b). Patient study where gradual power delivery was applied for each ablation episode. (Maximum power = 30W)

3.2   Statistical Summary of Results

The estimated probability of coagulum occurring, P(coag), was modelled statistically by a logistic model, since many dose-response relationships have been found to follow a logistic sigmoid curve. This particular statistical model employed logit risk of coagulum as the dependent variable and the calculated *Coagulum Index* (C.I.) as the independent or predictor variable. Table I summarizes the relationship between C.I. and the estimated percentage probability of coagulum formation based on this logistic model of coagulum occurrence.[11]

Table 1. Coagulum Index (C. I.) and Corresponding Probability (%) of Coagulum Formation

C. I.	4	8	12	16	20	24
P(coag)%	2	10	32	69	91	98

In this data series (n=398 ablation episodes from 15 patient cases) derived from the REVELATION Tx U.S. clinical trials, it was found that the logistic model of risk of coagulum formation demonstrated a significant fit between C.I. and the estimated percentage probability of coagulum occurring (p<0.0001). Hence, from this analysis, a clear correspondence between C.I. and coagulum formation exists. Furthermore, a distinct threshold of C.I. $\geq$ 12 is obtained, beyond which the probability of coagulum formation increases significantly.[11]

3.3   Suggestions for Best Practice Based on these Findings

Thus, it appears that one possible mechanism of mitigating coagulum formation would be to have the REVELATION Tx catheter electrodes deliver RF power in such a way that the rise time of the power, and hence temperature curve, is more gradual and consistent. For example, when using the Radionics RFG-3E generator with a set maximum of 30W, one should commence with a lower power setting of 10W for the first 10 seconds or so, and then gradually adjust the knob manually on the RF generator to the set maximum of 30W, while still maintaining total RF delivery time at 60 seconds.[12]   When this technique was applied, it decreased coagulum formation, as is evident in the data shown in Figure 6(b). Hence, it is inadvisable to introduce a large amount of RF energy into tissue in a very short time window, in an attempt to heat tissue faster and deeper.   If our goal is to achieve deeper lesions, we have to look towards prolonging RF application duration for the answer.

One must also be cognizant of the characteristics of the other generators on the market. The Irvine Biomedical IBI-1500T has 4 user-selectable choices for controlling the power delivery ramp-up curve.[13]   The Osypka HAT300 Smart RF Generator incorporates "fuzzy logic" algorithms which appear to regulate power delivery rise time gradually.[14]   Finally, the battery-powered Medtronic CardioRhythm Atakr has no user override controls for power delivery application,[15] although a new model Atakr II with improved features and performance will be introduced commercially soon.   In comparison, the Radionics RFG-3E has a rather steep automatic ramp-up power curve; we recommend selecting the manual control mode which allows the user to manually increase power output during the delivery of RF energy.[12]

3.4   Summary of Clinical Data using Best Practice Methodology for Coagulum Reduction

It was important to ascertain how the absence of coagulum affects the clinical effectiveness of linear ablation.   Best practice methods guided by the Coagulum Index (C.I.) for coagulum reduction were applied during RF ablation in Phase II of the REVELATION Tx clinical trials, and not in Phase I. Progressing from Phase I to Phase II, we see almost a doubling of the percentage of patients (40% to 77%) who had greater than 50% reduction in AF episodes. A significant increase was also observed for patients who no longer had any AF episodes (100% reduction), from 30% in Phase I to 53% in Phase II.[16]

Table 2. Reduction of AF Episodes after 6 Months: Phase I and Phase II Clinical Data Comparison[16]

% Reduction of AF Episodes after 6 Months	Phase I (N=10)	Phase II (N=17)
>50% reduction	4/10 Pt (40%)	13/17 pt (77%)
100% reduction (no AF Episodes)	3/10 Pt (30%)	9/17 pt (53%)

It should be noted that the majority (6 out of 9) of the clinical test-sites in Phase II were newly enrolled sites, hence the improvement in clinical results were not simply due to more experience with the catheter ablation process by the clinical investigators. Therefore, the six-month follow-up clinical data strongly suggests that coagulum reduction enhances the quality of the resulting linear lesions. This improvement may be due to the eradication of impedance rises during RF ablation caused by the presence of coagulum, which in turn trigger the RF generator to shut-off energy delivery prematurely, thereby contributing to inadequate lesion depth.   Furthermore, when there is no resistive layer of coagulum between electrode and tissue, RF energy transfer is more efficient and lesion depth is increased.

SUMMARY

This chapter has introduced basic concepts regarding RF ablation biophysics, as well as typical features of RF generators and catheter-based RF energy delivery systems that are used clinically in cardiac electrophysiology laboratories. It also has addressed theoretical aspects and practical techniques pertaining to coagulum reduction during linear MAZE RF ablation procedure in the right atrium.

A novel quantitative parameter, the Coagulum Index (C.I.), has been derived from basic physical quantities that are measurable during RF ablation. In turn, the C.I. was used as a guide in the development of best practice methods for RF ablation. Specifically, excellent electrode-tissue contact, in combination with gradual RF power delivery to a maximum level of 30W to 35W, constitutes a sound prescription for best practice of RF ablation with the least probability of coagulum formation at the electrode site, without dependence on the cooling effect of irrigated ablation catheters.

Improved safety and effectiveness of right atrial MAZE RF ablation was attained by minimizing coagulum formation, as evidenced by comparing the REVELATION Tx U.S. Phase I and Phase II six-month clinical data.

While this analysis has been performed with the CARDIMA REVELATION Tx microcatheter system, it is envisaged that these insights can be extrapolated to procedures using other catheters for other RF ablation procedures as well. Furthermore, these results from right atrial MAZE ablation may portend to left atrium ablation procedures, where minimizing coagulum formation may decrease the risk of stroke and associated mortality.

ACKNOWLEDGMENTS

The author would like to thank Michael Pao, Mohsen Nasab, Kushal Vepa, Reynaldo Hilario, David Carner, Allan Abati, Harrison Stubbs and Diane Magary for their assistance in various aspects of this chapter, Phillip Radlick for his encouragement and support, and Gabriel Vegh for his vision of using microcatheters to create a better quality of life for AF patients.

APPENDIX A

MATHEMATICAL DERIVATION OF COAGULUM INDEX BY DIMENSIONAL ANALYSIS OF PHYSICAL PARAMETERS PERTINENT TO RF ABLATION

The passage of RF current, I, through cardiac tissue generates heat via molecular and ionic friction. This "resistive heating" takes place because cardiac tissue has an intrinsic impedance. Furthermore, an observable impedance rise during the ablation process may be attributed to one or more of the following influencing factors:

1. An intermittent or prolonged reduction in the integrity of electrode-tissue contact;
2. An increase in the resistivity of the tissue itself due to a decrease in ionic mobility (protein coagulation) during the heating process; or
3. Build-up of a resistive film of coagulum between the tissue and electrode surface.

A hypothesis was therefore formulated based on the notion of impedance rise as an indicator of coagulum formation. In the presence of an alternating RF current, I, the capacitive component of tissue impedance $Z(\Omega)$ comes into play. The mathematical treatment of this hypothesis begins with the definition of capacitive impedance:[17]

$$Z(\Omega) = 1/j\omega C$$
Eqn.[1]

where Ω or ohms is the unit for impedance,
C = electrical capacitance of the tissue, $j = \sqrt{-1}$,
$\omega = 2\pi f$, a constant term for a particular RF generator, assuming that the RF oscillator frequency, f, is stable and constant.

Now we define electrical capacitance, C, in terms of its fundamental *Systeme Internationale* (S.I.) units:[18]

$$C = A^2 / (Kg.m^2.s^{-4})$$
Eqn.[2]

where A, amperes, is the S.I. unit for current, I.

Capacitive impedance cannot be measured directly because the impedance on the RF generator readout includes inductive, capacitive and resistive components of impedance. Fortunately, we have discovered a proportional representation of capacitive impedance by dimensional analysis of the physical units defining the RF power delivery curve.

For each single-electrode catheter ablation event, the slope of the power curve can be calculated from a plot of *Power,* P(W) *vs. Duration,* t(s), where duration is the time taken for the sensed temperature to rise from baseline temperature (approximately 37°C) to target temperature (50°C to 55°C). Figure 5 shows a graphical log of a typical 60 second ablation episode. If the target temperature cannot be reached, then the duration is the time for the sensed temperature to reach the maximum temperature for that ablation episode.

This slope is mathematically defined as:

$$
\begin{aligned}
\text{Slope} \quad &= \text{Power/Time} \\
\text{Eqn.[3]} \\
&= (\text{Work Done/Time}) \,/\, \text{Time} \\
&= (\text{Force} * \text{Displacement}) \,/\, \text{Time}^2 \\
&= ((\text{Mass} * \text{acceleration}) * \text{Displacement}) \,/\, \text{Time}^2
\end{aligned}
$$

In S. I. units, Mass = Kg [kilogram], Length = m [meter], Time = s [seconds].

Substituting the units for acceleration as ms^{-2}, then a dimensional analysis of the units in Eqn.[3] show that the units for the slope of the power curve are:

$$
\text{Slope} \quad = (\text{Kg.m.s}^{-2}\,\text{m})/\text{s}^2
$$
Eqn.[4]

Rearranging and simplifying terms:

$$
\text{Slope} \quad = \text{Kg.m}^2.\text{s}^{-4}
$$
Eqn.[5]

An important observation is that Eqn.[5] has the same dimensional units as the denominator in the dimensional definition of capacitance C in Eqn.[2]. Hence, we can then formulate a proportional representation of tissue capacitance from the dimensional units:

$$
C \propto A^2 \,/\, \text{Slope}
$$
Eqn.[6]

Z, the capacitive impedance of tissue, can then be expressed as function of the power curve slope, by subisuting Eqn.[6] into Eqn.[1]. Hence, a *Relative Impedance* term can be calculated that is proportional to the capacitive impedance $Z(\Omega)$ of cardiac tissue in the presence of an alternating RF current, I(A):

$$
\textit{Relative Impedance} = k * \text{Slope} \,/\, I^2
$$
Eqn.[7]

where k is a proportionality constant which includes the $j\omega$ term, where j is a constant. In practice, since the same type of RF generator, the Radionics RFG-3E, was used throughout the CARDIMA REVELATION Tx U.S. multicenter study, the RF frequency is also a preset, constant value and ω therefore is also constant. Therefore, for practical purposes, the proportionality constant k is set to unity in the calculation. The results discussed in Section 3 showed a close correspondence between this calculated value and the probability of coagulum formation at the ablation electrode site. Hence, the term *"Coagulum Index"* (C.I.) was given to this quantity. We therefore finally arrive at:

$$Coagulum\ Index = Slope\ /\ I^2$$

$$C.I. = (P/t)\ /\ I^2$$
$$Eqn.[8]$$

The slope of the power curve for each ablation episode can be conveniently measured from the duration t (seconds) taken to reach target temperature, as well as the power P(W) and current I(A) recorded at that time. Hence, C.I. is a practical quantity that can be easily calculated from the data records of individual ablation episodes. The units for *Coagulum Index* are therefore $W.s^{-1}.A^{-2}$.

REFERENCES

1. Schoenmakers CCW, CE marking for medical devices - A handbook to the medical device directives: Medical Device Directive 93/42/EEC; The Active Implantable Medical Device Directive 90/396/EEC, Piscataway: IEEE Press, 1997.

2. Cosman ER, Rittman WJ, "Physical aspects of radiofrequency energy applications". In: Huang SKS, ed. Radiofrequency Catheter Ablation of Cardiac Arrhythmias - Basic Concepts and Clinical Applications, Armonk: Futura, 1994:13-23

3. Eick OJ, Wittkampf FH, Bronnenberg T, Schumacher B, "The LETR-Principle: A novel method to assess electrode-tissue contact in radiofrequency ablation", J Cardiovascular Electrophysiology 1998; 9(11):180-1185.

4. Hindricks G, Haverkamp W, "Determinants of radiofrequency- induced lesion size - What are the important parameters to monitor during energy application?". In: Huang SKS, ed. Radiofrequency Catheter Ablation of Cardiac Arrhythmias - Basic Concepts and Clinical Applications, Armonk: Futura, 1994:97-121.

5. Neuman MR, "Therapeutic and prosthetic devices". In: Webster JG, ed. Medical Instrumentation - Applications and Design, Boston: Houghton Mifflin Company, 1978:655-656.

6. Yamauchi Y, Aonuma K, Oh J, Hachiya H, Kobaysahi I, Kano H, Korenaga M, "Difficulty in typical atrial flutter ablation depends on tricuspid valve-inferior vena cava isthmus anatomy", Circulation 1999; 100(18):I-652.

7. He DS, Sharma P, Wang XZ, Bosnos M, Marcus F, "Bio-battery signal predicts myocardial lesion formation and depth in vivo", J Interventional Cardiac Electrophysiology 1999; 3:69-77.

8. Cox J, Boineau J, Schuessler R, Ferguson B, Cain M, Lindsay B, Corr P, Kater K, Lappas D, "Successful surgical treatment of atrial fibrillation", JAMA 1991; 226(14):1976-1980.

9. Murgatroyd FD, Haines DE, Swartz JF, "Catheter ablation as a curative approach to the substrate of atrial fibrillation". In: Murgatroyd FD and Camm AJ, ed. Nonpharmacological Management of Atrial Fibrillation, Armonk: Futura, 1997:239-255.

10. Asirvatham S, "Can microcatheters produce linear lesions without sacrificing transmurality in the canine atrium?", Circulation 1999; 100(18):I-374.

11. Chan EKY, Vepa KP, Hacker VF, "Coagulum index predicts coagulum formation in right atrial linear maze RF ablation", Europace 2000; 1:D-50.

12. Radionics RFG-3E Lesion Generator Operating Instructions, 920-60-001 Rev. E, Burlington: Radionics, Inc., 1998.

13. IBI-1500T Cardiac Ablation Generator with Temperature Control - Operator's Manual, 75554 Rev. B, Irvine: Irvine Biomedical, Inc., 1999.

14. Sulzer Osypka HAT 300 Smart Radiofrequency Ablation System Version 2.0 - Instructions for Use, Grenzach-Wyhlen: Sulzer Osypka GmbH, 1997.

15. Medtronic CardioRhythm Atakr Ablation System Technical Manual 01970, San Jose: Medtronic, Inc., 1995.

16. Chan EKY, Abati AL, Vepa K, "Coagulum index predicts coagulum formation in right atrial linear maze Rfablation", PACE 2000;23(II):1856-1858.

17. Hayt WH, Kemmerly JE, Engineering Circuit Analysis, Third Edition, New York: McGraw-Hill, 1978:296.

18. The NIST Reference on Constants, Units, and Uncertainty, http://physics.nist.gov/cuu/Units/units.html

Chapter 19

COOLED RADIOFREQUENCY CATHETER ABLATION

George J. Juang, Walter L. Atiga*, Ronald D. Berger, Hugh Calkins
*Department of Medicine, Division of Cardiology, The Johns Hopkins University, Baltimore, Maryland, USA; *University of Pittsburgh, Pittsburgh, Pensylvania, USA.*

INTRODUCTION

During the past decade, radiofrequency catheter ablation has emerged as an important definitive approach to the treatment of most types of ventricular and supraventricular arrhythmias.[1,2] The development of temperature monitoring and closed loop temperature control of RF energy output was subsequently shown to facilitate RF catheter ablation and have been accepted into routine clinical practice.[3,4] Despite the remarkable safety and efficacy of RF catheter ablation as used in routine clinical practice, certain types of arrhythmias proved to be more refractory to attempts at catheter ablation. Most notable among these were atrial fibrillation, atrial flutter, and nonidiopathic ventricular tachycardia. For these arrhythmias, new tools to facilitate ablation of these arrhythmias were deemed necessary. Linear catheter ablation systems and ablation systems designed specifically to facilitate catheter ablation in the region of the pulmonary veins are being developed for atrial fibrillation.[5,6] In contrast, it was felt that ablation systems capable of creating deeper lesions were required to improve the efficacy of catheter ablation of atrial flutter as well as nonidiopathic VT. Cooling the tip of the ablation catheter was subsequently proposed as a potential solution to develop larger and deeper lesions during RF application.[7,8] The purpose of this chapter is to review the current understanding of the mechanism by which cooling of the ablation electrode facilitates creation of larger lesions as well as the results of animal and clinical trials which have employed cooled RF ablation technology.

L. Bing Liem and E. Downar (eds.), Progress in Catheter Ablation, 311-326.
© 2001 *Kluwer Academic Publishers. Printed in the Netherlands.*

1. BIOPHYSICS OF CONVENTIONAL RF ABLATION

Conventional radiofrequency ablation involves the delivery of an alternating electrical current at a frequency between 350kHz and 750 kHz from an electrode catheter positioned on the endocardium to a ground patch placed on the surface of the body.[9] The ground plate, or dispersive electrode, has a much larger surface area than the tip. Current density is thus focused on the tip. The flow of current from the active tip electrode occurs at a high frequency in alternating directions. Intense ionic agitation of the tissues only in very close proximity to the electrode tip results in resistive heating of the tissue. The tissue itself is the source of heat generation in contrast to a thermal probe where the resistive element is in the probe itself.

The power generated in watts is equal to the square of the total current (I) multiplied by the total resistance (R) when capacitive effects are neglected: Power = I^2R. Resistive heating of the tissue is due to the local power density (p) which is related to the local current density (j) and the resistance (R) according to $p=j^2R$. The current and power densities sharply decrease with increasing distance (r) from the electrode, falling by $1/r^2$ and $1/r^4$ respectively. The duration of time (T) power is applied also influences heat generation. Finally, the total energy applied (E) is power integrated over time. If power is constant, total energy E = PT = I^2RT.

Heating of the tissue surrounding the RF catheter tip is a two step process: resistive heating followed by conductive heating from the area of resistive heating to the surrounding myocardium (Figure 1). Resistive heating is significant only within the first millimeter of tissue extending past the ablation electrode. Conductive heat transfer is then responsible for further thermal injury up to several millimeters away. Lesion size is mainly due to the equilibrium reached by conductive heat generation and convective heat loss in the surrounding tissue. Convective heat loss occurs when surrounding blood flow cools the area of the lesion. The creation of significantly different lesion volumes may occur depending on the underlying heat transfer properties of the cardiac structures or the cooling effects of different rates of blood flow.

The heat created in tissues increases with time. The temperature rise generated by resistive heating plateaus quickly, within 10 seconds for a 1 mm electrode. The heating created by conduction manifests more slowly and plateaus within 200 seconds for a 1 mm electrode. A steady state thermodynamic equilibrium is reached when the net gain of energy delivered by conduction equals the net loss by convection, leading to no further lesion growth despite continued RF application. In the thermodynamic model proposed by Haines et al.[10] the steady-state myocardial temperature a distance r from the heat source depends linearly on the source temperature and falls by 1/r with distance.

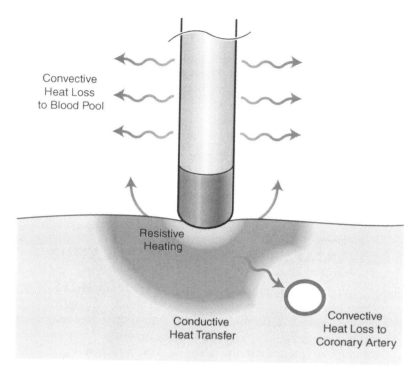

Figure 1. Schematic drawing of radiofrequency catheter ablation on the endocardium demonstrating zones of resistive and conductive heating and convective heat loss into the blood pool and coronary arteries. Reproduced with permission (9).

The success of RF ablation depends on tissue destruction with subsequent loss of electrical conductivity. Increasing temperatures lead to thermal injury, protein denaturation, and ultimately tissue coagulation and desiccation. Radiofrequency energy delivered at high current densities without increases in tissue temperature results in loss of cellular excitability. Once a temperature >43°C is reached, myocardial depolarization and loss of excitability occurs. At temperatures near 48°C (ranging from 43°C to 51°C) reversible loss of myocardial excitability occurs. At temperatures greater than 50°C irreversible damage ensues. The maximum temperature achievable is 100°C at which boiling creates steam within the tissues adjacent to the electrodes and coagulum formation on the catheter, followed by a significant loss of current delivered.[9] Sudden boiling can result in audible popping. The dramatic increase in impedance results in large decreases of current density and limits further lesion growth. The 100°C ceiling for tissue heating thus creates a theoretical maximal lesion size for a given size electrode.

Temperature monitoring during RF ablation reduces the incidence of coagulum formation and impedance rises. By using catheters equipped with internal thermistors placed near the tip, Langberg et al.[3] were able to successfully ablate accessory pathways at a mean temperature of 62±15°C. Transient interruptions occurred at temperatures of 50±8°C. Abrupt impedance rises were noted with temperatures rising to 95-100°C. A positive dose-response curve was seen for power versus temperature at any level of power applied. When power control versus temperature control was compared during ablation of paroxysmal supraventricular tachycardia, Calkins et al.[4] found a significant decrease in the incidence of abrupt impedance rises or coagulum formation when using temperature control. A coagulum occurred in 0.8% of RF applications undergoing temperature monitoring and 2.2% of those with power monitoring (P=0.006). Overall, there was a 2% versus 12% incidence of an impedance shutdown, temperature shutdown, or coagulum formation when using temperature versus power control (P=0.001).

2.   ADVANTAGES OF COOLED RF ABLATION

Although temperature monitoring can minimize the incidence of coagulum formation requiring catheter withdrawal and cleaning, the power applied is decreased and the lesion size becomes limited. Methods to increase lesion depth include using larger electrodes or cooling the electrode tip.[11] A larger electrode has the advantage of increasing the area for resistive heating while gaining increased convective cooling from the surrounding blood, leading to a longer duration of power and greater application of energy. In a dog thigh muscle model, 4- and 8-mm tip electrodes were bathed in flowing or stationary blood and placed parallel and perpendicular to the muscle. RF applications were performed with the electrode-tissue interface kept at a constant temperature of 60°C or at a tissue temperature of 90°C when measured 3.5 mm deep. The larger compared with the smaller electrodes developed higher tissue temperatures at depths of 3.5mm (90°±9°C vs 74±10°C) and deeper lesions (7.8±0.8 mm vs 6.6±0.5 mm) when the surface temperature was controlled and flowing blood bathed the muscle. When the cooling effect from flowing blood was removed, lower current, voltage and power requirements produced the same surface temperature and led to shallower lesions. When the internal tissue temperature at 3.5 mm was kept constant at 90°C, a lower temperature at the electrode-tissue interface developed using the 8 mm as compared to the 4 mm electrode (57°±3°C vs 65°±6°C). When the electrodes were placed parallel to the tissue plane and the surface temperature kept constant, the 8 mm tip produced high temperatures than the 4 mm tip at a 3.5 mm depth (69°±4°C vs 61°±4°C) and deeper lesions were produced (8.4 ±0.6 mm vs 7.2±0.6 mm). Thus cooling the electrode-tissue interface and using larger electrodes produce significantly larger lesions while maximizing the amount of power applied.[11]

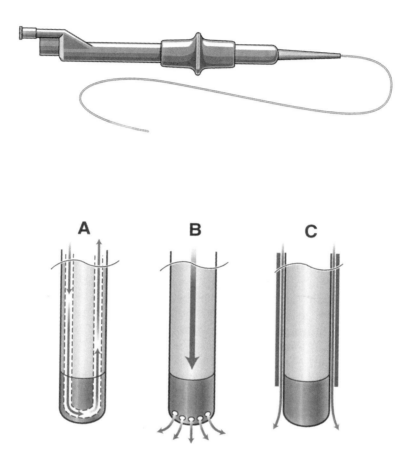

Figure 2. Schematic drawing of the Chilli ® Cooled Tip Catheter (above) and three different methods of cooling (below): (A) internal saline irrigation, (B) showerhead or sprinkler type, (C) external sheath irrigation.

Significant disadvantages of using larger electrodes make cooled tip RF ablation more appealing. Larger electrodes may decrease electrogram resolution and increase the difficulty of finding an optimum ablation site. Their stiffness and decreased compliance may reduce maneuverability of the catheter.[12] Cooling the tip of the RF ablation catheter using saline can decrease the size of the electrode while maintaining the advantages of larger lesions. Three methods have been proposed for achieving cooling: a showerhead where saline flows out of a porous tip, internal saline circulation, and external saline circulation from a sheath surrounding the tip (Figure 2). Demazumder et al.[13] reported that the internal mode of irrigation led to a somewhat smaller lesion when compared to the showerhead or sheath approach. The benefits of having a closed system include: (1) the patient does not receive any significant fluid boluses during the course of the procedure, and (2) the catheter tip may remain more stable on the endocardium with a less likelihood of dislodgement during RF application. However, a showerhead approach may lead to greater tissue irrigation and lower temperatures at the interface. Whether one system is more effective than another remains to be determined.

The most frequently used cooled tip electrode systems involve either internal irrigation or a sprinkler-type head coupled to a 4-mm electrode. Multiple other configurations are under active investigation. A screw-tip needle electrode, which allows intramural infusion of contrast and saline, has demonstrated efficacy in fluoroscopically isolating the ablated area in canines.[14] A 2-mm electrode was shown to develop larger lesions than a 5-mm electrode when placed perpendicularly to the canine thigh muscle preparation.[12] The 2-mm electrode delivered 49% more heating power to the tissue than the 5-mm, which shunted more current to the surrounding blood, decreasing the effective RF current. A long cooled saline/foam electrode was deployed across the tricuspid annulus-inferior vena cava isthmus in sheep.[15] The catheter consisted of two 2 cm long saline/foam electrode pockets separated by 1.5-mm, each pocket containing an 8-mm electrode. Internal cooling occurred through a double inner lumen at a saline infusion rate of 0.4mL/s. Power applied was 50 watts for 90 seconds, resulting in transmural lesions 15-35 mm in length, 5-6 mm in width and 1-2 mm in depth. The ability to create long linear lesions without gaps may result in higher success rates for atrial flutter and atrial fibrillation.

Currently only one cooled tip RF system is available commercially in the United States. The Chilli® Cooled RF Ablation System (Cardiac Pathways Corporation) is approved by the FDA for use in patients with non-idiopathic ventricular tachycardia.[16,17] The Chilli® Cooled RF system is a 7 French quadripolar catheter containing a 4-mm electrode tip and two internal cooling channels. In clinical applications,[16] cooling is achieved by pumping 0.6 ml/sec of saline to the tip of the catheter during RF applications. RF energy is generated initially at 25W with further increases to achieve an electrode temperature between 40°C and 50°C to a maximum of 50W for 60 to 180 seconds. Impedance rises to greater than 250 ohms or electrode temperatures greater than 65°C leads to automatic discontinuation of RF energy. In explanted human hearts, lesions up to 7 mm deep have been demonstrated by histology after ablation using the Chilli® system[18] (Figures 3,4). Some lesions were noted extending past 4-mm transmural scars into the epicardial fat and subepicardial myocytes. A second system has been employed in the therapy of atrial flutter. Jaïs et al.[19,20] used a showerhead-type irrigated tip catheter (Cordis Webster, Medtronic). Temperatures were maintained at 50°C with a power limit of 50W for 60 seconds. Cooling was achieved with saline pumped at a rate of 17 ml/min during RF application and 3 ml/min during all other times. Both the internal cooling and external showerhead systems have recently undergone clinical trials.

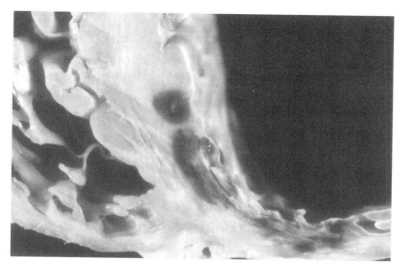

Figure 3A.   Heart from 64 year old man explanted 18 days post RF ablation.   Right ventricle, interventricular septum, and inferoseptal left ventricle is shown in short axis. An old myocardial infarction with white fibrotic tissue and thinning is seen in the inferoseptal left ventricle.   RF was applied to the dark brown areas resulting in coagulation necrosis and ecchymosis.   The most superior septal lesion extends 7 mm deep. Reproduced with permission.[18]

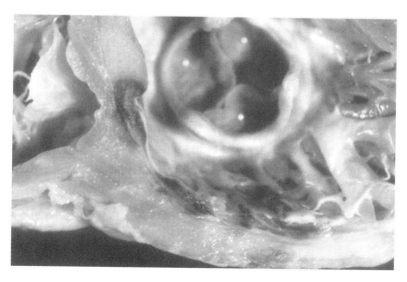

Figure 3B.   Left ventricular short axis of the base, inferior wall is at the bottom and interventricular septum is at the left. A bioprosthetic mitral valve is seen. The septal border of the old inferior myocardial infarction contains a large area of confluent lesions produced by cooled RF ablation. A transmural scar is seen on the inferior wall (5 o'clock position. Reproduced with permission.[18]

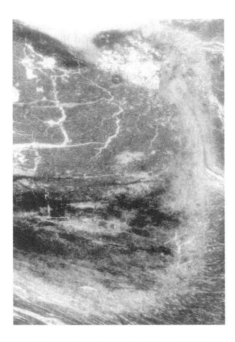

Figure 3C.   Hematoxylin and eosin stain of cooled RF ablation site at 33X magnification. Endocardium is seen at the top. Present around the lesion is organizing thrombus, a rim of granulation, coagulation necrosis and hemorrhage. The lesion is 7mm deep. Reproduced with permission.[18]

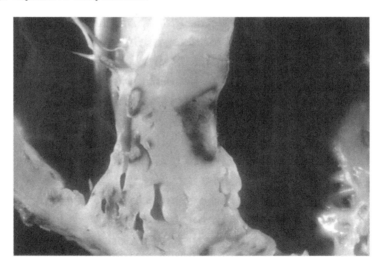

Figure 4. Heart from 33 year old man explanted 21 days post cooled RF ablation. Heart is viewed in the long axis with the left ventricle to the right. RF lesions can be seen on the right ventricular and left ventricular aspects of the interventricular septum. The maximal lesion depth is 7 mm. White areas are due to sarcoidosis. Reproduced with permission.[18]

3.   RESULTS OF TRIAL IN ANIMAL MODELS

Multiple in vitro and in vivo studies have validated the claim of larger and deeper lesion volumes with cooled RF ablation when compared with standard RF systems. In an ovine model, closed internal saline cooling with 30W RF energy applications was compared to standard RF energy delivered to keep the tip temperature slightly below 100°C.[21]   Energy applications continued for 60 seconds ceasing when temperature rises greater than 100°C or audible pops indicative of intramural gas formation occurred. The cooled tip lesions were threefold larger in volume than the standard lesions (1247 ± 521 mm³ vs 436 ± 177 mm³) (Figure 5).

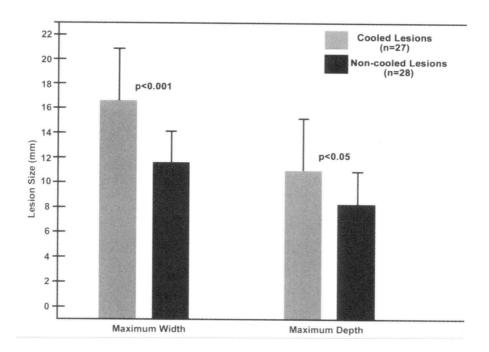

Figure 5.   Comparison of the dimensions of cooled (gray bars) versus standard (black bars) RF lesions. Reproduced with permission.[21]

This larger volume size was a direct result of the greater amount of power delivered in the cooled versus standard electrode (22.04 ± 4.51 W vs 6.10 ± 2.47 W). No impedance rises were seen in the cooled RF system. Nakagawa et al.[22] used a canine thigh muscle preparation to demonstrate that the lesions formed with RF were ellipsoid in character. Maximal lesion formation was found to again occur in a cooled tip group when compared to the voltage or temperature control groups. In the constant voltage (CV) group, the voltage was maintained at 66V. The standard temperature control group received voltages that maintained the tip thermistor at 80°C to 90°C without irrigation. A third CV group had 66V in the setting of saline irrigation through pores in the tip. All groups received 60 second RF applications. For the standard CV group, the maximal lesion diameter appeared on the tissue surface. The temperature-control group developed maximal lesion diameters 1.2±0.5 mm below the surface. The saline-irrigated group developed maximal lesion diameters 4.1±0.7 mm deep with significantly greater areas than surface areas (14.3±1.5 mm vs 10.1±1.3 mm, P<0.01). The total lesion volume in the saline-irrigated group was significantly greater than the temperature-control group, which was in turn significantly greater than the constant voltage group (700±217 mm^3 vs 275±55 mm^3 vs 135±33 mm^3) (Figure 6). In a porcine myocardium model, larger lesions were seen in vivo and in vitro using a cooled sprinkler-type RF ablation electrode when compared with standard RF electrodes. The incidence of cratering and disruption of myocardial tissue from steam formation was not significantly different between the two groups. No coagulum formation was noted in the cooled tip ablation.[23] These studies demonstrate that an important method of creating larger lesions is through the use of cooled RF ablation.

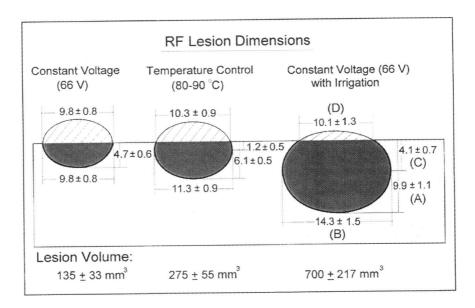

Figure 6. Lesion dimensions for constant voltage (left), temperature controlled (middle) and irrigated cooled RF (right) groups. Reproduced with permission.[22]

The greater effects of surface tissue cooling which allows longer RF application times may explain the differences in lesion size and volume among constant voltage, constant temperature, and cooled tip ablation groups. During the application of constant voltage, surface tissues are heated rapidly without allowing much time for convective cooling from flowing blood, resulting in the greatest lesion formation at the surface. Temperature control allows more gradual heating of the surface and a longer effective application time for RF energy, producing larger lesions than constant voltage. With the use of a cooled tip, surface temperatures are decreased dramatically due to the additive convective cooling of saline and blood. The longest effective durations of RF energy application and maximal development of lesion volumes are achieved with cool tip ablation.

Temperature monitoring during cooled RF application may be unreliable as a marker for determining the duration of RF application since the actual surface temperature is underestimated. Wharton et al. showed impedance rises may be minimized to less than 6.3% if tip temperatures are maintained less than 45°C.[24] A more accurate method for maximizing the delivered energy may be through maintaining a constant power of 50W for the internally irrigated tip[25] or 20W for a porous electrode tip (26). In the canine ventricle, Skrumeda et al.[26] examined the effects of different levels of power using porous tip catheters. Craters formed from the separation of myocardial layers due to steam were produced in 30-54% of ablations by irrigated tip RF at 50W. At 30W craters were only noted at 120 seconds and not seen when power was applied for only 30 seconds. Using 20W for 5 minutes and 10 minutes, no craters appeared. Coagulum formation only occurred using 50W but not at any other power setting. Recently Petersen et al.[27] directly examined the tissue temperatures and lesion volumes formed when a sprinkler head-type cooled tip was used in the setting of either temperature control or power control. Porcine left ventricle strips were excised and subjected to RF applications with temperature monitoring through fluoroptic fibers placed 2 mm through the endocardium. Using temperature control at both 80°C and 70°C produced lesions similar to power control at 40W. Significantly smaller lesions were formed with temperature control at 60°C. Notably, positive correlations between lesion volume and tissue temperature appeared. No correlations between lesion volume and peak electrode tip temperatures were seen. Monitoring internal tissue temperatures in patients is technically difficult. Current systems control both tip temperatures and power output.

The flow rate of saline coolant plays a role in determining the lesion size. Wong et al.[28] examined ovine left ventricles exposed to a constant internal saline rate of 0.3 ml/sec and 0.5 ml/sec while maintaining power at 20 W and compared lesions formed to either 20 W without flow or temperature control at 70° on the surface. Lesion volumes achieved were 79.6 mm^3 for 20 W without flow, 64.1 mm^3 for 20 W and 0.3 ml/sec flow, 47.5 mm^3 for 20 W and 0.5 ml/sec flow, and 28.6 mm^3 for temperature control. The use of irrigation thus allows for larger lesion formation than the use of temperature control. The optimum flow rate in human trials remains to be determined but may be less than the 0.6 ml/sec used currently in practice.

4.   CLINICAL TRIALS

Recent trials have demonstrated the effectiveness of cooled tip catheter ablation in treating ventricular tachycardia (VT)[16] and atrial flutter.[17,19,20] Calkins et al.[16] evaluated the effectiveness of cooled RF ablation in 146 consecutive patients enrolled in the Chilli® Cooled RF Ablation System clinical trial.   The Chilli® Cooled RF system is a 7 French quadripolar catheter containing a deflectable 4-mm electrode tip and 2-5-2-mm interelectrode spacing. Cooling is achieved by pumping 0.6 ml/sec of saline to the tip of the catheter through two internal cooling channels during RF applications.   RF energy is generated initially at 500 kHz and 25 W with further increases to achieve an electrode temperature from < 31°C to between 40°C and 50°C. A maximum of 50W for 60 to 180 seconds was delivered. Impedance rises to greater than 250 ohms or electrode temperatures greater than 65°C leads to automatic discontinuation of RF energy.   Enrollment criteria for the patients included documented sustained monomorphic VT with at least two episodes in the two months preceding enrollment, spontaneous VT which was stable and due to ischemic heart disease, and the failure of at least two antiarrhythmic agents in controlling VT.   The study was designed as a prospective randomized trial of catheter ablation versus pharmacological therapy. The randomized portion of the study was subsequently terminated after it was demonstrated that catheter ablation was superior to antiarrhythmic therapy.[29]   Calkins et al.[16] recently reported the overall results of cooled RF ablation in 146 patients who participated in this trial. The 146 patients enrolled all presented with structural heart disease. Ischemic heart disease was present in 119 patients (82%), 107 patients (73%) had an ejection fraction (EF) ≤35% with a mean of 31±13%. Only 1 person had noninducible VT, 37 patients (25%) had one inducible VT, 35 patients (25%) had two inducible VTs, and 70 patients (49%) had more than two inducible VTs. The clinical VT was inducible in 126 patients (89%). Acute catheter ablation defined as elimination of all inducible, mapable VTs at the conclusion of the procedure was successful in 106 (75%) patients with 26% of patients completely noninducible.   During 253±153 days of follow up 66 (46%) patients had recurrent sustained VT with a one year recurrence rate of 56%. Long-term survival was 75% at one year. Multivariate regression analysis revealed that the only predictors of survival were age less than 65 years and less than two types of inducible VT. Major complications occurred in 12 (8%) patients with 4 (2.7%) deaths from stroke, tamponade, valve injury, and myocardial infarction. It is notable that in only 1 patient was the cardiac tamponade associated with RF energy delivery. This patient presented with right ventricular dysplasia. During RF application at a site on the free wall aspect of the right ventricular outflow tract, the patient developed acute tamponade. No "pop" was heard during the RF delivery. The number of people experiencing major complications was not significantly greater than reported previously in various series which averaged from 5-12%. Because this trial did not randomize patients to Cooled versus standard RF ablation, it is not possible to precisely define the magnitude of benefit achieved by use of the Cooled RF ablation system. The results of this study were subsequently used to study the cost effectiveness of catheter ablation versus amiodarone for treatment of nonidiopathic VT. The results of this analysis revealed that catheter ablation was associated with a cost-effectiveness of $20,923 per quality-adjusted life-years as compared with amiodarone, which is within the range for accepted procedures in the United States.[30]

There have also been a number of clinical trials that have evaluated the safety and efficacy of cooled RF ablation for treatment of atrial flutter. Cooled tip ablation has proven to be as safe as standard RF ablation and may achieve isthmus block more expeditiously during atrial flutter ablations. Atiga et al.[17] divided a group of 59 patients with type I atrial flutter into two groups. One group underwent standard RF ablation and the second underwent cooled tip ablation with the Chilli system initially. After twelve unsuccessful attempts the groups crossed over. The endpoint was either successful bidirectional isthmus block or a total of 24 RF applications in all groups. Following the initial 6 RF applications a total of 25% patients in the cooled tip group and 23% in the conventional group achieved bidirectional isthmus block. After 12 total RF applications a significantly greater number of patients in the cool tip group achieved bidirectional block: 79% vs 55% in the conventional group. Importantly, no major complications such as death, tamponade, or pericardial effusion occurred in either group.

Jaïs et al.[20] randomized 50 patients to conventional (n=26) or irrigated-tip catheter (n=24) ablation of typical atrial flutter using a sprinkler-head system (Cordis Webster Thermocool D curve system, Medtronic). Temperatures were maintained at 50°C with a power limit of 50W for 60 seconds. Cooling was achieved with saline pumped at a rate of 17 ml/min during RF application and 3 ml/min during all other times. All patients in the irrigated-tip group underwent successful creation of bidirectional isthmus block and flutter termination while 22 (85%) patients in the conventional catheter achieved success within 21 RF applications. The 4 patients who failed conventional flutter ablation were then crossed over into the irrigated-tip group and were all treated successfully after 1 to 11 additional RF applications. Coronary angiograms performed on the first 30 enrolled patients were unchanged before and after the ablation procedure. After a mean follow-up of 5±2 months, no recurrences of flutter were noted except in one patient in the conventional arm who required additional ablation 2 days after his initial procedure. No procedural complications as a result of flutter ablation were noted for either group. Significant decreases in the number of RF applications required to achieve bidirectional block were found in the cooled-tip group: 13±10 applications for the conventional group, 5±3 applications in the irrigated-tip group (P=0.0003). The mean procedure duration was significantly decreased in the cooled tip group: 53±41 minutes for the conventional group and 27±16 minutes for the irrigated-tip group (P<0.0008). The total x-ray exposure time was significantly decreased in the cooled-tip group: 27±16 minutes for the conventional group versus 9±6 minutes for the cooled tip group (P=0.01). A second study by Jaïs et al.[19] focused on 13 (7.6%) of 170 patients in which conventional atrial flutter ablation failed to create bidirectional block due to gaps within the isthmus line. Using the same irrigated-tip catheter system, complete block was achieved in 12 (92%) of the 13 patients, 6 with only a single additional cooled RF application, 6 with an additional 2 to 6 applications. No complications were noted with the procedure. Cooled RF ablation in atrial flutter is as safe as conventional RF ablation and may be more effective in creating complete bidirectional block along the isthmus while decreasing procedural times and x-ray exposure.

CONCLUSION

Cooled RF ablation represents an important advance in catheter ablation technology as it allows for creation of larger and deeper lesions. Initial clinical studies suggest that despite the creation of larger and deeper lesions, catheter ablation of atrial flutter and nonidiopathic VT using cooled RF technology is not associated with a higher risk of complications as compared with standard RF ablation technology. There is also increasing evidence to suggest that cooled RF ablation improves the efficacy of catheter ablation of atrial flutter as well as nonidiopathic VT. These potential benefits suggest that ablation systems that incorporate cooled RF ablation technology are likely to become a standard tool for catheter ablation of these arrhythmias in the future.

REFERENCES

1. Calkins H, Sousa J, El-Atassi R, Leon A, Kou W, Kalbfleisch S, Morady F. Radiofrequency catheter ablation of accessory atrioventricular connections in 250 patients. Circulation. 1992;85:1337-1346.
2. Jackman WM, Wang X, Friday KJ, Roman CA, Moulton KP, Beckman KJ, McClelland JH, Twidale N, Hazlitt HA, Prior MI, Margolis PD, Calame JD, Overholt ED, Lazzara R. Catheter ablation of accessory atrioventricular pathways (Wolff-Parkinson-White syndrome) by radiofrequency current. N Engl J Med. 1991;324:1605-1611.
3. Langberg JJ, Calkins H, El-Atassi R Borganelli M, Leon A, Kalbfleisch SJ, Morady F. Temperature monitoring during radiofrequency catheter ablation of accessory pathways. Circulation. 1992;86:1469-1474.
4. Calkins H, Prystowsky E, Carlson M, Klein LS, Saul JP, Gillette P. Temperature monitoring during radiofrequency catheter ablation procedures using closed loop control. Circulation. 1994;90:1279-1286.
5. Calkins H, Hall J, Ellenbogen K, Walcott G, Sherman M, Bowe W, Simpson J, Castellano T, Kay GN. A new system for catheter ablation of atrial fibrillation. Am J Cardiol. 1999;83:227D-236D.
6. Lesh MD, Guerra PG, Roithinger FX, Goseki Y, Sparks PB, Diederich C, Nau WH, Maguire M, Taylor K. Novel catheter technology for ablative cure of atrial fibrillation. J Int Cardiac Electrophysiol. 2000;4(1):127-139.

7. Wittkampf FHM, Hauer RN, Robles de Medina EO. Radiofrequency ablation with a cooled porous electrode catheter. J Am Coll Cardiol. 1988;11:17.
8. Huang SKS, Cuenoud H, Tan de Guzman W. Increase in the lesion size and decrease in the impedance rise with saline infusion electrode catheter for radiofrequency catheter ablation. Circulation. 1989;80:II-324.
9. Dinerman JL, Berger RD, Calkins H. Temperature monitoring during radiofrequency ablation. J Cardiovasc Electrophysiol. 1996;7:163-173.
10. Haines DE, Watson DD, Verow AF. Electrode radius predicts lesion radius during radiofrequency energy heating. Validation of a proposed thermodynamic model. Circulation Research. 1990;67:124-129.
11. Otomo K, Yamanashi WS, Tondo C, Antz M, Bussey J, Pitha JV, Arruda M, Nakagawa H, Wittkampf FHM, Lazzara R, Jackman WM. Why a large tip electrode makes a deeper radiofrequency lesion: Effects of increase in electrode cooling and electrode-tissue interface area. J Cardiovasc Electrophysiol. 1998;9:47-54.
12. Nakagawa H, Wittkampf FHM, Yamanashi WS, Pitha JV, Imai S, Campbell B, Arruda M, Lazzara R, Jackman WM. Inverse relationship between electrode size and lesion size during radiofrequency ablation with active electrode cooling. Circulation. 1998;98:458-465.
13. Demazumder D, Kallash HL, Schwartzman D. Comparison of different electrodes for radiofrequency ablation of myocardium using saline irrigation. PACE. 1997;20:II-1076.
14. Hoey MF and Mulier PM. Fluoroscopic visualization of ventricular ablation after radiofrequency energy application with the saline electrode. Circulation. 1997;96(Supp 1):I-319.
15. Liem LB, Pomeranz M, Riseling K, Anderson S, Berry GJ. Electrophysiological correlates of transmural linear ablation. PACE. 2000;23:40-46.
16. Calkins H, Epstein A, Packer D, Arria AM, Hummel J, Gilligan DM, Trusso J, Carlson M, Luceri R, Kopelman H, Wilber D, Wharton JM, Stevenson W. Catheter ablation of ventricular tachycardia in patients with structural heart disease using cooled radiofrequency energy. J Am Coll Cardiol. 2000;35:1905-14.
17. Atiga WL, Worley SJ, Hummel J, Berger RD, Gohn DC, Mandalakas NJ, Kalbfleisch S, Halperin H, Donahue K, Tomaselli G, Calkins H, Daoud E. Prospective randomized comparison of cooled RF versus standard RF energy for ablation of typical atrial flutter. Submitted. 2000.
18. Delacretaz E, Stevenson WG, Winters GL, Mitchell RN, Stewart S, Lynch K, Friedman PL. Ablation of ventricular tachycardia with a saline-cooled radiofrequency catheter: Anatomic and histologic characteristics of the lesions in humans. J Cardiovasc Electrophysiol. 1999;10:860-865.
19. Jaïs P, Haïssaguerre M, Shah DC, Takahashi A, Hocini M, Lavergne T, Lafitte S, Le Mouroux A, Fischer B, Clementy J. Successful irrigated-tip catheter ablation of atrial flutter resistant to conventional radiofrequency ablation. Circulation. 1998;98:835-838.
20. Jaïs P, Shah DC, Haïssaguerre M, Hocini M, Garrigue S, Le Metayer P, Clémenty J. Prospective randomized comparison of irrigated-tip versus conventional-tip catheters for ablation of common flutter. Circulation. 2000;101:772-776.
21. Ruffy R, Imran MA, Santel DJ, Wharton JM. Radiofrequency delivery through a cooled catheter tip allows the creation of larger endomyocardial lesions in the ovine heart. J Cardiovasc Electrophysiol. 1995;6:1089-1096.
22. Nakagawa H, Yamanshi WS, Pitha JV, Arruda M, Wang X, Ohtomo K, Beckman KJ, McClelland JH, Lazzra R, Jackman WM. Comparison of in vivo tissue temperature profile and lesion geometry for radiofrequency ablation with a saline-irrigated electrode versus temperature control in a canine thigh muscle preparation. Circulation. 1995;91:2264-2273.
23. Petersen HH, Chen X, Pietersen A, Svendsen JH, Haunso S. Temperature-controlled irrigated tip radiofrequency catheter ablation: Comparison of in vivo and in vitro lesioni dimensions for standard catheter and irrigated tip catheter with minimal infusion rate. J Cardiovasc Electrophysiol. 1998;9:409-414.

24. Wharton JM, Wilber DJ, Calkins H et al. Utility of tip thermometry during radiofrequency ablation in humans using an internally perfused saline cooled catheter. Circulation. 1997;96(Suppl 1);I-318.
25. Nibley C, Sykes CM, McLaughlin G, Chapman T, Rowan R, Wolf P, Wharton JM. Myocardial lesion size during radiofrequency current catheter ablation is increased by intra-electrode tip chilling. J Am Coll Cardiol. 1995;25:293A.
26. Skrumeda LL, Mehra R. Comparison of standard and irrigated radiofrequency ablation in the canine ventricle. J Cardiovasc Electrophysiol. 1998;9:1196-1205.
27. Petersen HH, Chen X, Pietersen A, Svendsen JH, Haunso S. Tissue temperatures and lesion size during irrigated tip catheter radiofrequency ablation: An in vitro comparison of temperature-controlled irrigated tip ablation, power-controlled irrigated tip ablation, and standard temperature-controlled ablation. PACE. 2000;23:8-17.
28. Wong WS, VanderBrink BA, Riley RE, Pmeranz M, Link MS, Homoud MK, Estes NA 3rd, Wang PJ. Effect of saline irrigation flow rate on temperature profile during cooled radiofrequency ablation. J Interv Card Electrophysiol. 2000;4:321-6.
29. Wilber D, Epstein A, Kay GN, Stevenson W, Wharton JM, Carlson M, Gilligan D, Ellenbogen K, Stark S, Packer D, Estes NAM III, Wang P, Berger R, Calkins H. Radiofrequency ablation system for the treatment of ventricular tachycardia. PACE. 1997;20:1123
30. Calkins H., Bigger JT, Ackerman SJ, Duff SB, Wilber D, Kerr RA, Bar-Din M, Beusterien KM, Strauss MJ. Cost-effectiveness of catheter ablation in patients with ventricular tachycardia. Circulation. 2000;101:280-288.

Chapter 20

RADIOFREQUENCY ABLATION USING A POROUS TIP ELECTRODE

David M. Fitzgerald
Wake Forest University School of Medicine, Winston-Salem, North Carolina, USA

INTRODUCTION

Radiofrequency current was initially adapted for intracardiac catheter ablation using conventional diagnostic electrode catheters with a tip electrode 2 millimeters in length through which energy was delivered.[1] However, power output was limited due to sudden increases in system impedance associated with the development of coagulated blood on the ablation electrode.[2,3] In vitro studies of the thermodynamics of radiofrequency lesioning demonstrated that this sudden increase in impedance was related to local tissue overheating at the electrode – tissue interface and associated with surface tissue temperatures greater than 100 °C .[4] This increase in surface tissue temperature to the boiling point of water could result in coagulation of blood. With increase in the size and surface area of the ablation electrode, sudden elevations of impedance were seen less frequently allowing higher power delivery to the tissue.[5] Increasing the ablation electrode length from 2 to 4 millimeters markedly improved the efficacy and efficiency of the technique.[6] However, sudden increases in impedance and coagulum formation were still a limiting factor with use of higher power outputs. Tip thermometry was developed to try and limit impedance rises and coagulum formation while maximizing energy delivery.[7] By measuring tip temperature either inside the electrode or at its tip, power could be regulated to maintain temperature at a level that could result in tissue injury but not allow boiling of tissue water or blood. Unfortunately, sudden impedance elevations can still occur with temperature- controlled energy delivery and because energy is limited in response to temperature, deep heating of tissues may be limited, especially in areas with reduced blood flow or with the electrode embedded in trabeculated tissue.[8]

L. Bing Liem and E. Downar (eds.), Progress in Catheter Ablation, 327-341.
© 2001 *Kluwer Academic Publishers. Printed in the Netherlands.*

1.   IN VITRO STUDIES OF IRRIGATED CATHETERS

To maximize energy delivery and prevent sudden increases in impedance and coagulum formation, some degree of cooling of the electrode- tissue interface must be employed. Increasing ablation electrode size provides a larger area for convective cooling of the electrode by the blood.[9]   Alternatively, the electrode itself could be cooled actively by flushing saline through it. Using an electrode catheter with a central lumen through the 2 millimeter tip for saline irrigation, Wittkampf   et al. noted that higher radiofrequency energy outputs could be delivered without sudden increases in   impedance or coagulum formation.[10] Mittleman et al compared the use of a saline-irrigated lumened catheter (with an end hole and two side holes drilled into the 2 millimeter tip electrode) to a conventional 2 millimeter non-lumened tip electrode during radiofrequency energy application.[11] The irrigated electrode allowed delivery of higher energy outputs without impedance rise and created larger lesions when similar power outputs were applied.

A 5-millimeter long ablation electrode with a central lumen was then adapted for saline- irrigated energy delivery by   drilling 6 holes (0.4 millimeter in diameter) into the electrode 1 millimeter from the tip.   A thermistor was embedded in the tip electrode for temperature monitoring. Using a novel model for evaluation of the effects of different parameters on lesion size during radiofrequency ablation, Nakagawa et al described a series of experiments with this electrode comparing the effects of constant voltage radiofrequency energy delivery with and without irrigation and with temperature control using the internal thermistor to titrate voltage.[12]   An incision was made over the thigh muscle of a dog and the subcutaneous tissue pulled back to expose the muscle and form a cradle into which heparinized blood was circulated at 20 cc/minute and maintained at a temperature of 37 ° C.   Fluoroptic thermal probes were inserted into the tissue at depths of 3.5 and 7.0 millimeters from the surface to measure tissue temperature during energy application. During energy delivery through the irrigated electrode, room temperature saline was infused at 20 cc/minute.   The radiofrequency generator provided a constant voltage power output, which was delivered between the tip electrode of the ablation catheter and a surface patch.

The ablation protocol included conventional energy delivery at a constant voltage (66 volts) without irrigation or temperature control for 31 applications, a temperature control group with target temperature of 80-90 ° C (voltage modulated between 20-66 volts) without irrigation for 39 applications, and saline irrigation with constant voltage (66 volts) for 75 applications. No differences were noted in impedance between groups. However, in all 31 conventional applications at a constant voltage without irrigation or temperature control, an impedance rise > 10 ohms occurred at a mean of 11.6 seconds limiting further energy delivery. All of these impedance increases were associated with a thin coagulum on the ablation electrode. Audible popping sounds were associated with the impedance increase in 3/31 applications. With temperature control, tip temperature was maintained to 80-90 ° C and no impedance rises were noted. All 39 applications were delivered for 60 seconds. The mean power during energy delivery with temperature control was 18.3 ± 6.4 watts. With irrigation, 69/75 applications were maintained for the entire 60 seconds. In 6 applications, impedance increases were seen at 31-51 seconds and all were associated with an audible pop. No coagulum was found on the catheter upon inspection after these sudden impedance elevations. The mean power during energy delivery was 50.6 ± 4.7 watts similar to conventional energy delivery but of longer duration.

Tip electrode temperature and temperature at tissue depths of 3.5 and 7.0 millimeters were analyzed for each method of energy delivery. With conventional constant voltage energy delivery, tip temperatures reached 100°C during all 31 applications. Because of the early rise in impedance during these applications, temperature at 3.5 millimeters was 62.1 ± 15.1 °C and at 7.0 millimeters, only 40.3 ± 5.3 °C . With temperature control, tip temperature was maintained at 80-90 ° C resulting in temperature at 3.5 millimeters of 67.9 ± 7.5°C and at 7.0 millimeters of 48.3 ± 4.8°C. With saline cooling using the irrigated electrode, tip temperatures were maintained at 38.4 ± 5.1 °C while temperature at 3.5 millimeters ranged 94.7 ± 9.1°C and 65.1 ± 9.7 °C at 7.0 millimeters.

Lesion geometry was ellipsoid in each mode but the center of the ellipse mirrored the temperature profiles described above (see Figure 1). With conventional constant voltage energy delivery, an ellipsoid lesion with maximal diameter of 9.8 ± 0.8 millimeters was measured at the surface. These lesions had a maximal depth of 4.7 ± 0.6 millimeters. With temperature-control, maximal width of the lesion was 11.3 ± 0.9 millimeters at a depth of 1.2 ± 0.05 millimeters from the surface. Maximal depth of the lesion was 6.1 ± 0.05 millimeters. With irrigation, maximal width of the lesion was 14.3 ± 1.5 millimeters at a depth of 4.1 ± 0.07 millimeters from the surface. Maximal depth was 9.9 ± 1.1 millimeters. Surface diameter of the lesions did not differ between groups but the lesion depth, maximal diameter, depth at maximal diameter and volume were greater with irrigation than with temperature- control or conventional energy delivery.

Analysis of temperature and impedance profiles associated with audible pops in the irrigated electrode group indicates that surface temperatures at the time of impedance rises were always below 100° C however, deeper tissue temperatures at 3.5 mm were greater than 100 °C suggesting that the impedance rise was related to release of steam from the deeper tissue rather than boiling of blood as in the conventional energy delivery group. Small craters were found at 5/9 sites of energy delivery associated with audible pops regardless of method of energy delivery.

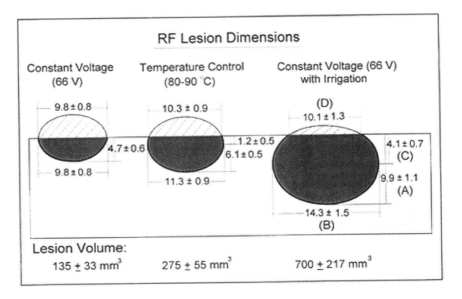

Figure 1. Diagram of lesion dimensions for the three groups studied. Values are expressed in millimeters (mean ± SD). **A** indicates maximal lesion depth; **B** , maximal lesion diameter; **C**, depth at maximal lesion diameter; and **D**, lesion surface diameter. Lesion volume was calculated by using the formula for an oblate ellipsoid by subtracting the volume of the "missing cap" (hatched area). (Reprinted with permission from Nakagawa H, et al. Circulation 1995;91:2264-2273.)

In another study, Nakagawa et al[13] used this same model to compare the effects of saline irrigation using tip electrode lengths of 5 millimeters and 2 millimeters. Constant voltage (50 volts) was delivered for 30 seconds during saline irrigation with each electrode positioned either perpendicular or parallel to the surface at a constant pressure. Similar temperature measurements were obtained using a fluoroptic probe at 3.5 and 7.0 millimeters below the surface. Of interest, in this series of experiments, the insulated electrode impedance was measured at each ablation site by substituting deionized water for blood in the cradle to create a high resistance barrier around the electrode and evaluate the impedance of the electrode-tissue interface only, without the influence of blood.

A total of 148 lesions were made in 11 dogs. No impedance increases > 10 ohms were noted. Because of saline irrigation, tip electrode temperatures remained below 53°C with all applications. In the perpendicular electrode orientation, 31 applications with the 2-millimeter electrode were compared to 32 applications with the 5-millimeter electrode. Impedance during energy delivery was higher with the 2 millimeter electrode (98 ± 8 vs 70 ± 9 ohms). Delivered power was lower with the 2 millimeter electrode (26 ± 2.1 vs 36.4 ± 5.0 watts). Interestingly, tissue temperatures at 3.5 and 7.0 millimeters were higher during constant voltage energy delivery with the 2 millimeter electrode than the 5 millimeter electrode resulting in lesions that were deeper (8.0 ± 1.0 vs 5.4 ± 0.9 millimeters) and wider (12.4 ± 1.4 vs 8.4 ± 0.9 millimeters).

During energy delivery with parallel electrode-tissue orientation, impedance was higher with the 2 millimeter electrode (101 ± 7 vs 76 ± 5 Ohms) resulting in a lower power delivery (25 vs 33 watts). Tissue temperatures at 3.5 and 7.0 millimeters were significantly higher with the 2 millimeter electrode (3.5 millimeter = 98 vs 79.8°C and 7.0 millimeter = 61 vs 55°C) despite the lower energy delivery. Lesions were deeper with the 2-millimeter electrode (7.3 vs 6.9 millimeters) but maximum diameters were similar (11.1 vs 11.3 millimeters).

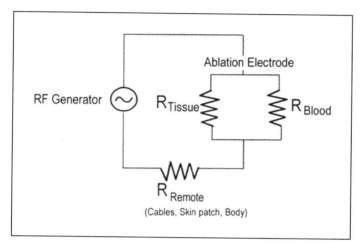

Figure 2. Circuit for RF ablation can be considered to have overall impedance consisting of nonablation electrode impedance (R_{remote}) produced by cables. Skin patch, and body, which is in series with impedance of ablation electrode consisting of electrode-tissue interface impedance (R_{tissue}) and electrode-blood interface impedance (R_{blood}) connected in parallel. (reprinted with permission from Nakagawa et al. Circulation 1998;98:458-465).

Of note, insulated impedance did not differ between the 2 and 5-millimeter electrodes in the perpendicular electrode-tissue interface (229 vs 228 ohms) where only the electrode tip was in contact with myocardium. However, in the parallel electrode-tissue orientation, insulated impedance was significantly higher with the 2 millimeter electrode (238 vs 187 ohms) since the surface area in contact with myocardium was larger with the 5 millimeter electrode. After measuring the various resistances of the components of the ablation circuit (see Figure 2) and calculating the voltage drop across these resistances, the effective power delivered to the tissue was calculated in each electrode configuration. In the perpendicular configuration (Figure 3), the 2 millimeter electrode resulted in 6.1 watts of energy to the tissue while the 5 millimeter electrode delivered only 4.1 watts. In the parallel configuration, similar power is delivered to the tissue with the 2 and 5 millimeter electrodes resulting in similar lesion diameters but because similar powers are delivered over different surface areas, the 2 millimeter electrode results in greater tissue temperatures and lesion depth due to the relatively higher current density. The larger ablation electrode allows more current to be shunted to the blood and decreases the effective voltage available for tissue heating.

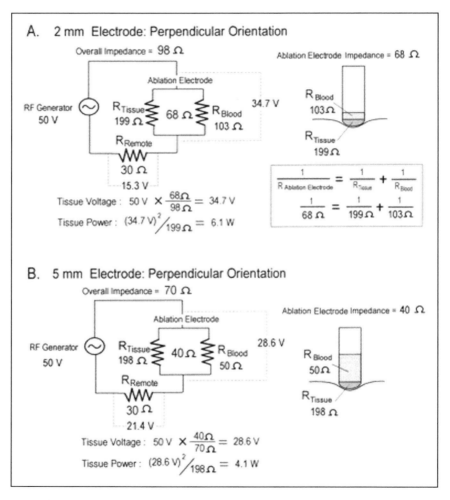

Figure 3. Estimation of tissue voltage and tissue power for 2 and 5 mm electrodes in perpendicular electrode-tissue orientation. (reprinted with permission from Nakagawa et al. Circulation 1998;98:458-465)

When the 5 millimmeter irrigated electrode was used in vivo in the canine left ventricle, temperature control (voltage varied by 30 – 80 volts to maintain temperature of 90 °C) without irrigation resulted in a sudden increase in impedance in 3/15 pulses.[14]   With irrigation and a constant voltage output of 90 volts, impedance rises were seen in 6/15 pulses. Lesion depth and diameter were significantly different when irrigaton was compared to temperature control (irrigation depth = 12.1 vs temperature control = 9.3 millimeter and irrigation diameter = 20.5 vs temperature control = 12.7 millimeter). Impedance rises with both temperature control and irrigation were associated with audible steam pops.

This catheter was also used in an in vivo study in dogs in which lesions were made in the coronary sinus near the lateral /anterolateral aspect of the coronary sinus and at the ostium / middle cardiac vein region.[15]   Constant voltage was applied at either 50 or 66 volts for 60 seconds. Coronary sinus venograms and coronary angiograms were obtained pre-ablation, immediately post-ablation, and at 6 days after ablation. Lesion size varied with voltage output with a smaller lesion diameter noted with 50 volt pulses (2.8 vs 7.6 millimeters). No impedance rises were noted with the 50-volt pulses while 3/18 pulses at 66 volts caused impedance rises. All impedance increases occurred with a tip electrode temperature of < 40°C and were associated with an audible popping sound. No thrombus was noted during inspection of the catheter electrode after an impedance rise. Coronary sinus venograms showed no evidence of occlusion post-ablation. Coronary angiograms exhibited no change in response to 50-volt pulses. However, 66 volt pulses resulted in segmental necrosis of the adventitia and media but not the intima of the neighboring segment of the left circumflex coronary artery in 8/18 pulses. Pathology of the lesions demonstrated epicardial damage of the left atrium and the left ventricle in 17/18 lesions in the 66-volt group but in only 1/10 of the 50-volt group. The lesions did not extend to the endocardium in either group.

Using a different irrigated catheter with a central lumen and open tip as well as 13 other .01 inch diameter holes along the length of the 4-millimeter tip electrode for efficient cooling, other investigators have reported similar findings.[16, 17]   When comparing irrigated radiofrequency ablation in a porcine preparation with this catheter set at a 60°C target temperature versus a conventional catheter with target temperature of 80°C, lesion volumes were larger with the irrigated catheter with no endocardial cratering or thrombus formation.[16] With the conventional catheter, 52% of applications resulted in coagulum on the catheter. In another study, using canine ventricular muscle for comparison of irrigated ablation versus both manual power delivery and temperature-controlled power delivery through a standard ablation catheter, irrigated catheters again resulted in larger lesions and infrequent coagulum formation compared to standard catheters.[17] Crater formation occurred more frequently with irrigated catheters particularly as power outputs were increased to ≥ 30 watts.

2.   CLINICAL EXPERIENCE WITH IRRIGATED ELECTRODES

The clinical experience with irrigated electrodes is limited.   Arruda et al described their use of an irrigated electrode (5 millimeter tip, with six .01 mm holes) in a small series of patients undergoing catheter ablation of posteroseptal or posterior accessory pathways.[18]   In nine patients, coronary angiograms were obtained pre- and post-ablation. In two patients, 70-80% narrowing of the distal right coronary artery was seen on angiography post-ablation. These patients had no ST segment changes and cardiac enzymes were not elevated. No specific treatment was applied. A follow-up angiogram at 6 months showed resolution of the narrowing. In one patient, the post-ablation angiogram showed complete occlusion of the distal right coronary artery with evidence of a small posterobasal infarction. This vessel was emergently opened with angioplasty. Follow-up angiogram showed a 60 % narrowing in this region at 6 months. A series of canine studies were done in which an intracoronary ultrasound probe was used to monitor the wall of the coronary artery opposite the ablation catheter during energy delivery through the irrigated catheter. Energy was terminated if changes in coronary artery wall thickness or echogenicity were seen. After demonstrating the efficacy of this technique of monitoring radiofrequency energy delivery through an irrigated electrode, it was employed in one patient. In this patient, an intacoronary ultrasound probe was used to monitor the right coronary artery during energy delivery through an irrigated catheter placed in the middle cardiac vein. In 2/3 applications of energy, arterial wall thickness began to increase and energy was interrupted at 34 and 44 seconds of energy delivery.   The posteroseptal pathway was successfully ablated.   The post-ablation angiogram showed no significant change in the caliber of the coronary artery. These findings suggest that radiofrequency lesioning with irrigated electrodes near coronary arteries could result in wall injury or occlusion and that monitoring of the coronary artery with an intracoronary ultrasound probe could warn of impending arterial injury.

This group of patients was expanded to include 90 patients who underwent catheter ablation of 95 accessory AV pathways in all locations using this irrigated electrode.[19] All patients has success but 3/90   (3%) patients had pericardial tamponade as a complication of the procedure. The location of the accessory pathway was right posterolateral, right anterolateral, and left lateral in each patient with tamponade. Steam pops were noted during energy delivery in each of these patients. Of note, in each patient with tamponade, the electrode was oriented perpendicular to the wall rather than parallel, and voltages > 80 volts were applied. This group of patients was compared to 875 patients treated with conventional electrode catheters where only 2 pericardial tamponades were noted (0.2%). Location of the accessory pathway in these patients was left lateral in one and posterolateral (in a branch of a posterolateral cardiac vein) in the other. Modulation of voltage output or total energy to < 80 volts and orienting the catheter in a parallel rather than perpendicular position on the annulus were entertained as possible methods to avoid tamponade using an irrigated porous electrode.

A novel electrode design made of stainless steel spheres that were sintered or fused together created a tip electrode with micropores between the sintered speres of 15-micron diameter (Figure 4).[20] This effectively allows saline cooling along the entire surface of the electrode, presumably with low saline flow rates (1.6- 5 cc/minute) when compared to irrigated electrodes used in other studies where saline flow rates of 15-60 cc/minute were evaluated. A thermocouple is embedded in the tip to monitor tip temperature but power delivery was manual adjusted and not controlled by tip temperature.

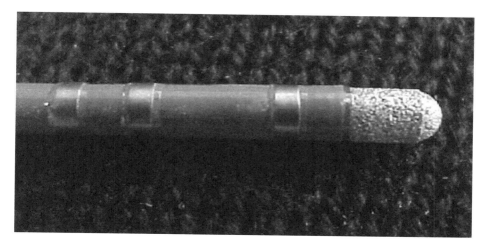

Figure 4. Porous irrigated tip catheter. Tip is made of fused steel spheres separated by small pores of approximately 15 microns in diameter through which saline exudes during irrigation. [20]

This electrode design was recently tested in a feasibility trial in 20 patients referred for treatment of supraventricular tachycardia. In six patients referred for catheter ablation of the AV node, success was achieved in a mean of 4.3 pulses. In five patients with accessory pathways (left free wall = 4, posteroseptal =1), 4.4 pulses were required for ablation. In five patients with AV nodal reentry, selective slow pathway modification was achieved with 5.0 pulses. In four patients with ectopic atrial tachycardia (right atrial in 3 and left atrial in 1), 10.8 pulses were required for ablation. A summary of the overall results is listed in Table 1. Overall, in this diverse group of patients, successful ablation was achieved using this catheter with a mean of 5.8 pulses per patient. A total of 116 pulses were delivered in the study. There were no sudden increases in impedance or audible steam pops noted during energy delivery. No thrombus was noted on the catheter electrode upon removal. In one patient, undergoing catheter ablation of the AV node, an intracardiac ultrasound catheter was placed to guide energy delivery on the septum. During energy delivery, a steam pop was visibly documented despite no change in recorded impedance or detection of an audible sound (see Figure 5).

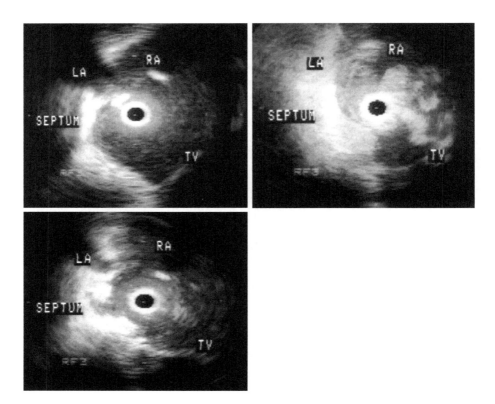

Figure 5. Intracardiac ultrasound images of a steam pop. A (top left). Cross-section image at the tricuspid valve showing the attatchment of the tricuspid valve leaflet to the muscular septum. The circle in the center is the ultrasound probe (12.5 megahertz). The ablation catheter tip is the echodense structure noted at 11:00 between the probe and the septum. B (top right). With energy application and tissue overheating, a sudden release of echodense gas bubbles occurs. C (bottom left). Sequelae of a steam pop. An irregular crater is now present on the endocardium of the muscular septum at the site of the steam pop.

This irrigated catheter prevented coagulum formation despite delivery of moderate power outputs (mean power = 40 watts). Although not compared to a conventional ablation catheter, these results imply that the efficiency of an ablation procedure may be improved using an irrigated catheter.

Table 1.   Summary data from Angecool Radiofrequency Ablation Catheter for Ablation of Supraventricular Arrhythmias. [20]

Ablation Parameter	Mean ± Standard Deviation	Range
Number of Pulses	5.8 ± 5.4	1 - 23
Power (watts)	40.1 ± 9.3	15 - 50
Impedance (ohms)	95.9 ± 9.3	80 - 118
Pulse Duration (seconds)	45.8 ± 29.6	3 - 201
Maximum Temperature (°C)	34.9 ± 9.7	20 - 70
Fluoroscopy Time (minutes)	20.2 ± 16.4	3.8 - 67
Total procedure Time (hours)	4.3 ± 2.9	0.9 - 11

More recently, Jais et al described use of an irrigated catheter (5 millimeter tip with central lumen and six pores of .1mm diameter) for ablation of atrial flutter in 13 of 170 patients who had failed ablation with conventional electrode catheters.[21]   Failure was defined as incomplete block in the cavo-tricuspid isthmus after > 21 conventional radiofrequency pulses had been delivered using a generator with maximal output of 50 watts. Using temperature-controlled energy delivery (target temperature of 50 °C) and a saline flow rate of 17 ml/minute, successful ablation was achieved in 12 patients.   In 6 patients only a single application of current was required to create complete bidirectional block in the cavo –tricuspid isthmus while in 6 patients 2-6 pulses were required. Maximum power output was limited to 50 watts with saline irrigation. No impedance rises were seen but one audible steam pop was detected which caused no adverse sequelae.   In one patient, despite delivery of 21 lesions using the irrigated electrode at maximal power outputs of 50 watts, atrial flutter could not be terminated.

3.   LIMITATIONS OF RADIOFREQUENCY ABLATION WITH IRRIGATED POROUS ELECTRODE

Irrigated ablation catheters can reduce the incidence of impedance rise associated with coagulum formation, but there is a potential for overheating, particularly the deeper subendocardial regions resulting in sudden steam formation with disruption and cratering of tissue as steam is released. Although steam pops occur during conventional radiofrequency energy delivery, the incidence may be higher with irrigation due to the more effective transfer of energy to the tissue and the abilty to deliver higher energies to the tissue without coagulum formation.[22,23] This is of concern particularly when lesions are created in the arterial circulation (left atrium, left ventricle) where a crater resulting from a steam pop could form a nidus for thrombus formation. or could result in perforation.

Factors associated with steam pops using irrigated catheters include use of voltages greater than 50 volts during constant voltage power delivery in one study[15] and voltage or power output and measured tip impedance at the end of the radiofrequency pulse in another study.[24]

In addition to steam popping, overheating of deeper tissues could potentially damage epicardial coronary arteries particularly if energy is delivered through the thin-walled atria or in the coronary sinus or its venous branches. Monitoring coronary arteries with intracoronary ultrasound at sites close to the irrigated electrode may provide information that could prevent damage to the coronary artery.[18] Intracardiac ultrasound has been used to monitor the effects of energy delivery through irrigated electrodes on the endocardium and to characterize tissue changes in response to energy delivery.[24,25] Steam pops and crater formation are readily detected with intracardiac ultrasound but myocardial tissue changes are seen only on occasion.

Steam pops may be avoided by applying a lower power to the tissue but delivering it over a longer time.[17,26,27] Skrumeda et al observed that although larger lesions could be created in vitro with irrigated energy delivery at 50 watts for 30 – 120 seconds, 30-50% of the pulses (depending on duration of the pulse) were associated with impedance rises and crater formation at autopsy.[17] Lowering the energy to 20 watts and prolonging energy delivery to 5-10 minutes prevented impedance rises and was associated with lesion volumes that were similar to 50 watt pulses delivered for 30 seconds. In a closed chest canine study, energy delivery through irrigated catheters placed in the coronary sinus was associated with injury if the neighboring coronary artery if voltage outputs of 60 volts were used. Delivering a lower energy of 40 volts for a longer duration (180 seconds) prevented injury to the nearby coronary artery but resulted in epeicardial lesion volumes similar to the 60 volts pulses.[27] In the canine thigh muscle preparation, limiting energy to 50 volts during saline–irrigated energy delivery prevented steam pops.[13] Alternatively, pulsing the radiofrequency current with short periods on and off, allows the superficial tissue along the electrode to cool during brief off periods while the deeper tissues demonstrate a gradually increasing temperature due to conduction of heat across the thermal gradient.[28]

CONCLUSIONS

The in vitro data show a clear benefit of irrigated catheters with regard to efficient energy transfer resulting in larger lesions and prevention of thrombus formation on the ablation electrode. The risk however, is that excessive heating of the tissue remote from the electrode may result in intracardiac explosions that could lead to perforation and tamponade, damage to neighboring vascular structures such as coronary arteries, or crater formation on the endocardium posing risk for thrombus formation and embolization. Clearly, more clinical experience is required to address safety issues with this form of lesioning particularly when applied to thin-walled atrial tissues, in the coronary sinus, or on the epicardium. The role of new monitoring techniques such as intracardiac ultrasound for evaluation of lesion extent and associated complications requires more study. However, the initial clinical results warrant expansion of clinical trials using irrigated catheters for radiofrequency ablation.

REFERENCES

1. Hoyt RH, Huang SK, Marcus FI, Roger S. Factors influencing transcatheter radiofrequency ablation of the myocardium. J. Applied Cardiol 1986;1:469-486.
2. Ring ME, Huang SK, Gorman G, Graham AR. Determinants of impedance rise during catheter ablation of bovine myocardium with radiofrequency energy. Pacing Clin Electrophysiol 1989;12:170-176.
3. Haines DE, Watson DD. Tissue heating during radiofrequency catheter ablation: A thermodynamic model and observations in isolated perfused and superfused canine right ventricular free wall. Pacing Clin Electrophysiol 1989;12:962-976.
4. Haines DE, Verow AF. Observations on electrode-tissue interface temperature and effect on electrical impedance during radiofrequency ablation of ventricular myocardium. Circulation 1990;82:1034-1038.
5. Langberg JJ, Lee MA, Chin MC, Rosenqvist M. Radiofrequency catheter ablation: The effects of electrode size on lesion volume in vivo. Pacing Clin Electrophysiol 1990;13:1242-1248.
6. Jackman WM, Wang X, Friday KJ, Fitzgerald DM, Roman C, Moulton K, Margolis PD, Bowman AJ, Kuck KH, Naccarelli GV, Pitha JV, Dyer J, Lazzara R. Catheter ablation of the atrioventricular junction using radiofrequency current in 17 patients: Comparison of standard and large-tip catheter electrodes. Circulation 1991;83:1562-1576.
7. Langberg JJ, Calkins H, El-Atassi R, Borganelli M, Leon A, Kalbfleisch SJ, Morady F. Temperature monitoring during radiofrequency catheter ablation of accessory pathways. Circulation 1992;86:1469-1474.
8. Peterson HH, Chen X, Pietersen A, Svendsen JH, Haunso S. Lesion dimensions during temperature-controlled radiofrequency catheter ablation of left ventricular porcine myocardium. Impact of ablation site, electrode size, and convective cooling, Circulation 1999;99:319-325.
9. Otomo K, Yamanashi WS, Tondo C, Antz M, Bussey J,Pitha JV, Arruda M,Nakagawa H, Wittkampf FHM, Lazzara R, Jackman WM. Why a large tip electrode makes a deeper radiofrequency lesion: Effects of increase in electrode cooling and electrode-tissue interface area. J Cardiovasc Electrophysiol 1998;9: 47-54.
10. Wittkampf FHM, Hauer RN, Robles de Medina EO. Radiofrequency ablation with a cooled porous electrode catheter. J Am Coll Cardiol 1988;11:17 (abstract)

11. Mittleman RS, Huang SKS, deGuzman WT, Cuenoud H, et al. Use of the saline infusion electrode catheter for improved energy delivery and increased lesion size in radiofrequency catheter ablation. Pacing Clin Electrophysiol 1995;18:1022-1027.

12. Nakagawa H, Yamanashi WS, Pitha J, Arruda M, Wang X, Ohtomo K, Beckman KJ, McClelland JH, Lazzara R, Jackman WM. Comparison of in vivo tissue temperature profile and lesion geometry for saline-irrigated electrode versus temperature control in a canine thigh muscle preparation. Circulation 1995;91:2264-2273.

13. Nakagawa H, Wittkampf FHM, Yamanashi WS, Pitha J, Imai S, Campbell B, Arruda B, Lazzara R, Jackman WM. Inverse relationship between electrode size and lesion size during radiofrequency ablation with active electrode cooling. Circulation 1998;98:458-465.

14. Nakagawa H, Yamanashi WS, Pitha J, Yong KC, Arruda M, Rome M, Wang X, Ohtomo K, Lazzara R, Jackman WM. Comparison of radiofrequency lesions in the canine left ventricle using saline irrigated electrode versus temperature control. J Am Coll Cardiol 1995;25:42A (abstract)

15. Nakagawa H, Yamanashi WS, Pitha J, Yong KC, Arruda M, Rome M, Wang X, Ohtomo K, Lazzara R, Jackman WM. Effective delivery of radiofrequency energy through the coronary sinus without impedance rise using a saline irrigated electrode. J Am Coll Cardiol 1995;25:293A(abstract).

16. Petersen HH, Chen X, Pietersen A, Svendsen JH, Haunso S. Temperature-controlled irrigated tip radiofrequency catheter ablation: Comparison of in vivo and in vitro lesion dimensions for standard catheter and irrigated tip catheter with minimal infusion rate. J Cardiovasc Electrophysiol 1998;9: 409-414.

17. Skrumeda LL, Mehra R. Comparison of standard and irrigated radiofrequency ablation in the canine ventricle. J Cardiovasv Electrophysiol 1998;9: 1196-1205.

18. Arruda M, Nakagawa H, Chandrasedaran K, Otomo K, Wang X, Beckman K, McClelland J, Gonzalez M, Widman L, Reynolds D, Lazzara R, Jackman WM. Radiofrequency ablation in the coronary venous system is associated with risk of coronary artery injury which may be prevented by use of intravascular ultrasound. J Am Coll Cardiol 1996;27:160A(abstract)

19. Nakagawa H, Imai S, Arruda M, Scholernkufer D, Freedoff F, Shah N, Beckman K, McClelland J, Gonzalez M, Otomo K, Lazzara R, Jackman WM. Prevention of pericardial tamponade during radiofrequency ablation of accessory pathways using a saline irrigated electrode. Pacing Clin Electrophysiol 1997;20; II-1068. (abstract)

20. Crossley GH, Fitzgerald D, Nakagawa H, Beckman K, Simmons T, Gonzalez M, Arruda M, Haisty WK, Savage S, Camp S, Jackman W. Novel low-flow irrigated-tip RF catheter prevents impedance rises. Pacing Clin Electrophysiol 1998;21:II-965. (abstract)

21. Jais P, Haissaguerre M, Shah DC, Takahashi A, Hocini M, Lavergne T, Lafitte S, Le Mouroux A, Fischer B, Clementy L. Successful irrigated-tip catheter ablation of atrial flutter resistant to conventional radiofrequency ablation. Circulation 1998; 98: 835-838.

22. Avital B, Morgan M, Hare J, Khan M, Lessila C. Intracardiac explosions during radiofrequency ablation: histopathology in the acute and chronic dog model. Circulation 1992;86: I-191. (abstract).

23. Rothman SA, Hsia H, Thome LM, Campo RA, Panas G, Buxton AE, Miller JM. 'Popping" during radiofrequency catheter ablation: an in vitro model – new observations. J Am Coll Cardiol 1998;31 (suppl A): 119A. (abstract)

24. Packer DL, Johnson SB. Predictors of impedance rise occurring during ablation with open, irrigation tip catheters in the canine ventricle. Circulation 1996;94:I-558 (abstract)

25. Johnson SB, Packer DL. Characterization of the tissue sequelae of the impedance rise occurring with ablation with an open, irrigation tip catheter. Circulation 1996;94 (supp I): I-494.

26. Arruda M, Tondo C, Otomo K, Pitha JV, Antz M, Bussey J, Nakagawa H, Lazzara R, Jackman WM. Radiofrequency current delivery in the coronary venous system using long pulse duration at low voltage prevents thermal injury to the adjacent coronary artery. Pacing Clin Electrophysiol 1996;19:II-713. (abstract)

27. Imai S, Nakagawa H, Yamanashi WS, Wittkampf FHM, Pitha JV, Campbell BW, McClelland JH, Beckman KJ, Arruda M, Lazzara R, Jackman WM. Avoidance of steam 'pop" during radiofrequency ablation. Circulation 1996;94: I-494 (abstract)
28. Nakagawa H, Wittkampf FHM, Imai S, Yamanashi WS, Holden M, Arruda M, Pitha JV, Lazzara R, Jackman WM. Pulsed current delivery combined with saline irrigation produces deeper radiofrequency lesions without steam "pop". J Am Coll Cardiol 1997;29 (suppl) : 374A. (abstract)

Chapter 21

RADIOFREQUENCY ATRIAL LINEAR ABLATION USING MICROCATHETERS

Sung H. Chun

Cardiac Arrhythmia and Electrophysiology, Stanford University, Stanford, California, USA

Microcatheters were initially developed for the purpose of electrophysiological mapping within the right coronary arterial system to locate right-sided accessory pathways. These included 2.2-French bipolar catheter manufactured by Viggo-Spectramed from Oxnard, California, and a 3-French fixed-wire design catheter with ten bipolar electrode pairs manufactured by Cardima, Inc. from Fremont, California. Both Elecath, Inc. and Mansfield/Boston Scientific, Inc. also had microcatheters applying a different design; they used an over-the-guide-wire system similar to the angioplasty approach, using 0.014-inch high-torque floppy angioplasty guide wire.[1] Unfortunately, for various reasons this application failed to gain popularity and none of these microcatheters received approval from the U.S. Food and Drug Administration (FDA).

However, with the new interest in ablation for atrial fibrillation, one particular design of microcatheter from Cardima, Inc. applied its technology in atrial linear ablation, specifically for the use of endocardial modified Maze procedure. Currently, this microcatheter system is being used for cardiac electrophysiologic mapping endocardially, within the coronary sinus venous system, as well as within the pulmonary venous system via left atrium. It was approved by the U.S. Food and Drug Administration (FDA), and was granted CE Mark in Europe for such mapping purpose. It is also being evaluated for the purpose of radiofrequency linear ablation in the right atrium. Based on the clinical data to date, one particular design, REVELATION™ Microcatheter System, was granted the CE Mark in Europe for radiofrequency ablation. Similar microcatheter design is under investigation in the United States for the same use.

L. Bing Liem and E. Downar (eds.), Progress in Catheter Ablation, 343-352.
© 2001 *Kluwer Academic Publishers. Printed in the Netherlands.*

1. TECHNICAL ASPECT OF MICROCATHETER SYSTEM

At the present time, Cardima, Inc. from Fremont, California is the only company manufacturing a microcatheter system for the cardiac electrophysiologic purpose. There are several designs available. For mapping microcatheters, outer diameter varies from 1.5 French (PATHFINDER mini™) to 3.3 French (REVELATION™) with number of electrodes from 4 to 16 per microcatheter. There is also an over-the-guide-wire design microcatheter for the mapping purpose (TRACER™) that goes over 0.010 inch guide wire. Two specific microcatheter designs are available for radiofrequency linear ablation in microcatheter system. REVELATION™ is a non-temperature sensing design with 8 electrodes, each electrode of 3mm in length with an overall working electrode length of 38mm, and REVELATION™ Tx is a 3.7 French temperature sensing version with 8 electrodes, each electrode of 6mm in length with an overall working electrode length of 62mm. Each electrode uses the thermocouple just proximal to the electrode (centered between electrodes) for temperature feedback and control of radiofrequency energy in order to maintain a preselected thermocouple set temperature (Figure 1). All above microcatheters essentially share the same basic design of multiple coil electrodes and a laminated platinum tip to prevent injury to the tissue (Figure 2).

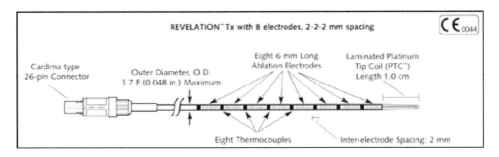

Figure 1: Diagram of Cardima REVELATION™ Tx 3.7F microcatheter

The current microcatheter system set up utilizes a guiding catheter to introduce microcatheter to a desired position within the endocardial space. Any commercially available guiding catheter with an intraluminal diameter of 5 French can be used. Tuohy-Borst type adapter or rotating hemostatic valve with the side arm (RHV) is connected to the guiding catheter hub to infuse continuous heparinized saline drip. The principle of operation of the current microcatheter system is the same as other currently marketed electrode recording and ablation catheters. The microcatheter is linked to a switchbox which in turn links to a standard ECG recorder, a pacing stimulator, and the RF generator (Figure 3).

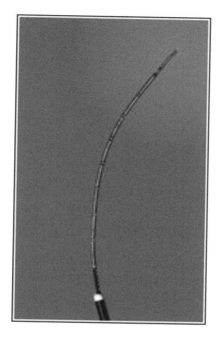

Figure 2: Picture of Cardima REVELATION™ Tx 3.7F microcatheter

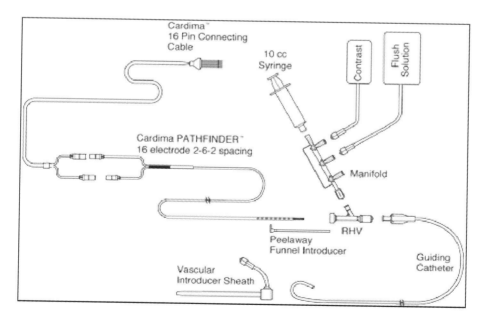

Figure 3: Cardima microcatheter system set-up diagram

2.   EXPERIMENTAL DATA

Series of *in vivo* experiments were carried out to test microcatheter system's performance. In an earlier study by Keane, et al,[2] eight goats with acutely induced atrial fibrillation underwent right atrial radiofrequency ablation using a non-deflectable flexible octapolar ablation microcatheter (PATHFINDER™-Cardima, Inc.). Using 8 French guiding catheter, a microcatheter was aligned along five predetermined right atrial linear trajectories that connected orifices of the superior vena cava to inferior vena cava, the tricuspid annulus, and the coronary sinus. Atrial fibrillation was non-inducible in all eight goats after the ablation. Histology analysis confirmed transmural lesions were achieved.

Two studies compared microcatheter radiofrequency ablation performance to that of standard radiofrequency ablation catheters.

Schneider, et al[3] conducted an in vivo study using 22 sheep, investigating efficacy of three different multipolar ablation catheters. In eleven sheep, 3.3 French microcatheter with 8 electrodes (3 mm length with 2 mm interelectrode spacing) (Cardima, Inc.) was placed in their right atria via the internal jugular vein and linear radiofrequency ablation was performed. This was a non-temperature sensing microcatheter; electrodes were connected consecutively in pairs and radiofrequency energy was applied for 60 seconds using 10-20 watts per application. In 7 sheep, a steerable 7 French ablation catheter with four 6-mm electrodes (EPT) was inserted using same approach. In remaining 4 sheep, a steerable 7 French ablation catheter with four 5-mm electrodes (Bard) was placed via the internal jugular vein. Both 7 French ablation catheters were temperature sensing; each radiofrequency energy application was in temperature controlled unipolar setting with target temperature of 70°C for 60 seconds. Lesions created with the microcatheter had depth of 0.8 ± 0.9 mm, width of 2.9 ± 2.6 mm, and length of 10.8 ± 9.4 mm, whereas lesions from the 7 French ablation catheter had depth of 3.3 ± 1.8 mm, width of 6.1 ± 3.4 mm, and length of 16.1 ± 10 mm. This comparative study showed that the microcatheter without temperature-sensing ability created narrower lesions whereas the 7 French temperature controlled ablation catheters were able to create deeper lesions, thus higher chance of achieving transmural lesions.

Another study by Jumrussirikul, et al[4] compared 3.7 French temperature-sensing microcatheter (REVELATION™ Tx, Cardima, Inc.) to a 7-French quadripolar electrode catheter (RF Marinr, Medtronic Cardiorhythm) in ten dogs. Microcatheter was placed in the right atrium in six dogs via femoral vein; with a target temperature of 50°C, radiofrequency power output up to 50 watts was delivered for 60 seconds to each electrode sequentially. In remaining four dogs, a 7-French quadripolar catheter was placed in the right atrium via femoral vein; with a target temperature of 60°C, radiofrequency power output between 0.5-50 watts was delivered for 60 seconds at a time. After each radiofrequency application, the catheter tip was withdrawn 5 mm for another radiofrequency application until each targeted line was completed. Each catheter position was evaluated with electrogram amplitude and pacing threshold just prior to and immediately after each ablation. These linear lesions were compared four weeks post-ablation. Microcatheter system lesion dimensions were as follows: length 29.6±14.9 mm; width 2.6±0.9 mm; and depth 2.4±0.8 mm. The 7 French ablation catheter lesions were length 25±11.2 mm, width 4.9±0.9 mm, and depth 2.1±0.5 mm. Using microcatheter, eleven of 24 lesions were transmural (45%) in depth, and 18 of 24 lesions were continuous (75%) (Figure 4). With 7 French ablation catheter, six out of sixteen lesions were transmural in depth (37%), and six of 16 lesions were continuous (37%) (Figure 5). Unlike the previous study, microcatheter performed superior to the 7 French ablation catheter in creating transmural and continuous lesion.

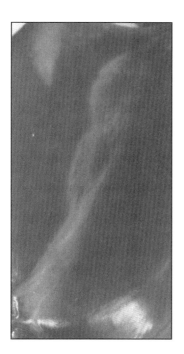 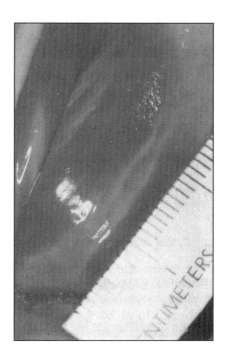

Figures 4 and 5. Figure 4 (left): Endocardial lesion created with conventional radiofrequency catheter system. Note its discontinuous lesion formation. Figure 5 (right) Endocardial lesion created with Cardima Revelation™ Tx radiofrequency Microcatheter system. Note its narrow and continuous lesion formation. (Reprinted with permission from PACE)

There are several potential explanations for different findings with these two studies. Most importantly, the study by Schneider, et al used a non-temperature sensing microcatheter. Perhaps the non-temperature controlled radiofrequency application resulted in less effective, non-transmural lesions. Previous studies have shown importance of temperature controlled radiofrequency application for an optimal ablation.[5-7] Secondly, Schneider, et al did not evaluate microcatheter positioning with electrogram amplitude and pacing threshold; they also did not assess effectiveness of each radiofrequency application with comparison of these two parameters, electrogram amplitude and pacing threshold, pre- and post-ablation.   Experiments by several investigators correlated effective lesion formation to reductions in electrogram amplitude and pacing threshold.[8-10]   This was also verified by Jumrussirikul, et al's study.[4]   In their study, post-ablation pacing threshold of ≤1 mA and electrogram reduction of ≥ 50% served as predictors of transmural lesion formation.   It is possible that the microcatheter positioning in Schneider's experiment did not have adequate contact with endocardial tissue to create optimal lesions.   More positive result using microcatheters by Jumrussirikul, et al may in part be due to the fact that their microcatheter was temperature-sensing and thus each radiofrequency application was temperature controlled.   The reason why the 7 French ablation catheter had less continuous lesions (37% vs 75% for microcatheter) is probably because it was not a multipolar linear ablation catheter and each line had to be achieved by the point-by-point ablation technique.

One important data that is not available with a microcatheter radiofrequency ablation is the correlation between transmural lesion formation to the alteration of electrophysiologic properties of the atrial tissue.   Even though it is well accepted that a transmural lesion formation correlates to achievement of conduction block across the lesion, actual interruption of electrophysiologic property and verification of conduction block across a lesion have not been directly shown using a microcatheter.[8]   Although a thinner lesion may serve as an advantage by causing less interruption and thus better preservation of overall electrophysiologic property in the atrium, it has not been proven that decrease in width of lesion still results in complete conduction block across such lesion.   However, one study did provide an indirect evidence that such conduction block can be achieved using a microcatheter system.   An experiment by Keane, et al showed that in acute atrial fibrillation model of eight goats, such atrial fibrillation was non-inducible after multiple linear ablations in the right atrium using microcatheters, suggesting that electrophysiologic interruptions across these linear lesions were achieved.[2]

It is important to note that all animal experiments, including those mentioned above as well as our own experience, repeatedly demonstrated that the current microcatheter system is safe to use at least in the right atrium and in the coronary sinus venous system.   There was no structural damage to the endocardial tissue, endovascular system, or tricuspid annulus, and no perforation of atrial wall or endocardial membrane was observed.   No significant thrombus or coagulum formation was noted when proper set up was applied with adequate continuous flushing of heparinized saline through the guiding catheter.[2-4]

3. EVALUATION OF CURRENT MICROCATHETER SYSTEM

3.1 Advantages

Based on animal experiments and our own experience with the current microcatheter system, several potential advantages and disadvantages can be identified.

The most apparent potential advantage of the microcatheter system is its size and flexibility. Due to its thin diameter as well as flexible material and design, it can be shaped to the surface that comes to contact with. In addition, its flexible and thin design suits well in accessing narrow space such as the coronary sinus venous system and the pulmonary venous system.

Its multipolar design of the microcatheter system is ideal for linear ablation. As seen from the study by Jumrussirikul, et al,[4] this multipolar microcatheter system is superior to the conventional quadpolar ablation catheters in creating a more continuous linear lesion.

The lesions created by the microcatheter system is significantly narrower in width than the conventional 7 French ablation catheters. At least in theory, thinner yet transmural lesions may mean achieving alterations of conduction with minimal impact on the overall electrophysiologic integrity of the tissue.

3.2 Disadvantages

There are several potential disadvantages using the current microcatheter system.

Its flexible and thin design can actually work against achieving optimal tissue contact in certain locations. This is especially true in the distal portion of the microcatheter that tends to curve away from the tissue. This can usually be resolved by minimizing the microcatheter tip that gets deployed out of the guiding catheter.

Another potential disadvantage of the microcatheter is the difficulty in positioning over the isthmus between the tricuspid annulus and the inferior vena cava. This most likely is due to the fact that the current microcatheter is so flexible that it cannot generate enough pressure against the floor of the right atrium to achieve adequate contact throughout "ridges and valleys" along such isthmus.

Unlike the conventional 7 French steerable ablation catheters, the current microcatheter is non-steerable that requires a guiding catheter. This can potentially be cumbersome for two reasons. The guiding catheter requires a continuous heparinized saline infusion set up that the conventional ablation catheter does not need. Also, different locations within the atrium may require differently shaped guiding catheter for optimal positioning; this would mean exchanging to a new guiding catheter in the middle of the procedure as well as incurring more cost.

One important issue regarding the current microcatheter system is the potential risk of thrombus and coagulum formation. This is an issue that is universally important to all radiofrequency ablation catheter technology; fortunately, the current microcatheter system thus far proved to be quite safe in this regard. Even though the guiding catheter lumen is a potential source of thrombus formation, this has not been a problem as long as an adequate continuous infusion of the heparinized saline is maintained. The coil design of each electrode could potentially be more thrombogenic when compared to the conventional 7 French smooth electrode tip. However, as mentioned earlier extensive animal data as well as human data proved that such coil design did not increase thrombogenicity, perhaps because of very thin diameter.

4.   HUMAN ATRIAL LINEAR ABLATION DATA

Based on promising animal study results, human atrial linear ablation clinical trials using radiofrequency microcatheter were performed. Because of relatively small number of patients enrolled as well as only short-term follow up data available at the present time, discussion of these clinical trials will be brief. First, a ten patient feasibility study was conducted at three centers in the United States. All enrolled patients had history of paroxysmal atrial fibrillation with at least two episodes per month, and were refractory to two or more antiarrhythmic agents. In all ten patients, the REVELATION™ Tx radiofrequency microcatheter (Cardima, Inc.) was used to create linear lesions in the right atrium only. Pre and post ablation data showed a significant decrease in atrial electrogram amplitude as well as increase in pacing threshold from each electrode. Pacing threshold rose from an average of 5.28mA (SD=0.84) to 9.90mA (SD=1.49) (p<0.01); atrial electrogram amplitude decreased from an average of 1.25mV (SD=0.12) to 0.72mV (SD=0.09) (p<0.01). One patient with pre-existing sinus node dysfunction experienced worsening sinus node dysfunction after the procedure and required a permanent pacemaker implant. There were no other major complications. At one month follow-up, six out of nine patients had less recurrence of atrial fibrillation when compared to the month prior to the procedure. Three other patients had an increase in the number of episodes of symptomatic atrial fibrillation during the month following the procedure as compared to the month prior to the ablation. One patient was noncompliant and had inadequate data to analyze. At six month follow-up, seven patients had adequate data to analyze. Three patients had >80% reduction in symptomatic atrial fibrillation episodes; one patient had 70% reduction; and three patients had no change in recurrence rate. No long-term adverse effect was noted.

Currently, there are two on-going multi-center clinical trials assessing safety and efficacy of right atrial linear ablation using a radiofrequency microcatheter technique, one in the United States and one in Europe. The United States clinical trial, Phase II, involves ten medical centers, enrolling similar patients as the Phase I study. Same Revelation™ Tx radiofrequency microcatheter (Cardima, Inc.) is being used. Eighteen patients have been enrolled thus far, ten males and eight females. As with the Phase I study result, these patients had statistically significant increase in intracardiac electrogram amplitudes as well as reduction in pacing thresholds when post-ablation values were compared to pre-ablation values, suggesting effective transmural ablation. Phase one and phase two outcome data were combined for below analysis. At one month follow-up (n=24 patients) five patients (21%) had >80% reduction in AF episodes, eight patients (33%) had 50-79% reduction, seven patients (29%) had less than 50% reduction, and four patients (17%) had no reduction in AF episodes. At three month follow-up (n=15 patients) nine patients (60%) had >80% reduction in AF episodes, one patient (7%) had between 50-79% reduction, three patients (20%) had <50% reduction, and two patients (13%) had no reduction in AF episodes. Mean procedural time up to now is 323 minutes (minimum 210 minutes; maximum 555 minutes) with mean fluoroscopy time of 79 minutes (minimum 5.5 minutes; maximum 202 minutes). As with the Phase I study, Phase II study thus far has been safe with only one patient experiencing sinus node dysfunction post-ablation that required a permanent pacemaker implant. No other serious adverse event such as stroke or death was noted. Of note, majority of these patients required conventional "non-micro" radiofrequency ablation catheter to create a linear lesion along the isthmus between tricuspid annulus and inferior vena cava because of difficulty positioning REVELATION™ Tx radiofrequency microcatheter (Cardima, Inc.) along this trajectory.

In Europe, six centers are involved in a similar protocol as the United States clinical trial; in Europe, REVELATION™M radiofrequency microcatheter (Cardima, Inc.) is being used which does not have a temperature control feature. Of the 48 patients enrolled, in one month follow-up 25 patients (52%) had >80% reduction in AF episodes, five patients (10%) had between 50-79% reduction, seven patients (15%) had <50% reduction, and eleven patients (23%) had no reduction in AF episodes. At three month follow-up (n=45 patients), 21 patients (47%) had >80% reduction in AF episodes, nine patients (20%) had between 50-79% reduction, four patients (9%) had <50% reduction, and eleven patients (24%) had no reduction in AF episodes. Virtually all patients required conventional "non-micro" radiofrequency ablation catheter to create a linear lesion along the isthmus between tricuspid annulus and inferior vena cava. One death occurred 36 days post-ablation which was thought to be unrelated to the procedure. No other adverse event was reported.

In summary, radiofrequency microcatheter appears to be effective in creating transmural lesions in most locations within the human right atrium. It also appears to be safe to use at least within the human right atrium. Technical improvement may be ncessary to achieve linear ablation in the isthmus between tricuspid annulus and inferior vena cava. Most importantly, to achieve ultimate goal in elimination of atrial fibrillation recurrence in these patients will most likely depend on determination of ideal location(s) to ablate, e.g. left atrium and pulmonary veins, as well as further advancement in ablation technology. It is very possible that radiofrequency microcatheter system may play an important role in achieving these goals in the near future.

REFERENCES

1. Lesh, Michael Techniques for Localization and Radiofrequency Catheter Ablation of Right Free Wall Accessory Pathways Chapter 95, Cardiac Electrophysiology: From Cell to Bedside, second edition, edited by Zipes & Jalife, pg1078-1092
2. Keane D, Guerrero L, Ettelson L, McGovern BA, Garan H, Ruskin JN Right Atrial Multipolar Catheter Ablation of Atrial Fibrillation in a Pace-Induced Goat Model J Am Coll Cardiol 1997;Suppl:32A (abstract)
3. Schneider MAE, Ndrepepa G, Richter T, Vallant A, Gayk U, Henke J, Zrenner B, Karch MR, Erhardt W, Schömig A, Schmitt C Efficacy to perform atrial linear radiofrequency lesions: an experimental histologic comparison European Heart Journal Vol 20, Abstr. Suppl. Aug/Sep 1999, pg 234
4. Jumrussirikul P, Atiga WL, Lardo AC, Berger RD, Halperin H, Hutchins GM, Calkins H. Prospective Comparison of Lesions Created Using a Multipolar Microcatheter Ablation System with Those Created Using a Pullback Approach with Standard Radiofrequency Ablation in the Canine Atrium. Pacing Clin Electrophysiol 2000;23:203-213.
5. Langberg JJ, Calkins H, el-Atassi R, Borganelli M, Leon A, Kalbfleisch SJ, Morady F. Temperature Monitoring During Radiofrequency Catheter Ablation of Accessory Pathways. Circulation 1992;86:1469-1474.
6. Calkins H, Prystowsky E, Carlson M, Klein LS, Saul JP, Gillette P. Temperature Monitoring During Radiofrequency Catheter Ablation Procedures Using Closed Loop Control. Atakr Multicenter Investigators Group. Circulation 1994;90:1279-1286.
7. Strickberger SA, Daoud EG, Weiss R, Brinkman K, Bogun F, Knight BP, Bahu M, Goyal R, Man KC, Morady F. A Randomized Comparison of Fixed Power and Temperature Monitoring During Slow Pathway Ablation in Patients With Atrioventricular Nodal Reentrant Tachycardia. J Interv Card Electrophysiol 1997;1:299-303
8. Gepstein L, Hayam G, Shpun S, Cohen D, Ben-Haim SA. Atrial Linear Ablations in Pigs. Chronic Effects on Atrial Electrophysiology and Pathology. Circulation 1999;100:419-426.
9. Liem LB, Pomeranz M, Riseling K, Anderson S, berry GJ. Electrophysiological Correlates of Transmural Linear Ablation. Pacing Clin Electrophysiol 2000;23:40-46.
10. Azegami K, Satake S, Okishiege K, Sasano T, Ohira H, Yamashita K. Monitoring the Local Electrogram at the Ablation Site During Radiofrequency Application for Common Atrial Flutter. Jpn Circ J 1998;62:559-564.

Chapter 22

RADIOFREQUENCY LINEAR ABLATION USING LOOPED MULTIPOLAR CATHETERS

Boaz Avitall, Arvydas Urbonas, Dalia Urboniene, Scott C. Millard
The University of Illinois at Chicago, Chicago, Illinois, USA

INTRODUCTION

The goal of catheter-based ablation of atrial fibrillation (Afib) should be safe minimal tissue destruction allowing for the restoration of sinus rhythm under autonomic nervous system control combined with recovery of atrial mechanical transport to prevent the development of a thromboembolic event and provide hemodynamic benefits for the patient. Because the atrial chambers are globular, elastic, and only a few millimeters thick, we hypothesized that a catheter system that creates adjustable loops which create dynamic contact with the atrial walls is most likely to be able to adapt to the atrial structure and create good contact for ablating and recording. This chapter summarizes our experience using a catheter technology that was designed to create linear contiguous lesions in both atria.

A catheter system with 24 4-mm ring electrodes that can create loops in the atria was the initial prototype (Figure 1). The electrodes can be used to record electrical activity and deliver radio frequency (RF) power for ablation. In 33 dogs, 82 linear lesions were generated using 3 power titration protocols: fixed levels, manual titration guided by local electrogram activity, and temperature-control. Bipolar activity was recorded from the 24 electrodes before, during, and after lesion generation. The lesions were created principally in 5 loop catheter positions as shown in Figure 2. Data was gathered regarding lesion contiguity, transmurality, and dimensions; the changes in local electrical activity amplitude; the incidence rate of rapid impedance rise and desiccation or char formation; and rhythm outcomes. Catheter deployment usually requires <60 seconds. Linear lesions (12-16 cm in length and 6 ± 2 mm wide) can be generated in 24-48 minutes without moving the catheter. Effective lesion formation can be predicted by a marked decrease in the amplitude of bipolar recordings (67±34%). Splitting

L. Bing Liem and E. Downar (eds.), Progress in Catheter Ablation, 353-376.
© 2001 *Kluwer Academic Publishers. Printed in the Netherlands.*

or fragmentation of the electrogram and increasing pacing threshold (3.1 ± 3.3 mV to 7.1 ± 3.8 mV, p<0.01) are indicative of effective lesion formation. Impedance rises and char formation occurred at 91 ± 12 °C. Linear lesion creation did not result in the initiation of Afib, however, atrial tachycardia was recorded after the completion of the final lesion in 3 of 12 hearts. When using temperature-control, no char was noted in the left atrium (LA), while 8% of the right atrial (RA) burns had char.

Based on these results we have concluded that the adjustable loop catheter, which forces the atria to conform around the catheter, is capable of producing linear, contiguous lesions up to 16 cm long with minimal effort and radiation exposure. Pacing thresholds, electrogram amplitude and character are markers of effective lesion formation. Although Afib could not be induced after the completion of the lesion set, sustained atrial tachycardia could be induced in 25% of the hearts. In an effort to increase the efficiency of the ablation system we evaluated and reported on the use of a loop catheter with 14 12-mm long coil electrodes 2 mm apart (Figures 1,2) equipped with two thermistors, which were positioned at the two edges of each coil. The power is regulated to the maximal temperature measured between the two thermistors.[1]

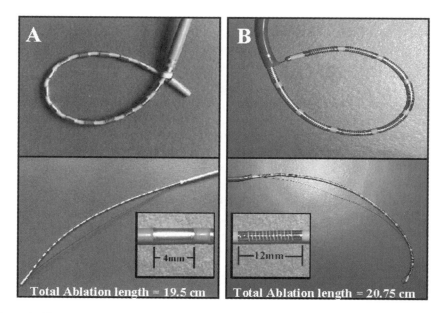

Figure 1. Ring and coil electrode ablation catheters. A = ring electrode ablation catheter, B = coil electrode ablation catheter.

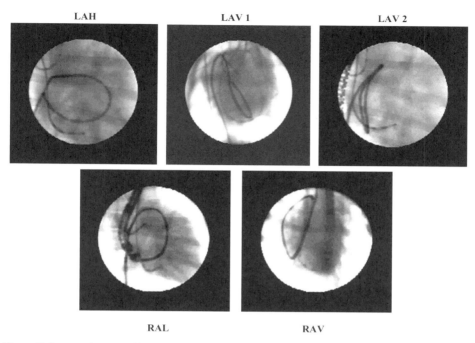

Figure 2. Loop catheter positions. LAH = circular left atrial lesion above the mitral valve identified as "left atrial horizontal", LAV 1 and LAV 2 = vertical left atrial lesions connecting the mitral valve and the top of left atria, bisecting the pulmonary veins laterally and medially, RAL = anteromedial loop connecting the tricuspid ring, superior vena cava (SVC) and inferior vena cava (IVC), RAV = right atrial vertical loop, connecting the SVC, IVC and lateral right atrial wall.

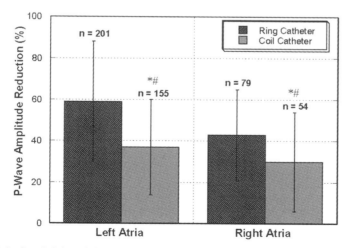

Figure 3. Left and right atrial P- wave reduction after radiofrequency lesions. *p<0.01 vs coil electrodes, # p<0.05 vs pre-ablation.

This catheter system was found to be effective and efficient when compared to the 24 4-mm ring type electrodes that were used in an earlier version of the technology.[2] Although temperature monitoring has been shown to be essential for the prevention of over heating and char formation,[3,4] we have reported on the use of local electrogram amplitude reduction as a marker for transmural lesion creation with the 12 mm long coil electrodes.[5] In this study the R-wave reduction of greater than 50% was a marker of transmural lesion formation (Figure 3), an example of which is shown in Figure 4. In several instances regional tissue isolation or marked decremental conduction was recorded after the creation of several linear lesions in the LA. Example of such tissue isolation is shown in Figure 5 were a segment of the LA has been isolated from the rest of the atria, which was still in Afib. Distal coronary sinus isolation is shown in Figure 6.

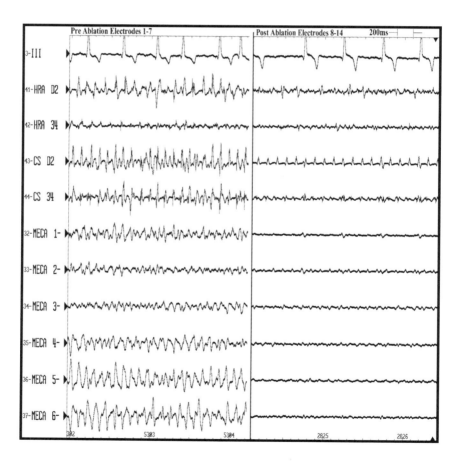

Figure 4 (A&B). Pre/post ablation 12mm P- wave reduction (9210 - lesion 1). A (left panel) = pre-ablation electrodes 1-7, B (right panel) = post-ablation electrodes 8-14

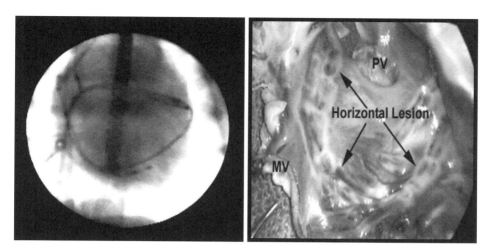

Figure 4 (C&D). C (left panel) = X-ray position of the loop catheter, D (right panel) = gross pathology of the lesion.

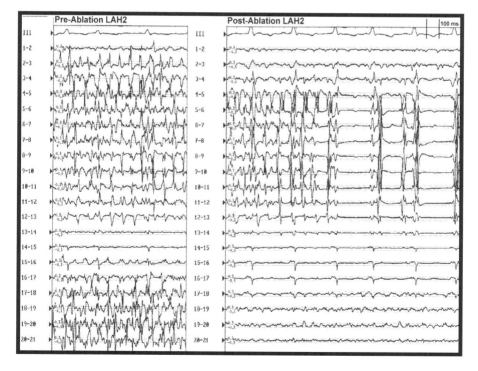

Figure 5. Local electrogram activity pre/post ablation: LAH2 position (lesion 2) High level conduction block in isolated left atrial tissue. A (left panel) = pre-ablation LAH 2, B (right panel) = post-ablation LAH 2.   See also Figures 5 C-E (next page).

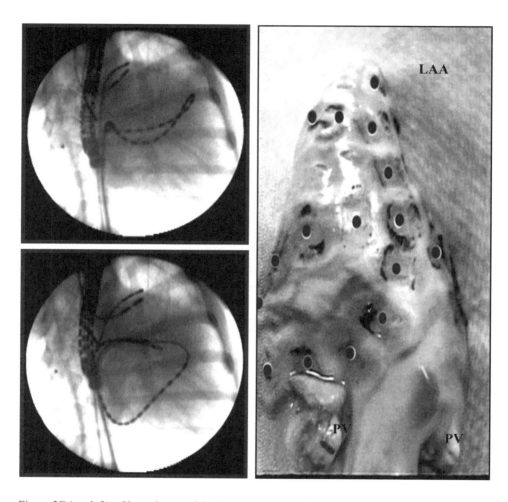

Figure 5C (top left) = X- ray image of the loop catheter in LAH 2 position, D (bottom left) = X-ray image of the loop catheter in LAH 1 position, E (right panel) = gross anatomy of the lesion in LAA (left atrial appendage), PV = pulmonary vein. See also Figures 5 A&B (previous page).

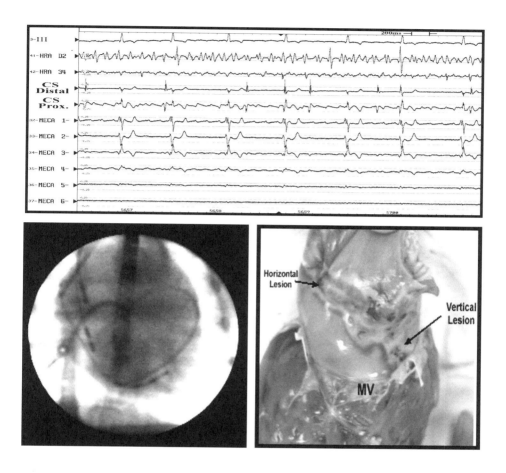

Figure 6. Example of the coronary sinus disconnection from the rest of the atria post-ablation. A (top panel) = electrogram showing distal coronary sinus isolation from the rest of the right atrium, B (lower left) = X –ray image of the loop catheter in LAH, C (lower right) = gross anatomy of the left atrium, showing horizontal and vertical lesions.

1.   LINEAR LESION EFFICACY AND OUTCOMES

The creation of incomplete linear lesions promotes the initiation of atrial tachycardia in every case in which skipped lesions were created.[6]   Although skipped lesions do not result in the induction of Afib in the normal dog atria, these lesions placed in the RA resulted in the induction of an incessant type atrial tachycardia that could not always be terminated with over-drive pacing. Furthermore, in dogs with chronic Afib induced with rapid pacing, linear lesions in both atria resulted in 83% conversion of the Afib. However, in 33% of the dogs, sustained atrial tachycardia, which could be terminated by overdrive pacing (Figure 7), was induced with burst pacing.[7,8]

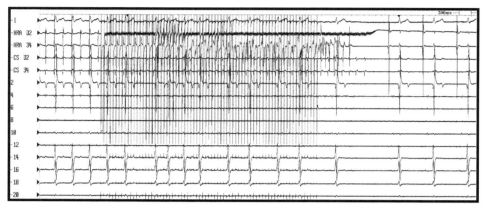

Figure 7. Conversion after burst pacing from HRA D2. HRA D2 = Quadripolar distal tip in high right atrium.

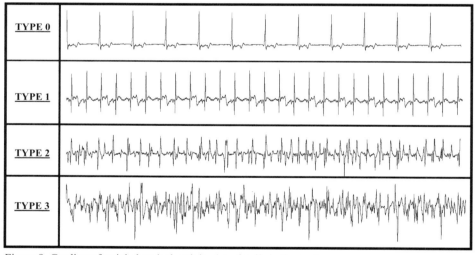

Figure 8. Grading of atrial electrical activity (see details in the text).

These results imply that lesion creation for the ablation of Afib must be kept to a minimum and that the lesions have to be contiguous and transmural terminating at a non-conductive barrier. While noncontiguous and transmural lesions have been shown to promote atrial tachycardia the ablation of Afib does not require contiguous and transmural lesions.[9] In the identification of the atrial tissues that promote Afib in the rapid pacing dog model we hypothesized that linear lesions placed at regions of maximal fractionated electrical activity (Fx) will cause generalized changes in the rate and character of the Afib. These lesions would eventually lead to the termination of Afib, and imply localized dominance of these regions. In dogs with chronic Afib, induced by the rapid pacing dog model, atrial mapping and linear contiguous lesions were placed in the regions of maximal Fx activity. The hetrogenicity of localized electrical activity was divided into 4 types: Type 0 – normal sinus rhythm (NSR) or atrial tachycardia, Type 1 – atrial flutter or tachycardia, Type 2 – high voltage Afib with no baseline fractionation, Type 3 - Afib with baseline fractionation (as shown in Figure 8).

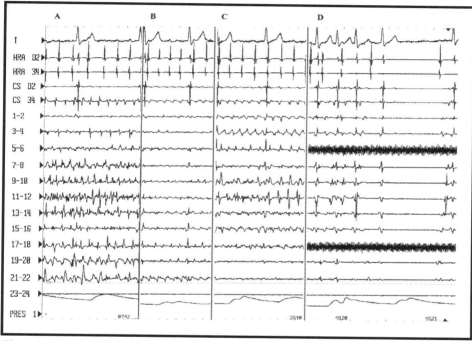

Figure 9. 24-pole recording/ablation catheter recording positioned above mitral valve and under the PVs. A = electrical activity is continuous and fractionated (Fx), especially in electrodes 7-14, which is under the left superior PV, HRA and CS are organized. B = after completion of LA sub-PV lesion, the amplitude of the electrical activity decreased, C = catheter was then placed in a vertical position bisecting the roof of the atria and showing highly Fx activity in electrodes 13-18, D = the Afib Fx activity decreased and converted to discrete electrogram activity followed by NSR during RF delivery to electrodes 17.

In these dogs, LA lesions connecting the pulmonary vein (PV) and the mitral valve were associated with sudden termination of local electrical activity of types 3 to 1 or 0 and were regionalized to the PV. Based on this study we can conclude that regionalized linear lesions targeted at Fx localized recorded activity cause global changes in Afib electrical activity, which lead to the termination of Afib (an example of Afib activity and termination during LA linear lesion is shown in Figure 9 and the localized depolarization organization that it is often a prelude to conversion as shown in Figure 10). This finding implies localized dominance for these regions in driving the Afib. The common characteristic of these regions (in 66%) was Afib of Type 3. Thus, the identification of highly Fx local electrical activity provides a mappable target for regionalized ablation, the majority of which is under the PVs.[10] The Fx activity that was recorded in the dog model was found to be similar to the activity that was mapped in humans with Afib whose local atrial electrical activity was mapped in the operating room prior to mitral valve replacement and the creation of the MAZE operation for the treatment of chronic Afib.[11,12]

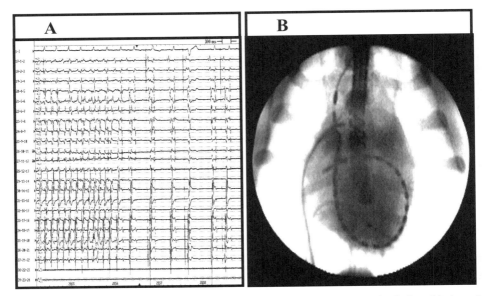

Figure 10. Spontaneous conversion from Afib to NSR with 24-ring electrode during ablation of electrode 10 at the LAH position as shown in the fluoroscopic image. A = electrogram, B = fluoroscopic image of the catheter position.

We further hypothesized that non-linear analysis of the local electrogram activity in the coronary sinus and RA appendage will predict the efficacy of linear lesions placed in either atria in order to ablate Afib. Two nonlinear dynamic measurements were calculated; the Lyapunov exponent (LE) and the correlation dimension (CD) on 5 second notch filtered signals from a catheter in the coronary sinus (CS) and the high right atrium (HRA) pre and post ablation. CD was calculated using the Grassberger Procaccia algorithm. The correlation dimension, which is a predictor of the complexity of a system, steadily decreased post ablation of each lesion. Initially, CD = 1.63 ± .65, LE =.121 ± .05 and post ablation of each lesion CD decreased by .255 ± .19 and LE decreased by .025 ± .014. Upon achieving NSR, CD = .281 ± .033 and LE = .006 ± .006. Thus there is evidence that nonlinear dynamic measurements are good predictors of the organization of atrial electrograms from Afib to NSR after consecutive generation of linear lesions. CD and LE may be used to define the efficacy of each linear lesion.[13]

2. CHRONIC OUTCOME OF ATRIAL FIBRILLATION ABLATION IN THE RAPID PACING DOG MODEL

Twenty-nine dogs were in spontaneous Afib for 6 month prior to ablation and were monitored for 6 months after the ablation. In 7/29 (24%) the Afib was converted to normal sinus rhythm (NSR) with lesions that were placed in only left or right atria. In 6/7 dogs the lesions were placed in the LA and only 1/7 in the RA. In 4/7, the rhythm was converted to atrial tachycardia, and in 2/7 dogs only one lesion was needed to convert the Afib. In 26/29 dogs the Afib was converted to NSR or to atria tachycardia which could have been converted with overdrive pacing. Only 3 dogs (7%) could not be converted with linear lesions in both atria. The number of lesions that were placed to conversion of Afib to either NSR or atrial tachycardia was 5 ± 2 lesions. In 15/21 (73%) dogs LA linear lesions resulted in Afib conversion to atrial tachycardia and only 6/21 (27%) RA lesion resulted in the conversion of the Afib to atrial tachycardia. The conversion rate to either NSR or atrial tachycardia was similar with the use of 4-mm rings (92%) and 12-mm coil electrodes (87%). However, acutely, the 12-mm coil electrode multi-electrode loop catheter design is more likely to convert the Afib to atrial tachycardia (60% vs. 42%) and similar differences were noted with the non-conversion. Only 5 dogs post 4-mm multi-electrode loop catheter ablations were followed for 6 months, and all the dogs(100%) were in NSR at the terminal study. 7/10 (70%) dogs post 12-mm multi-electrode loop catheter ablation were in NSR, 1/7 (10%) - in overdrivable atrial tachycardia, 1/7 (10%) - in sustained atrial tachycardia and 1/7 (10%) in Afib. The 6 month combined chronic rhythm outcome is 80% in NSR, and 7% (one dog) in each of the other rhythm states (Table 1).

Table 1. Acute and chronic heart rhythm outcome using 4-6-mm ring and 12-mm coil multi-electrode loop catheters

	4 – 6-mm		12-mm		Combined	
	Acute	**Chronic**	**Acute**	**Chronic**	**Acute**	**Chronic**
NSR	7/14 (50%)	5/5 (100%)	4/15 (27%)	7/10 (70%)	11/29 (38%)	15/15 (80%)
OdrAfltr	3/14 (21%)		4/15 (27%)	1/10 (10%)	7/29 (24%)	1/15 (7%)
NSR/Afltr	3/14 (21%)		5/15 (33%)	1/10 (10%)	8/29 (28%)	1/15 (7%)
Afib	1/14 (7%)		2/15 (13%)	1/10 (10%)	3/29 (10%)	1/15 (7%)

NSR = normal sinus rhythm, OdrAfltr = overdrivable atrial flutter, Afltr = atrial flutter, Afib = atrial fibrillation.

3.   THE LINEAR LESION LOCATION AND CONVERSION

Of the 26 dogs that the Afib was converted: 12 had LA vertical and sub-PV lesions which connected the mitral valve ring to the dome of the atria in the anterior posterior position, 5 had only LA horizontal type lesion encircling the pulmonary veins above the mitral ring, 9 had RA lesions that resulted in conversions (1 - RA isthmus, and 8 - RA loop connecting the tricuspid valve anteriorly to the RA appendage, superior vena cava (SVC), and SVC to inferior vena cava (IVC).

4.   ATRIAL FIBRILLATION PREVENTION BY LINEAR LESIONS

More recently we investigated whether linear atrial lesions provide protection from Afib in two sets of dogs. One group (7 dogs, 35 ± 3 kg) previously had chronic Afib due to rapid atrial pacing, but was converted to normal sinus rhythm (NSR) after the creation of linear lesions. This group is referred to as "Afib" dogs. The other group (5 dogs, 30 ± 4 kg) included "Normal" dogs in NSR in which linear lesions have been created. Rapid-pacing pacemakers were implanted in 7 mongrel dogs. Rapid atrial pacing was maintained for 56 ± 9 days. Spontaneous sustained Afib was recorded after 21 ± 8 days. The dogs maintained spontaneous Afib for 178 ± 64 days as verified by weekly rhythm evaluations via surface electrocardiogram (ECG) and telemetry from the intracardiac leads. Creation of linear lesions was performed in both groups of dogs using a loop catheter capable of creating expanding loops in both atria. The catheter has fourteen 12-mm coil electrodes. Radiofrequency energy was delivered through each electrode. Power was titrated with automatic temperature control to attain an average target temperature of $70°$ C for 60 seconds. In the 7 Afib dogs NSR was attained after 5 ± 2 lesions were placed in LA and 2 ± 1 in RA. In 5 Normal dogs linear lesions were placed in the LA (3 ± 1) and RA (2 ± 1) using the loop catheter. Post linear lesions rhythm status was monitored weekly via surface ECG and telemetry from the intracardiac pacing leads. After 6 months of recovery, arrhythmia inducibility was tested with burst pacing (10 times at 50 msec cycle length for 5 sec). In the Afib group: after the termination of burst pacing 2 dogs remained in NSR, 4 dogs exhibited atrial tachycardia, and 1 dog had nonsustained Afib. In the Normal dogs: a run of nonsustained atrial tachycardia was induced in 1 dog (Table 2).

Table 2. Re-induction of Afib with rapid pacing (6 months after linear lesions)

		Post Burst	1 week	2 weeks	3 weeks	1 month
Afib dogs	NSR	2	0	1	0	0
(Paced 31±8 days)	Afltr	4	0	1	4	1
	Afib	1	7	5	3	6
NSR dogs	NSR	4	2	0	0	0
(Paced 34±5 days)	Afltr	1	2	3	3	2
	Afib	0	1	2	2	3

NSR = normal sinus rhythm, Afltr = atrial flutter, Afib = atrial fibrillation, Burst = burst pacing (10 times at 50 msec cycle length for 5 sec).

RA rapid pacing at 400 B/M was initiated in both groups for 33 ± 7 days. Rhythm was evaluated daily during rapid pacing and 2 weeks after the pacemaker was turned off. After the creation of linear lesions and 5 ± 1 weeks of repacing rapidly, Afib and atrial tachycardia were induced in all the dogs. As shown in Table 3, within 3 days of cessation of pacing, none of the Normal dogs were in Afib, and 2 of the Afib group remained in Afib.

Table 3. Rhythm outcomes after stopping rapid atrial pacing post linear lesions

		15 minutes after repacing termination	3 days after repacing termination	1 week after repacing termination	2 weeks after repacing termination
	NSR	2	4	4	4
Afib Dogs - 7	Afltr	2	1	1	2
	Afib	3	2	2	1
	NSR	0	2	4	5
NSR Dogs – 5	Afltr	2	3	1	0
	Afib	3	0	0	0

Within 2 weeks, all of the Normal dogs returned to NSR and 1 dog, from the Afib group, remained in Afib (examples of Afib conversions to NSR are shown in Figures 11,12, and 13). Based on the result from this preliminary study it was concluded that rapid pacing induced sustained Afib in all paced dogs within 1 month of rapid pacing without the linear lesions. The linear lesions were highly effective in ablating the Afib in this model. During the 6 month of post linear lesions recovery, no Afib was recorded in both groups. In the Afib group, burst pacing for 5 seconds (10 times), NSR returned immediately in 2/7, and in 4/7 Atrial tachycardia was induced, and only 1/7 had sustained Afib. In the Afib dogs, after 4 weeks of rapid re-pacing only 2/7 had sustained Afib following linear lesion placement. Linear lesions in the LA and RA prevented the re-initiation of sustained Afib in all of the NSR dogs. Only one NSR dog had non-sustained atrial tachycardia. Linear lesions did not prevent induction of Afib in both sets of dogs as a result of rapid pacing. Constant rapid repacing resulted in SHORT LIVED (1-2 weeks) Afib and atrial tachycardia in both groups. It is concluded that linear lesions protect the atria from the induction of sustained Afib.[14]

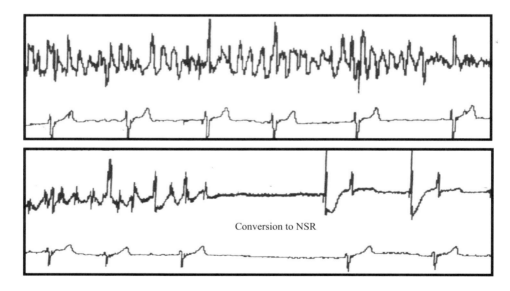

Figure 11. Examples of Afib conversion to NSR. A = Afib dog 24 weeks post Afib ablation and 4 weeks of rapid pacing, B = the same Afib dog converted to NSR immediately after cessation of rapid pacing.

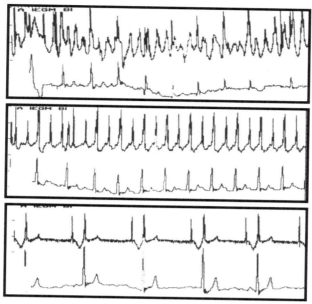

Figure 12. Sequential conversion to atrial flutter (Afltr) and NSR. A = NSR dog 6 months post linear lesions ablation and after 4 weeks of rapid pacing, which caused Afib, B = the same NSR dog 3 days after cessation of rapid pacing converted to Afltr, C = the same NSR dog 1 week after cessation of rapid pacing converted to NSR.

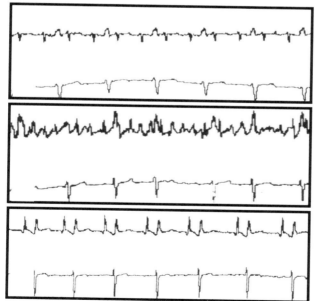

Figure 13. Conversion from Afltr to Afib and NSR. A = Afib dog 24 weeks post Afib ablation with linear lesions, Afltr was induced 2 weeks of rapid repacing, B = in the same Afib dog after 3 weeks of rapid repacing the Afltr had degenerated to Afib, C = after 3 days of cessation of rapid pacing in the same dog spontaneous conversion to NSR is seen.

5.   STUDIES OF LEFT ATRIAL MECHANICAL FUNCTION

Though the primary goal of RF ablation of Afib is to achieve NSR, the restoration of LA mechanical function is an important secondary goal. We have evaluated the LA mechanical function pre and post linear lesion creation using standard transthoracic echocardiography and pulsed Doppler techniques. Two groups of 6 dogs were studied: 1) Normal = healthy dogs in NSR and 2) Afib = dogs with chronic Afib for 6 months due to rapid atrial pacing for 57 ± 14 days. In both groups, long linear lesions were created in the LA and RA with an expanding loop catheter. Rhythm: NSR was restored with linear lesions in the 6 Afib dogs. In 10/12 dogs, overdriveable reentry type atrial tachycardia was inducible after ablation; however, all dogs maintained NSR 6 months post ablation. **LV and valvular function**: LV function was preserved in both sets of dogs. Moderate mitral regurgitation was present in 50% of the Afib dogs before ablation. At 6 months post ablation 2 of 5 Afib dogs had only mild MR. **LA systolic area**: LA systolic area was significantly larger before ablation in the Afib group compared to NSR group (12 ± 1.7 vs. 10 ± 1.3 cm^2, p<0.032). The atria decreased in size and reached a plateau within 2 months post ablation. The atrial size was similar in both groups and was significantly smaller than before ablation (Figure 14). **Doppler echocardiography**: No active LA contraction was recorded in the Afib group prior to conversion to NSR, but within 2 days post ablation there was recorded LA active contraction with the maximal velocity of the transmitral "A"wave of 0.21 ± 0.24 m/s. A-wave amplitude was reduced by 43% from 0.7 ± 0.2 m/s to 0.4 ± 0.08 m/s in the Normal dogs 2 days post ablation. Atrial mechanical function was recorded within 2 months post ablation and was not statistically significant between the 2 groups (Figures 15-17).[15-17] The equal recovery suggests that the chronic Afib in this rapid pacing dog model is not a pathological injury to the atria; but rather, an electrical remodeling. After 6 months of recovery, there was no evidence of thrombus or intracardiac trauma.

Based on these data it was concluded: Significant acute reduction in LA mechanical activity was noted in the first week post ablation in all dogs. This finding is supportive of post ablation need for anticoagulation to prevent strokes. With the lesion set described in this paper, LA mechanical activity recovery was completed 2 months post ablation, reaching 71%-80% of the pre-ablation state.[17] These results were noted despite the lesion endocardial surface area of 12-15 cm2 suggesting that the LA appendage, which was not ablated, may be the principal factor in the preservation of atrial contribution to transmitral flow.

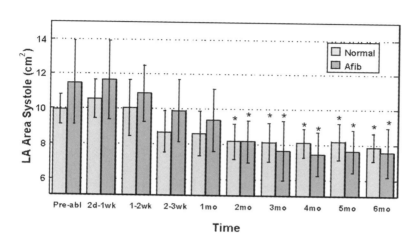

Figure 14. Changes of the LA systolic area from pre-ablation to up to 6 months post-ablation in Normal **and Afib dogs.** * p<0.05 vs. Afib Pre-abl and 2d-1wk.

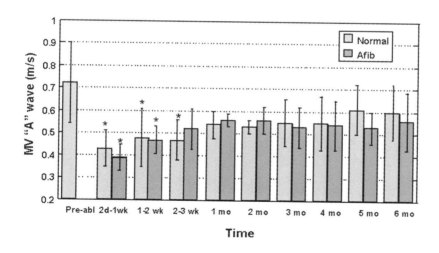

Figure 15. Changes of the maximal velocity of the transmitral "A" wave from pre-ablation to up to 6 months post-ablation in Normal and Afib dogs.   * p<0.05 vs. Normal Pre-abl.

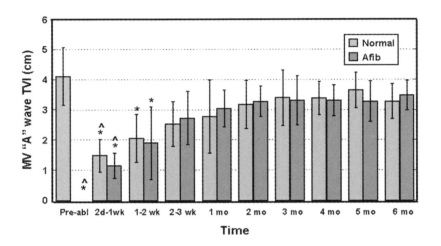

Figure 16. Changes of the integrated velocity of the late transmitral diastolic flow – time velocity integral (TVI) of "A" wave from pre-ablation to up to 6 months post-ablation in Normal and Afib dogs. * $p<0.05$ vs. Normal Pre-abl, ^ $p<0.05$ vs. Normal and Afib 2,3,4,5,6mo.

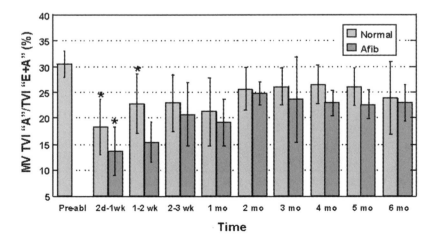

Figure 17. Changes of the late atrial contribution to the total diastolic filling from pre-ablation to up to 6 **months post-ablation in Normal and Afib dogs.** * $p<0.05$ vs. Normal Pre-abl.

6. GROSS AND HISTOLOGICAL FINDINGS

6.1 Histopathology

The evaluation of Afib ablation in this model was further extended into the histopathological charactristics of the lesions and chronic atrial function with the use of the 4-mm ring type ablation catheter. The linear lesions were composed of thin, dense, bead-like individual lesions protruding from both the endocardial and epicardial surfaces (as shown in Figure 18). These individual lesions fused into one contiguous rigid cord, which was sharply different from the surrounding tissue. The average size of each bead was 6 x 7 mm, with the maximal length of the lesion up to 16 cm (LA circular lesion around the pulmonary veins). The lesions transected the atria dividing them into distinct regions, some of which were completely isolated. Histologically, the lesions were characterized by extensive cartilage formation, proliferation of connective tissue, fibrosis and the presence of chronic inflammatory cells on the epicardial site. Among these changes some interrupted areas of relatively healthy myocardium were observed. From the endocardial side, lesions were totally covered with endothelium, and there was no sign of clot formation. The linear lesions that were created with the 12-mm coil electrodes are shown in Figures 19 and 20. The lesions are contiguous and unlike the lesions that were created with the 4mm ring electrode, the lesions are flat and were less calcified. The long-term organization of the RF lesion includes fibrosis, extensive formation of cartilage, and proliferation of connective tissue resulting in the formation of rigid transmural structures within the atria. Such structures have the potential to restrict atrial mechanical function. Complete endothelization of lesions reduces the danger of thrombogenesis.[9]

LA lesion dimensions in the Afib and Normal groups included length = 19 ± 4, 17 ± 4 cm; diameter = 8 ± 0.9, 7m ± 1 mm; and total lesion area = 15 ± 4, 12 ± 3 cm^2 (p = NS between groups). A higher percentage of transmural and contiguous lesions were created in the Afib dogs versus the Normal dogs (transmural = 91 ± 10% vs. 65 ± 22%; contiguous = 100 ± 11% vs. 91 ± 31%). Calcification was palpable in 30 ± 24% vs. 53 ± 37% of lesions in the Afib and Normal groups, respectively. On histological exam, the lesions consisted primarily of fibrous tissue, but calcium was noted in 30-50% of the linear lesions.[14]

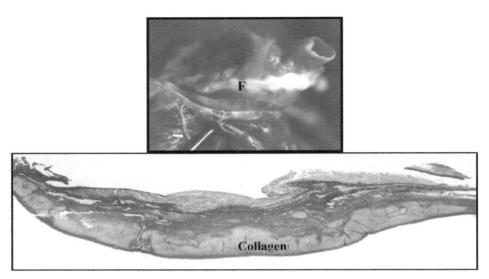

Figure 18 (see Color Plate 23). Histopathology of the Afib ablation linear lesions created with the 4-mm ring type ablation catheter. F = fibrous tissue.

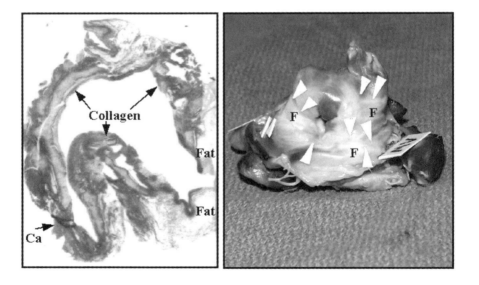

Figure 19 (see Color Plate 24). Histopathology of the Afib ablation linear lesions created with the 12-mm coil electrodes. Ca = calcium, F = fibrous tissue.

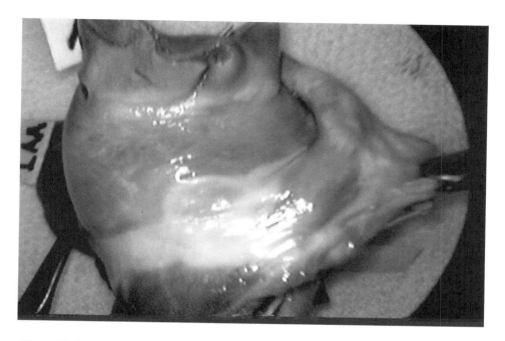

Figure 20. Gross pathology 6 months post-ablation of the LA circular lesions created with the 12-mm coil electrodes.

7. THE LOOP CATHETER DESIGN EVALUATION

7.1 Lesion Generation

The loop catheter design is an effective tool to create long contiguous and transmural linear lesions.

The design was modified to 12-mm coils that increased the efficiency of the system.

In the multiple studies in the acute and chronic dog model in NSR and chronic Afib we have proven that this catheter technology is capable of creating long (16-19 cm) linear lesions and ablating Afib with 83-90% efficacy rate.

7.2 Conformation of lesion adequacy

Reduction of greater than 50% in the amplitude of bipolar recordings of local electrical activity and temperature of 70 degrees C provides a measure of lesion contiguity and transmurality.

Incomplete lesions that are either nontransmural, noncontiguous, or both result in the formation of atrial tachycardia.

The most important lesions to ablate rapid pacing induced Afib were the set of LA lesions, where the total conversion to either NSR or atrial tachycardia occurred in 15/21 (73%); whereas, only 6/21 (27%) of RA lesions resulted in the conversion. Linear lesion sets placed in both atria following the ablation of Afib or atrial ablation in NSR was found to prevent rapid pacing induced Afib from sustaining in 92% of the dogs.

7.3   Tissue localization for the site of ablation

g. Identification of highly Fx local electrical activity provides a mappable target for regionalized ablation, the majority of which is under the PVs.

7.4   Histopathology

h. Analysis of the linear lesions 6 months later revealed that the lesions are completely endothelialized, and include fibrosis, extensive formation of cartilage, and proliferation of connecting tissue resulting in the formation of rigid transmural structures within the atria.

7.5   Mechanical function

i. LA mechanical function revealed significant acute 43% reduction in LA mechanical activity in the first week post ablation in all dogs.

j. LA mechanical activity recovery was completed 2 months post ablation, reaching 71%-80% of the pre-ablation state. These results were noted despite the lesion endocardial surface area being of 12-15 cm^2.

8.   FUTURE TECHNIQUES FOR THE ABLATION OF ATRIAL FIBRILLATION

The goal of catheter-based ablation of Afib should be safe minimal tissue destruction allowing the restoration of NSR under autonomic nervous system control combined with recovery of atrial mechanical transport to prevent the development of a thromboembolic event and provide hemodynamic benefits for the patient.

The amount of tissue ablated should be the minimum necessary to convert and maintain the atria in NSR while allowing for effective recovery of atrial transport. To justify exposing the patient to this procedure, the recovery of atrial mechanical function after the procedure is imperative. Theoretically, ablating the majority of the atrial tissues can terminate Afib, however, if mechanical function is not restored, the risk of thromboembolic stroke will remain requiring continuous anticoagulation. Furthermore, other than rate control, no mechanical benefit will be provided to the patient. If this is the outcome of a catheter-based Afib intervention, AV node modification or AV node or His ablation followed by permanent pacer insertion and continued anticoagulation may be a more appropriate therapy for those highly symptomatic patients whose medical therapy has failed. Such an approach presents with minimal acute risk and often is rewarding.[18]

In this chapter we have summarized the effort made to date in the development and testing of the loop catheter design, and the development of methodology for the effective ablation of Afib in experimental models. To date other than the ablation of focal source of Afib, which thus far appears feasible, the ablation of both persistent and chronic Afib has been associated with mixed results and numerous complications. It is thought that the initial source of chronic Afib is focal atrial depolarization and the ablation of such foci will prevent the induction of chronic Afib. Currently we have no data to support this hypothesis, however, it is now well established that in patients with paroxysmal Afib, the attempt to map and ablate the source of arrhythmia could be very rewarding for a follow-up period of 11 months. We believe that with an appropriate ablation catheter technology coupled with rapid electroanatomical mapping systems (i.e. 3D intracardiac echocardiography and electrical mapping, 3D guidance systems) it may be possible to reproduce the MAZE type atrial lesions. This goal does not exclude the use of other energy forms to create the desired lesions such as laser, CRYO, ultrasound and others. However, it remains to be seen if linear lesions in the human atria provide the long-term protection from re-initiation of Afib in the face of continued cellular degeneration and decoupling.

REFERENCES

1. Avitall B, Helms R, Koblish J, Sieban W, Kotov A, Gupta G. The creation of linear contiguous lesions in the atria with an expandable loop catheter. JACC 1999; 33(4):972-984.
2. Gupta G, Millard S, Urbonas A, Helms R, Avitall B. The creation of linear lesions to ablate atrial fibrillation: 12-mm coil electrodes vs. 4-mm ring electrodes. PACE 1998; 21(4 Pt2):804A.
3. Haines D. The biophysics of radiofrequency catheter ablation in the heart: the importance of temperature monitoring. PACE 1993;16:587-591.
4. Avitall B, Kotov A, Helms R. New monitoring criteria for transmural ablation of atrial tissues. Circulation 1996; 94(8):I-904A.
5. Avitall B, Helms R, Kotov A, Sieben W, Anderson J. The use of temperature versus local depolarization amplitude to monitor atrial lesion maturation during the creation of linear lesions in both atria. Circulation 1996; 94(8):I-904A.

6. Avitall B, Helms R, Chiang W, Perlman B. Nonlinear atrial radiofrequency lesions are arrhythmogenic: a study of skipped lesions in the normal atria. Circulation 1995; 92(8):I-265A.
7. Avitall B, Gupta G, Bharati S, Helms R, Kotov A. Atrial fibrillation in the chronic dog model: the long term success and failure. Circulation 1997; 96(8):I-382A.
8. Avitall B, Kotov A, Helms RW, Gupta GN, Bharati S. Transcatheter ablation of chronic atrial fibrillation in the canine rapid atrial pacing model: is the cure worse than the disease? JACC 1997; 29(2 Supplement A):32A.
9. Avitall B, Gupta G, Bharati S, Helms R, Kotov A. Are transmural contiguous lesions essential? Post atrial fibrillation ablation: lesion morphology vs. outcome. JACC 1998;31(4 Pt2):367A.
10. Avitall B, Kotov A, Bharati S, Helms R, Gupta G. Mapping of atrial fibrillation: directed localized ablation of fractionated local electrical activity confers conversion. Circulation 1997; 96(8):I-382A.
11. Avitall B, Hartz R, Bharati S, Krajacic A, Helms R, Perlman B. The correlation of local histology with fractionated local electrical activity during atrial fibrillation in patients undergoing the Maze procedure and mitral valve replacement. PACE 1996; 19(4 Pt2):725A.
12. Avitall B, Bharati S, Kotov A, Helms RW, Gupta GN. Histopathologic similarities between the human mitral disease chronic atrial fibrillation and the canine rapid pacing model of chronic atrial fibrillation. PACE 1997; 20(4 Pt2):1139A.
13. Gupta G, Helms R, Kotov A, Bharati S, Avitall B. Chaos analysis predicts stepwise changes in the character of atrial fibrillation prior to termination by the creation of linear lesions. Circulation 1997; 96(8):I-259A.
14. Avitall B, Urbonas A, Millard S, Helms R. Do linear lesion provide protection from induction of atrial fibrillation? PACE 1999; 22(4 Pt2):893A.
15. Avitall B, Helms R, Chiang W, Kotov A. The impact of transcatheter generated atrial linear radiofrequency lesions on atrial function and contractility. PACE 1996;19(4 Pt2):698A.
16. Avitall B, Urbonas A, Gupta G, Millard S, Helms R. Intra-atrial ultrasound pre and post linear lesions: alterations in atrial mechanical function. Circulation 1998; 98(17):I-643A.
17. Urbonas A, Urboniene D, Gupta G, Helms R, Millard S, Avitall B. Time course of atrial rhythm and mechanical recovery following the creation of linear lesions in the left and right atria in normal dogs vs. chronic atrial fibrillation model dogs. PACE 1998; 21(4 Pt2):963A.
18. Feld GK, Fleck RP, Fujimura OP et al. Electrophysiology/pacing: control of rapid ventricular response by radiofrequency catheter modification of the atrioventricular node in patients with medically refractory atrial fibrillation. Circulation 1994; 90:2299-2307.

Chapter 23

Epicardial Mapping and Ablation to Treat Sustained Ventricular Tachycardia

Mauricio Scanavacca, André d'Avila, Eduardo Sosa
Heart Institute, University of São Paulo Medical School, São Paulo, Brazil

INTRODUCTION

Recurrent sustained ventricular tachycardias (VT) present well-established functional characteristics.[1] However, the same can not be said about the anatomic substrates responsible for their mechanisms.[2,3] The lack of knowledge about the spatial organization and the anatomical location of critical portion of the VT circuit limits the success of the radiofrequency (RF) catheter ablation which essentially depends on a good contact of the catheter with the crucial portion of the VT circuit.[4,5]

In post myocardial infarction (post MI) VT, the reentrant circuits are frequently intramyocardial but may involve subendocardial and subepicardial layers of the ventricular wall.[2,3] Conventional RF endocardial pulses are efficient to interrupt and cure most mapable VT related to an endocardial circuit.[4-11] However, one of the reasons for standard endocardial pulses of RF to fail is the presence subepicardial circuits.[12-15]

Therefore, in order to improve the results of catheter ablation to treat VT, an epicardial mapping and ablation technique that could be performed in the EP laboratory would be highly desirable. In this chapter we will describe this novel approach recently introduced by our group.[16-18]

L. Bing Liem and E. Downar (eds.), Progress in Catheter Ablation, 377-387.
© 2001 *Kluwer Academic Publishers. Printed in the Netherlands.*

1.   EXPLORING THE EPICARDIAL SURFACE IN THE ELECTROPHYSIOLOGY LABORATORY

The search for an alternative mapping and ablation technique in patients with mapable and recurrent VT was motivated for our unsatisfactory results observed, mainly, in patients with VT and chronic chagasic cardiomiopathy, the most frequent cause of VT in Latin-American countries.[19-26]

One of the hypotheses raised to explain our success rate of approximately 20% in this subset of patients was the presence of subepicardial circuits, as observed in some post inferior wall MI myocardial in which endocardial applications are not efficient.[27-29]

2.   THE EXPLORATION OF THE PERICARDIAL SAC: DOG MODEL

As the exploration of the pericardial sac could provide useful information for the comprehension of the chagasic VT mechanisms, we looked for the establishment of an animal experiment to perform the first procedures.

The dogs were anesthetized with sodium thiopental, intubated and ventilated maintained in the supine position. After trichotomy of the thoracoabodominal region the skin was infiltrated with 2% lidocaine. The puncture was performed at the subxiphoid region and the needle (Tuohy #18) guided by fluoroscopy and injection of iodinated contrast. The contrast media infusion marked the cardiophrenic ligament guiding the direction of the needle. The introduction of the needle in the pericardial space was confirmed by the infusion of contrast media. A 0.35-mm guide wire was then introduced and advanced inside the pericardial space till the lateral edge of the cardiac area. Afterwards, a 7F-catheter introducer was placed in the pericardial space. The aspiration of a normal pericardial fluid confirmed the absence of puncture accident. Finally, a regular deflectable catheter (Marinr #7F) was introduced.

In the first 5 animals tested, the pericardial space was reached without any puncture accidents as it could be observed after the sacrifice of the animal. Lesions at the coronary vessels on the surface of the parietal epicardium were not observed. In one dog, three independent pericardial punctures were successfully performed and the intrapericardial catheters could be manipulated without limitations. Both ventricles and atria could be extensive and easily explored during these procedures.

3.　PUNCTURE OF THE PERICARDIAL SAC IN HUMAN BEINGS WITHOUT PERICARDIAL EFFUSION

The initial protocol of investigation involving human beings was performed in chagasic patients with recurrent VT, refractory to pharmacological treatment and unsuccessful previous endocardial ablation. The study protocol was approved by Scientific and Ethical Committee of the University of São Paulo, Brazil and an Informed consent was obtained from the patients.

The procedure was performed in the EP Lab with the patient in a fasting state. Sedation was achieved with midazolam, fentanil and propofol. Lyncomicine, 600 mg IM, was administered 30 min before the procedure. Continuous arterial pressure monitoring was obtained trough a radial artery puncture.

Initially, two quadripolar catheters were introduced by puncture of the right femoral and jugular veins. The first catheter was positioned in the apex of the right ventricle and the second one in the coronary sinus. Programmed ventricular stimulation with 600 and 400 ms cycle lengths with up to 3 extra-stimuli was performed. VT was considered hemodinamically stable if systolic blood pressure (SBP) was maintained equal to or above 80 mmHg. If the VT was stable, the transthoracic pericardial puncture was performed using a Tuohy-#17 needle.

The technique of subxyphoid transcutaneous pericardial puncture was described by Krikornian and Hancock.[31] The adequate localization of the needle in the pericardial space was demonstrated by the infusion of contrast media inside the pericardial space under fluoroscopic guidance in the left anterior oblique projection. This projection was chosen because once the needle reaches the pericardial sac, the displacement of the guide wire (0,35) around the lateral edge of the heart confirms its intrapericardial position. Mapping can be then undertaken with a regular #7 Fr ablation catheter. After confirmation of no pericardial bleeding a fourth deflectable catheter (EPT #8F) was introduced by femoral artery puncture to left ventricle mapping to allow simultaneous epicardial and endocardial mapping. In this time, 5000 UI bolus of heparin followed by 1000 UI per hour were administered.

During stable VT we first performed epicardial mapping because the manipulation of the epicardial catheter is easier than that of the endocardial catheter. Once the best epicardial place was found, the endocardial catheter was placed in front the epicardial catheter, looking for the earliest endocardial activation site. In the first three cases, the earliest activation site was found in the posterolateral region of the left ventricle. In one patient epicardial fractionated electrograms were obtained with precocity of 140 ms in relation to the beginning of QRS in leads I, II, III and V1. The exploration of the endocardium in this region registered an electrogram with a precocity of 70 ms in relation to the peripheral QRS complex but 70ms later than the epicardial electrogram. We concluded from this initial observation that puncture and exploration of the epicardial surface of the heart could be safely accomplished. Thus, an extensive epicardial mapping could be carried out in the electrophysiology laboratory without complications and it could be used to guide positioning of the endocardial catheter.

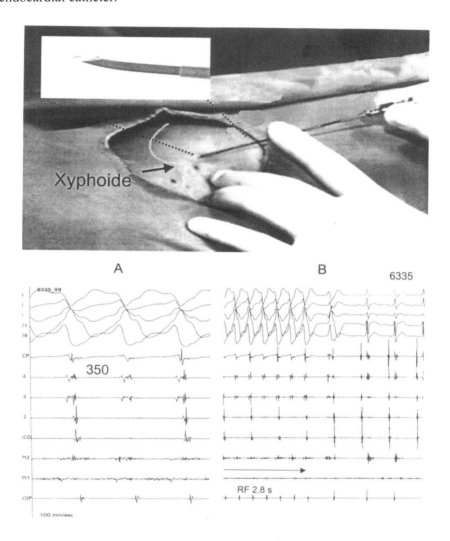

Figure 1 - A regular needle used for epidural anesthesia (shown in details in the left superior corner) is utilized during transthoracic puncture according to the technique described by Kirkorian to drain epicardial effusions. In the lower panels A and B, continuous electrical activity can be seen in the distal mapping electrode (epi 1). A pulse of RF interrupts VT within 2.8 seconds rendering it noninducible. Shown are electrocardiographic leads I to V6 and electrograms obtained from the coronary sinus (SCP, 4, 3, 2, SC distal) and from the right ventricular apex (VDP).

4. ENDOCARDIAL ABLATION GUIDED BY EPICARDIAL MAPPING

It was clear that endocardial RF ablation could be guided by epicardial mapping but the question of whether an endocardial application would destroy a subepicardial circuit remained unanswered. On the other hand, in case a standard endocardial application was unsuccessful, safety of an epicardial RF application was unclear.

In order to answer the first question four patients with chagasic cardiomiopathy and recurrent VT. In these cases VT was considered predominantly related to an epicardial circuit when mapping showed the earliest electrogram located in the epicardial surface and the local stimulation caused concealed entrainment with a return cycle similar to the tachycardia cycle length. The pacing maneuvers were performed as described by Stevenson *et al.*[4] The application of RF from the endocardium surface was anatomically guided towards the distal electrode of the epicardial catheter. In two patients VT were predominantly subepicardial as entrainment was obtained by the epicardium pacing but not by the endocardium. Several RF applications through the endocardium interrupted the VT, in general after 30 sec from the beginning of the application, but VT was always reinduced.

In one patient there was RV perforation during the puncture, the bleeding was self-limited and slight (< 50 ml) and did not prevent the continuation of the procedure. Echocardiograms performed within 24 hours of the procedure and on discharge from hospital did not show pericardial effusion.

We learned from this observation that some circuits are really subepicardial and that isolated conventional endocardial RF applications may not be able to destroy them. We also had our first complication (pericardial effusion), due to the puncture of the right ventricle, which was easily controlled and without hemodinamic consequences.

With these observations, it became clear that to ablate epicardial mural circuits successfully, we would have to perform applications in the epicardial surface of the heart.

5. EPICARDIAL MAPPING AND ABLATION

In order to established the usefulness of this procedure, 20 consecutive patients with chagasic cardiomiopathy and recurrent VT were then studied. The mean LV ejection fraction at the echocardiogram was greater than or equal to 55% in 8 patients and less than 55% in 12 patients. Fifty-six VTs (mean of 3 morphologies/patient) were induced by programmed right ventricular stimulation. In four patients the induced VT caused important hemodynamic disorders and could not be mapped.

Epicardial mapping and ablation were performed initially, to avoid endocardial manipulation and systemic anticoagulation. The endocardial mapping was performed when isolated epicardial mapping was unsuccessful. The criterion to determine the epicardial circuit was the presence of concealed entrainment with perfect return cycle, performed in the area with earliest presystolic and mid diastolic electrogram. When the epicardial capture was not possible using pulses of up to 15 mA and 3.5 ms, thermomapping was performed with RF application at 60^0 for 10s. When interruption of VT during this RF pulse was obtained, the circuit was classified as an epicardial circuit. When not, an endocardial mapping was then performed using the precocity of the epicardium electrogram as reference to move the catheter in its direction, searching for presystolic, middiastolic or continuos activity during VT.

The circuit was defined as endocardial by the demonstration of concealed entrainment with perfect return cycle during endocardial stimulation and the consequent interruption of VT during the application of RF pulse at a temperature of 70^0 C during at least 30s. According to these criteria, epicardial circuits were observed in eight patients, endocardial in two patients and epicardial and endocardial in three patients. The RF application was prolonged for 60 s and two or three additional pulses were applied near the pulse that interrupted the VT. Using this method there was interruption of VT without reinduction in 82% of the cases.

Four patients showed hemopericardium during puncture of the pericardial sac, in two after systemic anticoagulation to perform the simultaneous epicardial and endocardial mapping. There was no cardiac tamponade; neither did they motivate the interruption of mapping and ablation. In these cases, the blood was removed from the pericardial sac and infused to the systemic circulation through an IV line. Two patients showed electromechanical dissociation as a consequence of prolonged VT mapping. Both showed an LVEF less than 30. Four patients complained of chest pain in the two days subsequent to epicardial mapping and improved after the introduction of non-hormonal anti-inflammatory drugs. One patient with RF application close to the posterior ventricular branch of the circumflex artery showed chest pain associated to supra elevation of the ST segment. The peak of CK-MB reached 35 UI, but Q wave MI was not present. Coronariography showed occlusion of the distal portion of the circumflex artery. The echocardiogram at the discharge from hospital showed slight pericardial effusion without hemodynamic impairment in one patient. In the control after one month the echocardiogram did not show effusion or pericardial thickening.

During a follow-up period of 8-month, nine patients (69%) remained without recurrence. Amiodarone (200 to 400 mg/day) was given to all patients.

6.   EPICARDIAL MAPPING AND ABLATION IN ISCHEMIC CARDIOMYOPATHY

In reentrant post MI VT, 20 to 40% of the patients remained with inducible VT after endocardial ablation.[4-11]   One of the possible reasons for that is the presence of subepicardial circuits unreachable by standard endocardial RF. These circuits have already been demonstrated during intra-operative epicardial mapping in the patients with inferior infarct.[27-29]   Due to the similarity of the morphological aspects of VT in patients with chagasic cardiomiopathies and those with inferior infarction, we thought that epicardial mapping and ablation could contribute to obtain better results in post MI VT related an old inferior myocardial infarction as it did for chagasic VT.

From October 1996 to February 1999, 16 consecutive patients with inferior myocardial infarction and recurrent VT were submitted to an attempt of transthoracic epicardial ablation. In two patients, endocardial ablation had already been tried, without success. One of the patients had incessant VT and the other, with ICD, received several shocks due to acceleration of VT during the attempt of interruption with pacing. Ten patients were males, with an average age of 56±15 years and mean LV ejection fraction of 50±12% at the echocardiogram. The episodes of VT started between 8 and 108 months after myocardial infarction. Thirteen patents presented with occlusion of the right coronary artery and in three the obstructive lesions involved the left coronary artery. Ventriculography showed inferior akinesia or slight dyskinesia in 15 patients and a large inferior aneurysm in one patient. A total of 30 sustained VTs were induced during the EP study. Due to hemodynamic intolerance 12 VTs could not be mapped. In 14 patients it was possible to map at least one well-tolerated VT with an average cycle of 415±48 ms. Seven VTs were interrupted and not reinduced after epicardial RF applications (39%). The thermomapping was the better technique to select the place of application on the epicardium. The selected electrogram for application of thermomapping had the average precocity of 87±13 ms before the beginning of the QRS complex. The complete RF applications (60 degrees during 60s) had an average potency of 35±16 W, mean temperature of 56±10 degrees Celsius and impedance of 118±15 Ohms. The average time for the end of the procedure was 210±16 min and the time of fluoroscopy was 22±4 min (pulsed fluoroscopy at 7 charts/sec). The procedure was well tolerated in all patients and no increase in the CK-MB curve was observed. All the seven patients who had VT interrupted by epicardial applications remained without VT recurrence after an average of 14±2 months of follow-up, but just two were out of antiarrhythmic drugs.[32]

After this observation, we concluded that possible post MI epicardial adherence did not prevent epicardial mapping. We also confirmed the high prevalence of epicardial circuits in these selected patients and that they could be safely ablated by an epicardial RF application.

7.   EPICARDIAL MAPPING AND ABLATION IN CHILDREN.

Idiopathic sustained VT is the most frequently VT observed in health young people.[32-35]   RF catheter ablation is effective to ablate idiopathic VT in approximately 85% of these patients. In the remaining, subepicardial localization of the circuits could limit RF ablation. In young children, RF ablation rarely is indicated as first line treatment. In general it is indicated just in case of incessant VT, refractory to antiarrhthmic drugs.

Recently a 1-year-old child with drug refractory incessant VT was referred to our hospital with cardiac failure. Endocardial ablation had been tried unsuccessfully. EKG showed sustained VT with a right bundle branch block morphology and SÂQRS axis deviated upwards. After trying endocardial ablation through the transeptal approach, we observed that the best pacemapping was obtained in the posterobasal region of the left ventricle. At this place, there was no precocity in relation to the peripheral QRS complex and a RF pulse at 60^0 C for 30s was applied without success. Due to the deterioration clinical condition of the patient, we decided to perform a transthoracic epicardial mapping despite his young age.

The puncture of the pericardial sac was performed without difficulty through the subxiphoid approach. The contrast injection confirmed the position of the needle inside the pericardial space. A metallic probe of 0.35 mm was introduced, followed by 7F-catheter introducer. Mapping was performed with a Marinr # 7F catheter. The catheter was guided to the posterobasal region towards the catheter positioned in the endocardium and a successful epicardial RF ablation was performed (Figure 2). After 10 months of follow-up, the child persisted in sinus rhythm and ventricular function was reestablished.[33]

After this first observation, the epicardial ablation procedure was repeated with success in other two children. One of them presented incessant VT, the other paroxistic VT with frequent recurrence. In both endocardial RF attempt had failed and we concluded that epicardial VT ablation can also be safely performed in young patients as well.

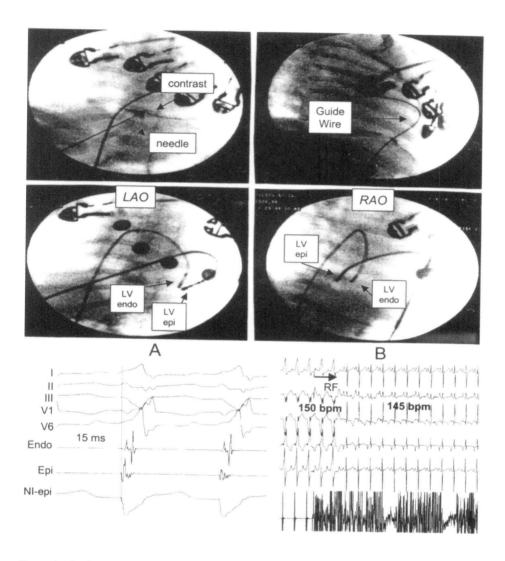

Figure 2 – In the upper panels, introduction of the mapping and ablation catheter in the pericardial space is shown. In the lower panels A and B, mapping and ablation of the VT in shown (see text for details).

CONCLUSIONS

Extensive epicardial mapping can be safely performed in the EP laboratory. The novel approach described in this chapter allows identification and RF ablation of epicardial VTs. The potential benefits derived from this approach seem to overcame the risks of damaging coronary arteries and it should be incorporated for those investigators dealing with VT on regular basis.

REFERENCES

1. Josephson ME. Recurrent ventricular tachycardia. In Josephson ME, Ed. Clinical Cardiac Electrophysiology. 2ND edition. Lea & Febiger, Philadelphia, 1993, pp.417-615.
2. de Bakker JMT, van Capelle FJL, Janse MJ, Wilde AA, Coronel R, Becker AE, Dingemans KP, van Hemel NM, Hauer RN. Reentry as a cause of ventricular tachycardia in patients with chronic ischemic heart disease: Electrophysiologic and anatomic correlation. Circulation 1988;589-606.
3. de Bakker JMT, van Capelle FJL, Janse MJ, van Hemel NM, Hauer RN, Defauw JJ, Vermeulen FE, Badder de Wekker PF. Macroreentry in the infarcted human heart: Mechanism of ventricular tachycardias with a focal activation pattern. J Am Coll Cardiol 1991;18:1005-1014.
4. Stevenson WG, Khan H, Sager P, Saxon LA, Middlekauff HR, Naterson PD, Wiener I. Identification of reentry circuit sites during catheter mapping and radiofrequency ablation of VT late after myocardial infarction. Circulation 1993;88:1647-1670.
5. Morady F, Harvey M, Kalbfleisch SJ, El-Atassi R, Calkins H, Langeberg JJ. Radiofrequency catheter ablation of ventricular tachycardia in patients with coronary artery disease. Circulation 1993;87:363-72.
6. Gonska BD; Cao K; Schaumann A; Dorszewski A; von zur Mühlen F; Kreuzer H. Catheter ablation of ventricular tachycardia in 136 patients with coronary artery disease: results and long-term follow-up. J Am Coll Cardiol 1994;24:1506-14.
7. Rothman SA; Hsia HH; Cossú SF; Chmielewski IL; Buxton AE; Miller JM. Radiofrequency catheter ablation of postinfarction ventricular tachycardia: long-term success and the significance of inducible nonclinical arrhythmias. Circulation 1997;96:3499-508.
8. Callans DJ; Zado E; Sarter BH; Schwartzman D; Gottlieb CD; Marchlinski FE. Efficacy of radiofrequency catheter ablation for ventricular tachycardia in healed myocardial infarction. Am J Cardiol 1998;15:429-32,
9. Trappe HJ, Klein H, Auricchio A, Wenzlaff P, Lichtlen PR. Catheter ablation of ventricular tachycardia: Role of the underlying etiology and the site of energy delivery. Pacing Clin Electrophysiol 1992;15:411-424.
10. Kottkamp H, Hindricks G, Chen X, Brunn J, Willens S, Haverkamp W, Block M, Breithardt G, Boorggrefe M. Radiofrequency catheter ablation of sustained ventricular tachycardia in idiopathic dilated cardiomyopathy. Circulation 1995;92:1159-1168.
11. Kim YH, Sosa-Suarez G, Trouton TG, O'Nunain SS, Oswaldo S, McGovern BA, Ruskin JN, Garan H. Treatment of ventricular tachycardia by transcatheter radiofrequency ablation in patients with ischemic heart disease. Circulation 1994;89:1094-1102.
12. Blanchard SM, Walcott GP, Wharton JM, Ideker RE. Why is catheter ablation less successful than surgery for treating ventricular tachycardia that results from coronary artery disease? Pacing Clin Electrophysiol 1994;17:2315-2324.
13. Wilber D, Kall J, Kopp D, et al: Catheter ablation of the mitral isthmus for ventricular tachycardia associated with inferior infarction. Circulation 1995;92:3481-3489.
14. Svenson RH, Littmann L, Gallagher JJ, Selle JG, Zimmern SH, Fedor JM, Colavita PG. Termination sequence of ventricular tachycardia with epicardial laser photocoagulation: A clinical comparison with patients undergoing successful endocardial photocoagulation alone. J Am Coll Cardiol 1990;15:163-170.
15. Arruda M, Otomo K, Pitha J, Schaer A, Tondo C, Antz M, Bussey J, Nakagawa H, Lazzara R, Jackman W. Epicardial left ventricular recordings and radiofrequency catheter ablation from the coronary veins: a potential adjunct approach for mapping and ablation of ventricular tachycardia. Pacing Clin Electrophysiol 1997;20:1075.

16. Sosa E, Scanavacca M, d'Avila A, Pilleggi F. A new technique to perform epicardial mapping in the electrophysiology laboratory. J Cardiovasc Electrophysiol 1996;7:531-536.
17. Sosa E, Scanavacca M, d'Avila A, Piccioni J, Sanchez O, Velarde JL, Silva M, Reolão B. Endocardial and epicardial ablation guided by nonsurgical transthoracic epicardial mapping to treat recurrent ventricular tachycardia. J Cardiovasc Electrophysiol 1998;9:229-239.
18. Sosa E, Scanavacca M, d'Avila A, Bellotti G, Pilleggi F. Radiofrequency catheter ablation of ventricular tachycardia guided by non-surgical epicardial mapping in chronic Chagasic heart disease. Pacing Clin Electrophysiol 1999;22:128-30.
19. Marin-Neto JA, Simões MV, Sarabanda AVL. Cardiopatia Chagasica. Arq Bras Cardiol 1999;72:264-280
20. Scanavacca M; Sosa E. Electrophysiologic study in chronic Chagas' heart disease. São Paulo Medical Journal 1995;113: 841-50.
21. Scanavacca M, Sosa E, Lee JH, et al. Tratamento empirico com Amiodarona da Taquicardia Ventricular Sustentada em Pacentes com Cardiopatia Chagásica Crônica. Arq Bras Cardiol 1990;
22. Sosa E, Scalabrini, Rati M, Bellotti G, Pileggi F. Successful catheter ablation of the origin of recurrent ventricular tachycardia in chronic chagasic heart disease. J Electrophysiol 1987;1:58-61.
23. Sternick EB; Sobrinho AL; Lisboa JC, et al. Transcoronary chemical ablation of ventricular tachycardia in a patient with chronic chagas cardiomyopathy. Arq Bras Cardiol 1992; 58:4, 307-10.
24. de Paola AA; Pinheiro Tavora MZ. Radiofrequency ablation of the sustained ventricular tachycardia in patients with structural heart disease. Arq Bras Cardiol 1996; 66:1:, 51-8.
25. Rosas F; Velasco V; Arboleda F, et al. Catheter ablation of ventricular tachycardia in Chagasic Cardiomyopathy. Clin Cardiol 1997; 20:2, 169-74.
26. Sosa E, Scanavacca M, Barbero Marciel M, Bellotti G, Jatene M, Pilleggi F, Jatene A. Surgical treatment of cardiac arrhthymias. In Cruz Filho FES, Maia IG,eds: Eletrofisiologia Clínica e Intervencionista das Arritmias Cardíacas. Editora Revinter Ltda, Rio de Janeiro, 1997. pp. 443-55.
27. Kaltenbrunner W, Cardinal R, Dubuc M, Shenasa M, Nadeau R, Tremblay G, Vermeulen M, Savard P, Pagé PL. Epicardial and endocardial mapping of ventricular tachycardia in patients with myocardial infarction. Is the origin of the tachycardia always subendocardially localized? Circulation 1991;84:1058-1071.
28. Littman L, Svenson RH, Gallagher JJ, Selle JG, Zimmern SH, Fedor JM, Colavita PG. Functional role of ventricular tachycardia. Observations derived from computerized epicardial activation mapping, entrainment, and epicardial laser photoablation. Circulation 1991;83:1577-1591.
29. Hadjis T, Stevenson WG, Friedman PL, Sager P, Saxon LA: Ventricular tachycardia after inferior wall myocardial infarction: Predominance of locations for critical slow conduction zones. J Am Coll Cardiol 1995;25:108A. Abstract 926-28.
30. de Paola AAV, Melo WDS, Távora MZ, Martinez EE. Coronary venous mapping in patients with sustained ventricular tachycardia. J Am Coll Cardiol 1997; 29:202A, Abstract 750-4.
31. Krikornian JG, Hancock EW. Pericardiocentesis. Am J Med 1978;65:808-816.
32. Sosa E, Scanavacca M, d'Avila A, Oliveira F, Ramirez AF. Nonsurgical transthoracic epicardial catheter ablation to treat recurrent ventricular tachycardia occurring late after myocardial infarction (submitted).
33. Sosa E, Scanavacca M, d'Avila A, Tondato F, Kunyoshi R, Elias J. Nonsurgical transthoracic mapping and ablation in a child with incessant ventricular tachycardia. J Cardiovasc Electrophysiol (in press).

Chapter 24

TRANSCATHETER CRYOABLATION

Paul Khairy, Marc Dubuc
Montreal Heart Institute, Montreal, Quebec, Canada

INTRODUCTION

Since its introduction in the mid-1980s as an experimental treatment for cardiac arrhythmias in animal models, radiofrequency (RF) catheter ablation has become the procedure of choice for a wide variety of clinical arrhythmias. While the extent of coagulation and tissue necrosis induced by RF current application depends on a variety of factors, lesions created by hyperthermia unavoidably involve a certain degree of tissue destruction that increases the risk of aneurysmal dilatation, myocardial perforation, and thromboembolic events. Over the past two decades, hypothermia has been employed in the surgical management of arrhythmias. Among the advantages of this alternative form of energy are its non-thrombogenicity and preservation of underlying tissue architecture. Recently, percutaneous cryoablation catheters have been devised and transcatheter cryoablation is emerging as a promising alternative to RF ablation.

In this chapter, we will review the mechanisms of tissue injury involved in cryoablation, its historical beginnings, and the insights gained from the cardiac cryosurgical experience with hand-held probes. A transvenous cryocatheter system will be detailed and animal experiments discussed. The advantages of catheter cryoablation over RF energy will be considered and the clinical experience thus far summarized.

1. MECHANISMS OF TISSUE INJURY

In the transcatheter cryoablation of cardiac arrhythmias, tissue-freezing temperatures are brought into contact with the endocardial surface by means of a

L. Bing Liem and E. Downar (eds.), Progress in Catheter Ablation, 389-407.
© 2001 *Kluwer Academic Publishers. Printed in the Netherlands.*

percutaneous steerable catheter. The objective of cryoablation is to render inactive all cells within a targeted area. While the actual mechanism of cell death is debated, cellular alterations are thought to involve three phases: freeze/thaw, hemorrhage and inflammation, and replacement fibrosis.[1]

In the freeze/thaw phase, rapid cooling of cells to subzero temperatures results in ice crystal formation. Crystals are initially produced in the extracellular matrix due to a larger number of nucleation sites[2] but subsequently form intracellularly as well. The density and size of ice crystals is a function of their proximity to the cryoenergy source, the tissue temperature, and freezing rate. While the crystals themselves do not seem to disrupt the integrity of the cellular membrane, they compress and deform adjacent nuclei and cytoplasmic components.[3,4] The earliest changes occur in mitochondria with predominantly central[5,6] irreversible damage.[7] Subsequent warming, referred to as the "thawing effect", is an integral part of the cryodestructive process.[2,8-10] During the warming cycle, small high-energy intracellular crystals enlarge and fuse, thereby conglomerating into larger crystals with potentially deleterious effects.

Hemorrhage[11] and inflammation[6] characterize the second phase of tissue destruction, and occur within 48 hours of thawing.[1] In order to re-establish the osmotic equilibrium disturbed by ice crystal formation, water gradually migrates from within myocardial cells, resulting in an increased intracellular solute concentration. The hyperosmotic state ensuing from this "solution effect" chemically damages cell membranes.[8] Subsequent restoration of the microcirculation to the previously frozen tissue results in oedema, with exudation of fluid across damaged microvascular endothelial cells and circumscribed ischemic necrosis. In the final phase of cryoinjury, replacement fibrosis occurs within weeks, forming a well-circumscribed dense lesion.[12]

2.   HISTORICAL BEGINNINGS

Since the early 1960s, following the development of an automated cryosurgical apparatus cooled by liquid nitrogen,[13] cryoenergy has been used to treat a variety of pathologies including cutaneous, gynecologic, prostatic, hepatic, ophthalmologic, neurosurgical, and oncologic disorders.[9,14-16] The production of controlled predictable myocardial lesions with cryoenergy was first described by Hass et al. in 1948 (Table 1).[17,18] Using carbon dioxide in the cooling process, the ability of hypothermia to produce a homogeneous, sharply-demarcated lesion free of intracardiac thrombosis was demonstrated. Cardiac transmural lesions were created without subsequent rupture or aneurysmal dilation. Absence of such complications and the maintenance of ultrastructural tissue integrity have been attributed to the remarkable resilience of collagen and fibroblasts to hypothermal injury.[19]

In 1964, Lister and Hoffman[20] reported the first study of cooling applied to specialized cardiac conductive tissue. A 4-mm "U"-shaped silver tube was sutured to the atrial septum near the His bundle. Passage of a cooling mixture composed of alcohol and carbon dioxide inhibited atrioventricular (AV) node function at -10^0C to -20^0C. Atrioventricular node function was altered by progressively decreasing the temperature, with PR interval prolongation progressing to a 5:1 block at -45^0C. Almost immediately after termination of the cooling process, AV conduction returned to its baseline state.

Table 1. **Historical Landmarks in Cardiac Cryoablation**

Year	Authors	Contribution
1948	Hass and Taylor[17]	Myocardial lesions produced by cryoenergy
1963	Cooper[13]	Development of cryosurgical apparatus
1964	Lister and Hoffman[20]	Cryoenergy applied to conductive tissue
1977	Harrison et al.[19]	Cardiac cryosurgery with hand-held probe
1991	Gillette et al.[21]	Transvenous cryocatheter in animals
1998	Dubuc et al.[22]	Steerable cryocatheter with recording and pacing electrodes
1999	Dubuc et al.[23]	Catheter cryoablation in man

3.   CARDIAC CRYOSURGERY

3.1   Atrioventricular Nodal Ablation

Cryosurgery with a hand-held bipolar electrode probe was first introduced for the management of cardiac arrhythmias in 1977 by Harrison et al.[19] Atrioventricular nodal ablation was carried out in 20 dogs and subsequently three patients with drug-resistant supraventricular tachycardias. During cardiac surgery with cardiopulmonary bypass, cryomapping with a nitrous oxide probe produced complete but reversible heart block in all patients by lowering the temperature in the His bundle area to 0^0C for 30 seconds. Permanent third degree AV block was then induced by cooling to -60^0C for 90 to 120 seconds, with a minimum of two consecutive freeze/thaw cycles. In 1980, the same group reported long-term follow-up of these three patients together with an additional 19 similar cases that had a variety of intractable supraventricular tachycardias.[24] Overall, successful AV block was achieved in 17 of 22 patients.

Several subsequent studies confirmed the clinical utility of applying cryoenergy in AV node ablation.[25-27] Surgical approaches not requiring an extracorporeal circulation were later proposed.[26,28,29] Bredikis[26] described a surgical technique using two atriotomy incisions allowing for the passage of the cryoprobe and a finger for digital palpation and identification of the surrounding anatomic landmarks. The appropriate position was subsequently confirmed by recording electrodes, cryomapping, or pressure-induced AV block. Complete AV block was successfully performed in 85% of 34 patients. The same group of investigators[28] later reported a success rate of 92% in a series of 72 patients. An alternate approach was proposed by Louagie et al.[29] with cryomapping and subsequent cryoablation performed using an epicardial approach via the right coronary fossa.

3.2   Accessory Pathways

Since its initial description in AV node-His bundle ablation, cryosurgical technology has been applied to the treatment of most types of arrhythmias with variable success. Gallagher and coworkers[30] reported the first two cases of cryosurgical ablation of accessory pathways in 1977. One patient had a left lateral accessory pathway successfully ablated by freezing at -60°C for 90 seconds. The second had a concealed septal accessory pathway with retrograde conduction. Cooling to 0°C was initiated at the earliest site of endocardial activation until reversible loss of VA conduction occurred. Following confirmation of the successful site, the pathway was then permanently ablated.

Several case series were subsequently reported.[31-36] The largest series[34] employed an epicardial approach in 105 consecutive patients with the Wolff-Parkinson-White syndrome: 74 with left lateral, 23 with posteroseptal, and 11 with right ventricular free wall accessory pathways. The technique involved dissection and mobilization of the AV fat pad with exposure and cryoablation of the AV junction at the site of AV pathways. All accessory pathways but one were successfully ablated with no incidence of AV block. Four patients required a second operation within the first few weeks for recurrence of AV pathway conduction, with one subject necessitating a third procedure. Recurrences occurred in patients thought to have subendocardial pathways protected by the warming effects of the circulating blood stream. In another series of 21 patients reported by Bredikis and Bredikis,[32] limitations in accessing left lateral and left posterior pathways were overcome by using a cryoprobe specifically designed to enter the coronary sinus, thus obviating the need for extracorporeal circulatory support. While 19 of the 21 patients were successfully treated by this approach, the coronary sinus was ruptured in two cases and required surgical ligation.

3.3   Ventricular Tachycardia

The first experience with surgical cryoablation of ventricular arrhythmias was reported by Gallagher et al. in 1978.[37] In a patient with scleroderma, a drug-resistant tachyarrhythmia originating from the anterior right ventricular free wall was ablated with three 90-second cryoapplications at -60°C. A second case of successfully ablated ventricular tachycardia was reported the following year in a patient with annular subaortic stenosis.[38]   Cryosurgery has since then been recognized as the treatment of choice in selected patients with incessant or life-threatening ventricular arrhythmias requiring definitive surgery.[14,25,39-42]   It has also been employed as an adjunct to other surgical modalities such as aneurysmectomy, subendocardial resection, encircling endocardial ventriculotomy, coronary artery bypass grafting, and valvular replacement[1] (see Chapter 32).

While no comparative prospective studies have examined the efficacy and safety of the various treatment modalities, impressive cure rates have been reported in case series of ventricular tachycardia surgically cryoablated.   In patients uniquely treated with cryosurgery, Caceres et al.[43] reported surgical and clinical cure rates of 79% and 93%, respectively, for refractory ventricular tachycardia following inferior myocardial infarction.   In a similar patient population, a surgical cure rate of 93% was noted in 14 patients who underwent cryoablation as an adjunctive treatment for ventricular tachycardia.[44]   These results compare favorably to other surgical modalities employed in the treatment of refractory ventricular tachycardia.[44-46]

3.4   Other Arrhythmia Substrates

Surgical cryoablation has also been employed in the management of various diverse rarer pathologies such as nodoventricular tachycardia,[47] sinoatrial reentrant tachycardia,[48] ventricular disabling bigeminy,[49] bidirectional bundle branch reentry tachycardia,[50] and fetal malignant tachyarrhythmias.[51]   It has also been employed in AV nodal modification procedures aimed at interrupting AV nodal reentrant tachycardias or arrhythmias with rapid nodal conduction, while preserving normal node function.[52-54]   Using hand-held cryoprobes, Holman et al.[55] successfully eliminated the dual AV nodal physiology previously demonstrated in three dogs.   Cox et al.[56] later applied this procedure in eight patients with recalcitrant AV nodal reentry tachycardia. Postoperatively, a single AV node conduction curve was noted in each patient and none required permanent pacing, although a right bundle-branch block was recorded in three cases. No AV node reentrant tachycardia was inducible and all patients remained symptom-free during a follow-up of up to five years.

3.5   Cryolesion Size

Animal studies with surgical ablation have shown that the size of the cryolesion depends on such factors as temperature of the cryoprobe and myocardium, diameter of the probe in contact with cardiac tissue, exposure time, and number of freeze/thaw cycles.[11,57-59] Longer application times and lower temperatures generally produce larger lesions, although lesion growth is halted after approximately five minutes.[4,8] Repeating the freeze/thaw cycle generates lesion dimensions larger than those obtained by a single cryoapplication of longer duration.[60,61] Thus, by varying such parameters, early cryosurgical experience demonstrated the ability of cryoenergy to produce predictable discrete electrophysiologically inert lesions that are sharply delineated from normal cardiac tissue.[10,59] Although cardiac cryoprobes are relatively sparingly used today, surgical cryoablation experience demonstrated important cryoenergy properties such as the ability to reversibly suppress conduction tissue and to produce electrophysiologically inert lesions while maintaining intact structural integrity.

4.   TRANSVENOUS CARDIAC CRYOABLATION

4.1   Animal Experiments

4.1.1   Original Transvenous Cryocatheters

The first animal study employing a transvenous cryocatheter was reported by Gillette et al. in 1991.[21] Complete AV block was produced in five miniature swine with an 11-French cryocatheter cooled by pressurized nitrous oxide. Cryothermia was applied for three minutes and repeated up to three times until a successful lesion was produced. Four of the five pigs maintained complete AV block for one hour while the fifth exhibited 2:1 AV block. Histologically, sharply demarcated hemorrhagic lesions were present acutely. The same group of investigators reported the histology of chronic six-week lesions in eight pigs two years later.[62] Successive three-minute cryoapplications were applied to the AV junction at -60°C by means of an 8 or 11-French cryocatheter. Long term AV block was maintained in five of the eight animals. At six weeks, discrete dense lesions with no signs of inflammation or thrombus formation were noted.

While these initial studies demonstrated the feasibility of cryolesion formation by means of transvenous catheters, limited success was likely attributable to catheter size, lack of steerability, and the absence of recording electrodes on the cryocatheter. Accurate placement of the cryolesion required using a separate second catheter with recording capabilities.

4.1.2   Steerable Cryocatheter with Recording and Pacing Electrodes

In 1998, we reported the first animal experiment using a steerable cryocatheter with recording and pacing electrodes (Figure 1).[22] A 9-French catheter with a 4-mm electrode tip using Halocarbon 502 (Freon®) as a refrigerant fluid was used to create right and left ventricular lesions in six dogs.

Cryoapplications with temperatures warmer than -30°C did not result in pathologically identifiable lesions. Histological analysis of acute cryolesions revealed sharply demarcated hemorrhagic lesions with contraction band necrosis and no evidence of thrombus formation. In another two dogs, reversible ice mapping of the AV node was attempted and successfully performed. The cryocatheter was positioned at the AV nodal junction where successive cryoapplications with progressively lower temperatures were effectuated. When high degree AV block or greater than 50% prolongation of the PR interval was achieved, the cryoapplication was stopped. In both cases, seconds after terminating the cooling process, 1:1 AV conduction resumed. Gross and microscopic pathological examinations revealed no evidence of lesion formation. In a subsequent experiment,[63] catheter cryomapping was more extensively studied and achieved in seven of eight dogs at a mean temperature of -40°C. Electrophysiological parameters of the AV node measured before, 20 minutes, 60 minutes, and up to 56 days after cryoapplication were not significantly different. Such parameters included sinus cycle length, AH interval, HV interval, Wenkebach cycle length, and effective refractory period of the AV node.

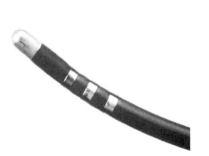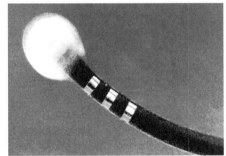

Figure 1. Transvenous cryocatheter electrode tip and ice ball formation. In panels A and B, the distal cooling electrode tip and three proximal ring electrodes are shown before (A) and after (B) ice ball formation in a water bath.

Chronic catheter cryoablation lesions were later characterized in a study of nine mongrel dogs sacrificed three and six weeks after the induction of lesions in right and left ventricles.[12] Well-demarcated stable lesions were observed following cryoapplications at a mean temperature of -55°C (Figure 2). No evidence of thromboembolic events was noted. Similar results were also obtained using 8.5-French cryocatheters in 6 dogs[64] and 7 pigs.[65]

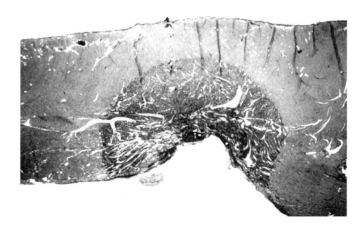

Figure 2 Low-power photomicrograph of a chronic lesion induced in a dog by catheter cryoablation on the right ventricular septum at a temperature of -55oC. Note the sharp smooth border clearly delineating cryoinjured tissue from normal surrounding myocardium. (Movat's staining).

4.1.3   Defining Optimal Freezing Parameters

In an attempt to better define optimal parameters for catheter cryoablation of the AV node, freezing was maintained at the lowest attainable temperature for five minutes (single freeze/thaw cycle) in six dogs (Group I) in the AV node area.[63] Subsequently, in the following six animals (Group II), the site of interest was frozen for five minutes and repeated a second time after a period of complete recovery to body temperature (double freeze/thaw cycle). Freeze/thaw cycles were performed at the sites previously identified by cryomapping, where temperatures warmer than –40°C had produced reversible high degree AV block. Chronic AV block was achieved in all six animals with double freeze/thaw cycles but in only one of the six dogs with single freeze/thaw cycles. Thus, double cycles were shown to be effective and superior to single cycles for AV nodal ablation. This finding was consistent with previous studies of liver, prostate, and skin demonstrating the production of larger lesions with more extensive tissue injury with double versus single freeze/thaw cycles.[9,15]

An additional property of cryotherapy was reported in the same study:[63] the ability to visualize formation of the "ice ball" by ultrasonic means. Using a 12.5-MHz rotating transducer mounted on a 6.2-French catheter, intracardiac ultrasound was performed in the six dogs that received double freeze/thaw cycles. Endocardial contact was confirmed by echocardiography and serial measurements were made to assess growth of the ice ball during cryoapplications. Intracardiac echocardiography clearly identified ice ball formation as a hypoechogenic density with a bordering hyperechoic rim and posterior accoustic shadowing (Figure 3). No evidence of microcavitation (gas formation) was observed during cryoapplication. The size of the ice ball was shown to continuously enlarge during the first three minutes of the freezing cycle and remain stable thereafter. Whether three minutes of cryoapplication is sufficient to obtain maximal results or an additional benefit is gained by further extending the procedure to a total of five minutes remains to be elucidated.

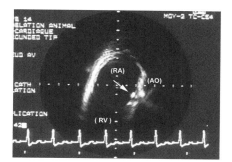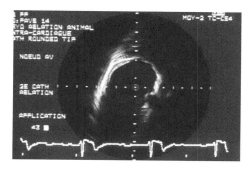

Figure 3. Intracardiac echocardiographic monitoring of ice ball formation during catheter cryoablation of the AV node in a canine heart. In panel A, the catheter situated in the right atrium is indicated by the arrow. At the bottom, ECG shows normal sinus rhythm. In panel B, following application of cryoenergy, the presence of an ice ball seen as a hypoechoic zone bordered by a hyperechoic rim with posterior shadowing. At the bottom, ECG shows complete AV block with ventricular escape rhythm. RA= right atrium, RV= right ventricle, AO= aorta.

4.2 The Transvenous Catheter Cryoablation System

As previously discussed, the basic cryoablation technique requires rapid freezing to temperatures considered lethal for cells, followed by a passive thawing process and repetition of the freeze/thaw cycle.[9,14,22,25,63] Cooling of the distal catheter tip in contact with endocardial tissue is effectuated as rapidly as possible. As cooling continues, freezing extends further into the tissue thereby establishing a temperature gradient. The lowest temperature and fastest freezing rate is generated at the point of contact with the cryocatheter tip, and slower tissue cooling rates are obtained more peripherally. While an effect on conduction tissue is observed with temperatures in the order of -20°C to -30°C, cryosurgical experience and animal studies with cryocatheters have shown that temperatures in the range of -40°C to -50°C are required to ensure cell death.[11,22,58,59,63] Tissue destruction is more definitely assured if the damaging freeze/thaw cycle is subsequently repeated.

In the first cryosurgical apparatus developed by Cooper in 1963,[13] probe cooling was produced by a change in the phase of nitrogen from a liquid to a gaseous state. Other principles such as the Joule-Thomson effect (whereby cooling is effectuated by expansion of a compressed gas after passage through a needle valve) or the Peltier effect (using thermoelectric cooling) have been incorporated in the design of cryoprobes.[9,14] As a wide range of devices have been developed, several methods of refrigeration and various cryogens including nitrogen, nitrous oxide, solid carbon dioxide, argon, and several fluorinated hydrocarbons have been used.[9]

We have previously described a transvenous cryocatheter system using Halocarbon 502 (Freon®) as a refrigerant fluid (Cryocath Technologies Inc., Montreal, Canada)[22] (Figure 4). More recently, another commercially available refrigerant fluid (Genetron® AZ-20) has been used. The cryocatheter consists of a hollow shaft with a closed distal end containing a cooling electrode tip and three proximal ring electrodes capable of recording and pacing. A central console containing refrigerant fluid releases the cryogen under pressure. The cooling fluid travels through the inner delivery lumen to the distal electrode that is maintained under vacuum. At the cryocatheter tip, the liquid cooling fluid is boiled. This accelerated liquid-to-gas-phase change results in rapid cooling of the distal catheter tip to temperatures as low as -60°C. Temperature is recorded at the distal tip by an integrated thermocouple device. The gas is then conducted away from the catheter tip via a vacuum return lumen and back to the console where it is collected and restored to its liquid state.

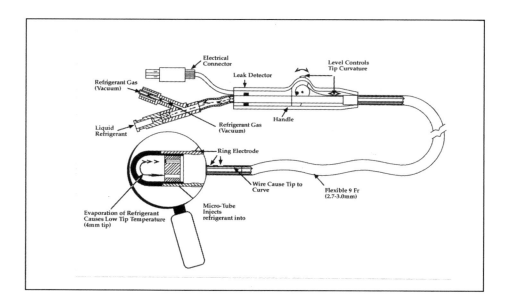

Figure 4. Catheter cryoablation system. From Dubuc et al.,22 J.Interv.Card.Electrophysiol. 1998;2:285-292. Please see text for a detailed description of the various components.

4.3   Catheter Cryoablation versus RF Ablation

4.3.1   Adhesiveness to Underlying Tissue

Transcatheter cryoablation has many potential advantages when compared to radiofrequency energy (see Table 2). In cryoablation, the hypothermia generated at the distal cooling electrode affords greater catheter stability, analogous to the adhesive effects encountered when a wet tongue makes contact with a frozen pole. This property may prove to be a significant advantage over RF energy, as ablation is performed in a continuously moving target with beat-to-beat variations. It may be particularly advantageous if the arrhythmogenic substrate is anatomically located at a site where contact is difficult to maintain.[22,23]

4.3.2   Characteristics of the Cryolesion and Non-Thrombogenicity

The actual lesion dimensions created by cryoablation appear to be similar to those produced by RF energy.[22,64] However, cryolesions are more homogeneous with clearer and smoother demarcations from underlying normal myocardium. In contrast, RF lesions are characterized by rougher more ragged edges. In addition to permitting greater control over the extent of the cryolesion, sharp borders are thought to be less arrhythmogenic.[12,63,64] Border zones with damaged yet viable cells may be at higher risk of undesired depolarisations. Given the greater control over the size and shape of the lesion by adjusting parameters in the freezing process, catheter cryoablation may prove useful in the management of arrhythmic substrates for which radiofrequency is of limited efficacy, such as ventricular arrhythmias, atrial fibrillation, and atrial flutter. For example, larger lesions may be produced by increasing the surface area of the catheter tip in contact with the endocardium or by decreasing the temperature at the catheter tip.[59]

Other significant benefits of cryoablation over RF energy include the absence of histologically identifiable thrombus formation, a finding confirmed by several studies.[12,21-23,62-64] The risk of subsequent embolic events is, therefore, effectively eliminated. Moreover, the dense cryolesion scar has no tendency to rupture or form aneurysms and ultrastructural tissue integrity is maintained.[19,24]

4.3.3   Cryomapping

Another major advantage of cryoablation compared to RF energy is the ability to reversibly suppress conduction tissue by varying the temperature at the catheter tip. While a functional effect is obtained at sub-lethal temperatures, complete recuperation to baseline electrophysiological properties is observed almost instantaneously upon termination of the cryoapplication, with no histologically identifiable damage produced.[22,63] Thus, by identifying the desired substrate prior to definitive ablation, the appropriate catheter placement site may be confirmed and creation of inappropriate lesions avoided. Reversible ice mapping may be particularly advantageous when considering ablating arrhythmogenic substrates located near critical sites such as the AV node, where a missed target lesion can have irreversible consequences.

Table 2. Advantages of Cryoablation Over Radiofrequency Ablation

Advantages	Clinical Implications
Adhesiveness to endocardial tissue	Greater catheter stability
Homogeneous sharply demarcated lesions	Non-arrhythmogenic
	More controllable lesion depth and volume
Non-thrombogenic	Decreased risk of subsequent embolization
Reversible suppression of conduction tissue	Predict successful site
	Avoid unwanted lesions
	Ablation of high-risk substrates
	Possible use in AV nodal modification
Visualization by ultrasound	Real-time monitoring
	Confirm endocardial contact
	Define optimal freezing parameters

4.3.4   Visualisation by Ultrasound

A further distinct advantage of cryoablation over RF ablation is the ability to visualize ice ball formation by ultrasonography (Figure 3). Providing a continuous real-time image of the freezing process was a major technological advancement in cryosurgical technique, renewing interest in visceral cryosurgery in the 1990s.[9] Monitoring of the freeze/thaw cycle and frozen tissue volume by ultrasound contributed to rapid improvements in hepatic and prostatic surgery. Intracardiac imaging by intravascular ultrasonography has already been employed in monitoring the catheter cryoablation procedure, and has confirmed appropriate contact between the catheter tip and endocardium.[23,63] It is proving to be a useful tool in better defining optimal freeze/thaw cycle lengths. Moreover, by offering an alternative means of visualising catheter placement, it may potentially reduce fluoroscopy exposure time.

4.4 Clinical Experience and Future Prospectives

Given the relative inexperience with transvenous catheter cryoablation when compared to RF energy, its use is limited by obstacles that new technologies face. The lower procedural efficacy initially observed is being overcome by modifying the original devices and designing new systems with different configurations and catheter tips and more efficient energy transport systems capable of creating lower tissue temperatures in larger areas. With the aid of ultrasonic guidance, animal experiments, and clinical studies, optimal procedural settings regarding duration of the freeze/thaw cycle, size of the catheter tip, and required cryomapping and ablation temperatures are in the process of refinement.

In August 1998 at the Montreal Heart Institute, the first patient underwent catheter cryoablation with successful AV node ablation for refractory atrial fibrillation. Complete AV block was successfully performed in ten patients acutely using double freeze/thaw cycles at an average temperature of -58.1±5.4°C.[23] Eight of the ten patients remained in complete AV block after an average follow-up of 128.5±56.8 days. Cryomapping was successfully performed in all patients with underlying sinus rhythm at the time of the procedure. Moreover, intracardiac ultrasound visualization of the cryolesion growth was also realized. No complications were noted. Thus, cryoablation of the AV node was shown to be both feasible and safe in man.

In summary, cryoablation affords many advantages over RF energy, including greater catheter adherence, absence of thrombus formation, the ability to produce reversible effects on conduction tissue, visualization by echocardiography, and clearly delineated more controlled lesion formation. Catheter cryoablation has been studied extensively in animal models and has been used safely and effectively in man. Its potential as an alternate form of therapy to RF energy is promising, although its specific role in the management of the various arrhythmias remains to be defined. Clinical studies using cryoablation in the treatment of supraventricular tachycardias (Figure 5) are ongoing in Canada and the United States. The investigational use of cryoablation in the treatment of atrial flutter, atrial fibrillation and ventricular tachycardia will be explored in the near future. In addition, other potential non-arrhythmic uses of transvenous catheter cryoenergy in cardiology are currently under investigation in such areas as the prevention of restenosis post-coronary angioplasty and direct myocardial revascularization.

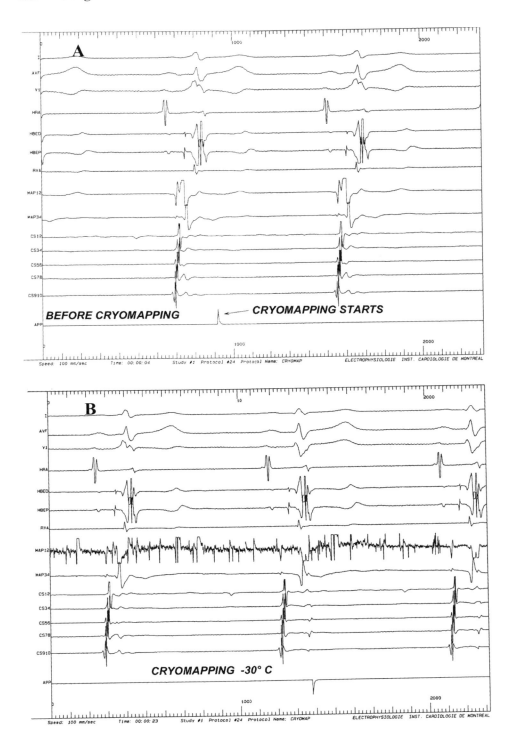

Figure 5 A+B

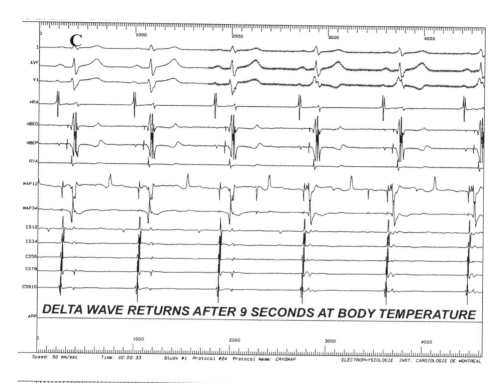

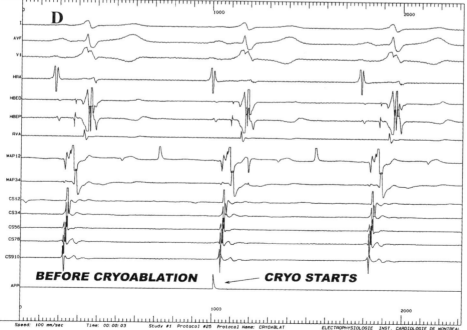

Figure 5 C+D

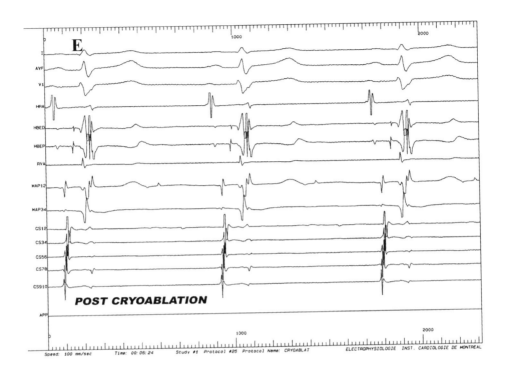

Figure 5. Cryomapping and cryoablation of an AV accessory pathway. The intracardiac and surface ECG of a patient with a left lateral accessory AV pathway with anterograde preexcitation (Wolff-Parkinson-White) in whom we successfully cryomapped and cryoablated the pathway. (A) Before cryomapping, left lateral AV preexcitation is present with a delta wave on the surface ECG on the intracardiac electrogram recorded by the distal pair of electrodes. On the cryoablation catheter (Map 12) positioned at the left lateral AV ring, atrial and ventricular components are fused. (B) After a few seconds at -300C, anterograde block in the accessory pathway is obtained as demonstrated by loss of preexcitation on the second beat. Typically, during cryoapplication, electrical noise appears on the intracardiac recording due to ice ball formation on the catheter tip. (C) Preexcitation resumed 9 seconds after cooling fluid injection was turned off showing reversibility and successful cryomapping when the catheter tip returns to body temperature. (D) Since cryomapping was successful, this site was chosen for cryoablating the pathway (see bipolar recording of the cryoablation catheter, Map 12). (E) Loss of preexcitation and normalized QRS post-successful cryoablation at -600C. Surface ECG leads: I= lead I, AVF = lead AVF, VI= lead VI. Intracardiac electrograms: HRA= high right atrium, HBED= His bundle distal, HBEP= His bundle proximal, RVA=right ventricular apex. Bipolar recordings on the cryoablation catheter between distal tip and first ring electrode (Map 1-2) and between ring 3 and 4 (Map 3-4), bipolar recordings of the coronary sinus distal (CS 1-2) to proximal (CS 9-10), APP= Signal showing when application starts

REFERENCES

1. Lustgarten DL, Keane D, Ruskin J. Cryothermal ablation: mechanism of tissue injury and current experience in the treatment of tachyarrhythmias. Prog.Cardiovasc.Dis. 1999;41:481-498.
2. Budman H, Shitzer A, Dayan J. Analysis of the inverse problem of freezing and thawing of a binary solution during cryosurgical processes. J.Biomed.Eng. 1995;117:193-202.
3. Whittaker DK. Mechanisms of tissue destruction following cryosurgery. Ann.R.Coll.Surg.Engl. 1984;66:313-318.
4. Gill W, Fraser J, Carter DC. Repeated freeze-thaw cycles in cryosurgery. Nature 1968;219:410-413.
5. Iida S, Misaki T, Iwa T. The histological effects of cryocoagulation on the myocardium and coronary arteries. Jpn.J.Surg. 1989;19:319-325.
6. Mikat EM, Hackel DB, Harrison L, Gallagher JJ, Wallace AG. Reaction of myocardium and coronary arteries to cryosurgery. Lab.Invest. 1977;37:632-641.
7. Tsvetkov T, Tsonev L, Meranzov N, Minkov I. Functional changes in mitochondrial properties as a result of their membrane cryodestruction. II. Influence of freezing and thawing on ATP complex activity of intact liver mitochondria. Cryobiology 1985;22:111-118.
8. Mazur P. Cryobiology: the freezing of biological systems. Science 1970;16:939-949.
9. Baust J, Gage AA, Ma H, Zhang C-M. Minimally invasive cryosurgery- technological advances. Cryobiology 1997;34:373-384.
10. Markovitz LJ, Frame LH, Josephson ME, Hargrove WC. Cardiac cryolesions: factors affecting their size and a means of monitoring their formation. Ann.Thorac.Surg. 1988;46:531-535.
11. Holman WL, Ikeshita M, Douglas JMJ, Smith PK, Cox JL. Cardiac cryosurgery: effects of myocardial temperature on cryolesion size. Surgery 1983;93:268-272.
12. Rodriguez-Santiago A, Dubuc M, Talajic M, Roy D, Thibault B. Percutaneous catheter cryoablation in dogs: chronic lesions characterization. Can.J.Cardiol. 1999;15: 102D.
13. Cooper I. Cryogenic surgery: a new method of destruction or extirpation of benign or malignant tissue. N.Engl.J.Med. 1963;268:743-749.
14. Ott DA, Garson AJ, Cooley DA, Smith RT, Moak J. Cryoablative techniques in the treatment of cardiac tachyarrhythmias. Ann.Thorac.Surg. 1987;43:138-143.
15. Berth-Jones J, Bourke J, Eglitis H, Harper C, Kirk P, Pavord S, et al. Value of a second freeze-thaw cycle in cryotherapy of common warts. Br.J.Dermatol. 1994;131:883-886.
16. Pease GR, Wong STS, Roos MS, Rubinsky B. MR image-guided control of cryosurgery. J.Magn.Res.Imag. 1995;5:753-760.
17. Hass GM, Taylor CB. A quantitative hypothermal method for the production of local injury of tissue. Arch.Pathol. 1948;45:563
18. Taylor CB, Davis CB, Vawter GF, Hass GM. Controlled myocardial injury produced by a hypothermal method. Circulation 1951;3:239
19. Harrison L, Gallagher JJ, Kasell J, Anderson RH, Mikat E, Hackel DB, et al. Cryosurgical ablation of the A-V node-His bundle: a new method for producing A-V block. Circulation 1977;55:463-470.
20. Lister JW, Hoffman BF. Reversible cold block of the specialized conduction tissues of the anaesthetized dog. Science 1964;145:723-725.
21. Gillette PC, Swindle MM, Thompson RP, Case CL. Transvenous cryoablation of the bundle of His. Pacing.Clin.Electrophysiol. 1991;14:504-510.
22. Dubuc M, Talajic M, Roy D, Thibault B, Leung TK, Friedman PL. Feasibility of cardiac cryoablation using a transvenous steerable electrode catheter. J.Interv.Card.Electrophysiol. 1998;2:285-292.
23. Khairy P, Rodriguez-Santiago A, Talajic M, Tardif J-C, Thibault B, Roy D, et al. Catheter cryoablation in man: early clinical experience. Can.J.Cardiol. 1999;15:173D.
24. Klein GJ, Sealy WC, Pritchett EL, Harrison L, Hackel DB, Davis D, et al. Cryosurgical ablation of the atrioventricular node-His bundle: long- term follow-up and properties of the junctional pacemaker. Circulation 1980;61:8-15.

25. Garratt C, Camm AJ. The role of cryosurgery in the management of cardiac arrhythmias. Clin.Cardiol. 1991;14:153-159.
26. Bredikis J. Cryosurgical ablation of atrioventricular junction without extracorporeal circulation. J.Thorac.Cardiovasc.Surg. 1985;90:61-67.
27. Camm J, Ward DE, Spurrell RA, Rees GM. Cryothermal mapping and cryoablation in the treatment of refractory cardiac arrhythmias. Circulation 1980;62:67-74.
28. Bredikis JJ, Bredikis AJ. Surgery of tachyarrhythmia: intracardiac closed heart cryoablation. Pacing.Clin.Electrophysiol. 1990;13:1980-1984.
29. Louagie YA, Guiraudon GM, Klein GJ, Yee R. Closed heart cryoablation of the His bundle using an anterior septal approach. Ann.Thorac.Surg. 1991;51:616-619.
30. Gallagher JJ, Sealy WC, Anderson RW, Kasell J, Millar R, Campbell RWF, et al. Cryosurgical ablation of accessory AV connections. Circulation 1977;55:471-479.
31. Guiraudon GM, Klein GJ, Gulamhusein S, Jones DL, Yee R, Perkins DG, et al. Surgical repair of Wolff-Parkinson-White syndrome: a new closed-heart technique. Ann.Thorac.Surg. 1984; 37:67-71.
32. Bredikis J, Bredikis A. Cryosurgical ablation of left parietal wall accessory atrioventricular connections through the coronary sinus without the use of extracorporeal circulation. J.Thorac.Cardiovasc.Surg. 1985;90:199-205.
33. Rowland E, Robinson K, Edmondson S, Krikler DM, Bentall HH. Cryoablation of the accessory pathway in Wolff-Parkinson-White syndrome: initial results and long term follow up. Br.Heart J. 1988;59:453-457.
34. Guiraudon GM, Klein GJ, Sharma AD, Milstein S, McLellan DG. Closed-heart technique for Wolff-Parkinson-White syndrome: further experience and potential limitations. Ann.Thorac.Surg. 1986;42:651-657.
35. Watanabe S, Koyanagi H, Endo M, Yagi Y, Shiikawa A, Kasanuki H. Cryosurgical ablation of accessory atrioventricular pathways without cardiopulmonary bypass: an epicardial approach for Wolff-Parkinson- White syndrome. Ann.Thorac.Surg. 1989;47:257-264.
36. Lee AW, Crawford FAJ, Gillette PC, Roble SM. Cryoablation of septal pathways in patients with supraventricular tachyarrhythmias. Ann.Thorac.Surg. 1989;47:566-568.
37. Gallagher JJ, Anderson RW, Kasell J, Rice JR, Pritchett ELC, Gault JH, et al. Cryoablation of drug-resistant tachycardia in a patient with a variant of scleroderma. Circulation 1978;57:190-197.
38. Camm AJ, Ward DE, Cory-Pearce R, Rees GM, Spurrell RAJ. The successful cryosurgical treatment of paroxysmal ventricular tachycardia. Chest 1979;75:621-624.
39. Krafchek J, Lawrie GM, Roberts R, Magro SA, Wyndham CR. Surgical ablation of ventricular tachycardia: improved results with a map-directed regional approach. Circulation 1986;73:1239-1247.
40. Page PL, Cardinal R, Shenasa M, Kaltenbrunner W, Cossette R, Nadeau R. Surgical treatment of ventricular tachycardia. Regional cryoablation guided by computerized epicardial and endocardial mapping. Circulation 1989;80:I124-I134.
41. Ott DA, Garson A, Cooley DA, McNamara DG. Definitive operation for refractory cardiac tachyarrhythmias in children. J.Thorac.Cardiovasc.Surg. 1985; 90:681-689.
42. Guiraudon GM, Thakur RK, Klein GJ, Yee R, Guiraudon CM, Sharma A. Encircling endocardial cryoablation for ventricular tachycardia after myocardial infarction: experience with 33 patients. Am.Heart J. 1994;128:982-989.
43. Caceres J, Werner P, Jazayeri M, Akhtar M, Tchou P. Efficacy of cryosurgery alone for refractory monomorphic sustained ventricular tachycardia due to inferior wall infarction. J.Am.Coll.Cardiol. 1988;11:1254-1259.
44. Hargrove WC, Miller JM, Vassallo JA, Josephson ME. Improved results in the operative management of ventricular tachycardia related to inferior wall infarction. Importance of the annular isthmus. J.Thorac.Cardiovasc.Surg. 1986;726-732.
45. Miller JM, Kienzle MG, Harken AH, Josephson ME. Subendocardial resection for ventricular tachycardia: predictors of surgical success. Circulation 1984;69:624-631.
46. Cox JL. The status of surgery for cardiac arrhythmias. Circulation 1985;71:413-417.

47. Silka MJ, Kron J, Cutler JE, Wilson RA, Cobanoglu A. Cryoablation of medically refractory nodoventricular tachycardia. Pacing.Clin.Electrophysiol. 1990;13:908-915.
48. Kerr CR, Klein GG, Guiraudon GM, Webb JG. Surgical therapy for sinoatrial reentrant tachycardia. Pacing.Clin.Electrophysiol. 1988; 11:776-783.
49. Vermeulen FE, van HN, Guiraudon GM, Defauw JJ, Elbers HR, de BJ, et al. Cryosurgery for ventricular bigeminy using a transaortic closed ventricular approach. Eur.Heart J. 1988;9:979-990.
50. Andress JD, Vander ST, Huang SK. Bidirectional bundle branch reentry tachycardia associated with Ebstein's anomaly: cured by extensive cryoablation of the right bundle branch. Pacing.Clin.Electrophysiol. 1991;14:1639-1647.
51. Assad RS, Aiello VD, Jatene MB, Costa R, Hanley FL, Jatene AD. Cryosurgical ablation of fetal atrioventricular node: new model to treat fetal malignant tachyarrhythmias. Ann.Thorac.Surg. 1995;60:S629-S632
52. Nitta T, Ikeshita M, Asano T, Terada K, Akiyama H, Tanaka S. Perinodal cryomodification for supraventricular tachycardia. Nippon.Kyobu.Geka.Gakkai.Zasshi. 1995;43:344-349.
53. Szabo TS, Jones DL, Guiraudon GM, Rattes MF, Perkins DG, Sharma AD, et al. Cryosurgical modification of the atrioventricular node: a closed heart approach in the dog. J.Am.Coll.Cardiol. 1987;10:389-398.
54. Klein GJ, Guiraudon GM, Perkins DG, Sharma AD, Jones DL. Controlled cryothermal injury to the AV node: feasibility for AV nodal modification. Pacing.Clin.Electrophysiol. 1985;8:630-638.
55. Holman WL, Ikeshita M, Lease JG, Smith PK, Lofland GK, Cox JL. Cryosurgical modification of retrograde atrioventricular conduction. Implications for the surgical treatment of atrioventricular nodal reentry tachycardia. J.Thorac.Cardiovasc.Surg. 1986;91:826-834.
56. Cox JL, Holman WL, Cain ME. Cryosurgical treatment of atrioventricular node reentrant tachycardia. Circulation 1987;76:1329-1336.
57. Hunt GB, Chard RB, Johnson DC, Ross DL. Comparison of early and late dimensions and arrhythmogenicity of cryolesions in the normothermic canine heart. J Thorac Cardiovasc Surg. 1989;97:313-318.
58. Peiffert B, Feldman L, Villemot JP, Verdier J. Cryosurgery in ventricular tachycardia. Value of myocardial hypothermia in the extension of the depth of cryogenic lesions. Chirurgie. 1992;118:137-143.
59. Klein GJ, Harrison L, Ideker RF, Smith WM, Kasell J, Wallace AG, et al. Reaction of the myocardium to cryosurgery: electrophysiology and arrhythmogenic potential. Circulation 1979;59:364-372.
60. Stewart GJ, Preketes A, Horton M, Ross WB, Morris DL. Hepatic cryotherapy: double-freeze cycles achieve greater hepatocellular injury in man. Cryobiology 1995;32:215-219.
61. Gage AA, Guest K, Montes M, Caruana JA, Whalen DAJ. Effect of varying freezing and thawing rates in experimental cryosurgery. Cryobiology 1985;22:175-182.
62. Fujino H, Thompson RP, Germroth PG, Harold ME, Swindle MM, Gillette PC. Histologic study of chronic catheter cryoablation of atrioventricular conduction in swine. Am.Heart J. 1993;125:1632-1637.
63. Dubuc M, Roy D, Thibault B, Ducharme A, Tardif JC, Villemaire C, et al. Transvenous catheter ice mapping and cryoablation of the atrioventricular node in dogs. Pacing Clin Electrophysiol. 1999;1488-1498.
64. Rodriguez LM, Leunissen J, Hoekstra A, Korteling BJ, Smeets JL, Timmermans C, et al. Transvenous cold mapping and cryoablation of the AV node in dogs: observations of chronic lesions and comparison to those obtained using radiofrequency ablation. J Cardiovasc Electrophysiol. 1998;9:1055-1061.
65. Hoekstra A, de LC, Nikkels PG, Korteling BJ, Bel KJ, Crijns HJ. Prediction of lesion size through monitoring the 0 degree C isothermic period following transcatheter cryoablation. J Interv Card Electrophysiol. 1998;2:383-389.

Chapter 25

PHOTOABLATION OF VENTRICULAR ARRHYTHMIAS
Past Results and Future Applications to Ventricular and Other Arrhythmias

Robert H. Svenson, Robert Splinter, Laszlo Littmann, George P. Tatsis
Carolinas Heart Institute, Charlotte, North Carolina, USA

INTRODUCTION

Ablation of cardiac arrhythmias began originally as a joint venture between cardiac surgeons and electrophysiologists. The demise of electrophysiologic surgery for arrhythmias associated with the Wolff-Parkinson-White syndrome, AV nodal re-entry, atrial flutter, and for the creation of AV block began with DC shock ablation and reached its peak with radiofrequency (RF) catheter ablation. In contrast, the demise of primary surgery for post-infarction ventricular tachycardia (PIVT) was not the result of catheter ablation techniques, but the development and widespread use of implantable devices. The mortality, morbidity and recurrence rates following PIVT surgery, while improving over time, could not compete with the extremely low morbidity and mortality associated with AICD implants, particularly the newer systems who's implantations are not dissimilar from a pacemaker implant. Furthermore, with the availability of current devices, it is difficult to accept even a low, but potentially fatal recurrence rate following PIVT surgery, while an AICD could guarantee survival.

At this particular time, the only commercially available catheter energy source for ablation of PIVT is RF. There is a vast literature on using RF for PIVT ablation. Nonetheless, across the broad spectrum of interventional electrophysiologists, RF ablation is rarely used as primary therapy for PIVT. Radiofrequency catheter ablation tends to be reserved for patients with incessant VT and for patients receiving frequent shocks from their AICD. This latter group constitutes an ever-growing population of patients who are experiencing dramatically, in some cases, the downside of the device rather than a cure.[1]

409

L. Bing Liem and E. Downar (eds.), Progress in Catheter Ablation, 409-423.
© 2001 *Kluwer Academic Publishers. Printed in the Netherlands.*

Why is catheter ablation not typically considered as primary therapy for PIVT? To answer this we need to look at what we have learned from the surgical and catheter ablation experience of PIVT. From the surgical mapping and ablation experience we have learned that re-entrant circuits are not consistently in the endocardial one-third of the ventricle but may be intramural and epicardial. Furthermore, the three dimensional arrhythmogenic matrix, i.e. the area of slow conduction capable of supporting re-entry, is usually large and transmural providing ample opportunity to support induction of many "non-clinical VT's".[2-12] From the RF catheter ablation experience we have also learned a number of important electrophysiologic criteria predicting a high ablation success rate for those "targeted" PIVT's with re-entrant circuits accessible from the endocardium.[13-18] If low amplitude mid-diastolic potentials and concealed entrainment cannot be identified from endocardial catheter studies, it implies that either the catheters can't find them or they are not on the endocardial surface. Moreover, ablating a "clinical" or "targeted" PIVT is not the same as a cure. The problem with RF is that nobody really knows for sure how deep RF lesions are when applied to an area of fibrosis in the beating human heart, even with the newer cooled tip catheter devices. Certainly no one has ever shown the ability of RF to generate transmural lesions in such an area.

It is our hypothesis that light energy offers the possibility of achieving a significant improvement over RF and other energy sources in curing and palliating patients with PIVT. It may have an important role in other arrhythmias as well. This hypothesis is based on the long-term cure rates from our surgical experience using both epicardial, and endocardial radiation,[19-21] and on experimental work by us and others[22-31] as well as on the results of early human clinical trials.[32-34] This hypothesis is supported by the dramatic developments in diode laser technology.

1.   LASER-TISSUE INTERACTION

Radiofrequency lesions depend on resistive heating with current density falling off with the fourth power of the distance from the RF catheter electrode, and on passive heat transfer from the tip and from within the tissues. In contrast, thermal lesions from lasers, particularly the continuous wave lasers at various wavelengths (790 to 1064 nm), are caused by direct photon absorption deep in the tissue with a small contribution of passive heat transfer from within the heated volume.[35,36] Therefore, the deeper the photon penetration (a function of the absorption and scattering coefficients and the mean scattering angle) the deeper the lesion. There are certain fundamental differences, however, in lesion development between non-contact (low power density) and contact myocardial irradiation (high power density).

<u>Low power density non-contact irradiation</u>: Clinical applications in this mode were confined to the intraoperative application of the Nd:YAG laser (1,064 nm) for treatment of PIVT. In experimental work, lesion dimensions correlate well with the Monte Carlo simulation of the light distribution within the myocardium based on the measured optical properties of the tissue.[37-40] At power densities of 150-500/cm^2, as employed in our surgical experience, transmural photocoagulation usually required irradiating both the endocardial and epicardial surfaces. However, lesion depths of 6-7 mm could commonly be obtained (unpublished observations based on histology of myocardial sections through irradiated areas). Using this method intraoperatively we achieved an 89% ten-year cure rate in survivors.[20] No patient had a recurrence after two years. Of the 5 patients with inducible or spontaneous PIVT, 3 of the 5, in retrospect, had epicardial reentrant circuits. These three patients occurred very early on in our experience before the significance of the functional role of the epicardium in PIVT was appreciated. We attributed this excellent long-term cure rate to the fact that we could obtain transmural photocoagulation and that we irradiated a large area of potentially arrhythmogenic myocardium not just map-directed sites during inducedVT.

<u>High power density contact irradiation</u>: Catheter applications of laser photocoagulation for PIVT require direct or near direct fiber contact with the endocardial surface to eliminate blood scattering and absorption. In contrast to non-contact applications, with power densities of 150-500 w/cm^2, direct tissue contact with a fiber of 400 to 600 micron diameter results in power densities of 12-16 kw/cm^2. One would assume that increasing the power densities by a factor of 500 or more would result in the immediate vaporization of tissue. Therefore, it was difficult to understand from a theoretical point of view the early pioneering work of Vincent et al who showed that large transmural lesions could be created in the canine LV without perforation or burning of the endocardial surface.[28,29]

Further studies from our laboratory confirmed the early work of Vincent et al as well as additional studies that helped us to understand this seemingly paradoxical phenomenon. At power densities greater than 10 kw/cm^2 the light distribution in the tissue becomes "anomalous", i.e. it does not behave according to the light distribution predicted and verified experimentally for the measured optical properties of the tissue at lower powers.[41-43] Indeed, quite remarkable phenomena are observed.

In normal canine LV myocardium, with direct fiber contact at 1064 nm and high power densities, an epicardial temperature of 60^0 can be reached within 1-10 seconds.[23,24,36,44] The initial lesion is very narrow (1-2 mm) and cylindrical in shape. As additional energy is delivered the lesion rapidly expands in width so that by 40 to 60 seconds a fully transmural lesion of 1-3 cm^3 is achieved (Figure 1). The myocardial target zone for PIVT, however, is not "normal myocardium;" rather it is a region with extensive myocardial fibrosis containing regions of surviving myocardial fibers. This altered matrix must affect the energy distribution regardless of the energy source. This has not been well worked out for RF. Studies from our laboratory with the Nd:YAG laser actually show a more favorable light distribution (photocoagulation profile) in scarred myocardium compared with normal myocardium. Transmural lesions through infarcted myocardium can be achieved in as little as 10-40 seconds, but the extent of endocardial coagulation is much greater at shorter ablation times.[24] There are two important reasons for this. First, in scarred myocardium the scattering coefficient increases together with an increase in the mean scattering angle.[38,45] Second, collagen fibers themselves seem to act as light guides directing the photons along the longitudinal axis of the fiber.[46] Table I compares data of lesions in infarcted canine myocardium with those in normal myocardium. In just 15 seconds using 20 watts of power, 62.5% of the lesions were transmural, with endocardial surface coagulation of approximately 1 cm in diameter from the point of laser contact. In normal myocardium the endocardial surface lesion dimensions were much smaller.

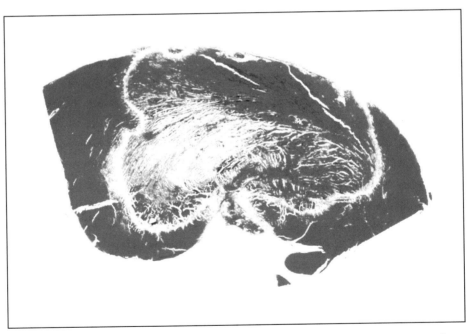

Figure 1. A fully transmural photocoagulation lesion of 14 mm depth (approximately 2.5 cm^3) was obtained in 40 seconds at a wavelength of 1064 nm. The duration of power application was 40 seconds. Note the relative sparing of the endocardial surface in normal myocardium due to cooling from circulating blood in contact with the endocardial surface. See also Color Plate 25.

TABLE I

CATHETER LV ENDOCARDIAL PHOTOCOAGULATION (300J)

	Infarct	Normal
Endocardial Surface Width	9.5 ± 2.0 mm n=8 $P<0.05$	2.9 ± 3.2 mm n=13
Lesion Depth	7.2 ± 2.7 $P<0.05$	12.3 ± 2.3
Transmural	62.5%	46%

With near-contact laser photocoagulation the situation is a little more problematic. Weber et al first published results using an optical fiber in a catheter in which the optical fiber was a few millimeters off the surface.[30] Blood was kept away between the fiber and the endocardial surface by a high flush rate of saline. Good-sized lesions were obtained, but crater formation was also observed. Similar phenomena were observed by others using a laser catheter in which the fiber was not in direct tissue contact. Perforations were observed leading to the mistaken conclusion that laser catheter ablation of PIVT may not be feasible.[47] The dynamics of the laser-tissue interaction under these conditions have not been well studied. The power densities at the surface are not known since saline can also cause alterations in the light path due to differences in the refractive index between saline and blood. Subsequent experimental work with Weber's device and some modifications of the optical fiber showed more promising results in photocoagulating myocardium in scarred infarcted areas in a canine model.[29]

2.   STUDIES COMPARING RF AND ND:YAG AND OTHER EXPERIMENTAL APPLICATIONS OF ND:YAG LASER ABLATION

There are few studies comparing RF and Nd:YAG lesions in the ventricle. Using direct-fiber tissue contact, Littmann et al demonstrated, at low and comparable total energies with RF, that laser lesions are larger with Nd:YAG than with radiofrequency.[27] Comparing 30 second temperature controlled lesions with RF (70^0c) and with Nd:YAG (30 watts) Weber et al found substantial differences in volume of coagulated tissue. Lesion volumes with Nd:YAG laser were approximately nine times larger than with RF.[48]

The safety and efficacy of catheter delivery of the Nd:YAG laser to various portions of the canine right atrium have been demonstrated by Weber et al.[49] Other experimental applications have also been reported. These applications include sinus node modification as a possible treatment for inappropriate sinus tachycardia,[50] modification of the AV nodal transmission for rate control during atrial fibrillation,[51] and ablation of the AV conduction system.[51-55]

3.   CLINICAL APPLICATION OF LASER CATHETERS FOR ABLATION

3.1   Post-infarction ventricular tachycardia

The feasibility of laser catheter ablation of PIVT was recently tested by us using a two-piece prototype device.[32] The first device was a 10F two-piece non-steerable system consisting of an outer guiding catheter of several pre-formed shapes together with an inner laser catheter. The device was evaluated in four patients with recurrent PIVT. The ablation was successful in only one patient due to lack of maneuverability of the device. However, one patient with two VT morphologies has been arrhythmia free without antiarrhythmic drugs for a period of eight years.

The second device was an 11.5F two-piece system consisting of an outer steerable guiding catheter and an inner 4.5F laser catheter. Four patients were treated with this device. Laser energy was delivered not just to mapped sites during VT, but also to sites showing slow conduction (paced stimulus to QRS interval>60 ms) and to areas with delayed potentials during sinus rhythm. All patients post-procedure were free of inducible sustained VT and to our knowledge have had no recurrences of arrhythmias in six years of follow-up. Three of the four patients had failed previous attempts at RF ablation.

Figure 2 is particularly important because it is the only known documentation of any energy source to create a transmural lesion through an area of scarred myocardium in the human heart. A standard quadripolar electrode catheter was placed in an epicardial vein via the coronary sinus over the posterolateral wall in a patient with a previous circumflex coronary infarction. Laser energy was delivered to the endocardial surface. The distance of the laser catheter placement was estimated to be 1.5 cm from the epicardium based on the known interelectrode distances of the catheter. During sinus rhythm delayed potentials were present on the epicardial electrogram. After 60 seconds of Nd:YAG laser delivery to the endocardium there was a significant reduction in electrogram amplitude and by 120 seconds, local epicardial activation was completely obliterated. We have no similar documentation for RF catheters including some of the new cooled tip designs.

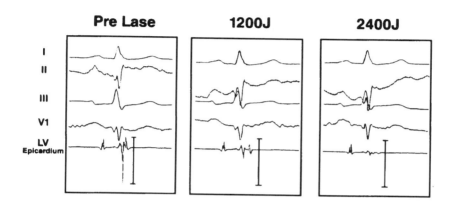

Figure 2. This is the only documented case of catheter transmural coagulation in the human heart. Epicardial potentials were recorded approximately 1.5 mm from the endocardial location of the laser catheter. Prior to delivery of laser radiation (wavelength 1064 nm) delayed potential in sinus rhythm were recorded from the epicardial surface. After 60 seconds (1200 Joules) there is marked reduction in electrogram amplitude. After 120 seconds (2400 Joules) there is complete obliteration of local activation under the epicardial recording site. The overlying atrial electrogram from the appendage is unaffected.

With our catheter device, endocardial lesion formation was extremely rapid. Laser energy was frequently delivered while pacing through the device at 20 ma output and with a 10 msec. pulse width at areas showing long stimulus to QRS intervals. Loss of capture occurred a mean of 4.5 ± 2.4 seconds from the onset of laser energy delivery. We have not been able to achieve similar results with RF. Long-term success was achieved because we could address the large three-dimensional arrhythmogenic matrix and all potential re-entrant sites, endocardial, intramural and epicardial. The total energy delivered via catheter (27.1 ± 13 kJoules) was similar to that delivered during intraoperative applications (27.9 ± 13 kJoules). There was no change in overall LV systolic function measured by echocardiogram or gated nuclear ventriculograms (EF pre $.34 \pm 7$ and post ablation $.35 \pm 8$). The size of the existing device was not feasible for routine clinical use because of the potential for damage related to the size and stiffness of the catheter. Current efforts are now underway to downsize this device into a 9 or 9.5F steerable system.

3.2   Application of Laser Energy to Other Forms of VT

Delivering laser energy by a single fiber in direct contact to non-scarred myocardium can result in a large area of thermal damage that potentially could lead to deterioration of LV function. Lesions in nonischemic hearts would be placed in wall segments which contribute to systolic function—unlike in PIVT. Moreover, the pattern of lesion evolution is not optimal since transmurality is achieved rapidly before the lesion expands in the lateral direction. In addition, there tends to be sparing of a large area of endocardium under the lesion (see Figure 1and Table 1). In order to apply this energy source for nonischemic VT's further experimental work will need to be done to modify the energy density profile on the endocardial surface. There are several possible approaches. First, the wavelength could be shortened below 1064 nm to one with a higher absorption in tissue water e.g. 980 nm. This would limit penetration into the tissue and keep the lesion more superficial. Second, the "duty cycle" of energy application could be altered. Instead of a continuous delivery of photons the delivery cycle could be modified so that energy would be delivered with short pulses, for example 0.01-0.3 seconds with pulse pauses of the same duration. This would reduce the total energy fluence rates in tissues deeper than 3-4 mm below that required to raise tissue temperatures to those necessary for coagulation. Another possible approach to this is suggested by recent studies using direct interstitial radiation[56]. An optical fiber that diffuses light 360 degrees around the axis of the fiber is placed into the tissue. The depth of the lesion depends on the depth of fiber penetration. Such a system may be capable of creating wider and shallower lesions without the risk of deleterious effects on ventricular function, particularly in cases where multiple lesions may be required.

Chagas disease VT may be an exception to this. In Chagas disease the ventricular re-entrant circuits are frequently epicardial and are usually located in the inferolateral wall. This wall segment is frequently severely hypokinetic or akinetic and may be aneurysmal.[57] This non-functioning wall segment is frequently interlaced with extensive scar tissue. Studies of the optical properties of fresh post-mortem hearts from patients with Chagas disease suggest that the 1064 nm Nd:YAG and other wave lengths with low water absorption may be useful in this disease.[58] Chagas disease is not a major problem outside the South American countries where 16 million people may be affected. In this region it presents a significant public health problem. However, there is a growing number of such patients in the United States due to the influx of Hispanic immigrants.

3.3   Application to Supraventricular Arrhythmias

Using a fiber-tissue near contact laser catheter, Weber et al have demonstrated the feasibility of using laser energy (Nd:YAG) for the ablation of atrial flutter and AV nodal re-entry tachycardia.[33,34] The advantage of using laser energy versus RF for these applications has still to be clearly demonstrated. It may potentially have some advantage in atrial flutter if it can be shown that lasers require fewer lesions for shorter periods of time resulting in a significant reduction in procedure time.

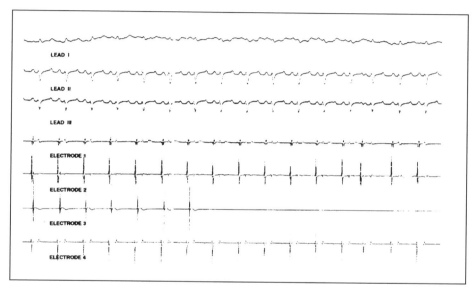

Figure 3. Electrical recordings were obtained from the right atrial appendage (electrode 1), right atrial freewall (electrode 2), left atrial appendage (electrode 3) and high right atrium (electrode 4). Fiber contact laser energy (1064 nm wavelength) is being delivered around the left atrial appendage, with abrupt loss of conduction (electrical isolation) to the left atrial appendage after 96 seconds.

3.4   Atrial fibrillation

The optimum approach to catheter or surgical ablation of this disease has still to be worked out regardless of the energy source. We recently conducted a canine study using direct epicardial fiber contact laser ablation of the atrium for creating lines of block and isolating both atrial appendages as well as isolating a separate area in the right ventricular freewall.[57] Figure 3 shows the electrical isolation of the left atrial appendage with abrupt loss of electrical activity. The lines of isolation or block were transmural and acceptably narrow (2-3 mm). Histology of a chronically isolated left atrial appendage is seen in Figure 4. Linear ablation rates were up to 5.4 cm/min were possibilities. This procedure is now under clinical evaluation in patients with atrial fibrillation undergoing mitral valve surgery (See Moosdorf, Rainer in this volume). The intraoperative application of this approach during atrial fibrillation may elucidate the requirements for a catheter based approach for the ablation of chronic atrial fibrillation. For example, the effect of isolating the pulmonary veins and creating other types of "MAZE" lines of block could be directly observed for their ability to terminate chronic atrial fibrillation—similar to our strategy for terminating PIVT intraoperatively.

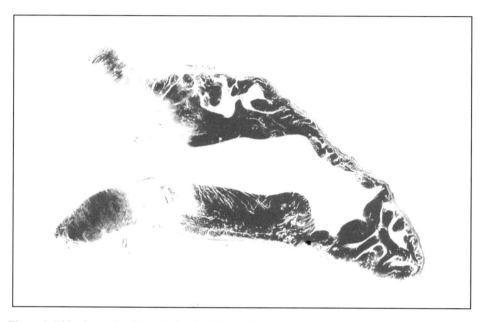

Figure 4. This shows the 2 week chronic lesion of the isolated left atrial appendage whose acute electrical isolation was shown in Figure 3. On re-study 2 weeks later electrical entrance and exit block was confirmed. A 2-3 mm wide area of fibrosis surrounded the entire atrial appendage. See also Color Plate 26.

4.   FUTURE DIRECTIONS

In spite of the fact that Vincent et al demonstrated the tremendous potential of the Nd:YAG laser for catheter ablation of PIVT in 1987, there has been little general interest in this modality both on the part of the medical device industry and the interventional electrophysiology community. There are several important reasons for this. Until recently, the Nd:YAG lasers available for clinical and experimental work were expensive large systems requiring external water-cooling and special electrical requirements. Radiofrequency generators by comparison were very small, easy to use, cheaper and a form of energy much easier to adapt to catheter systems. Two factors are beginning to reverse this trend. First, there is growing realization that RF and all of its catheter delivery system modifications is far from being an ideal energy source when deep lesions are required.[59,60] The second factor is the rapid changes in laser technology. Conventional Nd:YAG lasers are now much smaller and no longer require external cooling and complicated electrical connections. However, one of the most important advances is the development of diode laser technology. Diode laser technology now has made FDA approval of new wavelengths available for tissue coagulation (790 to 830 and 980 nm). These lasers are in many cases smaller and less expensive than 50 watt RF generators. Preliminary studies from our laboratory using diode lasers in the 790 to 830 nm range have shown comparable effects in normal and infarcted canine myocardium to those obtained with the Nd:YAG laser at 1064 nm wavelength unpublished observations. Initial studies with these wavelengths indicate the ability to achieve transmural photocoagulation in infarcted canine myocardium with epicardial temperatures reaching 60^0 in 55 ± 47 sec. at a depth of 12 ± 3.7 mm. These lasers, some of which are approved medical devices in the U.S. and elsewhere, are comparable in size and price to a 50 watt RF generator. These rapid advances in laser technology for tissue coagulation will make this a viable alternative to existing energy sources for safe and effective lesion formation.

SUMMARY & CONCLUSIONS

Light energy for PIVT both intraoperative and for catheter ablations experimentally and in preliminary human trials, has shown itself superior to RF. The application of light energy to other etiologies of VT and atrial arrhythmias will depend on catheter designs that alter the energy density profile in the tissue and/or selecting wavelengths that limit photon penetration of myocardial tissue. Rapid advances in diode laser technology will facilitate this goal, offering a range of FDA approved wavelengths that can be selected for their tissue specific effects.

REFERENCES

1.   Sears JR, Samuel F., Conti JB, Curtis AB, Saia T, Foote R, Wen F. Affective Distress and Implantable Cardioverter Defibrillators: Cases for psychological and behavioral interventions. PACE 1999;22:1831-1834.
2.   Svenson RH, Gallagher JJ, Selle JG, et al. Neodymium YAG laser photocoagulation: A successful new map-guided technique for the intraoperative ablation of ventricular tachycardia. Circulation 1987;76:1319-1328.
3.   Svenson RH, Littmann L, Gallagher JJ, Selle JG, Zimmern SH, Fedor JM, Colavita PG. Termination of ventricular tachycardia with epicardial laser photocoagulation: A clinical

comparison with patients undergoing successful endocardial photocoagulation alone. J Amer Coll Cardiol 1990;15:163-170.

4. Littmann L, Svenson RH, Gallagher JJ, Selle JG, Zimmern SH, Fedor JM, Colavita PG. Functional role of the epicardium in postinfarction ventricular tachycardia: observations derived from computerized epicardial activation mapping, entrainment, and epicardial laser photoablation. Circulation 1991;83:1577-1591.

5. Svenson RH, Littmann L, Splinter R, Selle JG, Gallagher JJ, Tatsis GP, Linder KD, Seifert KT. Application of lasers from arrhythmia ablation. In: Cardiac Electrophysiology; From Cell to Bedside. Zipes, D.P., Jalife, J. (eds) Philadelphia: W. B. Saunders, 1990.

6. Kaltenbrunner W, Cardinal R, Dubuc M, et al: Epicardial and endocardial mapping of ventricular tachycardia in patients with myocardial infarction. Is the origin of the tachycardia always sub-endocardially localized? Circulation 1991;84:1058-1065.

7. Lacroix D, Flug D, LeFranc P, et al. Intraoperative computerized mapping of ventricular tachycardia; differences between anterior and inferior myocardial infarctions. Pacing Clin Electrophysiol 1996;19(2):628.

8. Pfeiffer D, Moosdorf R, Svenson R, et al. Epicardial Neodymium:YAG laser photocoagulation of ventricular tachycardia without ventriculotomy in patients after myocardial infarction. Circulation 1996;94:3221-3225.

9. Moosdorf R, Pfeiffer D, Sneider C, et al: Intraoperative laser photocoagulation of ventricular tachycardia. Am Heart J 1994;127:1133-1138.

10. DeBakker J, Coronel R, Tasserion S, et al. Ventricular tachycardia in the infarcted Langendorff-perfused human heart: role of arrangement of surviving cardiac fibers. J Am Coll Cardiol 1990;15:1594-1607.

11. DeBakker JMT, van Capelle FJL, Janse MJ, et al. Reentry as a cause of ventricular tachycardia in patients with chronic ischemic heart disease: electrophysiolgic and anatomic correlation. Circulation 1988;77:589-606.

12. De Bakker JMT, van Capelle FJL, Janse MJ, et al. Reentry as a cause of ventricular tachycardia in patients with chronic ischemic heart disease: Electrophysiologic and anatomic correlation. Circulation 1988;77:589-606.

13. Borggrefe M, Willems S, Chen X, et al. Catheter ablation of ventricular tachycardia using radiofrequency current. HERZ 1992;17:171-178.

14. Stevenson WG, Khan H, Sager P, et al. Identification of reentry circuit sites during catheter mapping and radiofrequency ablation of ventricular tachycardia late after myocardial infarction. Circulation 1993;88:1647-1670.

15. Stevenson WG, Sager PT, Natterson PD, Saxon LA, Middlekauff HR, Wiener I. Relation of Pace Mapping QRS Configuration and Conduction Delay to Ventricular Tachycardia Reentry Circuits in Human Infarct Scars. J Am Coll Cardiol 1995;26:481-488.

16. Morady F, Harvey M, Kalbfleisch SJ, et al. Radiofrequency catheter ablation of ventricular tachycardia in patients with coronary artery disease. Circulation 1993;87:363-372.

17. Gonsak B-E, Cao K, Schauman A, et al. Catheter ablation of ventricular tachycardia in 136 patients with coronary artery disease. Results and long-term follow-up. J Am Coll Cardiol 1994;24:1056-1514.

18. Stevenson W. Ventricular tachycardia after myocardial infarction: From arrhythmias surgery to catheter ablation. J Cardiovasc Electrophysiol 1995; 6:942-950.

19. Svenson RH, Littmann L, Gallagher JJ, Selle J, Zimmern S, Fedor J, Marroum M-C, Seifert K, Tatsis GP, Linder K. Laser modification of the myocardium for the treatment of cardiac arrhythmias: Background, current results, and future possibilities. From: Lasers in Cardiopulmonary Medicine and Surgery. Abela G. (eds). Kluwer, Boston, Massachusetts, 1990.

20. Svenson R, Selle J, Littmann L, Gallagher J, Colavita P, Zimmern S, Fedor J, Wu G. Long-term arrhythmia outcome following intraoperative photoablation of ventricular tachycardia. PACE 1996;19:627.

21. Svenson RH, Gallagher JJ, Zimmern SH, Fedor J, Harbold N, Elliott C, Hall D, Austin K, Thomley A, Wilson BH, Selle J. Intraoperative Nd:YAG laser photocoagulative ablation of

ventricular tachycardia: observations relevant to transcatheter ablation techniques. J Amer Coll Cardiol 1987;9:249A.

22. Svenson, RH, Littmann L, Linder K, Tatsis GP, Splinter R, Seifert K, Marroum M-C, Chuang CH. Myocardial Nd:YAG laser photocoagulation as a function of irradiated surface area: method for reaching deep arrhythmogenic foci. Lasers Surg Med 1989;9:10.

23. Splinter R, Littmann L, Svenson RH, Brucker G, Tuntelder JR, Thompson M, Chuang CH, Tatsis GP. Epicardial ther-mography during in-vivo endocardial laser photocoagulation. Lasers Surg Med 1992;4:19-20.

24. Svenson RH, Littmann L, Splinter R, Tatsis GP, Chuang CH. Current status of lasers for arrhythmia ablation. J Cardiovasc Electrophysiol 1992;3:345-353.

25. Littmann L, Svenson RH, Brucker G, Splinter R, Chuang CH, Tuntelder JR, Dezern K, Thompson M, Tatsis GP. Percutaneous Neodymium: YAG laser photoablation of ventricular tachycardia: a canine feasibility study. Circulation 1992;86:I-192.

26. Littmann L, Svenson RH, Chuang CH, Splinter R, Kempler P, Norton HJ, Tuntelder JR, Thompson M, Tatsis GP. Neodymium:YAG contact laser photocoagulation of the in vivo canine epicardium: dosimetry, effects of various lasing methods, and histology. Lasers Surg Med 1993;13:158-167.

27. Littmann L, Svenson RH, Brucker G, Chuang CH, Splinter R, Dezer K, Tuntelder JR, Thompson M, Tatsis GP. Comparative study of the efficacy and safety of transcatheter radiofrequency ablation and contact Neodymium:YAG laser photoablation of the left ventricular endocardium in dogs. PACE 1993;16:859.

28. Vincent A, Fox J, Benedict B, et al. Laser catheter ablation of simulated ventricular tachycardia. Lasers Surg Med 1987;7:421-425.

29. Vincent A, Fox J, Knowlton K, et al. Catheter directed Neodymium:YAG laser injury of the left ventricle for arrhythmia ablation; dosimetry and hemodynamic, hematologic and electrophysiologic effects. Laser Sur Med 1989;9:446-453.

30. Weber H, Enders S, Keiditisch E. Percutaneous Nd:YAG laser coagulation of ventricular myocardium in dogs using a special electrode laser catheter. Pacing Clin Electrophysiol 1989;12:6, 899-910.

31. Weber HP, Heinze A, Enders S, Ruprecht L, Unsold E. Laser catheter coagulation of normal and scarred ventricular myocardium in dogs. Laser Surg Med 1998;22:109-119.

32. Svenson, R., Colavita, P., Zimmern, S., Gallagher, J., Fedor, J., Littmann, L., Brucker, G. Laser catheter ablation of ventricular tachycardia: a human feasibility study. PACE 1996;19:611.

33. Weber HP, Kaltenbrunner W, Heinze A, Steinbach K. Laser catheter coagulation of atrial myocardium for ablation of atrioventricular nodal reentrant tachycardia. First clinical experience (see comments) Eur Heart J 1997;18:3,487-495, Mar.

34. Weber HP, Heinze A. Laser catheter ablation of atrial flutter and of atrioventricular nodal reentrant tachycardia in a single session. Eur Heart J 1994;15:8,1147-1149.

35. Splinter R, Semenov SY, Nanney G, Littmann L, Tuntelder JR, Chuang CH, Svenson RH, Tatsis GP. Myocardial heat distribution under cw Nd:YAG laser irradiation in vitro and in vivo situations: theory and experiment. Appl Optics 1995;3:391-399.

36. Splinter R, Semenov SY, Nanney G, Littmann L, Tuntelder JR, Chuang CH, Svenson RH, Tatsis GP. Rate dependency of myocardial temperature distribution under cw Nd:YAG laser irradiation in vivo situations: practice and theory. Laser Surg Med 1994;6:4.

37. Splinter R, Littmann L, Keijzer M, Tuntelder JR, Chuang CH, Thompson M, Svenson RH, Tatis GP. Predicting cw Nd:YAG photocoagulation lesion size in myocardium from Monte Carlo light simulations. Proc ASME, Advances in Biological Heat and Mass Transfer, HTD 189/BED 18:75-78, 1991.

38. Splinter R, Svenson RH, Littmann L, Tuntelder JR, Chuang CH, Tatsis GP, Thompson M. Optical properties of normal, diseased, and laser photocoagulated myocardium at the Nd:YAG wavelength. Lasers Surg Med 1991;11:117-124.

39. Splinter R, Littmann L, Svenson RH, Keijzer M, Tuntelder JR, Chuang CH, Thompson M, Tatsis GP. Can cw Nd:YAG photocoagulation lesion dimensions in myocardium be predicted by Monte Carlo light propagation simulations? J Clin Eng 1992;17:409-418.

40. Splinter R, Svenson RH, Littmann L, Chuang CH, Tuntelder JR, Thompson M, Tatsis GP, Keijzer M. Computer simulated light distributions in myocardial tissues at the Nd:YAG wavelength of 1064 nm. Lasers Med Sci 1993;8:15-21.
41. Svenson RH, Splinter R, Littmann L, Chuang CH, Tuntelder JR, Thompson M, Dezern KR, Tatsis GP, Raja MYA. Low power density vs. high power density photocoagulation of ventricular myocardium for cardiac arrhythmias. Observations supporting non-linear tissue optics. IEEE Engineering Med Biol 1992;2: 318-129.
42. Splinter R, Svenson RH, Littmann L, Chuang CH, Tuntelder JR, Thompson M, Dezern KR, Tatsis GP, Raja MYA. Non-linear optical phenomena in contact fiber laser-photocoagulation of myocardium. IEEE Engineering Med Biol 1992;2: 316-317.
43. Splinter R, Raja MYA, Svenson RH, Anomalous optical behavior of biological media: modifying the optical window of myocardial tissues. Proc SPIE 1996;2671:125-131.
44. Splinter R, Svenson RH, Littmann L, Brucker GG, Chuang CH, Tuntelder JR, Dezern KR, Thompson M, Nanney GA, Tatsis GP. Myocardial temperatures during in vivo endocardial Nd:YAG laser irradiation. J Clin Laser Med Surg 1995;13:61-68.
45. Splinter R, Littmann L, Marroum MD, Svenson RH, Tuntelder JR, Chuang CH, Tatsis GP, Thompson M. Optical changes in myocardial tissue due to cw Nd:YAG irradiation. Proc IEEE 1990;12:1113-1114.
46. Splinter R, Raja MYA, Svenson RH. Laser induced light guides in tissue under high irradiance. Lasers Surg Med 1997;Suppl 9:2.
47. Hindricks G, Haverkamp W, Gulker H, Kramer T, Russel U, Teutemacher H, Borggrefe M, Breithardt G. Perkutane endokardiale Nd-YAG-Laserapplikation: Experimentelle Untersuchungen zur Ablation ventrikulren Myokards. Z Kardiol 1991;80:673-680.
48. Weber HP, Heinze A, Enders S, Ruprecht L, Unsold E. Laser versus radiofrequency catheter ablation of ventricular myocardium in dogs: A comparative test. Cardiology 1997;88:4,346-352.
49. Weber HP, Heinze A, Enders S, Ruprecht L, Unsold E, Catheter-directed laser coagulation of atrial myocardium in dogs., Eur Heart J 1994;15: 7, 971-80.
50. Littmann L, Svenson RH, Gallagher JJ, Bharati S, Lev M, Linder KD, Tatsis GP, Nichelson C. Modification of sinus node function by epicardial laser irradiation in dogs. Circulation 1990;81:350-359.
51. Littmann L, Svenson RH, Tomcsanyi I, Hehrlein C, Gallagher JJ, Bharati S, Lev M, Splinter R, Tatsis GP, Tuntelder JR. Modification of atrioventricular nodal transmission properties by intraoperative neodymium: YAG laser photocoagulation in dogs. J Amer Coll Cardiol 1991;17:797-804.
52. Obelienius V, Knepa A, Ambartzumian R, Markin E, Koshelev E, Transvenous ablation of the atrioventricular conduction system by laser irradiation under endoscopic control. Lasers Surg Med 1985;5:469-74.
53. Littmann L, Svenson RH, Chuang CH, Bharati S, Lev M, Kempler P, Splinter R, Tuntelder JR, Tatsis GP. Selective elimination of retrograde conduction by intraoperative Neodymium:YAG laser photocoagulation in dogs. J Am Coll Cardiol 1993;21:523-530.
54. Littmann L, Svenson RH, Chuang CH, Kempler P, Splinter R, Tuntelder JR, Tatsis GP. Catheterization technique for laser photoablation of atrioventricular conduction from the aortic root in dogs. PACE 1993;16:401-406.
55. Weber HP, Heinze A, Enders S, Ruprecht L, Unsold E, Mapping guided laser catheter ablation of the atrioventricular conduction in dogs. Pacing Clin Electrophysiol 1996;19:176-87.
56. Ware DL, Boor P, Yang CJ, Gowda A, Grady JJ, Montamedi. Slow intramural heating with diffused laser light – A unique method for deep myocardial coagulation. Circulation 1999;99:1630-1636.
57. Sosa E, Scanavacca M, D'Avila A, Piccioni J, Sanchez O, Velarde JL, Silva M, Reolao B, Endocardial and epicardial ablation guided by nonsurgical transthoracic epicardial mapping to treat recurrent ventricular tachycardia. J Cardiovasc Electrophysiol 1998;9:229-239.
58. d'Avila A, Splinter R, Scanavacca M, Svenson R, Sosa E, Ramirez, JAF. Laser Irradiation of Chagasic Heart. Feasibility study on the potential for deep laser photocoagulation in chagasic

hearts with diffuse myocardial damage. Brazilian Journal of Medical and Biological Research. (submitted for publication).

59. Svenson R, Splinter R, Moosdorf R, Selle J, Kassell J. Regional atrial electrical isolation. Lines of block created by laser photocoagulation: A possible intraoperative approach to atrial fibrillation. PACE 1999;22: 774.

60. Petersen HH, Chen X, Pietersen A, Svendsen JH, Haunso S. Tissue temperatures and lesion size during irrigated tip catheter radiofrequeny ablation: An in vitro comparison of temperature controlled irrigated tip ablation, power-controlled irrigated tip ablation, and standard temperature-controlled ablation. PACE 2000;23:8-17.

Chapter 26

TRANSCATHETER MICROWAVE ABLATION

L. Bing Liem and Dany Berubé*
*Cardiac Arrhythmia and Electrophysiology, Stanford University, Stanford, California, and *AFx Inc., Fremont, California, USA*

INTRODUCTION

Microwave energy was considered an attractive alternative source for tissue heating because it involves a fundamentally different process from radiofrequency energy.

In terms of their general physical properties, "radio" wave and microwave represent two of the many spectrums of electromagnetic radiation frequency. Radio waves occupy roughly the frequency range between 100 kHz to 100 MHz while microwaves represent the higher frequency spectrum between 500 MHz to 100GHz. All forms of electromagnetic sources are useful in delivering energy and signals to distant sites and are therefore used extensively in communication technology. It has also been applied in medical technology in the form of localized hyperthermic ablative therapy for cancer and other disorders.[1-10] A specific utility of radiofrequency energy application is in the local ablation of brain and cardiac tissue where a limited size of tissue destruction is desired. In this scope of its use, radiofrequency energy is used as an electrical rather than electromagnetic tool. When applied directly to tissue, attenuated current at frequencies between 300 and 1000 kHz produces a resistive form of heat.[11,12] Thus, the tissue closest to the electrode, with highest electrical density produces the highest amount of heat while adjacent tissue is heated by passive transfer of heat[13]; producing controlled but limited tissue necrosis. Microwave heating, on the other hand utilizes its radiation property. The microwave antenna radiates an electromagnetic field into the tissue and this field raises the energy of the dielectric molecules by conductive and displacement currents,[14,15] generating oscillatory movement of water molecules, resulting into frictional form of

L. Bing Liem and E. Downar (eds.), Progress in Catheter Ablation, 425-442.

heating. Based on such premise, microwave energy has the potential of heating deeper tissue and creating larger ablative lesions.

Thus, heating with microwave method is expected to overcome the limitations encountered with radiofrequency ablation. Several computer modeling and in-vitro studies have shown that lesions created by microwave ablation can indeed be larger than expected from radiofrequency ablation.[16-19] However, the application of this energy form in animal tissue had not been accomplished easily. Some in-vivo studies have shown microwave ablation lesions that are larger than the average RF lesion[20-24] while others showed just the opposite results.[25] In view of limited direct comparative data, it would be difficult to make any conclusive statement with respect to microwave advantages, although some preliminary data appear to support the expectations from microwave ablation. This chapter discusses the overall data on the use of microwave energy for cardiac tissue ablation with emphasis on its utility in transcatheter application.

1.   RATIONALE FOR USING MICROWAVE ENERGY

The assumption that catheter ablative procedure using radiofrequency energy has been unsuccessful in the treatment of scar-related ventricular tachycardia was mainly due to the inability to create large and deep enough lesions, prompted the search for alternative energy sources. Such assumption was supported by the notion that surgical approach utilizing cryoablation of such substrate was more successful. Of the various alternative energy sources, microwave was thought to be an ideal candidate because its radiative form of delivery is expected to be less dependent on contact and able to overcome barriers, such as necrotic tissue without overheating the tissue surface. Favorable results of experimental and clinical data on the use of microwave energy for tissue hyperthermia[17,26-28] further supported the rationale for using this energy for cardiac tissue. However, delivery of microwave energy through cardiac catheters turned out to be a great challenge. Although effective and safe tissue destruction could be achieved, the extent of transcatheter cardiac ablation using microwave energy was limited by suboptimal early antenna and cable prototypes.[22,29,30] Thus, the utility of microwave as a form of alternative energy, at least for the treatment of ventricular tachycardia, was later questioned.

Another rationale for using microwave energy relates to its potential practicality. Because theoretically microwave energy delivery is not limited to a certain electrode size, linear ablation using this form of radiating energy can be accomplished quicker and safer. Unlike radiofrequency ablation, in which optimal energy delivery is limited by electrode size, such as, typically, 8-mm long; microwave ablation can be achieved with antennas of much greater length. With the growing interest in performing catheter-based maze procedure in the left atrium, microwave ablation was again considered as a potentially ideal method of practical, effective, and safe procedure. So far, there are limited data on the performance of microwave linear ablation.

There are other characteristics of microwave ablation that may be of clinical significance.   Owing to its more gradual heating effect,[19,31,32] application of microwave ablation can potentially be easier to titrate, which offers a few potential advantages. If deep tissue heating can be accomplished cumulatively over time, ablation can be performed with a low energy setting, avoiding overheating of the antenna and damage to the endocardial surface. If endocardial damage and coagulum formation could indeed be reduced or eliminated, catheter ablation within the left atrium and ventricle could be attempted with greater freedom and confidence.

2.   BASIC CONCEPTS IN MICROWAVE ABLATION AND IN-VITRO DATA

2.1   Technical Considerations

Similar to the method achieved with radiofrequency and laser ablation, tissue destructive effect of microwave ablation is achieved through thermal injury. However, the mechanism of electromagnetic heating using microwave is fundamentally different from radiofrequency, which utilizes resistive heating method, or laser, which uses photocoagulation mechanism.   In microwave ablation, high-frequency electromagnetic waves are transmitted through a cable and antenna directly to the tissue and causes dielectric oscillation of water molecules, which in turn creates frictional kinetic energy and heat.[33,34]

At the tissue level, this bioenergetic process depends on several variables.[33-37] The rate of heating and tissue distribution of microwave energy are a function of antenna radiation pattern and energy absorption rate, which in turn is influenced by tissue conductive properties and dielectric constant (permittivity) and blood flow. As the microwave field is propagated through the tissue medium, energy is absorbed by the medium and converted into heat.   The rate of absorption of microwave electromagnetic energy by a medium is related to the water content of the medium. Thus, cardiac muscle and blood, which have high water content, would absorb more energy than, for instance fat and desiccated tissue. In tissue with low water content, microwave energy would be minimally absorbed and its radiation would result in deep penetration without significant loss. In this respect, microwave ablation has the advantage of potentially reaching deeply seated muscle and overcoming intervening fat or other tissue with low water content. Energy absorption by tissue is also known as the specific absorption rate (SAR), which is expressed in watts/weight.

Thus, optimal delivery of microwave energy takes advantage of the differences in tissue absorption rate of the electromagnetic energy, which is expressed as tissue dielectric constant or relative permittivity.   While it is recognized that there is also some variability in tissue conductivity and permitivity even within any given tissue, there is more striking differences among various types of tissue.[34,36,37]   Fat tissue has a low permitivity while muscle and blood have high permittivity and are more susceptible to microwave heating. Thus, as mentioned earlier, microwave electromagnetic energy delivery to the target muscular tissue would be impeded by intervening tissue with low dielectric constant and in theory, direct contact to target tissue would not be necessary either. However, it should be noted that in the case of intracardiac ablation, significant amount of microwave energy might be lost to the layer of intervening circulating blood (which has a high relative permittivity) in the case of poor contact.

From the delivery point of view, there are also many variables to be considered. Effectiveness of microwave energy transmission would depend on its delivery apparatus, which is technically more complex than radiofrequency energy delivery system. For example, the coaxial cable must be energy efficient and appropriately tuned to tissue impedance to avoid large energy reflection. To assure conservation of energy, early prototype coaxial cable design was thick, bulky and impractical for manipulation.   Impedance matching was also suboptimal, causing significant reflected energy, which would then result in poor forward energy delivery and over heating of the catheter shaft.

There are also differences in the pattern and depth of heating between the two available microwave frequencies, 915 MHz and 2,450 MHz.   In theory heating can be accomplished at a greater depth using the lower frequency (915 MHz).   However, lower frequency energy has also been known to have disadvantages, such as overheating of the surface and more widespread heating. The higher-frequency source (2,450 MHz) provides more controlled heating and allows for smaller antennae and is, therefore considered to be more suitable for cardiac ablation. Both types of frequency have been used for cardiac ablation and data from some in-vitro studies have showed little or no difference in lesion size generated by the 915 MHz microwave generator frequency as compared to that produced by the 2450 MHz source.[19,31]

Delivery of microwave energy also depends on the type of antenna. Several types of antennae have been described. While most published studies utilized either the helical-coil or monopolar design other prototypes have also been tested.[19,22,29,38-41] While it is still not clear whether there is significant advantages of one type over the other, it would be important to note that the pattern of radiation differs among the various designs. Such consideration may be of some importance in specific application of microwave ablation. It is also noteworthy that the orientation of antenna with respect to the tissue is a critical determinant for ablation efficacy. If the antenna is positioned at an angle with the tissue surface, significant electromagnetic energy might be lost to surrounding circulating blood because it has relative permittivity that is similar to the target muscle tissue.

In terms of its catheter design, microwave ablation system is markedly different from radiofrequency system. One example is the recording mechanism. In microwave ablation catheter, energy is conducted through a special component that is separate from the pacing and recording electrodes. While this feature offers the advantage of recording ability during ablation, it also has technical disadvantages. The additional electrode components add to the bulk of the catheter and the electrodes themselves might interfere with the delivery of microwave energy if placed on the antenna. Similarly, temperature-monitoring element is commonly placed separate from the antenna to avoid direct microwave heating of its metallic components. Thus, the temperature feedback reflects a temperature near but not at the target tissue and must be interpreted accordingly.

2.2   In-Vitro Data

In-vitro studies on microwave ablation reported the feasibility of a certain prototype and measurement of lesion size that is produced by the particular system and, in some cases, reported comparative study with radiofrequency ablation.[18,19,22,32,40-44]

Using a helical coil antenna resonating at the 2,450 MHz frequency, Wonnell et al[18] studied the effect of microwave ablation on a tissue-equivalent gel phantom model and compared the results with those produced by radiofrequency system. The effect of various contact angles was assessed. It was noted that heating patterns from radiofrequency electrodes dropped of much more abruptly than those of microwave's and that when the heat sources were well coupled to the tissue, the effect of microwave ablation was significantly larger than that of radiofrequency. It was also appreciated that heating pattern was significantly affected by the angle between energy source and tissue surface.

In a study assessing characteristics of tissue heating and injury, Whayne et al[19] reported the effects of microwave catheter ablation on isolated porcine right ventricles. The performance of monopolar and helical-coil antennas and 915 MHz and 2450 MHz frequencies were compared. In addition, 915-MHz monopolar antenna system was compared with radiofrequency ablation using 4-mm tip electrode. Comparison of the two frequencies showed no differences in terms of radial temperature profile and lesion dimensions (averaging 7.5 mm in width and 4.5 mm in depth). The two antenna designs also produced similar results except for lesion depth, which was slightly greater with the helical antenna. Overall, the lesions produced from microwave ablation were similar in depth and width to those produced by radiofrequency ablation. However, the time course of lesion formation was much longer with microwave ablation.

While radiofrequency energy reached its peak after 60 seconds or less, microwave ablation effect continued to rise even beyond 600 seconds. Hence it was concluded that with an effective system, microwave ablation would have the potential for creating larger lesion.

The data from in-vitro study performed by Yang et al[20] on ventricular myocardium also confirmed the findings of prior studies with respect to the gradual effect of microwave ablation. The study was performed using helical-coil antenna with 2,450 MHz frequency at varying degree of power and duration. Lesion volume was noted to have a parallel increase with increasing power up to 80 watts and also with ablation duration measured up to 180 seconds. It was noted that the increase in lesion volume was mainly due to increase in lesion depth rather than lesion width or length. Another in-vitro study using an electrode ball tip with 2,450 MHz frequency also showed the correlation between duration of ablation and lesion depth.[39]

The efficacy of a long helical-coil antenna design that was intended for linear lesion ablation was assessed in-vitro in terms of its forward and lateral heating pattern.[22,44] The heating pattern from the helical antenna with 2,450 MHz frequency was noted to correlate with the width and length of the antenna. With this antenna design, however, lesion depth was less than with other prototype described earlier. In a study using a monopole antenna design,[32] it was found that lesion produced by microwave ablation increased in volume with increasing power delivery and duration of ablation but it was also noted that the lesions had greater width than depth. Other investigators reported that pulsing energy delivery produced more uniform temperature gradients and spared the endocardium.[45]

The performance of other antenna designs has also been reported.[38] The lesions produced by three similar antenna designs were described. The antenna consisted of a center and outer conductors with a split dipole, cap-slot, or cap-choke tip, which can be used for electrical recording. Mean lesion volumes were noted to correlate linearly with the power delivered and the degree of contact between tissue and the antenna. With respect to its dimension, average lesion depth (5.4 mm) was also noted to be less than its width (6.9 mm) or length (8.7 mm) using highest energy of 35 watts. Catheter orientation also affected temperature distribution, with perpendicular orientation being the most effective.

Recently, the effects of microwave power, ablation duration, catheter orientation, and degree of antenna-tissue contact on temperature distribution in a phantom tissue using a long helical antenna were assessed (Figure 1, courtesy of Afx Inc. Fremont, California). It was also found that there was a strong influence of ablation duration and delivered power on depth of temperature change (Figures 2 and 3). The helical antenna, as previously described, was more effective when positioned parallel to the tissue surface. At an angle of 30-degrees or greater, there was minimal effect of ablation (Figure 3). However, the effect of ablation was evident in the absence of contact, with the antenna being up to one millimeter away from the surface (Figure 4).

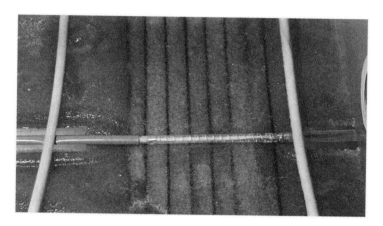

Figure 1. In-vitro study of a helical microwave ablation antenna on a tissue-phantom model. Eight probes are distributed at 5-mm apart as well as at 2-mm depth increments.

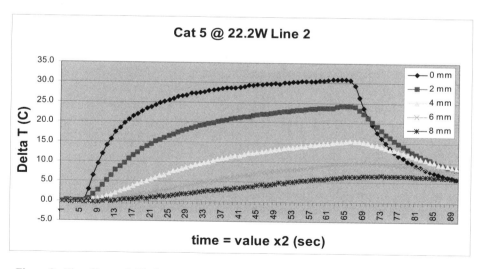

Figure 2. The effects of ablation over time at the various depth within the tissue phantom model

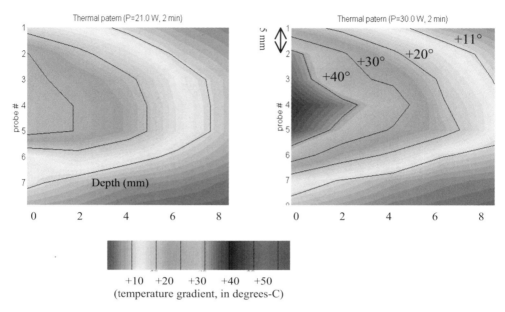

Figure 3. The effect of delivered power on temperature pattern. On the left panel, with 11-watt power, a 20-degree temperature gradient (resulting in a tissue temperature of 57^0 C, the point of irreversible damage) was only noted up to 4-mm depth; however (right panel) with 30-watt power, it reached 7-mm depth. At this power, tissue in contact with the midportion of the antenna reached 77^0 C. See also Color Plate 27.

The rise in temperature was gradual and reached a plateau between 90 to 120 seconds (at which point the ablation was terminated). At 22-watt power shown, even after 120 seconds lesion depth (of 15^0 C temperature gradient) was only at 6 mm. Deeper lesion can be achieved (Figure 3) with higher power, such as 30 watts. At this power, the highest temperature gradient (at the surface and closest to the antenna) was noted to be at 40^0 C, which would produce tissue temperature near 80^0 C, the point of endocardial damage and charring.

The effect of antenna-to-tissue angle was significant with this antenna design whereby at 30^0 or greater angle no effective tissue heating was achieved (Figure 4). Such differential effects may greatly influence the result of ablation, especially when a long antenna is used for linear ablation.

With respect to antenna contact with tissue, we found that while close parallel orientation of the antenna to tissue surface was crucial, complete contact was not necessary. With the antenna at 1-mm removed from tissue surface, heating could still be accomplished, although its depth was diminished (Figure 5). As shown, even though the depth thermal gradient was obviously less than when the antenna was in complete apposition, tissue heating by 20^0 C, which would be sufficient to produce irreversible damage, could be achieved at 4-mm depth when the antenna was 1-mm removed from the surface.

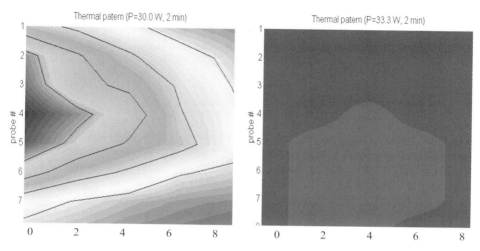

Figure 4. The effect of the angle between antenna and tissue on thermal distribution is shown above. Microwave application at 30 watts with parallel contact on the right panel produced a thermal pattern with effective ablation depth of 7 mm, while application of 33 watts at 30^0 angle produced no effective ablation. Both ablations were performed for 2 minutes. Units of temperature profile, probe configuration (vertical axis) and depth measurement (horizontal axis) are the same as in Figure 3. See also Color Plate 27.

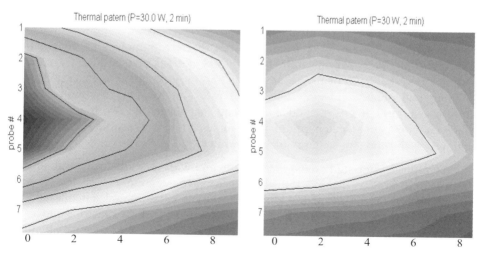

Figure 5. The effect of incomplete contact is shown above. The left shows thermal gradient pattern of complete contact between antenna and tissue surface. The effect of removing the antenna 1-mm away from the surface on thermal gradient distribution is shown on the right panel. Legend for thermal gradient is the same as in Figure 3. The horizontal axis represents depth of lesion. The vertical axis represents the length of antenna. See also Color Plate 27.

These findings may have clinical importance when using this antenna prototype because one can not be sure of the degree of contact and the angle between the antenna and tissue surface especially if such antenna design is to be applied for linear ablation in the atria.

3.   IN-VIVO DATA

There are now several published in-vivo data on microwave ablation using various types of antenna and catheter design and energy source. The studies were performed mainly to assess feasibility, efficacy, and safety of the technology. Langberg et al showed that microwave ablation using helical antenna with 2,450 MHz frequency can produce atrioventricular (AV) block in canines without causing any arrhythmia acutely; although one dog died six days after the ablation.[29] In that study, microwave ablation was applied with 50-watt power for an average of 114 seconds. In another study, Ikeda et al reported that microwave ablation applied to the canine's ventricular myocardium produced ventricular tachyarrhythmia when applied for longer than 90 seconds.[39,46] Microwave energy was delivered at 2,450 MHz frequency using an electrode ball tip. The size of lesion produced correlated with duration ablation and when ablation was applied for longer than 120 seconds, the coagulation layer extended to the epicardium in all of the animals. In their study, Yang et al also reported the safety and efficacy of microwave ablation for AV junction ablation in 11 dogs.[20] The investigators also used 2,450 MHz microwave generator and a helical antenna design. The lesion showed discrete homogenous coagulation necrosis with sharp margins from the adjacent normal myocardium. Lin et al also reported the result of their study using specially designed antenna consisted of inner and outer conductor with 2,450 MHz microwave generator. Using titration energy delivery method, they found that reversible AV block could be achieved with an average energy of 120.6 joules while irreversible AV block was achieved with an average energy of 188.1 joules.[30]

We reported our study using helical antenna with forward-firing and lateral-firing pattern in dogs using 2,450 MHz microwave generator.[22,47,48] We showed the safety and feasibility of the clinical prototype catheter and antenna and its efficacy in producing AV block and bi-directional block at the tricuspid cavo isthmus. We noted that, using such antenna design, after 60-second ablation, lesion depth was limited to 5-mm while its shape corresponded to antenna's length (Figure 6).

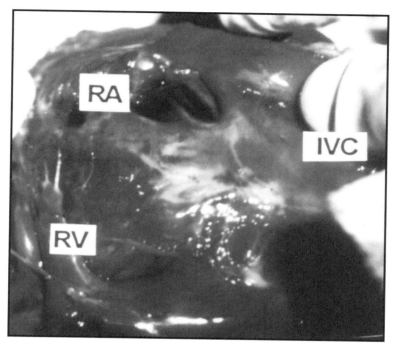

Figure 6. Shown here is the result of microwave ablation of the isthmus between the tricuspid annulus and the inferior vena cava using a helical antenna. Note the linear shape of the lesion (pale endocardial surface) and the absence of charring, coagulum, or other signs of endocardial surface overheating.

It should be noted that when efficacy of energy delivery is not optimal, attempts at overcoming it by delivering more power could result in overheating of endocardial surface (Figure 7). Overall, the lesions created with microwave ablation were noted to be homogenous with clean demarcated borders (Figure 7).

In a study comparing microwave and radiofrequency ablations, other investigators[25] also noted that microwave ablation created lesion with limited depth and width and that the overall lesion dimensions were less than those produced by radiofrequency ablation. In this study using a helical antenna and 915 MHz frequency, the authors also suspected that lesion depth correlated with catheter stability. However, in another study using monopolar antenna and 2,450 MHz frequency, microwave ablation was effective at producing transmural lesions in ventricular myocardium.[21]

Thus, microwave ablation appears to be safe and can be applied using catheter technique. It has also been shown to be effective at producing AV block and may also be suitable for the treatment of atrial flutter. With respect to the size of the lesion, the results were not uniform. While some investigators reported deep and transmural lesions in the ventricle, others reported lesions with depth of only 5 mm. The variations in in-vivo data with respect to lesion depth may be caused by several variables, including those noted in the in-vitro studies. The impact of specific catheter and antenna design may also play an important role and further comparison study is needed.

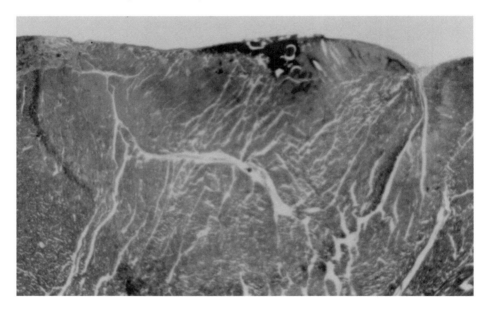

Figure 7.   Shown above is a photograph of low-power microscopic magnification of tissue histology (using trichrome stain) of a canine atrioventricular junction after microwave ablation. The lesion was 6-mm deep and had a clean border. However, a small coagulum was noted on the endocardial surface, which was probably produced by overheating as energy was delivered at a high power (90 watts) to overcome the ineffective early prototype catheter system.

4.   CLINICAL DATA

As most of microwave ablation systems are still in the pre-clinical stage, there is very limited published data on the clinical utility of microwave ablation for the treatment of arrhythmia. Furthermore, because microwave ablation is expected to offer some advantages over using radiofrequency modality, most investigators are attempting to use microwave technology for more complex arrhythmia such as ventricular tachycardia, difficult atrial flutter cases and atrial fibrillation. The assumption that microwave ablation would be effective for discrete targets such as AV junction and AV nodal or accessory pathway reentry arrhythmias, and the fact that such applications are not the aim of microwave ablation, they are not being pursuit. Unpublished data on the use of microwave ablation for AV junction (Figures 8 and 9) and tricuspid cavo isthmus showed the efficacy of this modality for these substrates in human although no comparison was made against radiofrequency energy.

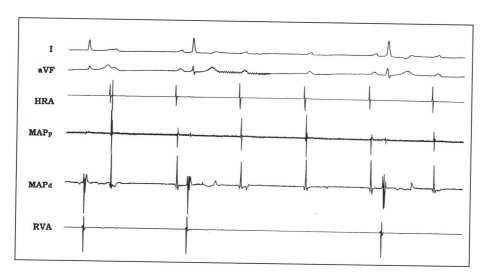

Figure 8. This figure shows the result of AV junction ablation using microwave energy. Surface ECG leads I and aVF are shown along with intracardiac recording from the high right atrium (HRA), microwave catheter (MAP p and MAPd) and the right ventricular apex (RVA). High-grade AV block was accomplished after 54 seconds of application of microwave energy. During ablation, the electrogram was never disturbed (MAPd) because the recording electrodes were separate elements from the microwave antenna (courtesy of Dr. Anthony Nathan, St.Bartholomew Hospital, London, UK).

An interesting observation that was noted during microwave ablation of the AV junction was the absence of rapid junctional tachycardia prior to the development of heart block (Figure 9). In all cases, only a few slow junctional beats were noted and heart block gradually developed with progressive slowing of the junctional escape rate. This phenomenon maybe attributed to the more gradual fashion of microwave heating as compared to radiofrequency ablation. Its mechanism and potential advantages deserve further investigation.

Application of microwave energy for ablation of reentry ventricular tachycardia is not being pursued extensively because enthusiasm in that field has been generally low and because its management with ICD therapy had proved to be very effective. Thus, the main application of microwave ablation has been focused mainly on the management of atrial fibrillation.

The challenges in the application of this new modality for atrial fibrillation are numerous. In terms of catheter technology, the requirement is beyond the concept of delivering the energy effectively through the conduit and out into the tissue. Efficacy of preventing atrial fibrillation propagation in the left atrium is likely dependent on the transmurality and location of the linear ablation as well as its inclusion of the proximal portion of the pulmonary veins. Since many of these factors are still largely unknown, it would be useful to first assess the feasibility, efficacy, and practicality of the technology per se. Thus, microwave ablation should first be applied directly to the targets and in this case, the electrophysiologist must again learn from the arrhythmia surgeon.

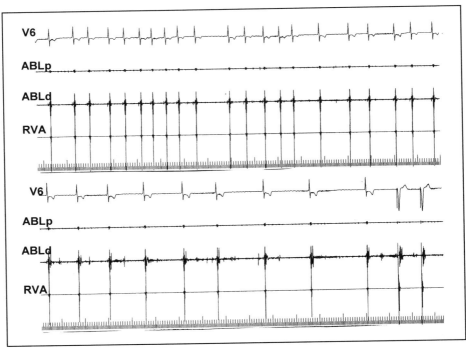

Figure 9. Shown here is the gradual development of complete heart block during microwave ablation. The two tracings are continuous recordings taken during microwave application printed on paper at 12.5 mm/sec speed. Surface ECG lead V6 is shown along with intracardiac recording from the proximal and distal bipolar electrodes of the microwave catheter (ABLp and ABLd, respectively) and from the right ventricular apex (RVA). The ventricular rate was noted to gradually slowed from a baseline rate of 120/minute to less than 40/minute, at which time ventricular pacing was applied at a rate of 60/minute. Note the absence of rapid junctional tachycardia that is usually observed with radiofrequency ablation.

Clinical data on the application of microwave ablation directly in the –open-heart procedure have been published recently.[49,50] Microwave ablation was applied using specially designed applicator for intraoperative technique directly to the left atrial endocardium during cardioplegia in chronic atrial fibrillation patients undergoing mitral valve and coronary artery bypass surgeries. Linear ablation was performed with direct visual guidance from the posterior mitral vale annulus and carried on to the entrances of the left inferior pulmonary vein, left superior pulmonary vein, right superior pulmonary vein and right inferior pulmonary vein, in that order. The ablation portion of the procedure took an average of 15 minutes to complete. The chronic success rate was 64% and 71% in the patients with mitral valve surgery and coronary artery bypass graft, respectively. Atrial transport was noted to be intact in those patients who maintain sinus rhythm.

CONCLUSION

Microwave energy produces tissue hyperthermia by direct radiation method and is therefore an attractive alternative source for myocardial ablation. The method of energy delivery is also markedly different from radiofrequency technology and therefore the progress of microwave ablation has been slow. Many factors must be considered in the design of a microwave catheter such that energy is delivered efficiently without significant loss in the coaxial tubing and without significant reflected energy due to poor tuning. Several antenna designs have been proposed and the results have varied. It appears that antenna orientation with respect to tissue surface is important. Catheter contact, although in theory should be of less importance than with radiofrequency, remains a significant factor for effective heating. So far, in-vitro and in-vivo data have been promising and confirm the promise of microwave utility. Clinical data remains lacking mainly because microwave ablation is intended for ablation of complex arrhythmia, which would require special antenna design, which in itself may reduce the efficacy of microwave delivery. Clinical data from the surgical procedure showed that microwave ablation is indeed practical and effective. Thus, microwave ablation, in concept, is a potentially useful tool for the creation of complex ablation.

REFERENCES

1. Christensen DA and Durney CH. Hyperthermia production for cancer therapy: a review of fundamentals and methods. J Microw Power, 1981;16(2):89-105.
2. Durney C and Christensen D, Hyperthermia for cancer therapy, in Biological Effects and Medical Applications of Electromagnetic Energy, O. Gandhi, Editor. 1990, Prentice Hall: Englewood Cliffs, NJ. p. 439-477.
3. Bolmsjo M, Sturesson C, Wagrell L, et al. Optimizing transurethral microwave thermotherapy: a model for studying power, blood flow, temperature variations and tissue destruction [see comments]. Br J Urol, 1998;81(6):811-816.
4. Cooper KG, Bain C, and Parkin DE. Comparison of microwave endometrial ablation and transcervical resection of the endometrium for treatment of heavy menstrual loss: a randomised trial. Lancet, 1999;354(9193):1859-1863.

5. D'Agostino HB and Solinas A. Percutaneous ablation therapy for hepatocellular carcinomas [comment]. AJR Am J Roentgenol, 1995;164(5):1165-1167.
6. Kigure T, Harada T, Satoh Y, et al. Microwave ablation of the adrenal gland: experimental study and clinical application. Br J Urol, 1996;77(2):215-220.
7. Montorsi F, Guazzoni G, Colombo R, et al. Transrectal microwave hyperthermia for advanced prostate cancer: long- term clinical results. J Urol, 1992;148(2 Pt 1):342-345.
8. Okada S. Local ablation therapy for hepatocellular carcinoma. Semin Liver Dis, 1999;19(3):323-328.
9. Satoh T, Seilhan TM, Stauffer PR, et al. Interstitial helical coil microwave antenna for experimental brain hyperthermia. Neurosurgery, 1988;23(5):564-569.
10. Sneed PK, Gutin PH, Stauffer PR, et al. Thermoradiotherapy of recurrent malignant brain tumors. Int J Radiat Oncol Biol Phys, 1992;23(4):853-861.
11. Erez A and Shitzer A. Controlled destruction and temperature distributions in biological tissues subjected to monoactive electrocoagulation. J Biomech Eng, 1980;102(1):42-49.
12. Organ LW. Electrophysiologic principles of radiofrequency lesion making. Appl Neurophysiol, 1976;39(2):69-76.
13. Haines DE and Watson DD. Tissue heating during radiofrequency catheter ablation: a thermodynamic model and observations in isolated perfused and superfused canine right ventricular free wall. Pacing Clin Electrophysiol, 1989;12(6):962-976.
14. Durney C, Electromagnetic field propagation and interactions with tissue, in An Introduction to the Practical Aspects of Clinical Hyperthermia, S. Fields and J. Hand, Editors. 1990, Taylor and Francis: New York, NY. p. 793-816.
15. Durney CH. Interactions between electromagnetic fields and biological systems. Ann N Y Acad Sci, 1992;649:19-34.
16. Mechling JA and Strohbehn JW. A theoretical comparison of the temperature distributions produced by three interstitial hyperthermia systems [published erratum appears in Int J Radiat Oncol Biol Phys 1987 Jun;13(6):949]. Int J Radiat Oncol Biol Phys, 1986;12(12):2137-2149.
17. Satoh T, Stauffer PR, and Fike JR. Thermal distribution studies of helical coil microwave antennas for interstitial hyperthermia. Int J Radiat Oncol Biol Phys, 1988;15(5):1209-1218.
18. Wonnell TL, Stauffer PR, and Langberg JJ. Evaluation of microwave and radio frequency catheter ablation in a myocardium-equivalent phantom model. IEEE Trans Biomed Eng, 1992;39(10):1086-1095.
19. Whayne JG, Nath S, and Haines DE. Microwave catheter ablation of myocardium in vitro. Assessment of the characteristics of tissue heating and injury. Circulation, 1994;89(5):2390-2395.
20. Yang X, Watanabe I, Kojima T, et al. Microwave ablation of the atrioventricular junction in vivo and ventricular myocardium in vitro and in vivo. Effects of varying power and duration on lesion volume. Jpn Heart J, 1994;35(2):175-191.
21. Watanabe H, Hayashi J, Sugawara M, et al. Experimental application of microwave tissue coagulation to ventricular myocardium. Ann Thorac Surg, 1999;67(3):666-671.
22. Liem LB, Mead RH, Shenasa M, et al. In vitro and in vivo results of transcatheter microwave ablation using forward-firing tip antenna design. Pacing Clin Electrophysiol, 1996;19(11 Pt 2):2004-2008.
23. VanderBrink BA, Gilbride C, Aronovitz MJ, et al. Safety and efficacy of a steerable temperature monitoring microwave catheter system for ventricular myocardial ablation [In Process Citation]. J Cardiovasc Electrophysiol, 2000;11(3):305-310.
24. Vanderbrink BA, Gu Z, Rodriguez V, et al. Microwave ablation using a spiral antenna design in a porcine thigh muscle preparation: in vivo assessment of temperature profile and lesion geometry. J Cardiovasc Electrophysiol, 2000;11(2):193-198.
25. Jumrussirikul P, Chen JT, Jenkins M, et al. Prospective comparison of temperature guided microwave and radiofrequency catheter ablation in the swine heart. Pacing Clin Electrophysiol, 1998;21(7):1364-1374.

26. Bostwick DG and Larson TR. Transurethral microwave thermal therapy: pathologic findings in the canine prostate. Prostate, 1995;26(3):116-122.

27. Hodgson DA, Feldberg IB, Sharp N, et al. Microwave endometrial ablation: development, clinical trials and outcomes at three years. Br J Obstet Gynaecol, 1999;106(7):684-694.

28. Sulser T. [Benign prostatic hyperplasia: prostatectomy and alternatives]. Ther Umsch, 1995;52(6):383-392.

29. Langberg JJ, Wonnell T, Chin MC, et al. Catheter ablation of the atrioventricular junction using a helical microwave antenna: a novel means of coupling energy to the endocardium. Pacing Clin Electrophysiol, 1991;14(12):2105-2113.

30. Lin JC, Beckman KJ, Hariman RJ, et al. Microwave ablation of the atrioventricular junction in open-chest dogs. Bioelectromagnetics, 1995;16(2):97-105.

31. Dudar TE and Jain RK. Differential response of normal and tumor microcirculation to hyperthermia. Cancer Res, 1984;44(2):605-612.

32. Thomas SP, Clout R, Deery C, et al. Microwave ablation of myocardial tissue: the effect of element design, tissue coupling, blood flow, power, and duration of exposure on lesion size. J Cardiovasc Electrophysiol, 1999;10(1):72-78.

33. King R, Trembly B, and Strohbehn J. The electromagnetic field of an insulated antenna in a conducting or dielectric medium. IEEE Trans Microwave Theory Technol MTT, 1983;31:574-582.

34. Johnson C and Guy A. Nonionizing electromagnetic wave effects in biological materials and systems. Proc IEEE, 1972;60:692-709.

35. Guy A. Analysis of electromagnetic fields induced in biological tissues by thermographic studies on equivalent phantom model. IEEE Trans Microw Theory Tech MTT, 1972;19:205-214.

36. Lin J, Microwave propagation in biological dielectrics with application cardiopulmonary interrogation, in Medical Applications of Microwave Imaging, L. Larsen and J. Jacobi, Editors. 1986, IEEE Press: New York, NY. p. 47-58.

37. Lin J, Engineering and biophysical aspects of microwave and radiofrequency radiation, in Hyperthermia, D. Watmough and W. Ross, Editors. 1986, Blackie and Sons: Glasgow, UK. p. 42-75.

38. Lin JC. Catheter microwave ablation therapy for cardiac arrhythmias. Bioelectromagnetics, 1999;Suppl(4):120-132.

39. Ikeda T, Sugi K, Enjoji Y, et al. Relation between the size of lesions and arrhythmias produced by microwave catheter ablation with a special electrode device. Jpn Circ J, 1994;58(3):214-221.

40. Shetty S, Ishii TK, Krum DP, et al. Microwave applicator design for cardiac tissue ablations. J Microw Power Electromagn Energy, 1996;31(1):59-66.

41. Nevels RD, Arndt GD, Raffoul GW, et al. Microwave catheter design. IEEE Trans Biomed Eng, 1998;45(7):885-890.

42. Lin JC and Wang YJ. The cap-choke catheter antenna for microwave ablation treatment. IEEE Trans Biomed Eng, 1996;43(6):657-660.

43. Gu Z, Rappaport CM, Wang PJ, et al. A 2 1/4-turn spiral antenna for catheter cardiac ablation. IEEE Trans Biomed Eng, 1999;46(12):1480-1482.

44. Berube D and Liem L. Microwave catheter ablation for the treatment of atrial flutter. in Surgical Applications of Enrgy. 1998. San Jose, CA: The International Society for Optical Engineering.

45. Haugh C, Davidson ES, Estes NA, 3rd, et al. Pulsing microwave energy: a method to create more uniform myocardial temperature gradients. J Interv Card Electrophysiol, 1997;1(1):57-65.

46. Ikeda T, Sugi K, Fukazawa H, et al. [An experimental study of catheter ablation using microwave energy via coaxial electrode catheter]. Kokyu To Junkan, 1993;41(10):981-985.

47. Liem LB, Mead RH, Shenasa M, et al. Microwave catheter ablation using a clinical prototype system with a lateral firing antenna design. Pacing Clin Electrophysiol, 1998;21(4 Pt 1):714-721.

48. Liem LB and Mead RH. Microwave linear ablation of the isthmus between the inferior vena cava and tricuspid annulus. Pacing Clin Electrophysiol, 1998;21(11 Pt 1):2079-2086.

49. Knaut M, Spitzer SG, Karolyi L, et al. Intraoperative microwave ablation for curative treatment of atrial fibrillation in open heart surgery--the MICRO-STAF and MICRO-PASS pilot trial. MICROwave Application in Surgical treatment of Atrial Fibrillation. MICROwave Application for the Treatment of Atrial Fibrillation in Bypass-Surgery. Thorac Cardiovasc Surg, 1999;47 Suppl 3:379-384.

50. Spitzer SG, Richter P, Knaut M, et al. Treatment of atrial fibrillation in open heart surgery--the potential role of microwave energy. Thorac Cardiovasc Surg, 1999;47 Suppl 3:374-378.

Chapter 27

PULMONARY VENOUS ABLATION USING CIRCUMFERENTIAL ULTRASONIC ENERGY

Robert A. Schweikert, Ennio Pisano**, Rafaelle Fanelli**, Domenico Potenza**, Pietro Santarelli**, Walid Saliba, Douglas Packer[†], David Wilber[‡], Andrea Natale

*The Cleveland Clinic Foundation, Cleveland, Ohio, USA; **Casa Sollievo della Sofferenza, San Giovanni Rotondo, Italy; [†]Mayo Clinic Foundation, Rochester, Minnesota, USA; [‡]University of Chicago, Chicago, Illinois, USA.*

1. ATRIAL FIBRILLATION ABLATION: RATIONALE FOR PULMONARY VEIN ISOLATION

Atrial fibrillation is frequently encountered by clinicians, however the treatment of this condition remains frustrating. Antiarrhythmic drug therapy has had only modest efficacy and has been associated with significant morbidity and even increased mortality. Catheter-based ablation or modification of the atrioventricular node has been used for ventricular rate control; however this approach does not address the ongoing atrial fibrillation and its potential complications of thromboembolism and atrioventricular dyssynchrony.

There is a need for a safe and effective treatment for atrial fibrillation. As with other arrhythmias, knowledge of the mechanisms of initiation and maintenance of atrial fibrillation has been crucial for the development of treatment strategies. The presence of simultaneous multiple wandering reentrant wavelets within the atria has been the most widely accepted hypothesis for the maintenance of atrial fibrillation.[1] This theory led initially to surgical atrial compartmentalization to interrupt the wandering wavelets, "herding" the electrical activity through a maze,[2] but this method requires open-heart surgery. More recently, percutaneous catheter-based method has been developed for the

L. Bing Liem and E. Downar (eds.), Progress in Catheter Ablation, 443-453.

strategical placement of linear endocardial lesions.[3] However, at the present time this method is limited by very long procedure times and low efficacy.

Recently, investigators have reported that the majority of episodes of atrial fibrillation are initiated by focal firing from within the pulmonary veins.[4-6] This led to the development of percutaneous catheter-based methods to map and ablate these focal sites within the pulmonary veins. However, standard mapping techniques and radiofrequency ablation delivered with point lesions have been limited by technical difficulties, significant complications, and long procedure times with high recurrence rates.

These limitations have led investigators to consider an anatomically guided ablation procedure with the goal of electrically isolating the pulmonary veins from the atrium. This method would prevent atrial fibrillation because any focal triggers firing from within the pulmonary veins would not be able to exit the pulmonary veins and reach the atrium (Figure 1). This approach ideally requires a circumferential lesion at the ostium of the pulmonary vein. Catheter-based delivery of single-point radiofrequency lesions around the circumference of the pulmonary vein has been attempted with mixed results. Overall, it has been technically quite difficult, even with the assistance of newer mapping techniques.

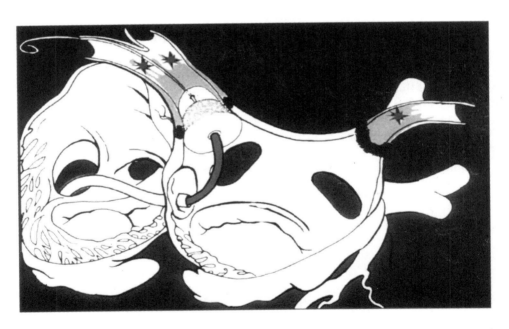

Figure 1: Schematic diagram of atria and pulmonary veins illustrating the concept of isolation of the focal initiators of atrial fibrillation.

The need for a more effective approach to pulmonary vein isolation has become quite evident. One alternative approach is the use of ultrasound energy, which has been previously used for cardiac ablation,[7-9] and appears to produce deeper and more uniform tissue necrosis than radiofrequency energy.[10] Recent animal studies have demonstrated the feasibility and safety of a system that delivers circumferential ultrasonic lesions to the ostia of the pulmonary veins for the purpose of electrical isolation of the pulmonary veins from the atrium.[11, 12] We have recently initiated the experimentation in human subjects of this through-the-balloon circumferential ultrasound vein ablation (CUVA) system (Atrionix, Inc., Palo Alto, CA).

1.1   Methodology for the CUVA System

Instrumentation in this series varied based upon the operator preference. In 18 patients it consisted of a custom-made 7 French 16-electrode catheter, with 8 distal electrodes positioned in the coronary sinus and 8 proximal electrodes floating in the high right atrium. The distance between the 2 sets of electrodes was 7 centimeters. This catheter was used for recording, pacing and internal atrial defibrillation when required. A 4 French bipolar esophageal catheter (CardioCommand, Inc., Tampa, FL) was positioned in the mid-esophagus via the nares to record from the posterior wall of the left atrium. A 7 French octapolar-recording catheter (Boston Scientific EP Technology, Sunnyvale, CA) was placed in the pulmonary vein via transseptal access. This catheter was used for mapping of the atrial premature contraction foci and confirmation of complete conduction block at the junction of the left atrium and pulmonary vein. Several multielectrode mapping catheters were placed in the remaining 12 patients.

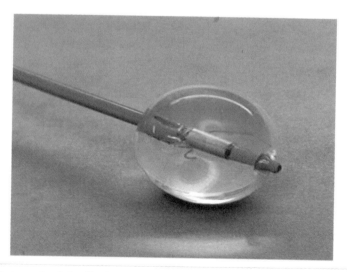

Figure 2: Photograph of the distal portion of the CUVA catheter system showing the ultrasound transducer located centrally within the inflated balloon. Note the two thermocouples within the balloon that provide temperature data for the balloon-tissue interface.

Ablation using the ultrasound balloon system was performed in every pulmonary vein ostium that was larger than 5mm and showed evidence of a sleeve of atrial muscle (manifest by sharp, discrete electrical potentials within the vein), or in pulmonary veins showing firing that triggered the initiation of atrial fibrillation. The ultrasound ablation system consists of a catheter (0.035-inch diameter lumen) with a distal balloon housing a centrally located ultrasound transducer (Figure 2). This transducer converts the high frequency electrical signals from the generator into acoustic energy that is conducted through the balloon wall into the target tissue.

The ultrasound ablation system was deployed into the pulmonary vein using a 12 French sheath that was advanced into the target vein over a deflectable catheter previously placed into the vein. The deflectable catheter was then removed, and a contrast venogram was obtained through the 12 French sheath. A guidewire was then advanced through the sheath into the target pulmonary vein, and the ultrasound ablation system was then advanced over this guidewire to the ostium of the target pulmonary vein (Figure 3, Panel A). In a few instances, preformed 12 French sheaths were used to advance the guidewire directly into the pulmonary vein. Based upon the operator preference, a double transseptal puncture was also used to avoid catheter exchanges for mapping and ablation purposes.

Once the ultrasound ablation system was introduced into the target pulmonary vein and the balloon deployed, a contrast venogram was obtained to demonstrate complete occlusion of the vein with the balloon (Figure 3, Panels B, and C). Ablation system performance and tissue heating was monitored and confirmed by thermocouples on the balloon and the ultrasound transducer. The ultrasound generator was set to a frequency based upon the resonant frequency of the specific transducer, which ranged from 7 to 9 megahertz (MHz). During ablation the energy was adjusted to achieve an interface temperature of 60 to 70 degrees Centigrade. The duration of ablation was two minutes, followed by an additional minute with the balloon inflated. The balloon was then deflated.

After ablation, the ultrasound system was removed and a multielectrode catheter was repositioned into the ablated pulmonary vein. Once entry block into the pulmonary vein was confirmed, a venogram of the ablated pulmonary vein was repeated to exclude acute thrombosis or stenosis. Following the procedure, anticoagulant therapy with warfarin was initiated. The patients were monitored intensively with Holters and an event recorder. All patients underwent spiral computerized tomographic scanning with contrast both before and 3 months after the procedure to assess for development of pulmonary vein stenosis or other structural abnormalities.

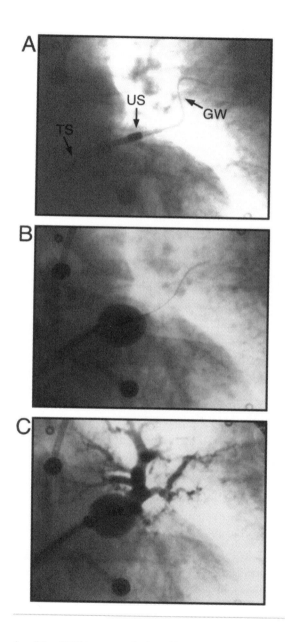

Figure 3: Radiographs of the CUVA system deployed in the left superior pulmonary vein. Panel A: CUVA system deployed through a transseptal sheath into the pulmonary vein over a guidewire. Panel B: CUVA system deployed into the ostium of the pulmonary vein with the balloon inflated. Panel C: Pulmonary venogram with CUVA system balloon inflated. Note that there is complete occlusion of the pulmonary vein, which verifies proper contact between the balloon and the pulmonary vein. TS = transseptal sheath, US = ultrasound transducer, GW = guidewire.

2.   PATIENT POPULATION

Thirty patients were enrolled and underwent ultrasound ablation. The mean age was 54 ± 13 (range, 25 – 69) years. The gender distribution was 13 (43%) male and 17 (57%) female. Twenty patients had no known structural heart disease, six patients had a history of hypertension, one patient had a dilated cardiomyopathy, two patients had valvular heart disease, and 1 patient had coronary artery disease. The mean left ventricular ejection fraction was 56 ± 7 (range, 45 – 70) %. All patients had highly symptomatic atrial fibrillation.

Twenty-five patients had paroxysmal atrial fibrillation, four patients had persistent atrial fibrillation, and one patient had chronic atrial fibrillation. The patients failed a mean of 2.5 ± 1.5 (range, 1 – 6) antiarrhythmic drugs. Fourteen patients failed amiodarone therapy.

2.1   Acute and Follow Up Results

Of the 30 patients, 28 underwent ablation with the Atrionix ultrasound ablation system alone. In one case, a few radiofrequency lesions were required to complete isolation of a pulmonary vein ostium that was larger than the diameter of the balloon. In another case, stable deployment of the CUVA system in the right inferior pulmonary vein could not be achieved, and radiofrequency energy was used. The mean follow up for these patients is 29 (range 5.6 – 50) weeks. Overall, 77 veins were ablated. The mean number of veins ablated per patient was 2.6 ± 0.8. Ninety percent of the patients had their left superior pulmonary vein ablated and 96% had their right superior pulmonary vein ablated. In three patients all four pulmonary veins were isolated.

A total of 495 ultrasonic lesions were delivered, with a mean of 15.4 ± 12.1 (range 3 – 39) ablations per patient and 6.8 ± 7.4 (range 1 – 35) ablations per pulmonary vein. The mean procedure time was 361 ± 181 (range 135 – 705) minutes. The mean fluoroscopy time was 91 ± 46 (range 37 – 188) minutes.

Acute success, defined as electrical isolation of the treated pulmonary veins at the end of the procedure using only the Atrionix ablation system, was achieved in 27 of 30 (90%) patients. Chronic cure was obtained in 16 of 30 (53%) patients, and control of atrial fibrillation with previously ineffective drugs occurred in 9 of 30 (30%) patients. Five patients had recurrence of atrial fibrillation with no improvement.

2.2   Complications

Complications of the procedure included transient myocardial ischemia secondary to air embolism in 1 patient, asymptomatic right hemidiaphragm paralysis in 1 patient, and cerebellar stroke in 1 patient. Only the stroke required intervention.

Transient air embolism is related to access methods and should be limited with better sheaths and improved technique. The right hemidiaphragm paralysis is the result of ablation within the right superior pulmonary vein causing damage to the phrenic nerve which courses just anterior to this structure. This complication could be reduced with better awareness of the potential for this complication and perhaps high-output pacing to exclude diaphragmatic stimulation when ablating in this region. The ischemic stroke is a potential complication of any procedure that involves instrumentation of the left-sided chambers. No evidence of thrombus was seen in the left atrium or near the ablated pulmonary veins in this patient. The patient had reported nearly daily paroxysms of atrial fibrillation. The presence of a pre-existing intracardiac thrombus could not be excluded, as a pre-procedural transesophageal echocardiogram was not performed. It was subsequently learned that the patient had not been consistently taking anticoagulation therapy prior to the procedure. More strict attention to reducing the thromboembolic risk with adherence to anticoagulation guidelines and the performance of pre-procedural transesophageal echocardiogram may help reduce such a serious complication in the future.

No patients had symptoms suggestive of pulmonary vein stenosis. Twenty patients underwent spiral computerized tomographic scanning of the chest with contrast at the three-month post-procedure follow up visit. There was no evidence of pulmonary vein stenosis in these patients.

2.3   Limitations

The CUVA system appeared to be able to achieve acute electrical isolation of the target pulmonary veins in the majority of patients. Electrical isolation of the pulmonary veins via delivery of circumferential ostial lesions avoids the problem of mapping the pulmonary vein triggers as required with focal ablation methods. In addition, ultrasonic lesions in the ostial region of the pulmonary veins may reduce the incidence of pulmonary vein stenosis that has been observed with radiofrequency energy.

Our early experience with the CUVA system has demonstrated that practical and technical issues may limit the efficacy of this approach. There are significant design and methodological limitations of the present system, and there has been difficulty with proper assessment of the pulmonary vein and left atrial anatomy with conventional imaging systems.

The initial design of the CUVA system appeared to have the following limitations. The system may be difficult to deploy, particularly to the inferior pulmonary veins. This seemed to be primarily due to poor torque control of the catheter shaft and the absence of a deflectable tip. The impact of this limitation is attenuated by the fact that the majority of the trigger sites originate from the more accessible superior pulmonary veins. The system can be difficult to align correctly at the ostium of the pulmonary vein without buckling of the catheter, even with the additional support of an extra stiff guidewire. Incorrect alignment may result in an eccentric energy delivery with nonuniform lesion depth around the circumference of the pulmonary vein (Figure 4). This problem may not occur with a more rigid catheter.

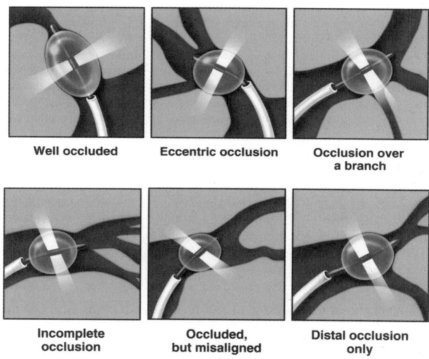

Figure 4: These diagrams illustrate anatomical variants of the pulmonary vein that may affect proper delivery of ultrasound lesions. Top Panel A (from the left): Proper occlusion and alignment of the ultrasound through-the-balloon ablation system. Note that the transducer is aligned parallel to the main axis of the pulmonary vein which optimizes the direction of the delivered ultrasonic lesion. Also note that the vein is occluded optimally with good contact of the midportion of the balloon with the pulmonary vein. The next diagram shows eccentric occlusion of the pulmonary vein with misalignment of the catheter resulting in the transducer not being parallel to the main axis of the pulmonary vein. The next diagram shows complete occlusion of the pulmonary vein distally, with the midportion of the balloon over a proximal branch. Bottom Panel B (from the left): Incomplete occlusion of the pulmonary vein with the ultrasound balloon due to the larger size of the vein. The next diagram shows occlusion of the pulmonary vein with the system misaligned. The next diagram shows complete occlusion with the distal portion of the balloon. However, there is not complete occlusion with the more proximal portion of the balloon, at the site of energy delivery.

The size of the target pulmonary vein had a significant effect on the performance of the CUVA system. In at least two patients, the balloon was of inadequate size for occlusion of the pulmonary vein and delivery of an effective ultrasonic lesion. Also, overinflation of the balloon resulted in suboptimal tissue interface temperature and possibly an ineffective lesion. This required delivery of the ultrasound lesion more distally in the pulmonary vein, which may not isolate more proximal triggering foci. Even with complete pulmonary vein occlusion with the balloon, it was difficult to consistently achieve adequate tissue interface temperature with pulmonary vein ostia larger than 2.0 cm. Investigators have recently demonstrated dilatation of the ostium and proximal portion of the pulmonary veins responsible for triggering atrial fibrillation [13]. Larger balloon sizes with the appropriate power to deliver effective lesions will be necessary in future designs of the CUVA system.

The initial design for the sheath used with the CUVA system had significant limitations. Delivery of the CUVA system to the target pulmonary vein with this sheath required a very meticulous approach to avoid air entry into the sheath secondary to inadequate sealing of the valve. Removal and introduction of catheters via the sheath had to be performed under water using a large basin, which was quite cumbersome. Obviously, an improvement in the design of the sheath is essential. Inability to deliver effective lesions due to the suboptimal temperature achieved was observed when proper transducer alignment to the main axis of the vein could not be obtained (Figure 4). Improvements in the catheter design and/or in the amount of available power may overcome this problem. In a few instances, we encountered a problem with a defective ultrasound transducer, which resulted in inability to deliver effective lesions despite proper system deployment and pulmonary vein occlusion. Improvements in quality control and a better understanding of the ultrasound transducer technology are clearly important.

Retrospective analysis of pulmonary vein angiograms obtained before, during and following ablation with the CUVA system have indicated a several anatomical and methodological issues that represent potential limitations to the delivery of effective lesions (Figures 4). There is presently no reliable method for determining the location of the true ostium of the pulmonary vein, which may result in delivery of lesions beyond the ostium, especially when independent branches take off from a funnel-shaped vein opening. Also, occlusion of the balloon over a proximal branch may result in incomplete isolation. The use of newer intracardiac ultrasound imaging devices may offer the opportunity to apply more precisely and effectively the ultrasound lesions [14]. It is important to realize that the CUVA system is designed specifically for ablation of the pulmonary veins and cannot be used to target other triggering sites, which may include the region of the posterior left atrium near the Marshall's vein remnant, as well as the right atrium and vena cavae.

Some of the patients in this series did not have documented triggering beats at the time of the procedure. However the majority of these patients have had no recurrence of atrial fibrillation since the ultrasound ablation. This implies that these patients had elusive pulmonary vein triggers that were quiescent during the procedure. The ability to achieve empirical pulmonary vein isolation is an important strength of this technique, as it does not rely upon the often-unpredictable frequency of firing of the triggers. In this respect, ablation and isolation of all four pulmonary veins appeared feasible and safe with this ultrasound ablation system.

CONCLUSIONS

In spite of these limitations, the CUVA system was able to deliver effective circumferential ultrasonic lesions to the pulmonary vein ostia in most patients. Therefore, blocking the spread of electrical activity from the pulmonary vein triggers to the left atrium with empirical circumferential ultrasonic lesions in the pulmonary veins appears to be feasible. This approach may become an important new tool for the treatment and prevention of atrial fibrillation. Future generations of the CUVA system should address the aforementioned technical and methodological limitations, so that therapy can be delivered more effectively. Further studies are necessary to determine the long-term efficacy and safety of this promising technique.

REFERENCES

1. Moe GK. On the multiple wavelet hypothesis of atrial fibrillation. Arch Int Pharmacodyn 1962; 140:183.
2. Cox JL, Schuessler RB, Lappas DG, Boineau JP. An 8 1/2-year clinical experience with surgery for atrial fibrillation. Ann Surg 1996; 224:267-73; discussion 273-5.
3. Jais P, Shah DC, Haissaguerre M, et al. Efficacy and safety of septal and left-atrial linear ablation for atrial fibrillation. Am J Cardiol 1999; 84:139R-146R.
4. Chen SA, Hsieh MH, Tai CT, et al. Initiation of atrial fibrillation by ectopic beats originating from the pulmonary veins: electrophysiological characteristics, pharmacological responses, and effects of radiofrequency ablation. Circulation 1999; 100:1879-86.
5. Haissaguerre M, Jais P, Shah DC, et al. Spontaneous initiation of atrial fibrillation by ectopic beats originating in the pulmonary veins. N Engl J Med 1998; 339:659-66.
6. Natale A, Pisano E, Beheiry S, et al. Ablation of right and left atrial premature beats following cardioversion in patients with chronic atrial fibrillation refractory to antiarrhythmic drugs. Am J Cardiol 2000; 85:1372-1375.
7. Zimmer JE, Hynynen K, He DS, Marcus F. The feasibility of using ultrasound for cardiac ablation. IEEE Trans Biomed Eng 1995; 42:891-7.
8. He DS, Zimmer JE, Hynynen K, et al. Application of ultrasound energy for intracardiac ablation of arrhythmias. Eur Heart J 1995; 16:961-6.
9. He DS, Zimmer JE, Hynynen K, et al. Preliminary results using ultrasound energy for ablation of the ventricular myocardium in dogs. Am J Cardiol 1994; 73:1029-31.

10. Hynynen K, Dennie J, Zimmer JE, et al. Cylindrical ultrasonic transducers for cardiac catheter ablation. IEEE Trans Biomed Eng 1997; 44:144-51.
11. Wilber DJ, Arruda M, Wang ZG, Patel A. Circumferential ablation of pulmonary vein ostia with an ultrasound ablation catheter: acute and chronic studies in a canine model. Circulation Supplement 1999; I100:I373.
12. Asirvatham S, Johnson SB, Wahl MR, Packer DL. Circumferential lesion creation in the pulmonary veins using ultrasound energy in dogs (abstr). Circulation 1999; 100:I-65.
13. Lin WS, Prakash VS, Tai CT, et al. Pulmonary Vein Morphology in Patients With Paroxysmal Atrial Fibrillation Initiated by Ectopic Beats Originating From the Pulmonary Veins : Implications for Catheter Ablation. Circulation 2000; 101:1274-1281.
14. Arruda M, Wang ZG, Patel A, et al. Intracardiac echocardiography identifies pulmonary vein ostea more accurately than conventional angiography (abstr.). J Am Coll Cardiol 2000; 35:110A.

Chapter 28

CURRENT PROGRESS OF ABLATION OF FOCAL ATRIAL FIBRILLATION

Shih-Ann Chen

Division of Cardiology, Department of Medicine, National Yang-Ming University School of Medicine and Taipei Veterans General Hospital, Taipei, Taiwan

INTRODUCTION

Atrial fibrillation (AF) is the most common sustained arrhythmia in clinical practice. Antiarrhythmic drugs can be associated with several side effects such as proarrhythmia and an increase in mortality. Catheter ablation of the AV junction with pacemaker implantation can facilitate ventricular rate control, however, the atrial tissues still have the possibility to become fibrillation, thus the but thromboembolic risk is unchanged and atrial systole is not restored. Catheter-based maze procedure is time consuming, also with high recurrence rate. Recently, several reports have demonstrated that most paroxysmal AF is initiated by ectopic beats from the thoracic veins or atria, and radiofrequency catheter ablation can effectively cure AF.[1-11] These ectopic foci include pulmonary veins (PVs), superior vena cava (SVC), ligament of Marshall, cristal terminalis, coronary sinus, and atrial wall.[1-11]

Several critical points would be summarized and emphasized in this chapter to facilitate the rapid progress of focal ablation of AF.

1. CHOICE OF PATIENTS FOR FOCAL ABLATION TECHNIQUE

Because this focal ablation technique is still under investigation, thus the criteria used to select patients for focal ablation of the ectopic beats initiating AF vary in different laboratories. In most laboratories, only the patients with atrial

L. Bing Liem and E. Downar (eds.), Progress in Catheter Ablation, 455-461.

premature beats related to bursts of rapid repetitive atrial depolarization or initiation of AF were considered to be eliminated by radiofrequency ablation. However, the issue about ablating the single atrial premature beat which is not clearly defined to be related to AF is still controversial. In the present stage, the patients who have very frequent episodes of symptomatic paroxysmal AF, without significant structural heart disease, refractory to several antiarrhythmic drugs would be the best candidates. The selection criteria may become loose if the new device can prove its safety and efficacy.

2.   HOW TO DO A SIMPLE AND DELICATE MAPPING

Several important issues about mapping need further discussion. First, the anatomical variations of the PVs, especially their junction with the left atrium, and their branching patterns should be considered. The left PVs (superior and inferior PVs) are often (around 20-30%) known to have a common opening into the left atrium, and trifurcation of the PVs (where the right middle lobe vein and the left lingual lobe vein open separately into the left atrium rather than join the upper PVs) is not rare.[12-17] Several studies also demonstrated dilatation of PV ostium in patients with atria arrhythmias originating from PVs.[18-20] Second, this laboratory and others also reported 5-37 % ectopic beats initiating AF originating from non-PV area.[6,8-11] Thus, simultaneous mapping of multiple PVs using regular size, micro size, Ring, Basket, or Lasso of multielectrode catheters around the ostium and the distal PVs, also the SVC, coronary sinus, cristal terminalis, and Marshall vein would be easy to observe the accurate activation pattern of focal AF (Figure 1).[21,22]

In some patients associated with typical atrial flutter, a multipolar electrode catheter can be positioned around the tricuspid annulus to record the right atrial activation in the lateral wall and the low right atrial isthmus simultaneously.

Additionally, intracardiac ultrasound imaging during the procedure, and spiral CT and MR angiography before the procedure would be useful to precisely delineate the veno-atrial junction area in comparison with angiographic localization.[23-25] Recently, non-contact mapping system has demonstrated the simple and high efficacy in localizing the ectopic focus for initiating focal AF.[26,27]

3.   CHOICE OF TARGET SITES AND PROCEDURE END POINT

There are some limitations using the ablation technique with a "point" lesion to eliminate the AF initiator. These include the possible stenosis inside the pulmonary vein, and the unpredictable electrophysiologic characteristics of AF initiator make the difficulty in inducing depolarization of focal triggers and the poor definition of ablation endpoint.[18]

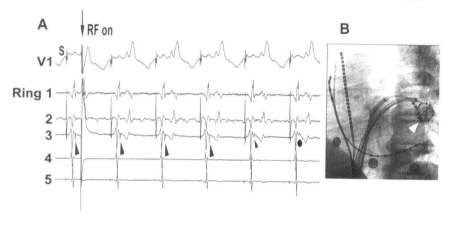

Figure 1. Use of ring catheter mapping of left inferior pulmonary vein (PV) ostium. Application of radiofrequency energy at one point (Ring-3) (arrow in Panel B) eliminated the PV potential (in the Ring 2 and Ring 3 recordings) and disconnected PV and left atrium. Arrows in panel A denoted the PV potential; dot in panel A denoted loss of the PV potential. (From Demonstration in New Deli Batra Heart Center)

Circumferential,[28] segmental, or discrete radiofrequency lesion around the PV (or SVC) ostium, with disconnection between PV (or SVC) and atrial tissues can create a conduction block barrier, thus the rapid PV (or SVC) depolarization can not conduct to the left (right) atrium via the PV (or SVC) ostium (Figure 1).

For the patients with focal AF from ligament of Marshall, it is necessary to disconnect the ligament with the atrial tissues or CS.[10,11] However, the current ablation technique using the endocardial approach only showed a moderate success rate. The other alternative approach using the epicardial ablation technique may improve the success rate. For the atrial foci, the presumed target sites with the earliest activation or unipolar QS pattern would be the optimal ablation sites.[6,29]

4.   RECURRENCE, SAFETY AND COMPLICATION

The success rate of focal ablation may depend on the number of ectopic foci initiating AF. In general, the acute success rate in AF patients with a single ectopic focus is around 90-95%, however, the success rate my decrease to 50-70% in patients with multiple AF initiators.[1-11] Recently, we found the success rate may be higher in patients with ectopic foci from the right atrial area, including SVC and cristal terminalis; maybe most of these foci initiate the typical type of focal AF (burst depolarization from the ectopic focus with normal substrate).[6-8]

Compared to other types of supraventricular tachycardia, the incidence of early (around 25-40%) and late (around 20-50%) recurrent AF after initially successful ablation is still high.[2,3,7,9-11] The long-term follow-up results obtained from point, segmental, or circumferential ablation technique may provide more information to decrease the recurrence. In addition, improvement of the mapping techniques and ablation devices may also decrease the recurrence rate.

Major complications may include cerebral emboli, cardiac perforation, and PV stenosis. The issue of anticoagulation therapy before, during, and after the ablation procedure is concerned. The follow-up methods and definitions of PV stenosis or narrowing may bias the results. Using the angiographic definition of stenosis (vessel narrowing >50%), Jais et al found PV stenosis was <5% in the long-term follow-up.[30] Yu et al used transesophageal echocardiography to assess the effects of RF ablation on PV, and found 30-40% of the ablated PV had increase of PV flow velocity.[31] Application of radiofrequency energy inside the PV or SVC can cause the problem of symptomatic PV stenosis with pulmonary hypertension or SVC syndrome.[30,31] Application of radiofrequency energy with lower power and lower preset temperature around the PV ostium may decrease the risk of PV stenosis.[30] However, correlation between the patients' symptoms of pulmonary hypertension (during rest and exercise) and degree of narrowing or stenosis (by transesophageal echocardiography, CT or MR angiography) need further assessment.

CONCLUSION

Further clinical trials are needed for evaluation of immediate and long- term safety and efficacy of the standard radiofrequency ablation technique or use of new device. The long-term result will provide the new therapeutic modality for cure of paroxysmal AF, and even for cure of chronic AF.[32-34]

Table 1. Critical Points in Focal Ablation of AF

Patient selection criteria

With or without other cardiovascular diseases

Drug refractory or not

Frequent or rare atrial premature beats with AF initiation

Anatomy of thoracic veins

Understanding the anatomic variations of PVs using PV angiography, ICE, CT or MRI

Interpretation of electrical signals

True depolarization or far-field potentials

Understanding the unusual electrophysiologic properties

4. Ablation technique

Electrophysiologic approach – nonprovocative AF as the end-point

Anatomic approach – discrete, segmental, or circumferential ablation with veno-atrial conduction block as the end-point

Optimal energy parameter with minimal complication

5. Prevention of recurrence

Improve the mapping technique

Simultaneous multiple electrode catheters in multiple PVs and other thoracic veins

Ring, Lasso, or Basket catheter to contact whole venous wall

Ensite image system

Improve the ablation device

　　balloon ablation with circumferential lesion

REFERENCES

1. Jais P, Haissaguerre M, Shah DC, et al. A focal source of atrial fibrillation treated by discrete radiofrequency ablation. Circulation 1997; 95: 572-576.
2. Haissaguerre M, Jais P, Shah DC, et al. Spontaneous initiation of atrial fibrillation by ectopic beats originating in the pulmonary veins. New Engl J Med 1998;339:659-666.
3. Wharton JM, Vergara I, Shander G, et al. Identification and ablation of focal mechanisms of atrial fibrillation. Circulation 1998; 98:I-18 (abstract).
4. Lau CP, Tse HF, Ayers GM. Defibrillation guided mapping and radiofrequency ablation of focal atrial fibrillation. J Am Coll Cardiol 1999;33:1217-1226.
5. Hsieh MH, Chen SA, Tai CT, et al. Double multielectrode mapping catheters facilitate radiofrequency catheter ablation of focal atrial fibrillation originating from pulmonary veins. J. Cardiovasc Electrophysiology.1999;10:136-144.
6. Chen SA, Tai CT, Yu WC, et al. Right atrial focal atrial fibrillation – electrophysiologic characteristics and radiofrequency catheter ablation. J Cardiovasc Electrophysiol 1999;10:328-335.
7. Chen SA, Hsieh MH, Tai CT, et al. Initiation of atrial fibrillation by ectopic beats originating from the pulmonary veins --- electrophysiologic characteristics, pharmacologic responses, and effects of radiofrequency ablation. Circulation 1999;100:1879-1886.
8. Tsai CF, Tai CT, Hsieh MH, et al. Paroxysmal atrial fibrillatio initiated by ectopic beats originating in the superior vena cava: electrophysiologic findings and radiofrequency ablation results. Circulation 2000;102:67-74.
9. Natale A, Pisano E, Beheiry S, Richey M, Leonelli F, Fanelli R, Potenza M, Tomassoni G. Ablation of right and left atrial premature beats following cardioversion in patients with chronic atrial fibrillation refractory to antiarrhythmic drugs. Am J Cardiol 2000;85:1372-1377.
10. Hwang C, Wu TJ, Doshi RN, Peter CT, Chen PS. Vein of Marshall cannulation for the analysis of electrical activity in patients with focal atrial fibrillation. Circulation 2000;101:1503-1508.
11. Tai CT, Hsieh MS, Tsai CF, Lin YK, Yu WC, Lee SH, Ding YA, Chang MS, Chen SA. Differentiating the ligament of Marshall from the pulmonary vein musculature potentials in patients with paroxysmal atrial fibrillation: electrophysiological characteristics and results of radiofrequency ablation. PACE 2000 (in press).
12. Michelson E, Salik JO. The vascular pattern of the lung as seen on routine and tomographic studies. Radiology 1959; 73: 511-526.
13. Cory RAS, Valentine EJ. Varying patterns of the lobar branches of the pulmonary artery. Thorax 1959;14:267-280.
14. Hislop A. Reid L. Fetal and childhood development of the intrapulmonary veins in man-branching pattern and structure. Thorax 1973;28:313-319.
15. Rosse C, Caddum-Rosse P. The Lungs. In: Rosse C, ed. Hollinsheads Textbook of Anatomy. Philadelphia, PA: Lippincott-Raven Publications, 1997:441-462.
16. Chen SA, Hsieh MH, Tsai CF, et al. Right middle lobe and left lingular branch of the superior pulmonary vein masquerading as inferior pulmonary vein-A pitfall in ablation of focal atrial fibrillation originating from pulmonary vein. Circulation 1999 (abstract).
17. Johnson CT, Zhong GW, Kall JG, et al. Morphometry and relationships of human left atrial anatomic structures. PACE 1998;21:816 (abstract).
18. Silvaram CA, Asirvatham S, Sebastian C, et al. Transesophageal echo abnormalities of pulmonary veins in atrial tachycardia originating from pulmonary veins. PACE 1998;21:888. (abstract).
19. Chiba N, Nakagawa H, Yoshioka K, et al. Dilatation of the pulmonary veins in patients with idiopathic atrial fibrillation. Circulation 1998, 98, I-702 (abstract).

20. Lin WS, Prakash VS, Tai CT, et al. Pulmonary vein morphology in patients with paroxysmal atrial fibrillation initiated by ectopic beats originating from the pulmonary veins implications for catheter ablation. Circulation 2000;101:1274-1281.
21. Haissaguerre M, Jais P, Shah DC, et al. Spontaneous initiation of atrial fibrillation by ectopic beats originating in the pulmonary veins. New Engl J Med 1998;339:659-666.
22. Guerra PG, SippensGroenewegen A, Mlynash M, et al. Esophageal and coronary sinus sequences predict the pulmonary vein origin of atrial activation. Circulation 1999;100 (suppl):I-653 (abstract).
23. Wahl MR, Roman-Gonzalez J, Asirvatham S, et al. Spatial fusion of ultrasound with computed tomographic imaging of the heart to facilitate 3D mapping. PACE 2000;23:626 (abstract).
24. Tsao HM, Tai CT, Lin YK, et al. An unperceived pulmonary vein: role of right middle pulmonary vein for catheter ablation of paroxysmal atrial fibrillation. Circulation 2000 (abstract).
25. Mangrum JM, Mounsey JP, DiMarco JP, Haines DE. Intracardiac echocardiography-guided, anatomically-based ablation of focal atrial fibrillation originating from pulmonary veins. PACE 2000;23:625 (abstract).
26. Schneider MAE, Ndrepepa G, Zrenner B, et al. Noncontact mapping-guided catheter ablation of atrial fibrillation associated with left atrial ectopy. J Cardiovasc Electrophysiol 2000;11:475-479.
27. Friedman PA, Grice S, Munger TM, et al. Spot Welding the Trigger in Focal Atrial Fibrillation Ablation. J Cardiovasc Electrophysiol 2000 September (in press).
28. Lesh MD, Diederich C, Guerra PG, Goseki Y, Sparks PB. An anatomic approach to prevention of atrial fibrillation: pulmonary vein isolation with through-the-balloon ultrasound ablation (TTB-USA). Thorac Cardiovasc Surg 1999;47(suppl):347-351.
29. Chen SA, Tai CT, Hsieh MH, et al. Recognition and catheter ablation of left atrial non-pulmonary vein dependent focal atrial fibrillation. PACE 1999; 22: 46 (abstract).
30. Jais P, Shah D, Haissaguerre M, et al. Pulmonary vein patency after radiofrequency ablation. PACE 1999; 22: 738 (abstract)
31. Yu WC, Hsu TL, Cheng HC, et al. Focal stenosis of pulmonary vein after application of radiofrequency energy in patients with paroxysmal atrial fibrillation. J Cardiovasc Electrophysiol 2001 (in press).
32. Chen SA, Tai CT, Hsieh MH, et al. Radiofrequency catheter ablation of atrial fibrillation initiated by spontaneous ectopic beats. Europace 2000;2:99-105.
33. Chen SA, Tai CT, Tsai CF, et al. Radiofrequency catheter ablation of atrial fibrillation initiated by pulmonary vein ectopic beats. J Cardiovasc Electrophysiol 2000;11:218-227.
34. Chen SA, Tai CT, Hsieh MH, et al. Radiofrequency catheter ablation of atrial fibrillation initiated by spontaneous ectopic beats. Current Cardiology Reports 2000;2:322-328.

Chapter 29

USE OF CARDIOPULMONARY SUPPORT FOR CATHETER ABLATION OF HEMODYNAMICALLY-UNSTABLE VENTRICULAR TACHYCARDIA

Paolo Della Bella, A.L. Bartorelli, N. Trevisi
Institute of Cardiology, University of Milan, Milan, Italy

INTRODUCTION

Endocardial catheter activation mapping and pacing techniques have been extensively investigated in the last years to guide the choice of the ablation site of postinfarction ventricular tachycardias (VT).[1-3] Although a reasonable success rate can be achieved by radiofrequency (RF) catheter ablation of monomorphic hemodynamically tolerated VT, a more widespread applicability of this technique is prevented by the hemodynamic intolerance of the spontaneously occurring or induced VT,[4,5,18,19] that can be related either to the fast rate of the arrhythmia or to a compromised ventricular function. Worsening of myocardial ischemia due to a diseased coronary anatomy may add a further load during prolonged ventricular tachycardia.[6] The elective institution of a percutaneous venoarterial cardiopulmonary support (pCPS) has been extensively used in the cardiac catheterization laboratory during hisk-risk coronary angioplasty procedures where a low cardiac output state related to myocardial ischemia can be foreseen.[7,8]

On the other hand, the use of cardiopulmonary support has also been described in the setting of cardiogenic shock or even refractory ventricular tachicardia or ventricular fibrillation due to drug toxicity or in the acute phase of myocardial infarction.[9-13] Since the pCPS is able to provide an auxiliary output during short - lasting and transient low-output states, we began recently to investigate the feasibility of using this system to support hypotensive VT.

L. Bing Liem and E. Downar (eds.), Progress in Catheter Ablation, 463-478.

In this chapter the use and the limitations of the pCPS to allow conventional catheter mapping and ablation of hemodynamically intolerated VT are presented and discussed.

1.   PATIENT SELECTION

The frequent occurrence of fast VT causing hemodynamic collapse in patients with an implanted automatic cardioverter defibrillator is a common cause of the so-called "excessive ICD therapy" and leads to deterioration of the quality of life in these patients and sometimes to low acceptance of this therapy despite its potential life-saving effect.[14-17,25] RF catheter ablation of VT is considered a useful adjunctive form of therapy to reduce the incidence of shock treatement,[16,17] but only slow and tolerated tachycardias can be adequately mapped.[18] The use of pCPS may enhance the efficacy of this procedure even on the faster VTs.

A different setting where a pCPS - supported RF catheter ablation may be beneficial -and sometimes may be viewed as the only feasible solution- is represented by true emergencies, following acute myocardial infarction or after cardiac surgery where the frequent occurrence of VT causes a prolonged state of hemodynamic compromise. In this setting, treatment with an ICD has a limited role because of the need for frequent therapies, and sometimes even a vigorous antiarrhythmic therapy can be ineffective or cause a deterioration of the hemodynamic status. The abolition of the VT mechanism in these patients is mandatory.

2.   METHODS OF PCPS INSTITUTION[24,35]

2.1   Preliminary Assessment

A preliminary assessment by echo-Doppler of the carotid arteries is mandatory to exclude patients with major occlusion who could be at risk of cerebrovascular damage. Similarly a significant occlusive disease of the iliac and femoral arteries must be excluded by non-invasive evaluation before undertaking the procedure. Severe aortic valvular insufficiency is a relatively important controindication to any pCPS because of the increased regurgitation flow leading to increased diastolic ventricular pressure.

Preexististing coagulopathy adds a major hemorragic risk because of the need for marked anticoagulation and the use of large-bore cannulas.

In addition of the above mentioned, the finding of fresh thrombi within the left ventricle is a strict contraindication to any procedure where handling of catheters within the chamber is considered.

2.2   Cannula Insertion Technique

Following femoral arterial and venous access catheterization by the standard percutaneous Seldinger technique, full systemic heparinization with 300 U/kg is administered.

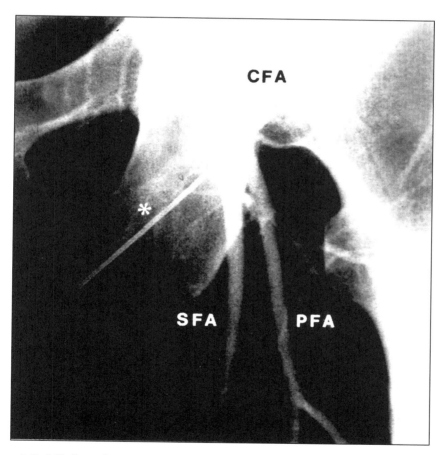

Figure 1. Left iliofemoral angiogram. A needle marker (asterisk) is placed on the patient skin along the groin crease to estabilish the relationship between puncture site and femoral artery bifurcation and to allow appropriate cannulation of the superficial (SFA) or common femoral artery (CFA) rather than the profunda femoris artery (PFA).

An iliofemoral angiogram is performed to assess the level of femoral artery bifurcation and the anatomical suitability of large – bore cannulas insertion (Figure 1). Progressive femoral vessel dilatations are performed to allow insertion of the cannulas. Under fluoroscopic guidance, multiple side-holed arterial (15F) and venous (17F) cannulas are positioned over a 0.038'' extra-stiff Amplatz (Mansfeld Scientific, Boston) "J" tip guide-wire at the proximal common iliac artery or distal abdominal aorta, and at the right atrial – inferior vena cava junction, respectively (Figure 2). The extra-stiff wire reduces the risk of vascular injury while advancing the cannulas into tortuous iliofemoral vessels. All air is carefully purged from the arterial and venous line prior to institution of pCPS.

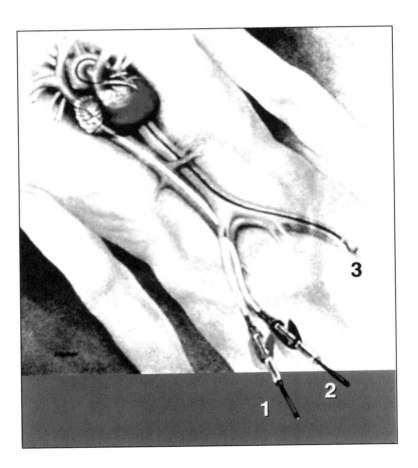

Figure 2. Percutaneous insertion of the arterial (1) and venous (2) cannulae. The arterial cannula is advanced to the proximal common iliac artery or distal abdominal aorta, while the venous cannula is placed above the junction between the right atrium and the inferior vena cava. A left percutaneous femoral approach (3) is used for electrophysiologic study and ablation. The iliofemoral side with the most suitable anatomy for CPS cannula placement is usually chosen.

2.3   pCPS System[20-24]

The pCPS system consists of a centrifugal non-occlusive pump in series with a polypropilene hollow fiber membrane oxygenator combined with a heat exchanger. Venous blood is actively aspired from the right atrium and inferior vena cava by the centrifugal pump. The blood then passes through the heat exchanger and membrane oxygenator and returns into the iliac artery and distal abdominal aorta of the patient (Figure 3). The system achieves flow rates of 1 to 6 L/min and allows retrograde perfusion of the mesenteric, cerebral and coronary circulation. The procedure is performed under deep sedation or anesthesia by the usual cardiac catheterization staff, a cardiac anesthesiologist and a perfusionist. An activated clotting time (ACT) > 350" is assured before pCPS is begun. Initiation of pCPS reduces preload and systemic vascular resistances,[35,36] therefore fluid administration is required in most patients to maintain arterial pressure. During pCPS arterial pressure, capillary wedge pressure, oxygen saturation, electrolyte values and ACT are monitored. At the end of the ablation procedure, the flow rate is progressively reduced over a period of 3 to 5 minutes before termination of the bypass. A cell saver is used to transfuse the blood remaining in the perfusion circuit. Cannulas are percutaneously removed when the ACT is between 150 and 200 seconds and the hemostasis is achieved using a mechanical groin clamp for 2-3 hours.

3.   ELECTROPHYSIOLOGIC PROCEDURE[26-31]

Programmed ventricular stimulation is performed, according to standard techniques, from the right ventricular apex or different left ventricular sites, while the pCPS is on stand-by.

Following the induction of VT, assessment of the hypotensive state is obtained within 30 seconds. In case of an average pressure of 50 mmHg or less, the CPS is turned on and the pump speed is gradually increased to provide an average pressure of 70 mmHg or more.

Activation mapping can therefore be carefully analyzed during ventricular tachycardia, moving the catheter to endocardial areas displaying diastolic activity. Validation of the diastolic electrograms can be searched by performing pacing manouvres, although the risk of inducing acceleration to ventricular flutter or fibrillation increases at shorter cycles, which are more frequently encountered during untolerated ventricular tachycardias.

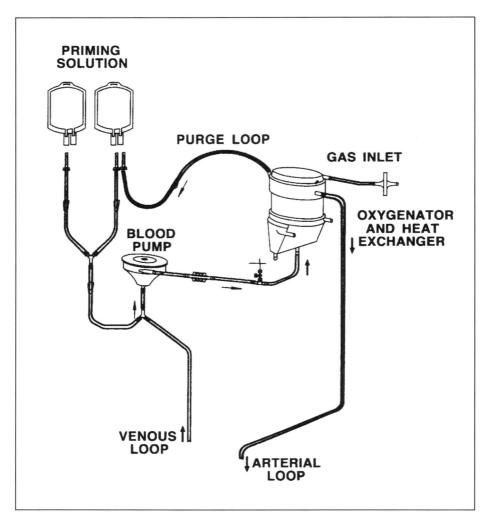

Figure 3. Diagram of the cardiopulmonary bypass support components and circuit. The venous blood is aspirated by a centrifugal pump, propelled through the heat exchanger and the membrane oxygenator and returned to the patients. Volume, crystalloid or blood products can be introduced through the priming line.

Delivery of RF current under thermal control is performed on the target site to obtain termination of the induced tachycardia; the effectiveness of the ablation is checked by a repeat programmed stimulation protocol.

The cardiopulmonary support is turned off at the termination of the VT, when typically the resumption of sinus rhythm is followed by the immediate recovery of an adequate stroke volume and cardiac output. In some istances, however, a variable period of support may be needed to correct a transient hypotension related to a post-ischemic depressed ventricular function. For this reason, it is the attitude in our laboratory to have the ventricular tachycardia interrupted by rapid pacing after 20 minutes, and to allow sinus rhythm for 5 to 10 minutes before attempting to reinduce and map the tachycardia.

The overall duration of the cardiopulmonary assistance should not exceed two hours also to avoid hemolysis.

4.   CASE STUDIES

4.1   Case 1

A 60-year-old man was referred in an emergency situation to the Electrophysiology Laboratory because of very frequent (more than 30 in one day) episodes of fast ventricular tachycardia, causing hemodynamic deterioration and the need for DC shock to terminate the arrhythmia, refractory to high dose intravenous amiodarone, lidocaine and beta-blockers. The patient had suffered one year before an episode of anterior myocardial infarction that had evolved to a left ventricular aneurysm; recently –ten days before the onset of ventricular tachycardias- a blind aneurysmectomy had been performed.

Upon admission the patient was in sinus rhythm. During the first day ten episodes of untolerated VT requiring external cardioversion to restore sinus rhythm occurred. A repeated surgical ventriculotomy to perform a map-guided surgical resection was considered to carry an excessive risk. An emergency RF catheter ablation attempt supported by a percutaneous venoarterial extracorporeal circulation was undertaken.

Under general anesthesia the pCPS was instituted as previously described. During spontaneous sinus rhythm the pump was left on stand-by. A preliminary left ventriculography showed a markedly reduced left ventricular cavity, truncated at the site of plication of the aneurysm (Figure 4).

A 4 mm tip ablation catheter could be easily introduced in the left cavity by a retrograde approach. Programmed ventricular stimulation was undertaken from the right ventricular apex, allowing the induction by two extrastimuli of a monomorphic VT at the rate of 200/min. Due to the lack of pulse pressure during the induction of the arrhythmia, the pump speed was set to provide an output of 2-4 L/min allowing an average pressure of 75 mmHg.

Endocardial activation mapping could then be carefully performed, disclosing the presence of an area with low-amplitude fragmented potentials, extending along the surgical suture of the ventriculotomy to the inferoapical septum, where the local electrogram preceded the onset of the QRS by 134 msec. Due to a risk of VT acceleration, pacing manouvres to prove concealed entrainment were not performed and a first pulse of RF current (temperature: 70°, power: 60 W), was delivered on this site, achieving the first VT interruption after 25 seconds. Several RF current pulses were delivered during sinus rhythm at adjacent sites before attempting a repeat programmed stimulation protocol.

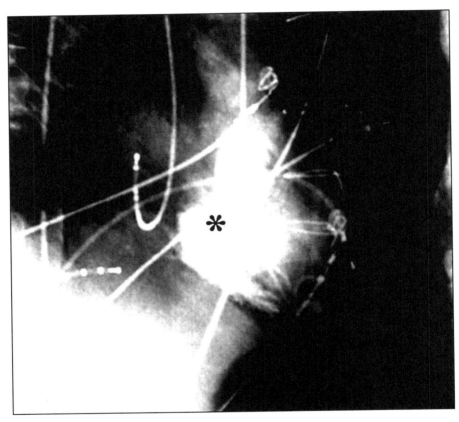

Figure 4. Left ventriculography (RAO projection) of the patient described in case report I. The ventricular cavity is small and appears truncated at the site of the aneurysmectomy as shown by the asterisk)

During the following course of the procedure three other morphologies of hemodynamically untolerated VT (rate: 200-240/min), could be induced by two extrastimuli. Diastolic activity could be consistently found along the suture line, where the delivery of a series of RF pulses enabled interruption of all the induced VTs (Figures 5-7).

In this case the cardiopulmonary support allowed careful conventional endocardial mapping of the left ventricle, showing that the line of suture was acting as the area of slow conduction shared by multiple VTs.

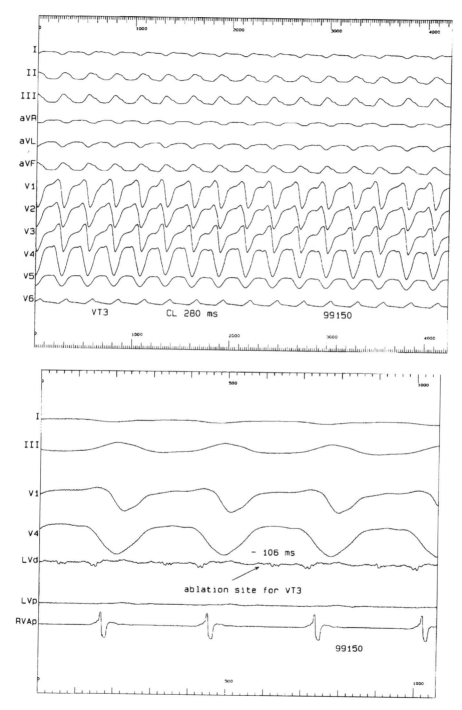

Figure 5 A+B

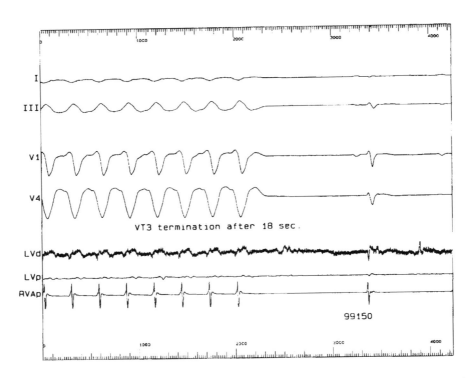

Figures 5A-C (Figures 5A and 5B are displayed on previous page; top and bottom panels, respectively). VT 3 morphology, ablation site and termination is shown (case report I). The procedure was supported by CPS flow (3 L/min), providing a mean arterial pressure of 70 mmHg.

After resumption of regular sinus rhythm a normal hemodynamic status allowed a rapid weaning from the cardiopulmonary support. Repeat programmed stimulation with a complete protocol (up to three extrastimuli) was performed one hour after and no further ventricular tachycardia was induced.

Regular sinus rhythm was documented in the following days and the patient could be discharged from the hospital without any arrhythmia recurrence.

4.2   Case 2

A 73-year-old man had an ICD implanted one year before because of recurrent sustained post-infarcton ventricular tachycardias causing hemodynamic collapse. In the last four months an increased frequency of VT recurrences caused even daily appropriate ICD discharges. The patient was therefore considered for RF catheter ablation as an adjunctive therapy to reduce the number of interventions.

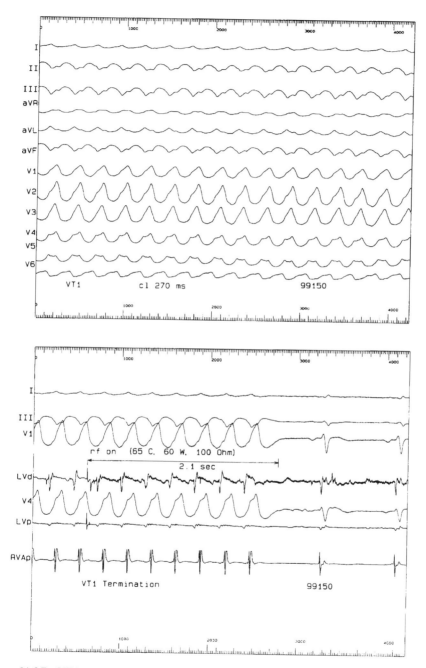

Figure 6A&B. VT1 morphology and termination is shown (case report 1)

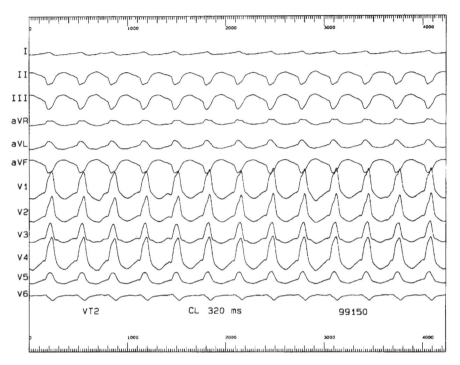

Figure 7. VT2 morphology is shown (case report 1). During VT2, mean arterial pressure (CPS flow = 3.2 L/min) was 70 mmHg.

Following the institution of venoarterial percutaneous cardiopulmonary support, programmed ventricular stimulation was undertaken to induce a sustained monomorphic VT at the rate of 180/min, with an arterial pressure of 40 mmHg; the cardiopulmonary support system was then instituted with an output of 3 L/min, allowing an average blood pressure of 75 mmHg.

During left ventricular mapping, an area with diastolic low amplitude and fragmented potentials was localized in the inferior septum, in the distal third toward the apex. Concealed entrainment could be proven at a site with a local electrogram preceeding of 80 msec the QRS onset. Delivery of RF current on this site caused VT interruption within 10 seconds. Ninety second pulses were sequentially delivered at this and at a closely (2 mm) related site to achieve prevention of inducibility of the target VT. The patient was kept under ECG telemetry the following 4 days. Sinus rhythm could always be documented. Following hospital discharge no further VT episodes could be documented upon interrogation of the ICD.

5.   COMPARISON WITH OTHER TECHNIQUES

Although newer mapping technologies have recently been introduced in the electrophysiology laboratory (non-contact mapping, electroanatomical mapping),[32-34] the concomitant institution of percutaneous venoarterial cardiopulmonary support is helpful in overcoming the limitation of conventional activation mapping techniques using a single catheter.

The use of electroanatomical mapping system[32] provides a reliable reconstruction of the anatomy of a given cardiac chamber coupled to the analysis of the superimposed activation pattern. This information can be obtained with the use of single catheter, but it requires a stable rhythm and a prologed time to define the map. The generation of voltage map during sinus rhythm by this system can be useful to delineate the contour of the infarcted myocardium, but it does not provide information of the functional role of these areas during a given VT.

On the other hand, an istantaneous global activation mapping of a virtually generated cardiac chamber can be visualized by the recently introduced non-contact mapping system.[33] This system requires only a few beats of tachycardia, and the analysis of the isopotential activation map of a given tachycardia can be performed subsequently during sinus rhythm after termination of the arrhythmia.

Furthermore, the system allows precise navigation of the ablation catheter to the endocardium to perform ablation lines aimed at the interruption of a reentry mechanism or to perform punctate lesions to abolish a focal mechanism.

Although suitable for the study and the treatment of unstable arrhythmias, the long – term reliability of this method requires further investigations. The precision to localize a critical area and to navigate the catheter to a target site decreases with the distance from the balloon catheter;[34] this issue becomes relevant in the presence of a dilated ventricle, likely to be found in these settings. Furthermore non-contact mapping requires the placement of two catheters in the ventricle.

A further potential advantage of the CPS aided conventional mapping and ablation technique is that it allows the evalutation of the VT termination during RF delivery; this fact, together with the possibility of studying any type of induced arrhythmia, provides a substantial degree of reliability of procedure outcome that cannot be offered by the aforementioned techniques.

6.   LIMITATION OF THE METHOD

The need for additional staff (perfusionist, anesthesiologist, stand-by surgery) attending to the procedure adds to the overall costs and organization problems of this approach.

An extensive occlusive disease of the ilio – femoral axis or the presence of aorto-femoral bypass consistute a major controindication to the procedure, but this limitation is also shared by others technique requiring catheterization with large sheats (non contact mapping).

The lack of adequate left ventricular venting causing an increase of diastolic pressure represents no more than a theoretical limitation of the partial venoarterial bypass, in the setting of hemodynamic support to an hypotensive VT.

The combination of increased oxygen consumption and diastolic pressure during VT and decreased coronary flow may lead to a deterioration of ventricular function and a troublesome low-output state after resumption of sinus rhythm and CPS interruption. For this reason, a prolonged VT time -even in spite of an apparent adequate arterial pressure- should be avoided by periodical VT interruptions followed by an interval in sinus rhythm.

REFERENCES

1. Stevenson WG, Sager PT, Friedman PL "Entrainment techniques for mapping atrial and ventricular tachycardias" J Cardiovasc. Electrophysiol. 1995; (6): 201-206
2. Stevenson WG, Khan H, Sager PT "Identification of reentry circuit sites during mapping and radiofrequency ablation of ventricular tachycardia late after myocardial infarction" Circulation 88: 1647-70
3. Morady F, Kadish SL, Rosentack WJ "Concealed entrainment as a guide for catheter ablation of ventricular tachycardia in patients with prior myocardial infarction " J Am Coll Cardiol 1988; 11: 1647-70
4. Stevenson WG, Friedman PL, Kocovic PL, Sager PT, Saxon LA, Pavri B "Radiofrequency catheter ablation of ventricular tachycardia after myocardial infarction" Circulation 1998; 98 (4): 308-14
5. Miller JM, Engelsein ED, Groh WJ, Olgin JE, al-Sheick T, Altemose GT "Radiofrequency catheter ablation for post-infarct ventricular tachycardia" Curr. Op Cardiol 1999; 14 (1): 30-5
6. Hoffmann J, Spann JA "Pressure-flow relation in coronary circulation" Physiol. Rev ; 70 (2), 1990
7. Guarneri EM, Califano JR, Shatz RA, Morris NB, Teirstein PS "Utility of standby cardiopulmonary support for elective coronary intervenctions" Catheter Cardiovasc Interv 1999; 46 (1): 32-5
8. Vogel RA "Cardiopulmonary bypass support of high risk angioplasty patients: registry result" J Interv Cardiol 1995; 8 (2): 193-7
9. Shawl FA, Domasky MJ, Wish MH, Davis M, Punja S, Hernandez TJ "Emergency cardiopulmonary bypass support in patients with cardiac arrest in the catheterization laboratory" Cathet Cardiovasc Diagn 1990; 19 (1): 8-12
10. Jasky BE, Lingle RJ, Overlie P, Favrot LK, Willms DC, Chillcott S, Dembitsky WP "Long – term survival with the use of percutaneous extracorporeal life support in patients presenting with acute myocardial infarction and cardiovascular collapse" ASAIO J 1999; 45 (6): 615-18
11. Nagao K, Hayashi N, Arima K, Ooiwa K, Kikushima K, Anazawa T, Ohtsuki J, Kanmatsuse K "Effects of combined emergency cardiopulmonary support and reperfusion treatment in patients with refractory ventricular fibrillation complicating acute myocardial infarction" Intern Med 1999; 38 (9): 710-16

12. Yoshikawa Y, Taniguchi S, Kawata T, Hamada Y, Kawachi K, Kitamura S "Life threatening ventricular tachyarrythmia after CABG in a patient with poor LV function – an experience with the implantable cardioverter-defibrillator" Nippon Kyobu Geka Zasshi (article in Japanese) 1997; 45 (8): 1122-26

13. Behringer W, Sterz F, Domanovits H, Schoerkhuber W, Holzer M, Foedinger M, Lagger AN "Percutaneous cardiopulmonary bypass for therapy resistant cardiac arrest from dygoxin overdose" Resuscitation 1998; 37 (1): 47-50

14. Bocker D, Breithhard G "Antiarrhythmic drugs or implantable cardioverter-defibrillator in heart failure: the "poor heart"." Am J Cardiol 1999; 83 (5B): 83D-87D

15. Cappato R "Secondary prevenction of sudden death: the Dutch Study, the Antiarrhythmics Versus Implantable Defibrillator Trial, the Cardiac Arrest Study Hamburg, and the Canadian Implantable Defibrillator Study" Am J Cardiol 1999; 83 (5B): 68D-73D

16. Strickberger SA, Man KC, Daoud EG, Goyal R, Brinkman K, Hasse C, Bogun F, Knight BP, Weiss R, Bahu M, Morady F "A prospective evalutation of catheter ablation of ventricular tachycardia as adjuvant therapy in patients with coronary artery disease and an implantable cardioverter-defibrillator" Circulation 1997: 96 (5): 1525-31

17. Stevenson WG, Friedman PL, Sweeney MO "Catheter ablation as an adjunct to ICD therapy" Circulation 1997: 96 (5): 1378-80

18. Callans DJ, Zado E, Sarter BH, Schwartzmann D, Gottlieb CD, Mrachlinski FE "Efficacy of radiofrequency catheter ablation for ventricular tachycardia in healed myocardial infarction" Am J Cardiol 1998; 82 (4): 429-32

19. Garan H "A perspective on the ESVEM trial and current knowledge: catheter ablation for ventricular tachyarrhythmias" Prog Cardiovasc Dis 1996; 38 (6): 457-62

20. Teirnstein PS "Cardiopulmonary support" Am J Cardiol 1992; 69 (15): 19F-21F

21. von Segesser LK "Cardiopulmonary support and extracorporeal membrane oxygenation for cardiac assist" Ann Thorac Surg 1999; 68 (2): 627-37

22. Sasako Y, Nakatani T, Nonogi H, Miyazaki S, Kito Y, Takano H, Kawashima Y "Clinical experience of percutaneous cardiopulmonary support" Artif Organs; 20 (6): 733-6

23. Orime Y Shiono M, Hata H, Yagi S, Tsukamoto S, Okumura H. Nakata K, Kimura S, Sezai A, Sezai Y "Clinical experience of percutaneous cardiopulmonary support: its effectiveness and limits" Aritf Organs 1998; 22 (6): 498-501

24. Bartorelli AL, Cossolini M, Crisci S, Glauber M, Valsecchi O, Zecchillo F, Rossi F, Alamanni F, Biglioli P "The role of mechanical circulatoryv support during percutaneous transluminal coronary angioplasty in high-risk patients" Anestesia Cardiotoracica & Circolazione Extracorporea 1995:1; 38-44 (article in Italian)

25. Naccarella F, Rolli A, Carboni A, Finardi A, Aurier E, Favaro L, Contini S, Gherli T, Caponi D, Maranga SS, Lepera G, Bartoletti A "Prospective clinical evalutation and follow-up of a cohort of consecutive VT/VF patients, using a staged-care protocol, including coronary arteriography, programmed electrical stimulation and cardiac surgery" G. Ital. Cardiol 1999; 29 (10): 1142-56

26. Kocovitz DZ, Harada T, Friedman PL, Stevenson WG "Characteristic of electrogram recorded at reentry circuit sites and bystanders during ventricular tachycardia after myocardial infarction" J Am Coll Cardiol 1999; 34 (2): 381-84

27. El-Shalakany A, Haddis T, Papageorgiou P, Epstein L, Josephson ME "Entrainment/mapping criteria for the prediction of termination of ventricular tachycardia by single radiofrequency lesion in patients with coronary artery disease" Circulation 1999; 99 (17): 2283-89

28. Bogun F, Knight B, Goyal R, Strickberger SA, Hohnloser SH, Morady F "Discrete systolic potentials during ventricular tachycardia in patients with prior myocardial infarction" J Cardiovasc Elecrophysiol 1999; 10 (3): 364-9

29. Ellison KE, Friedman PL, Ganz LI, Stevenson WG "Entrainment mapping and radiofrequency catheter ablation of ventricular tachycardia in right ventricular dysplasia" J Am Coll Cardiol 1998; 32 (3): 724-28

30. Saito J, Downar E, Doig JC, Masse S, Sevapsidis E, Shi MH, Chen TC, Kimber S, Harris L Mickleborough LL "Characteristics of local electrograms with diastolic potentials:

identification of different components of return pathways in ventricular tachycardia" J Interv Card Electrophysiol 1998; 2 (3): 235-45

31. Harada T, Aounuma K, Igawa M, Hachiya H, Oh JC, Tomita Y, Suzuki F, Nakagawa T "Catheter ablation of ventricular tachycardia in patients with right ventricular dysplasia: Identification of target sites by entrainment mapping techniques" Pacing Clin Electrophysiol 1998 21 (11Pt2): 2547-50

32. Varanasi S, Dhala A, Blank Z, Deshpande S, Akhtar M, Sra J "Electroanatomical mapping for radiofrequency ablation of cardiac arrhythmias" J Cardiovasc Electrophysiol 1999; 10 (4): 538-44

33. Schilling RJ, Peters NS, Davies DW "Feasibility of a non-contact catheter for endocardial mapping of human ventricular tachycardia" Circulation 1999; 99 (19): 2543-52

34. Schilling RJ, Peters NS, Davies DW "Simultaneous endocardial mapping in the human left ventricle using a noncontact catheter: comparison of contact and reconstructed electrograms during sinus rhythm" Circulation 1998; 98 (9): 887-98

35. Aroesty JM, Shawl FA "Chapter 24: Circulatory Assist Device" in Grossman W, Baim DS "Cardiac Cathetherization, Angiography and Intervention" 5th edition, Williams & Wilkins 1996 Baltimore, Maryland, USA, 1996: 421-62

36. Ronan JA, Shawl FA "Echocardiographic and hemodynamic changes during percutaneous cardiopulmonary bypass" in Shawl FA, ed "Supported complex and high risk coronary angioplasty" Boston, Dordrecht, London: Kluwer Academic Publisher, 1991:57

Part IV

Arrhythmia Surgery

Chapter 30

CURRENT STATUS OF SURGICAL TREATMENT FOR ATRIAL FIBRILLATION

Rainer Moosdorf
Department of Cardiovascular Surgery, Marburg, Germany

INTRODUCTION

Atrial fibrillation is one of the most common arrhythmias, which in major studies has demonstrated a prevalence of 0.4% to 1% in a general population.[1,2] It is considered to be even more frequent in the elderly[3,4] and especially in patients with mitral valve disease in up to 80%.[5,6] The main sequelae of atrial fibrillation are: an irregular ventricular rhythm, often associated with episodes of tachycardia, the loss of atrio-ventricular synchrony with subsequent hemodynamic deterioration and finally embolic complications due to the loss of atrial contractility. Any therapeutic approach must aim at the restoration of a normal sinus rhythm with regular atrio-ventricular conduction and a normal contractility of both atria.

1. ELECTROPHYSIOLOGICAL MECHANISMS

Mainly, there have been three mechanisms discussed for atrial fibrillation: a single automatic ectopic focus with an extremely high frequency, multiple ectopic foci with independent rates and intraatrial reentry circuits, inducing multiple wavelets. The unifocal origin had already been proposed by Rothberger in 1914[7] and has again been brought up Scherf in 1947, when he described an atrial tachycardia caused by the administration of Aconitine.[8] Clinically, this theory has been supported by successful focal ablation of atrial fibrillation, as by Haissaguerre[9] in 1994. However, there are convincing experimental data, demonstrating a persistent atrial fibrillation in all segments after subdivision of

481

L. Bing Liem and E. Downar (eds.), Progress in Catheter Ablation, 481-492.
© 2001 *Kluwer Academic Publishers. Printed in the Netherlands.*

the atrium, while, in case of an ectopic focus, one would expect one segment in fibrillation and the remaining ones with normal electrical activity.[10,11] After further subdivision, atrial fibrillation finally ceases in all of the remaining small tissue segments, which also disproves the multifocal theory, as abnormal electrical activity should have been found at least in some of them.[10] Under these aspects, local isolation or ablation seemed to be successful mainly in very rapid atrial tachycardia or special forms of atrial flutter, degenerating to atrial fibrillation. However, common atrial fibrillation is the result of multiple reentrant circuits. Early experimental studies in isolated hearts could already show, that anatomical obstacles as the orifices of the caval and pulmonary veins as well as different conduction properties, so called "unisotropy", of the atrial myocardium, due to fiber orientation and also pathologic changes, may act as the underlying substrate.[12-15] Finally, the use of a computerized endocardial mapping system in an experimental model by Allessie and associates[16] and especially the use of multipolar mapping arrays in an animal model and later on in patients by Cox and Boineau[17,18] confirmed the multiple wavelet theory on the basis of macroreentrant circuits, but without evidence of microreentrent circuits or focal automaticity.

2.   SURGICAL APPROACHES

Any therapeutic approach to atrial fibrillation should ideally aim at the restoration of a normal regular sinus rhythm, improvement of hemodynamics by a normal atrioventricular synchrony and alleviation of thrombembolic vulnerability. Medical therapy, if able to convert atrial fibrillation into a stable sinus rhythm, would fulfil all three criteria. However, in many patients it is only possible to limit rapid heart rate without influencing the basic risk factors. As well, established interventional therapies like AV-node ablation or modification are merely palliative procedures in restricting the ventricular rate but still leaving both atria in fibrillation. More invasive interventional approaches, creating long linear lesions in the right and also in the left atrium by radiofrequency current, have in recent reports[19] demonstrated the possibility of terminating atrial fibrillation, but are still associated with a number of complications and recurrences,[20] so that further developments by improved techniques have to be awaited.

2.1   Surgical Isolation of the Left Atrium

The surgical isolation of the left atrium was first reported by Williams and associates in 1980.[21] A standard left atriotomy was anteriorly extended across Bachmanns bundle to the left of the right fibrous trigon and also across the mitral valve annulus. Posteriorly it was extended transmuraly to the level of the coronary sinus and endocardialy to the left part of the interatrial septum, again crossing the mitral valve anulus. Additionally, a cryolesion was applied on both sides of the coronary sinus to ablate accompanying interatrial fibers. This surgical procedure was primarily intended for patients with automatic left atrial tachycardia, which could not be localized for focal ablation by intraoperative mapping. It also turned out to be effective in atrial fibrillation by restoring a normal sinus rhythm and atrioventricular conduction via the right atrium. However the isolated left atrium remained silent, or more frequently, in atrial fibrillation after the procedure, so that despite the restoration of a regular heart beat and a hemodynamic contribution of at least the right atrium, left atrial function remained impaired and vulnerability to thromboembolism still present. This procedure was a first step towards a curative therapy, but still left one of the three therapeutic requirements unfulfilled.

2.2 The Corridor Operation

The corridor operation was developed and published by Giraudon and associates in 1985.[22] Its principal concept is described by creating a strip of atrial tissue, connecting the sinoatrial and the atrioventricular node, isolated from the remainder of both atria. During long term follow-up, as reported by van Hemel and collegues,[23] sinus rhythm reappeared in the majority of patients, but however, especially left atrio-ventricular synchrony could not be re-established in any of the patients, with the left atrium silent or fibrillating, so that the heart remained hemodynamically restricted and still a source of thromboemboli. This may explain, why the corridor operation was not accepted on a broader basis.

2.3 The "MAZE" Procedure

Based on intensive electrophysiological studies in animals as well as in patients with supraventricular arrhythmias, Cox and colleagues developed and published a new method in 1991, called the "MAZE" procedure.[18,24,25] The underlying concept is a segmentation of both atria by specially placed incisions, including the amputation of both atrial appendages. The posterior part of the left atrium with the orifices of the pulmonary veins is totally isolated, while the remaining segments are still interconnecting with each other. The incision lines are interrupting the conduction of the underlying reentrant circuits but are still leaving a special route for propagation of the sinus node impulse to the AV-node and the ventricular myocardium. Moreover, the different interconnections between the created atrial segments allow for an electrical activation of the whole atrial myocardium except the pulmonary veins by multiple blind alleys, originating from the main conduction route. In contrast to the previously described corridor-procedure, this atrial MAZE does not only create a continuous conduction route between sinus- and AV-node but also prevents a propagation of the multiple wavelets and still allows a synchronous activation of the atrial segments. So this procedure should fulfil all the requirements for a curative approach in restoring sinus rhythm, atrial contractility and atrio-ventricular synchrony. The initial report of Cox[24] includes seven patients and all of them could be cured from atrial fibrillation without the necessity for further antiarrhythmic drugs. One patient developed an atrial flutter postoperatively, which was referred to an incomplete cryolesion, additionally being placed around the coronary sinus for ablation of its surrounding fibers. After catheter ablation of this remaining area, the patient also returned to a stable sinus rhythm. Besides the restoration of sinus rhythm, also a significant hemodynamic improvement could be demonstrated in all patients and be confirmed by echocardiographic findings of atrial contraction and the presence of an A-wave in doppler-flow, both for the tricuspid and the mitral valve, indicating a preserved atrial transport function. The major drawbacks of this initial MAZE-procedure were its demanding surgical technique and moreover the inappropriate response of the sinus node to exercise demands and the recurrence of left atrial dysfunction. As a consequence, the procedure was modified twice in avoiding incisions in close proximity to the sinus node region and consequently also modifying the other lines of block.[26,27] As a result, the chronotropic incompetence of the sinus node decreased from more than 70% in the first 32 patients after MAZE I to 14% in 47 patients after MAZE III. The improved sinus node function was also reflected in a decreased number of pacemaker requirements from 56% (MAZE I) to 25% (MAZE III). After the initial procedure, only 44% were in stable sinus rhythm, whereas 53% needed atrial pacing and 3% had a recurrence of atrial fibrillation. After the MAZE III-procedure 75% returned to normal sinus rhythm with a necessity for atrial pacing in only 25%. Analogously, the incidence of left atrial dysfunction decreased from 28% to 6%.[28-30]

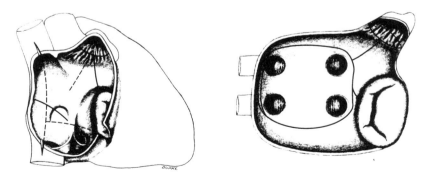

Figure 1: Schematic diagram of the MAZE III procedure. A (Left panel) Right atrial incisions. The free wall of the right atrium is removed. The broken lines represent the incisions over the free wall. B (Right panel). Left atral incisions. A view of the left atrium after removal of the interatrial septum. The broken line demonstrates the anterior amputation line of the left atrial appendage. The black spots in both diagrams show the location of the cryolesions.

While the MAZE I- and the MAZE II-procedure have indeed been limited to smaller series of patients, mainly performed by Cox, the MAZE III-procedure was rapidly adopted by other groups and mainly combined with mitral valve surgery,[31,32] but also with a closure of atrial septal defects and treatment of other concomitant heart diseases.[33,34] The published results of the different groups vary significantly with success rates between 67 and 100% concerning the restoration of sinus rhythm and 52 to 97% concerning the restoration of normal atrial function, especially in respect to the left atrium. However, comparison of these data is very difficult, as there are different indications, different follow up studies and time intervals and finally numerous modifications of the MAZE III procedure have been performed in order to simplify the procedure, as for example by using cryo- or radiofrequency lesions instead of the incisions and at the same time omitting one or another line of block.[35] Especially the electrophysiological background of missing incisions is oftentimes lacking.

3. CURRENT INDICATIONS FOR SURGERY

Indications for surgery are in first line influenced by the symptoms of the patient. Most of them complain about irregular and fast heart beat, oftentimes associated with a feeling of dizziness and also about fatigue, low exercise tolerance and dyspnea. Patients with paroxysmal atrial fibrillation may be more affected by these symptoms than patients with a chronic course and a certain adaptation. Another important point is the risk of thromboembolism and stroke.

In some articles,[28] a failed maximum medical therapy is considered a prerequisite for a surgical indication. However, there is a difference between lone atrial fibrillation and atrial fibrillation concomitant to a structural heart disease. In cases of **lone atrial fibrillation,** maximum medical therapy should precede considerations for surgery. However there may be young patients, in whom long term medication with certain antiarrhythmic drugs is associated with significant side effects and in whom surgery might be preferable. This is especially true for symptomatic patients with hemodynamic deterioration or after an episode of a cerebral ischemia from an embolic event. On the other hand, in elderly patients with generally limited exercise habits, even a failed medical conversion to sinus rhythm, but a sufficient control of the ventricular rate might be considered an appropriate therapy, compared to the perioperative risk. In the same way, only the threat of thrombembolic complications is not considered an indication, especially in the elderly group, as the risk of stroke must be calculated less than the risk of surgery.

In **cases of atrial fibrillation with concomitant structural heart disease**, indications for an adjunctive MAZE-procedure follow different guidelines. In general, the surgical procedure should aim at a complete restoration of the cardiac structures and the restoration of a normal atrio-ventricular function in order to offer the patients maximum benefit. It is well known that after only short episodes of atrial fibrillation in conjunction with a mitral valve disease or a septal defect, a normal sinus rhythm and atrial function may be restored just by repair.[33] However, after periods of more than three months, the probability of a recurrence is steadily increasing.[36] So in patients with a given surgical indication and paroxysmal or even chronic atrial fibrillation, a combined procedure should generally be considered. As in cases with lone atrial fibrillation, risk and benefit must of course be weight against each other. In some of the elderly high risk patients, restriction may be advised in favour of a shorter and simpler procedure. The same is true for cases with severely impaired left ventricular function or with an imminent high risk of surgery.

In general, the question of whether special risk factors may also influence the long term result of the MAZE-procedure, is still a matter of controversial discussion. Commonly, duration of the arrhythmia, left atrial diameter, cardiothoracic ratio and also age of the patient are seen as incremental risk factors for recurrence.[36] However the limits are varying significantly. So for example, the critical atrial diameter ranges from 40 to 80 mm and some others even propagate a MAZE-procedure in so called giant atria.[31] Even if strict guidelines may not be derived from the different observations, it should be taken into consideration, that especially combinations of those risk factors, as for example a long period of atrial fibrillation and a significantly increased atrial diameter will make a lon term success less likely, not only in respect to a stabile sinus rhythm but even more in respect to the recovery of atrial transport function.

Table 1
Results after different types of surgery for atrial fibrillation.

Authors	Surgical technique	No. pts.	Follow up	Sinus rhythm (%)	Pacemaker (%)	RA-Function (%)	LA-Function (%)
Cox (29)	MAZE I, II, III	164	3 mo-8.5 y	93	30.0*	98	86
Isobe (36)	MAZE III	30	8 mo-3.4 y	90	3.3	100	67
Kosakai (35)	MAZE III, modification	101	12 mo-3.1 y	82	4.0	88	73
v. Hemel (23)	Corridor	36	41 mo (mean)	69	13.0	72	0

* including patients with preoperative SA-nodal disease

4.   FUTURE TRENDS IN SURGERY

As already outlined, one restriction for a further expansion of the MAZE-procedure was its surgical complexity and as a consequence, the significant prolongation of cross clamp time. This has led to multiple modifications in terms of fewer incision lines and the use of different ablation techniques instead of cutting the tissue. Initial reports on the minimized MAZE-procedures, which partially are reduced to a right and left atrial incision, the isolation of the pulmonary veins and the amputation of the atrial appendages, show quite favourable results and are significantly less time consuming.[37] However, the missing lines of block are possibly leaving larger areas for wavelet propagation, so that even after restoration of sinus rhythm, parts of the atria may still not resume synchronous contraction and may also act as a source of atrial flutter. Some other groups have substituted a number of the intraatrial incisions by the application of cryothermia, radiofrequency current or laser energy.[35,38] One of the major problems in these simplifying approaches is the penetration depth of the energy used in different areas of the atria. If transmural lesions can be achieved, these procedures may significantly reduce the additional time required with similar results to the original MAZE-procedure. Our group has in 1998 performed a first laser-MAZE-procedure by reducing the incisions to the right and left atrial access and the amputation of the atrial appendages, while creating the other intraatrial lines of block by linear transmural laser lesions. By a number of experimental studies, we could determine the different energies needed for tissue penetration in the right and left atrium and we could also demonstrate, that by continuous cardioplegic perfusion, the lesion at the site of the coronary sinus near the mitral valve anulus would not create any thermal damage to the vessels. This is of major importance, as there is one report about a severe coronary obstruction in distance to a MAZE-procedure with typical cryoablation around the coronary sinus.[39] Meanwhile we have applied this procedure in another four patients with mitral valve disease and one ventricular septal defect and the first observation during follow up level those of the conventional MAZE operation. The main advantage of this new procedure is a significantly reduced cross clamp time, as the creation of the laser lines required a meantime of only fourteen minutes.

While most of the mentioned modifications of the MAZE-procedure were mainly aimed at simplifying the procedure from the surgical point of view, Cox and associates[40,41] have recently published a new development, which is called **radial approach**. While the incisions on the right side remain basicly the same, a totally different concept is presented for the left atrium. The right atrial appendage is no longer amputated and the atrial septal incision extends from the anterior limbus of the fossa ovalis inferoposteriorly down to the posterior interatrial septum, nearly opposite to the former incision of the MAZE-procedure. In the left atrium, the orifices of the pulmonary veins are no longer encircled as a whole but two separate lines are created superiorly and inferiorly, only connecting with the adjacent pulmonary vein orifices by deep cryolesions.

Both incisions end at the level of the mitral valve annulus, supported again by deep cryolesions. The new pattern of incisions pays especially more respect to the blood supply of the different atrial segments and allows a synchronous activation sequence. It may also be expected, that, by no longer isolating a major part of the posterior atrial wall, the transport function of the left atrium will be improved. This has been one of the limitations of the former MAZE-procedure,[42] another one being the increased fluid retention in the postoperative period.[43-45] This is addressed by the preservation of the right atrial appendage, as the atrial natriuretic peptide is mainly produced by the atrial appendages with the right one being predominant. The new design of the radial approach is based on the experiences with the MAZE-procedure and on extensive electrophysiological and anatomical studies of atrial activation sequences and coronary circulation. It may be expected that further improvements of the clinical outcome can be achieved with this new technique.[46,47]

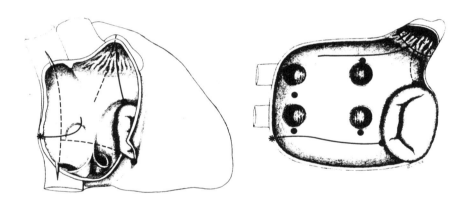

Figure 2: Schematic diagram of the radial approach. A (Left panel). Right atrial incisions. The free wall of the right atrium is removed. The broken lines represent the incisions over the free wall. B (Right panel). Left atral incisions. A view of the left atrium after removal of the interatrial septum. The broken line demonstrates the anterior amputation line of the left atrial appendage. The black spots in both diagrams show the location of the cryolesions. *Corresponding point of septal and inferior left atrial incision.

All of the currently existing procedures, as described above, are necessitating cardiopulmonary bypass. The ubiquitous efforts of minimally invasive surgery have also drawn the attention to a possible off pump procedure for atrial fibrillation. Cox and associates[48] have recently published first experimental data about a MAZE-procedure without cardiopulmonary bypass. By a special catheter based technique of duplicating the atrial wall at the site of the incisions, those may be performed from the outside without cardiac arrest and intracardiac access. However, this procedure can not be performed by a simple sternotomy, as the necessary manipulations for creating the lesions at the posterior wall of the left atrium would lead to severe hemodynamic impairment. So either the extension to a left-sided thoracotomy or, as primarily published, smaller bilateral thoracotomies are necessary to gain access to the target areas. At the moment, this procedure is very time consuming and still in an early experimental stadium. The approach may be further refined by newer techniques and also be supplemented by the use of laser- or thermal energy, so that it might become an interesting option especially for patients with lone atrial fibrillation and no necessity for concomitant open-heart surgery.

CONCLUSION REMARKS

Atrial fibrillation is the most frequent cardiac arrhythmia and associated with a significant morbidity. Medical therapy is in some instances able to convert it into stabile sinusrhythm but can in many cases, especially of long lasting chronic atrial fibrillation, only act as a palliative treatment in controlling the ventricular rate. Unregular heart beat, hemodynamic impairment and the risk of thrombembolism with the necessity of anticoagulation are remaining. The same is true for many of the interventional procedures as AV-node ablation or modification, as normal atrioventricular synchrony and atrial transportfunction cannot be restored. First results of more extensive, MAZE-like AV-ablations are more promising but still associated with variable success rates and the risk of complications. Surgical approaches like especially the MAZE-procedure have proven a high clinical effectivenes in not only restoring regular sinusrhythm but also atrioventricular synchrony and atrial transportfunction, thus leading to improved hemodynamics and a reduced risk of thrombembolism without special medication. These procedures should specially be considered in patients with concommittant heart disease and an indication for open heart surgery, but also in younger patients with lone atrial fibrillation, in whom significant side effects by medical therapy and an increasing comorbidity may be awaited. Newer developments like the radial approach or new minimal invasive off pump techniques may provide even better results and a lower risk. Surgery should be considered as part of the therapeutic options especially in case of medical failure or the necessity for open heart surgery, as it can be performed with an acceptable risk and success rate. The decision for any individual patient should be based on a close interaction between electrophysiologists and experienced cardiac surgeons, which will also stimulate the further development of surgical and interventional methods.

REFERENCES

1. Cameron A, Schwartz MJ, Kronmal R A, Kosinski A S; Prevalence and significance of atrial fibrillation in coronary artery disease (CASS Registry). Am J Cardiol 1988; 61:714-17.

2. Savage D D, Garrison R J, Castelli W P, et al; Prevalence of submitral (anular) calcium and ist correlates in a general population-based sample (the Framingham study) Am J Cardiol 1983; 51:1375-78.

3. Treseder A S, Sastry B S, Thomas T P, Yates M A, Pathy M S; Atrial fibrillation and stroke in elderly hospitalized patients; Age Aging 1986; 15:89-92.

4. Martin A, Benbow L J, Butrous G S, Leach C, Camm A J; Five-year follow-up of 101 elderly subjects by means of long-term ambulatory cardiac monitoring; Eur Heart J 1984; 5:592-96.

5. Hirosawa K, Sekiguchi M, Kasanuki H, et al; Natural history of atrial fibrillation; Heart Vessels 1987; suppl. 2:14-23.

6. Fisher C M; Embolism in atrial fibrillation. In: Kulbertus H E, Olsson S B, Schlepper M, eds; Atrial fibrillation. Hässle A B, Mohndal, Sweden 1982; 192-210.

7. Rothberger C J, Winterberg H; Über Vorhofflimmern und Vorhofflattern; Pfluegers Arch 1914; 160:42-90.

8. Scherf D; Studies on auricular tachycardia caused by aconitine administration; Proc Soc Exp Biol Med 1947; 4:233-39.

9. Haissaguerre M, Gencel L, Fischer B, Metayer P L, Poquet F, Marcus F I, Clementy J; Successful catheter ablation of atrial fibrillation; J Cardiovasc Electrophysiol 1994; 5:1045-52.

10. Garrey W E; Auricular fibrillation; Physiol Rev 1924; 4:215-50.

11. Engelmann T W; Refraktaere Phase und kompensatorische Ruhe in ihrer Bedeutung für den Herzrhythmus; Pfluegers Arch Ges Physiol 1894-95; 59:309-49.

12. Spach M S, Miller III W T, Geselowitz D B, Barr R C, Kootsey J M, Johnson E A; The discontinuous nature of propagation in normal canine cardiac muscle: evidence for recurrent discontinuities of intracellular resistance that affect the membrane currents; Circ Res 1981; 48:39-54.

13. Spach M S, Dolber P C; Relating extracellular potentials and their derivatives to anisotropic propagation at a microscopic level in human cardiac muscle: evidence for electrical uncoupling of side-to-side fiber connections with increasing age; Circ Res 1986; 58:356-71.

14. Moe G K; On the multiple wavelet hypothesis of atrial fibrillation; Arch Int Pharmacodyn 1962; 140:183-88.

15. Lewis T, Dury A N, Iliescu C C; A demonstration of circus movement in clinical flutter of the auricles; Heart 1921; 8:341-59.

16. Allessie M A, Bonke F I M, Schopmann F J G; Circus movement in rabbit atrial muscle as a mechanism of tachycardia. III. The "leading circle" concept: a new mode of circus movement in cardiac tissue without the involvement of an anatomical obstacle; Circ Res 1977; 41:9-18.

17. Boineau J P, Schuessler R B, Mooney C R, et al; Natural and evoked atrial flutter due to circus movement in dogs: role of abnormal atrial pathways, slow conduction, nonuniform refractory period distribution and premature beats; Am J Cardiol 1980; 45:1167-81.

18. Cox J L, Canavan T E, Schuessler R B, Cain M E, Lindsay B D, Stone C, Smith P K, Corr P B, Boineau J P; The surgical treatment of atrial fibrillation II. Intraoperative electrophysiologic mapping and description of the electrophysiologic basis of atrial flutter and atrial fibrillation; J Thorac Cardiovasc Surg 1991; 101:406-26.

19. Swartz J F, Pellersels G, Silvers J, Patten L, Cervantez D; A catheter-based curative approach to atrial fibrillation in humans; Circulation 1994;90 suppl:335.

20. Zhou L, Keane D, Reed G, Ruskin J; Thromboembolic complications of cardiac radiofrequency catheter ablation: a review of the reported incidence, pathogenesis and current research directions; J Cardiovasc Electrophysiol 1999; 10(4):611-20.

21. Williams J M, Ungerleider R M, Lofland G K, Cox J L; Left atrial isolation: a new technique for the treatment of supraventricular arrhythmias; J Thorac Cardiovasc Surg 1980; 80:373-80.

22. Defauw J J A M T, Guiraudon G M, van Hemel N M, Vermeulen F E E, Kingma J H, de Bakker J M T; Surgical therapy of paroxysmal atrial fibrillation with the „corridor" operation; Ann Thorac Surg 1992;53:569-71.

23. N M van Hemel, J J A M T Defauw, J H Kingma, W Jaarsma, F E E Vermeulen, J M T de Bakker, G M Guiraudon; Long-term results of the corridor operation for atrial fibrillation (Br Heart J 1994; 71:170-76).

24. Cox J L, Schuessler R B, ´Agostino Jr. H J D, Stone C M, Chang BC, Cain M E, Corr P B, Boineau J P; The surgical treatment of atrial fibrillation III. Development of a definitive surgical procedure; J Thorac Cardiovasc Surg 1991; 101:569-83.

25. Cox J L; The surgical treatment of atrial fibrillation; IV. Surgical technique; J Thorac Cardiovasc Surg 1991; 101:584-92.

26. Cox J L, Boineau J P, Schuessler R B, Jaquiss R D B, Lappas D G; Modification of the maze procedure for Atrial Flutter and Atrial Fibrillation; I. Rationale and surgical results; J Thorac Cardiovasc Surg 1995; 110:473-84.

27. Cox J L, Jaquiss R D B, Schuessler R B, Boineau J P; Modification of the Maze Procedure for Atrial Flutter and Atrial Fibrillation; II. Surgical technique of the maze III procedure; J Thorac Cardiovasc Surg 1995; 110:485-95.

28. Cox J L, Sundt III T M; The Surgical Management of Atrial Fibrillation; Annu. Rev. Med. 1997; 48:511-23.

29. Cox J L, Schuessler R B, Lappas D G, Boineau J P; An 81/2-Year Clinical Experience with Surgery for Atrial Fibrillation; Annals of Surgery 1996; Vol. 224 (3): 267-75.

30. Cox J L; Atrial transport function after the Maze procedure for atrial fibrillation: A 10-year clinical experience; Am Heart J 1998;136:934-36.

31. Yuda S, Nakatani S, Isobe F, Kosakai Y, Miyatake K; Comparative Efficacy of the Maze Procedure for Restoration of Atrial Contraction in Patients With and Without Giant Left Atrium Associated With Mitral Valve Disease; J Am Coll Cardiol 1998;31:1097-102.

32. McCarthy P M, Castle L W, Maloney J D, Trohman R G, Simmons T W, White R D, Klein A L, Cosgrove III D M; Initial experience with the maze procedure for atrial fibrillation; J Thorac Cardiovasc Surg 1993;105:1077-87.

33. Musci M, Pasic M, Siniawaski H, Lehmkuhl H, Edelmann B, Hetzer R; „Cox/Maze-III-Operation" als chirurgische Therapie des chronischen Vorhofflimmerns während Mitralklappen- und ASD-II-Operation; Z Kardiol 1998; 87:202-08.

34. Kobayashi J, Yamamoto F, Nakano K, Sasako Y, Kitamura S, Kosakai Y; Maze Procedure for Atrial Fibrillation Associated With Atrial Septal Defect; Circulation 1998;98:399-402.

35. Kosakai Y, Kawaguchi A T, Isobe F, Sasako Y, Nakano K, Eishi K, Kito Y, Kawashima Y; Modified Maze Procedure for Patients With Atrial Fibrillation Undergoing Simultaneous Open Heart Surgery; Circulation 1995;92, suppl II:359-64.

36. Isobe F, Kawashima Y; The Outcome and Indications of the Cox Maze III Procedure for Chronic Atrial Fibrillation with Mitral Valve Disease; J Thorac Cardiovasc Surg 1998; 116:220-27

37. Fieguth H G, Wahlers T, Borst H G; Inhibition of atrial fibrillation by pulmonary vein isolation and auricular resection--experimental study in a sheep model; Eur J Cardiothorac Surg 1997; 11(4):714-21.

38. Patwardhan A M, Dave H H, Tamhane A A, Pandit S P, Dalvi B V, Golam K, Kaul A, Chaukar A P; Intraoperative radiofrequency microbipolar coagulation to replace incisions of maze III procedure for correcting atrial fibrillation in patients with rheumatic valvular disease; Eur J Cardiothorac Surg 1997; 124(4):627-33.

39. Sueda T, Shikata H, Mitsui N, Nagata H, Matsuura Y; Myocardial Infarction after a Maze Procedure for Idiopathic Atrial Fibrillation; J Thorac Cardiovasc Surg 1996;112:549-50.

40. Nitta T, Lee R, Schuessler R B, Boineau J P, Cox J L; Radial Approach: A New Concept in Surgical Treatment for Atrial Fibrillation I. Concept, Anatomic and Physiologic Bases and Develeopment of a Procedure; Ann Thorac Surg 1999; 67:27-35.

41. Nitta T, Lee R, Watanabe H, Harris K M, Erikson J M, Schuessler R B, Boineau J P, Cox J L; Radial Approach: A New Concept in Surgical Treatment for Atrial Fibrillation. II. Electrophysiologic Effects and Atrial Contribution to Ventricular Filling; Ann Thorac Surg 1999; 67:36-50.

42. Feinberg M S, Waggoner A D, Kater K M, Cox J L, Lindsay B D, Pérez J E; Restoration of Atrial Function After the Maze Procedure for Patients With Atrial Fibrillation, Assessment by Doppler Echocardiography; Circulation 1994; 90: 285-92.

43. Perera S A, Frame R, Brodman R F, Zeballos G A, Hintze Th H, Panetta Th F; Atrial Natriuretic Peptide Replacement Therapy in Rats Subjected to Biatrial Appendectomy; J Thorac Cardiovasc Surg 1995;109:976-80.
44. Ki-Bong K, Chang-Ha L, Cheol-Ho K, Young-Joo C; Effect of the Maze procedure on the secretion of atrial natriuretic peptide; J Thorac Cardiovasc Surg 1998;115:139-47.
45. Fukushima K, Emori T, Shimizu W, Kurita T, Aihara N, Kosakai Y, Isobe F, Shimomura K, Kawashima Y, Ohe T; Delayed improvement of autonomic nervous abnormality after the Maze procedure: time and frequency domain analysis of heart rate variability using 24 Hour Holter monitoring; Heart 1997; 78:499-504.
46. Pasic M, Musci M, Siniawski H, Edelmann B, Tedoriya T, Hetzer R; Transient Sinus Node Dysfunction After the Cox-Maze III Procedure in Patients With Organic Heart Disease and Chronic Fixed Atrial Fibrillation; J Am Coll Cardiol 1998;32:1040-47.
47. Kawaguchi A T, Kosakai Y, Isobe F, Sasako Y, Eishi K, Nakano K, Takahashi N, Kawashima Y; Factors Affecting Rhythm After the Maze Procedure for Atrial Fibrillation; Circulation 1996;94 suppl II: 139-42.
48. Lee R, Nitta T, Schuessler R B, Johnson D C, Boineau J P, Cox J L; The Closed Heart MAZE: A Nonbypass Surgical Technique; Ann Thorac Surg 1999; 67:1696-702.

Chapter 31

UTILITY OF RADIOFREQUENCY ABLATION IN ATRIAL FIBRILLATION SURGERY

Teresa Santiago, Rosa Gouveia, Ana P. Martins, João Melo
Hospital de Santa Cruz, Linda-a-Velha, Portuga;

INTRODUCTION

Atrial fibrillation surgery is an evolving procedure. The maze operation, developed by James Cox,[1] has been the standard operation since the early nineties. However, the maze operation is a complex procedure with bleeding potential that always requires the use of cardiopulmonary bypass and a long myocardial ischemic time. Because of the complexity of the maze operation, different alternatives have been proposed aiming at simplifying the techniques and reducing the time and risks of the operation.[2-4] The final goal of each particular procedure is to create scars in the atrial wall in such a way that the initiators, the perpetuators or both mechanisms of atrial fibrillation will be eliminated.

Different physical agents can be selected to create these atrial scars. The most commonly used are radiofrequency, cryoablation, microwave and laser.

Our group has, since December 1996, selected to perform atrial fibrillation surgery using intraoperative radiofrequency catheter ablation. Our results are very satisfactory mainly in mitral patients with a left atrium smaller than 200 cubic-cm.[5] For optimal results to be achieved it is necessary to create full thickness scars. Unless these are obtained it will not be possible to assess which are the best operative techniques and to understand, to some extent, the underlying factors that lead to good results.

We present our current knowledge on the use of intraoperative endocardial radiofrequency catheter ablation for the treatment of chronic atrial fibrillation in mitral patients, acquired through in-vitro studies, experimental surgical radiofrequency ablation in animals and clinical cases. In order to avoid

L. Bing Liem and E. Downar (eds.), Progress in Catheter Ablation, 493-506.

cardiopulmonary bypass during experimental surgery in pigs, the radiofrequency applications were performed epicardially (with settings that had been previously studied in vitro using fragments of pig's atria) to assess its safety, namely when applied near the large caliber coronary arteries.

Samples were histologically assessed at all stages of the process to determine the depth of the lesions and correlate them with the radiofrequency settings that led to transmural lesions.

1. IN-VITRO EXPERIMENTAL STUDIES

1.1 Radiofrequency Settings and Types of Applications

When radiofrequency electrical currents are delivered to biological tissues the energy is converted into heat, according to the Joule effect, in the close vicinity of the active electrode where the density of current lines is highest. Heat is then transmitted to the remaining tissue by conduction and dissipated by convection. The temperature reached at different depths of the biological tissue is therefore dependent on the radiofrequency settings and the type of the application.

Most radiofrequency generators used in therapeutical ablation work under temperature control, i.e., the temperature is measured on the tissue's surface by means of sensors in the catheter, and power is delivered to the tissue until the temperature set by the user has been attained. In other words, the temperature on the catheter/myocardium interface does not exceed, within a predetermined error and over a certain time interval, the value set by the user.

Although the temperature at the surface is known and maintained around the set value throughout the ablation, the same does not apply to the temperature inside the tissue. In fact, the physical conditions at the tissue's surface are determined by the different forms of application: in endocardial applications during surgery the atria are cooled to around $30°$ C and there are heat exchanges between the endocardial and epicardial surfaces and the atmosphere; in epicardial applications off pump the atria is at body temperature and heat exchanges take place between the epicardium and the surrounding air, while the endocardial surface is being cooled by the circulating blood. In both cases the physical conditions at the point of radiofrequency application are different from those deeper into the myocardium. Although it might appear that the temperature inside the tissue is lower than at the surface, this is not necessarily true all along the depth of the tissue. Because power is applied, up to a set temperature, on a surface that is being cooled, electric current is conducted into areas of the tissue that are not being cooled hence raising its temperature to values that may be higher than those at the application surface. Deeper into the tissue the temperature will drop off to a value on the opposite surface that is likely to depend on the thickness of the myocardium and the physical conditions at that surface.

On the light of the above, and because it is believed that lesions are irreversible above 50° C we found it pertinent to study, in-vitro, the dependence of the temperatures measured sub-endocardially and sub-epicardially on the different settings of radiofrequency applications, and on the thickness of the atrial wall. We aim at determining the radiofrequency settings that lead to temperatures, on the myocardial surface opposite to the application surface, capable of producing permanent lesions.

1.2   In-vitro endocardial radiofrequency applications

The thickness of 14 human atria fragments from donors was measured at several points with a digitizer Pohemus B105A with an error of 1/3 mm. The digitizer was connected to a PC for data acquisition and processing.

T-type thermocouples were inserted sub-endocardially and sub-epicardially at those points and connected to a specially modified Meca APM Switch Box (EPT Technologies) for signal processing. The box was connected to a PC for data acquisition and real time graphics display of sub-endocardial and sub-epicardial temperature. Radiofrequency currents were then applied on the endocardial surface using a Thermaline catheter connected through a Meca Switch Box to a radiofrequency generator (EPT Technologies). The generator's RS output was connected to a portable PC and the variation of power, impedance and temperature (measured by the sensors in the catheter) were displayed in real time by means of an EPT graphics software. It was therefore possible to compare the variation in time of the temperature at the endocardium surface, with that of the temperatures measured simultaneously by the thermocouples placed sub-endocardially and sub-epicardially at several points of the atrial wall, whose thickness had previously been measured.

Figure 1A shows an example of the temperatures measured sub-endocardially and sub-epicardially during endocardial radiofrequency application at set temperatures of 70° C in three points where the atrial wall was 5.1, 3.4 and 3.1 mm thick. The sub- endocardial temperatures at those points are 5 to 10 °C higher than the set temperature which remains fairly constant throughout the application as can be seen in Figure 1B. The sub-epicardial temperatures vary between 50 and 66° C and are generally lower at points where the wall is thicker, as expected[*].

---

[*]However, this is not always true due to some imprecision in the depth of insertion of the thermocouples.

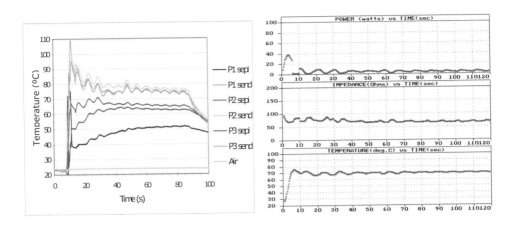

Figure1. A (Left panel) Sub-endocardial (send) and sub-epicardial (sepi) temperatures measured at three points of human atrial myocardium with thickness 5.1±0.3 mm (P1), 3.4±0.3mm (P2) and 3.1±0.3 mm (P3). B (Right Panel) Variation in time of power, impedance and temperature (measured on the endocardial surface) during an endocardial application of RF at a set temperature of 70° C.

Figure 2A shows a similar example for an application at set temperature of 80° C, in three points where the atrial wall was 4.6, 5.0 and 4.2 mm thick. The sub-endocardial temperatures are on average 10 to 15° C higher than the set value, which again remains fairly constant throughout the application (Figure 2B).

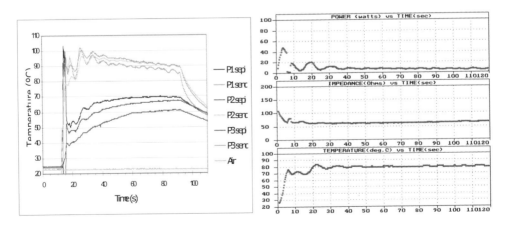

Figure 2. A (Left panel) Sub-endocardial (send) and sub-epicardial (sepi) temperatures measured at three points of human atrial myocardium with thickness 4.6±0.4 mm (P1), 5.0±0.3mm (P2) and 4.2±0.3 mm (P3). B (Right panel) Variation in time of power, impedance and temperature (measured on the endocardial surface) during an endocardial application of RF at a set temperature of 80° C.

The sub-epicardial temperatures vary from 60 to 70° C and are higher than the ones reached in the application at set 70° C on points where the atria have similar thickness. However, the sub-epicardial temperatures reach similar values to the ones of application at 70° C in points where the atria is thicker, confirming the notion that in the case of thicker atrial walls the set temperature needs to be higher if lesion forming temperatures are to be attained on the opposite surface.

However if, as is often the case in clinical ablation, the first application was aborted usually due to poor contact with the tissue, and a second application followed as soon as the temperature on the application surface was low enough for the generator to deliver power, the sub-epicardial temperatures reached higher values than they did when the intra-atrial tissue was at room temperature. In fact, the endocardial surface being in contact with the air cools down faster than the remaining tissue, and a temperature gradient exists between this surface and the inside of the tissue. When a second application starts the system applies power until the temperature at the surface is at the set value. Because the interior of the tissue was warmer than the surface its temperature will rise further to values that can be significantly higher than the set temperature.

Table I shows, for several wall thickness, the values (mean and standard deviation) of the sub-epicardial temperatures and the depth of the lesions in endocardial radiofrequency applications at set temperatures of 70 and 80° C when the intra-atrial tissue was at room temperature and when it was above 35° C. The latter always occurred after an aborted application and the temperature measured on the endocardial surface was lower than the values registered sub-endocardially and sub-epicardially.

In all applications the sub-endocardial temperatures were naturally higher than the sub-epicardial ones and had a maximum value of 87° C for applications at 70° C and of 97° C for applications at 80° C. In 8 out of 10 cases where they were available, sub-endocardial temperatures rose up to 15° C above the set values.

Eight lesions were histologically assessed (7 pertaining to applications at 70° C) and 7 were transmural. The other one at 80° C showed damage of the endocardium, and of the internal half of the myocardium (see histological assessment section).

Our data shows that endocardial radiofrequency applications in-vitro at 70° C lead to intra-tissue temperatures capable of producing transmural lesion in atria as thick as 6.4 mm. Rising the application temperature to 80° C can bring the intra-atrial temperatures closer to carbonization values, which will naturally impose an upper limit to the value of the application temperature, that will be lower than might be expected if sub-endocardial temperatures are not taken into consideration.

Table I

Set T (° C)	Initial tissue T (° C)	Atrial thickness (mm)	Sub-epicardial T (° C)	Sub-endocardial max. T (° C)	Lesion depth/wall thickness (mm)
70	≈ 23 (n=5) grad T≈0	1.7±0.3	67.5±10.9	87	1.35 /1.35
		3.2±0.7	69.9±2.7		2.50/2.50; 2.60/2.60
		4.1±1.4	59.9±6.4		3.25/3.25.
	>35 (n=3) grad T>0	3.0±0.7	79.8±5.9		2.00/2.00; 2.37/2.37.
		6.0±0.4	64.4±3.1		3.50/3.50
80	≈ 23 (n=3) grad T≈0	1.2±0.2	77.3±4.1	97	—
		4.6±0.8	75.4±5.9		2.37/3.5
	>35 (n=2) grad T>0	1.4±0.2	68.9±6.5*		—
		4.6±0.8	87.2±3.0		—

* In this particular case no record of the temperature at the endocardial surface is available and it was a typical case of an aborted application followed immediately by a successful one on a quite thin wall. It is therefore likely that the difference in temperature between the interior of the tissue and the endocardial surface, when the final application started was quite small which may explain the relatively low final values of the sub-epicardial temperatures.

It was also shown that consecutive endocardial applications can raise the intra-tissue temperatures (over which the surgeon has no information whatsoever) to values significantly higher than those of application, eventually risking tissue carbonization at set temperatures that seem perfectly safe. It should however be noted that the in-vitro experiments do not duplicate but are rather a simulation of the in-vivo applications. In fact, the micro-circulation that will certainly act as a cooling factor, is not reproduced in vitro. It is therefore possible that the conclusions drawn from the present in-vitro experimentation are slightly conservative regarding the temperatures of application. In other words, it is possible that slightly higher application temperatures, than the ones predicted in-vitro, will be needed in order to achieve intra-tissue temperatures capable of producing irreversible lesions.

2.   EXPERIMENTAL SURGERY

Pigs were chosen for experimental surgical radiofrequency application. In order to assess the safety of the procedures several radiofrequency applications were performed epicardially on a beating heart during surgery. Some applications were performed over the coronary arteries. All animals were operated under general anesthesia and orotracheal intubation. The animals were monitored by means of continuous ECG and central venous pressure. A thoracotomy was performed and the heart exposed by opening the pericardium in front of the phrenic nerve. Epicardial applications of radiofrequency at set temperatures of 80 and 85° C were performed on the left atrium of 10 pigs. In order to further establish the safety of the procedure, radiofrequency applications at 70° C were performed at the AV groove over the right coronary artery. The animal was then sacrificed and the coronary artery was histologically assessed.

3. SURGICAL ENDOCARDIAL RF ABLATION IN MITRAL PATIENTS

The knowledge acquired from in vitro or animal experiments is incomplete due to the limitations of the models. The in vitro experiments do not duplicate the micro-circulation of the atrial wall and the animal models have normal atria, without the histological alterations seen in mitral patients.

In order to overcome the above limitations we performed a radiofrequency application on the atrial wall of mitral patients and removed a small fragment for histological assessment. All the mitral patients, ages 47 to 75 (63.1±10.0) years, had concomitant atrial fibrillation and underwent valve surgery. All patients were submitted to bilateral isolation of the pulmonary veins using radiofrequency, as described previously by our group.[6,7]

After arresting the heart with cold cardioplegia and having reached a core temperature of 30° C, the left atrium was opened parallel to the inter-atrial septum, in front of the right pulmonary veins.

The initial opening was performed with scalpel, and the encircling lesion around the orifices of the pulmonary veins was completed applying radiofrequency catheter ablation at 70° C for 2 minutes.

Fragments of tissue were removed from the zone of ablation and histologically assessed.

4. HISTOLOGICAL EVALUATION

Histologically a transmural lesion induced by endocardial radiofrequency ablation, shows damage of the whole myocardium plus damage of the endocardium. The average thickness of the normal left atrial wall in humans is approximately 3mm and the composition of the sub-endocardial layer, at the endocardium/myocardium interface, varies between fibrous tissue (loose or dense) and adipose tissue (Figure 3 right side). However, both the thickness and the proportion of the three layers of the left atrial wall (endocardium, myocardium, epicardium) vary from person to person, depending not only on age but also on related diseases, both systemic (diabetes mellitus, hypertension, tumors) and cardiac (namely valvular). The thickness of the left atrial wall in patients with mitral valve pathology ranges from 1.7 to 5.3 mm. In these patients (Figure 3, left side), the endocardium is always thicker than in normal subjects, due to a higher content in elastic fibers and eventual smooth muscle hyperplasia. The thickness of the myocardium is also highly variable, due to myocite hypertrophy and fibrosis or lipomatosis of the interstitium. The thickness of the epicardium depends on its fat content.

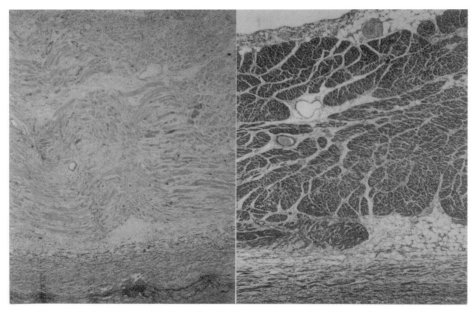

Figure 3. Left: Thickened left atrial wall from a mitral patient. Right: Atrial wall from a 60 years old normal subject. Note the adipose tissue at the endocardium/myocardium interface (elastic van Gieson × 40). See also Color Plate 28.

The samples were fixed in 10% buffered formalin, and fragments were serially taken from the whole line of radiofrequency application, in perpendicular sections, which included the whole thickness of the atrial wall. After paraffin embedding, 2μm cuts were done and then stained with histochemical dyes – haematoxylin/eosin, Gomori's trichrome, elastic van Gieson. The sections were analyzed under light microscopy by 2 observers. A metric eyepiece (with a precision of 0.025 mm) was used to measure the thickness of the left atrial wall, its layers and the lesions caused by radiofrequency.

We present the results pertaining to radiofrequency application in humans before the ones in animals and in-vitro due to their clinical importance, despite the fact that they were the last ones to be performed.

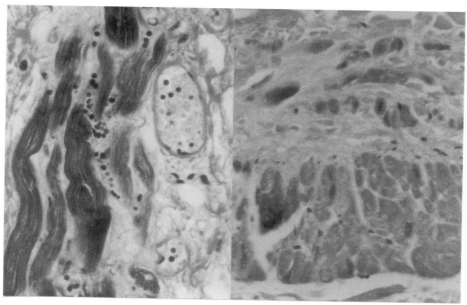

Figure 4. Left: Myocardium from a mitral patient with interstitial fibrosis and myocite hyperplasia. Right: The effect on the myocardium from a mitral patient of an endocardial radiofrequency application (Gomori's trichrome × 400). See also Color Plate 29.

4.1 "In Vivo": Endocardial RF Applications in Mitral Patients

Out of the 36 samples from ablations at 70° C that were evaluated, only 10 (females with mean age of 63 years [46 – 75 years]) were interpretable due to technical reasons (sample size, incorrect procurement, and inadequate inclusion). All the other fragments were excluded from the analysis. The lesions show (Figure 4, right side) damage of the muscle fibers, characterized by cytoplasm homogenization with total loss of cross striations, nuclear hyperchromasia and picnosis and ill defined cell membrane (histological features of coagulation necrosis). There is also thinning and collapse of the endocardial elastic fibers, loss of substance at the endocardium/myocardium interface that may be due to liquefaction necrosis of previous loose fibrous tissue or adipose tissue (Figure 5). The interstitium contains hemorrhagic foci.

The depth of the lesions varied from 0.200 to 2.000 mm (1.010±0.525 mm) in walls 1.25 to 4.5 mm thick (2.527±1.067 mm). Two lesions, observed in left atrial walls thinner than the average, were transmural without rupture of the wall. One of the transmural lesions measured 1.375 mm (the epicardium was spared) and occurred on a wall 1.7 mm thick. The other one measured 1.25 mm and the total wall thickness was 2.25 mm.

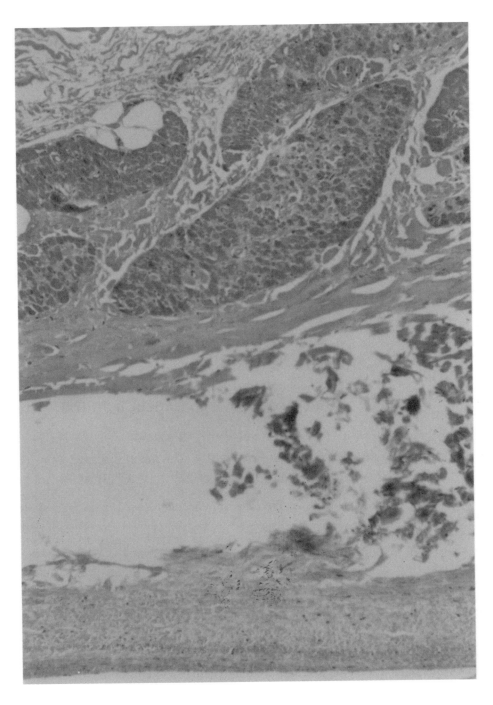

Figure 5. Transmural lesion induced by an endocardial RF application at 70° C in a mitral patient. Note the loss of tissue at the endocardium/myocardium interface (Gomori's trichrome × 40). See also Color Plate 30.

4.2   Epicardial Radiofrequency Applications in Pigs

Although highly variable in thickness, the porcine left atrial wall has a more homogeneous composition than the left atrial wall of mitral patients. Only 8 of the 12 samples of epicardial radiofrequency ablations observed in acute phase could be studied and showed lesions similar to the ones observed in humans. In epicardial radiofrequency applications the nerves and the large vessels of the epicardium did not show significant damage, except very scarce alterations of the adventitia of the last ones (Figure 6). Luminal thrombosis of the small vessels in the damaged areas was always observed.

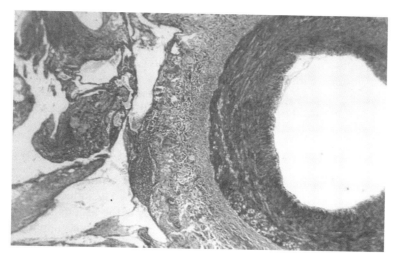

Figure 6. RF application at 70° C over the right coronary artery. The lesion is limited to the adventitia sparing the media and the endotelium. (Gomori's trichrome ×100). See also Color Plate 31.

4.3   "In Vitro": Endocardial RF Application in Fragments of Human Atria

Eight samples from the left atrium of heart valve donors (7 pertaining to applications at 70° C and 1 at 80° C) were histologically evaluated and the pathological characteristics were identical to the ones mentioned above, except for the absence of thrombosis of the interstitial small vessels (possibly related to the absence of circulation). All the 7 lesions obtained at 70° C were transmural reaching the endocardium, the myocardium and the whole of the epicardium. The lesions measured 1.350 mm to 3.500 mm (2.510±0.726 mm) and were induce in walls 2.5 to 6.4 mm (3.2±1.6 mm) measured with the digitizer before the radiofrequency application. The other sample, pertaining to an application at 80° C performed on a wall 4.6±0.4 mm thick (measured before the RF application), showed a non-transmural 2.370 mm deep lesion, that only damaged the endocardium (1.350 mm) and the inner half of the myocardium (2.040 mm).

The fact that the depth of the lesions measured under microscopy during histological evaluation is usually smaller than the value measured with the digitizer before the RF application, has to do with the retraction of the tissue due to the fixation of the samples in formalin, and also to shrinkage of the endocardial elastic fibers and loss of mostly adipose tissue during the radiofrequency application.

DISCUSSION

Our results from the in-vitro studies show that it is possible to obtain transmural lesions with endocardial applications at 70° C in atria as thick as 6.4 mm. However, it appears that the application temperature is not the sole factor that leads to deep lesions. Out of all the lesions histologically assessed the only non-transmural one occurred at 80° C and had a depth similar to the ones obtained at 70° C. The atrial wall composition may play an important role in the lesion formation.

Histological results from radiofrequency endocardial applications in mitral patients showed that the average depth of the lesions induced at 70° C was 1.010±0.525 mm on walls 2.527±1.067 mm thick at the lesions site, whereas the average depth of lesions induced in vitro by similar applications was 2.510±0.726 mm on walls of this thickness (the lesions were transmural). This means that the depth of the lesions induced in vitro on atrial fragments from human donors, is significantly higher than that of lesions similarly induced in mitral patients. We believe that the reasons for this are twofold: absence of micro-circulation in-vitro, and different histological composition of the atrial wall that shows severe pathology in many mitral patients and was normal in donors. In fact 2 transmural lesions were obtained in mitral patients with walls 1.700 and 1.250 mm thick, whereas in another patient with a wall 1.700 mm thick the depth of the lesion was only 0.850 mm.

Endocardial radiofrequency ablation can induce damage across the whole myocardial thickness without rupture of the atrial wall. The pathological features observed acutely are hemorrhage, coagulation and/or liquefaction necrosis of fibroelastic, adipose and muscular tissues. Thrombosis of the small vessels in the interstitium of the damaged areas was also observed. The chronic lesions are scars of dense fibrous tissue.

In epicardial applications in pigs, the nerves and the large vessels of the epicardium did not show significant damage, except very scarce alterations of the adventitia in the latter. Luminal thrombosis of the small vessels in the damaged areas was always observed, confirming the safety of intra-operative radiofrequency ablation when applied near large caliber arteries with blood circulating in its interior.

With the present radiofrequency delivery mode in which the electrical energy is converted into heat in the close vicinity of the active electrode due to active/dispersive electrodes geometry, the maximal lesion depth obtained was 2.0 mm in a 4.5mm wall. It is possible that radiofrequency set-ups with a different geometry will induce deeper lesions.

Our findings are in agreement with the results published in many clinical series and may explain some of the reported variability of the surgical results. To the best of our knowledge all published papers, up to the present, describe the treatment of atrial fibrillation with radiofrequency exclusively in mitral patients. Since the histological content varies from patient to patient it is logical to assume that this feature is the reason for such variability.

Because we believe that the thickness and the composition of the atrial wall are the major morphologic determinants to the depth of the lesion, further studies are required to achieve transmural scars during intra-operative radiofrequency catheter ablation. The development of a definitive treatment of atrial fibrillation with radiofrequency requires that the ideal ablation lines be defined. Until transmurality is achieved a scientific comparison between surgical techniques will remain a clinical challenge.

REFERENCES

1. Cox JL. The surgical treatment of atrial fibrillation. IV. Surgical technique. J Thorac Cardiovasc Surg 1991;101:584-92.
2. Graffigna A, Francesco P, Minzioni G, Salerno J, Viganò M. Left atrial isolation with mitral valve operations. Ann Thorac Surg 1992; 54: 1093-1098
3. Nitta T, Lee R, Schuessler RB, Boineau JP, Cox JL. Radial approach: a new concept in surgical treatment for atrial fibrillation I. Concept, anatomic and physiologic bases and development of a procedure. Ann Thorac Surg, 1999 Jan, 67: 27-35
4. Melo J, Adragão P, Neves J, Ferreira M, Pinto MM, Rebocho MJ, Parreira L, Ramos T. Surgery for atrial fibrillation using radiofrequency catheter ablation: assessment of results at 1 year. Eur J Cardiothorac Surg 1999; 15: 851-855.
5. Melo J, Adragão P, Neves J, Ferreira M, Timóteo A, Santiago T, Ribeiras R, Canada M. Endocardial and Epicardial Radiofrequency Ablation in the Treatment of Atrial Fibrillation with a new Intra-operative Device. Eur. J Cardiothorac Surg 18: 182-6, 2000
6. Melo J, Adragão P, Neves J, Ferreira M M, Calquinha MC, Santos A, Rebocho MJ. Surgery for atrial fibrillation using intra-operative radiofrequency ablation. Rev. Port. Cardiol. 17(4): 377-379 1998.

7.   Melo J, Adragão P, Neves J, Ferreira M, Rebocho M,. Teles R, Morgado F. Electrosurgical Treatment of Atrial Fibrillation with a New Intraoperative Radiofrequency Ablation Catheter. Thorac. Cardiov. Surg. 47 (suppl): 370-372, 1999.

Chapter 32

UTILITY OF MICROWAVE ABLATION FOR THE INTRAOPERATIVE TREATMENT OF ATRIAL FIBRILLATION

Stefan G. Spitzer, Michael Knaut*, Stephan Schüler*

*Institute of Cardiovascular Research and *Cardiovascular Institute, University of Dresden, Dresden, Germany*

INTRODUCTION

Atrial fibrillation (AF) is the most common atrial arrhythmia and is associated with significant symptoms and morbidity. Epidemiologic studies show that about 1% of the population is affected by AF with a distinct dependence on age reaching 7% in people older than 70 years.[1] The group of patients with high grade mitral valve defects represents the highest prevalence of AF reaching 80%. AF can cause a wide spectrum of clinical symptoms ranging from palpitations and tachycardias to diminished physical capacity, dyspnoea, dizziness, presyncopes, and syncopes. In addition, the risk of thromboembolic complication is distinctly increased in patients with AF, especially in those with mitral valve disease.[2] For these reasons, curative treatment of AF is one of the main challenges of today's electrophysiology. Many centers are working on an ideal treatment strategy, which should be effective, safe and easy to apply to ensure a widespread use. This chapter will focus on the substantial role of microwave energy in curative treatment of AF in heart surgery.

1.   SURGICAL TREATMENT OF ATRIAL FIBRILLATION

An ideal intraoperative strategy for curative treatment of AF would accomplish five goals:

L. Bing Liem and E. Downar (eds.), Progress in Catheter Ablation, 507-530.

1. Elimination of AF.
2. Restoration of sinus rhythm with chronotropic competence.
3. Maintenance of atrioventricular(AV)-synchrony.
4. Restoration of biatrial transport function.
5. Limitation of the risk of thromboembolism by elimination of blood stasis in both atria, thereby avoiding anti-coagulation.

The appropriateness of any ablative intervention needs to be judged against these five criteria.

The main strategy of the surgical techniques designed to eliminate AF was to reduce: (1) the critical number of reentrance circuits available to maintain the fibrillatory process, and (2) the surface area of both atria available to maintain the fibrillatory process.

1.1   The classic Maze procedure

The classic Maze procedure was based on the work of the Allessie group[3] on multiple reentrance circuits as the pathophysiological basis of AF. Cox and associates created first an electrical Maze which isolated the pulmonary veins and amputated both appendages. The additional interruption of reentrant circuits around the caval veins provided a single pathway conduction from the sinoatrial to the AV node guiding the activation from both atria along a single route.[5]

The Maze I concept (Figure 1) resulted in a chronotropic incompetence in about 34% of all patients requiring a post-operative pacemaker implantation.[4] The Maze II procedure thereby avoided the sinus node region by introduction of a transverse biatrial incision at the medial border of the superior vena cava displacing the atrial septotomy (Figure 2). This modified operation concept needed transection of the superior vena cava and the subsequent reconstruction with patch enlargement was necessary.

A total of 15 patients receiving this procedure needed a pacemaker implantation postoperatively in about 13%.[6] Therefore the Maze III procedure moved the transverse biatrial incision and atrial septotomy caudally and avoids bilateral incision in the superior vena cava thereby also avoiding patch reconstruction (Figure 3). Another advantage was the preservation of Bachmann's bundle which permitted more rapid activation of the left atrium and improved left atrial contractility.

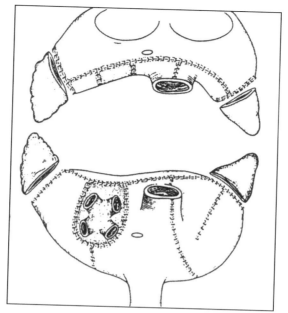

Figure 1. Maze I modification. Reproduced with permission from JL Cox.[4]

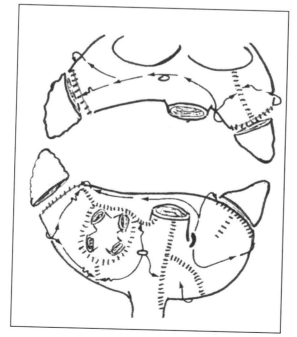

Figure 2. Maze II modification. Reproduced with permission from JL Cox.[6]

The incidence of prospective pacemaker implantation for latent sick sinus syndrome was about 14%.[7] The Maze III procedure has provided a technically complex but successful therapy for AF. One should also point out that in the group treated with the accepted Maze III concept, 58% of the patients suffered from paroxysmal AF and required no additional heart surgery. Obviously these were patients with relatively healthy hearts and a relatively high probability of restoration of sinus rhythm with a surgical technique.

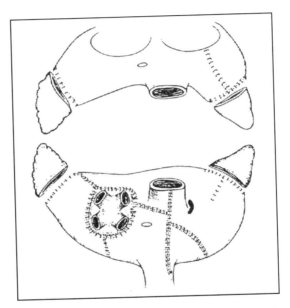

Figure 3. Maze III modification. Reproduced with permission from JL Cox.[7]

1.2   Modification of the MAZE III procedure

Besides the tremendous success, the classic Maze procedure is an extensive and time-consuming surgical technique. It has to be realised that the reported results represent the experience of the leading expert group for open-heart surgery of AF. The results of other centers have been reported considerably lower.[8]

The original Maze concept was based on the following premises:

1. AF is a micro-reentrant or small cycle-length micro-reentrant arrhythmia
2. multiple-reentrance circuits do exist at the same time in the atrium (transient in time and location)
3. initiation and termination of the multiple reentrant circuits occur spontaneously during the arrhythmia
4. circuits could be interfered by normal physiological / anatomic barriers.

The main reasons to alter the Maze-procedure are:

- decreasing the time required to perform the procedure,
- permitting application of a simpler procedure to a larger group of patients.

As early as 1992, Kosakai and colleagues[9] applied a modified Maze procedure using additional extensive cryoablation (Figure 4). By eliminating the longitudinal incision connecting the cavae an enhancement of the sinus node arterial supply was postulated.[9] Of the 70 patients operated 59 underwent this modified Maze procedure with mitral and frequently multiple valve operations.[10]

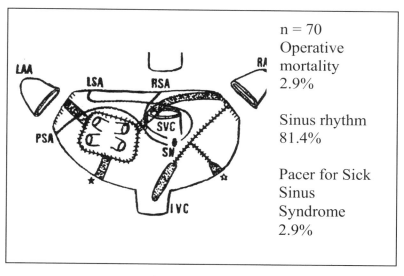

n = 70
Operative mortality 2.9%

Sinus rhythm 81.4%

Pacer for Sick Sinus Syndrome 2.9%

Figure 4. Kosakai modified Maze.[9] Areas of cryoablation at valvular annuli were close to the circumflex artery (closed asterisk) and the right coronary artery (open asterisk). LAA, left atrial appendage; RAA, right atrial appendage; SN, sinus node; LSA, left sinus node artery; RSA, right sinus node artery; PSA, posterior sinus node artery; SVC, superior vena cava; IVC, inferior vena cava.

For patients with mitral valve disease and where AF origin is presumed to be in the left atrium, a left atrial procedure was set up in 1996 by the group of Sueda.[11] The operation involved a pulmonary vein encircling incision and left atrial appendage amputation with linear cryolesions joining these to the mitral annulus (Figure 5). Of the 36 patients[12] with concurrent mitral valve operations reported, 25 required additional tricuspid and/or aortic valve procedures. (For patients undergoing tricuspid annuloplasty an additional cryoablation was applied to the right atrial septum).

Izumoto and colleagues modified the Maze procedure by substituting linear cryolesions for several incisions in both atria and the interatrial septum (Figure 6). In 1998 they reported of 87 patients receiving this modified operation concurrent with mitral valve or multiple valve procedures.[13,14]

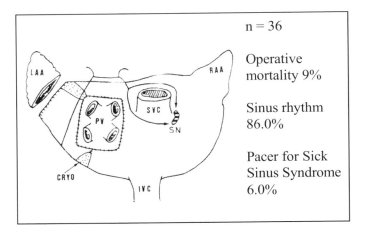

Figure 5. Sueda left atrial procedure.[11,12]   IVC, inferior vena cava; LAA, left atrial appendage; PV, pulmonary veins; RAA, right atrial appendage, SVC, superior vena cava; SN, sinus node. Reproduced with permission from   T Sueda.

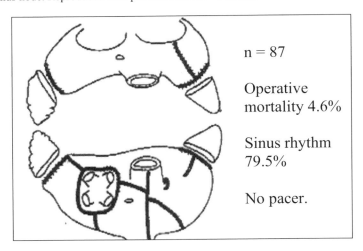

Figure 6. Izumoto's modified Maze.[13,14] Reproduced with permission from H Izumoto.

In 1997 an operative concept aiming at the elimination of anatomical determined left atrial anchor reentrant circuits was introduced by the group of Hindricks and Kottkamp. It involved the induction of continuous left atrial lesion lines between the pulmonary veins and the mitral annulus using radiofrequency energy.[15,16]   The concept based on the hypothesis that AF can no longer sustain in the case of elimination of all possible anatomically determined left atrial reentrant circuits (Figure 7). The experimental basis was the work of the Allessie group were Zarsse could show that AF was no longer inducible in Langendorff perfused rabbit model of biatrial dilatation following elimination of the anatomical determined atrial micro reentrant circuits.[17]

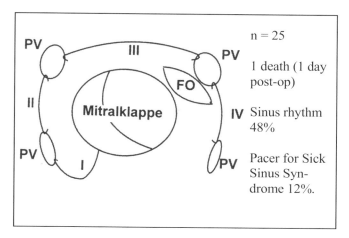

Figure 7. Schematic drawing of the left atrum (posterior view) and the geometry of the radio-frequency energy-induced left atrial lesions for treatment of AF. LAA, left atrial appendix; MV, mitral valve; LPV, left pulmonary vein; RPV, right pulmonary vein. Reproduced with permission from G Hindricks.[15,16]

The group of Melo introduced a technique using a new catheter for intraoperative radiofrequency ablation, in 1998.[18] Isolation of the bilateral pulmonary vein was achieved in 7±4 minutes. 44% of the 27 patients with one to three months follow-up regained normal sinus rhythm. No pacemaker implantation was required and no deaths occurred (Figure 8).

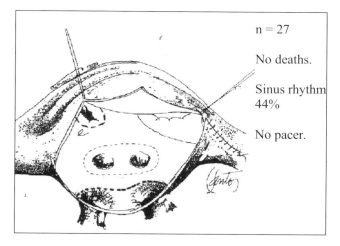

Figure 8. Intraoperative RF ablation using a new catheter. Reproduced with permission by J Melo.[18]

Despite the still open question, which lesion concept should be favoured in the future, there is no doubt that left atrial linear lesions are necessary for successful intraoperative treatment of AF.

The ideal ablation tool for intraoperative use therefore needs to meet the following requirements:

-    simple to use
-    safe and effective
-    long distance transmural linear lesion lines with few single applications.

2.   TECHNICAL BACKGROUND FOR CLINICAL USE OF MICROWAVE ABLATION DEVICES

The microwave region is between radio waves and infrared rays, wavelengths are in the decimeter to millimeter range. The manifold use of microwaves includes e. g. broadband communication, radar and heating of food (Figure 9*).

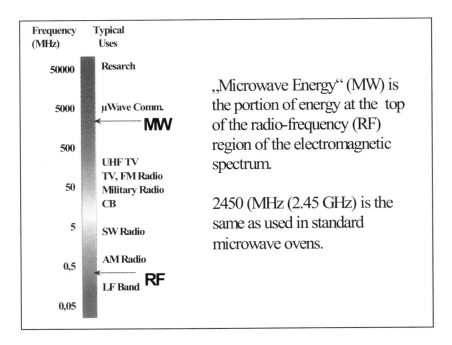

Figure 9. Electromagnetic spectrum and uses.

For medical use microwave technique focuses on hyperthermia and ablation of tissue by local heating of the tissue from the inside. Heat is produced by molecular vibrations and intramolecular oscillations that in turn are induced by microwaves directed at the tissue (dielectric heating) (Figure 10). Living tissue is destroyd when temperatures are above 48°C.[19]

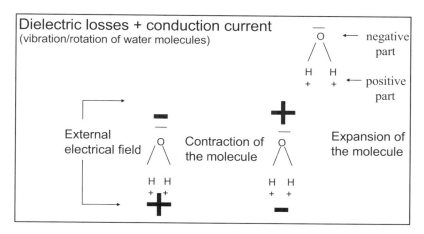

Figure 10. Scheme dielectric heating.

The principal components of a microwave ablation device are essentially a microwave generator, an antenna and a coaxial cable connecting the antenna to the generator. Microwave generators available and permitted by the Federal Communications Commission operate at 915 or 2450 MHz. Many different types of antennas have been designed and tested. The antenna has to be designed to have a good radiation efficiency and a good radiation profile in the tissue to ablate.[20-25] Antennas for cardiac ablation have been developed and tested for about ten years. Microwave technique is considered to be capable of effective and controlled heating of large tissue volumes without causing endocardial (epicardial) charring. Thus, it has the potential of creating long linear and transmural lesions as needed for preventing propagation of AF, or large and deep lesions as for ablation of ventricular tachycardias.[20,26-33] The construction of antennas has posed some problems. Historical devices had considerable loss of power and hence low power available for ablation. Those devices would not make therapeutic lesions, despite many ablations. Power losses resulted from high losses in the coaxial cable, power reflected back by the antenna through the transmission line, or selection of inappropriate material at the antenna area. Reflections at the antenna level generated heat in the shaft. New research work has brought about a new generation of microwave devices.

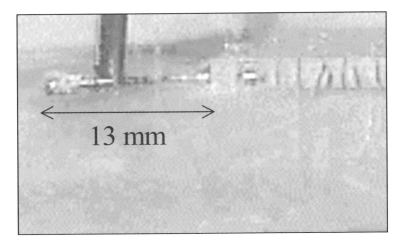

Figure 11. Deep lesion catheter.

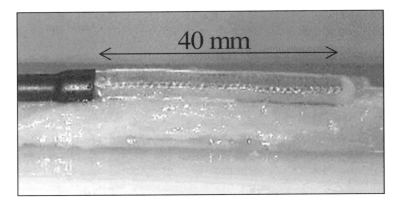

Figure 12. Tool for long linear lesions (ie. epicardial use).

There are antennas incorporated in catheters, flutter catheter with helical coil antenna for long linear lesions, deep lesion catheter with monopolar antenna for deep and circular lesions, and antennas as surgical tools for endocardial or epicardial use (Figures 11 and 12). One of them, the Lynx device, is being clinically tested.

2.1   Assessment of heating pattern

Numerical models were used to study the heating pattern in model tissue created by a model antenna under varying boundary conditions. Those models often use finite element methods that are well-suited for solving microwave problems and usually have certain symmetries to facilitate calculations. They are helpful for understanding the mechanism and for the design of antennas.[34-37]

Characteristic variables such as specific absorption rate (SAR) of microwave energy, temperature distribution, reflection losses, time course of lesion formation or lesion size are determined under varying settings by in vitro experiments (Figure 13a,b).

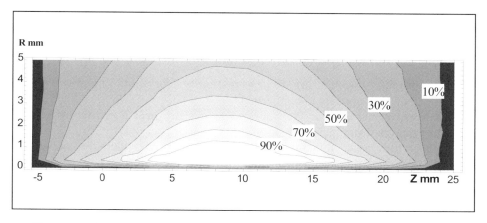

Figure 13a. The SAR pattern for Lynx device. Absorption of microwave energy into the tissue.

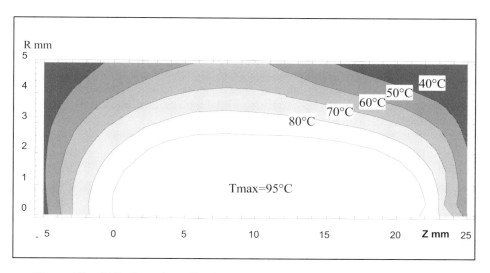

Figure 13b. SAR thermal profile for Lynx device. Increase of temperature as a consequence of microwave absorption.

Varying settings mainly refer to used power and application duration, frequency, antenna type and angle, and distance to the tissue. SAR and temperature measurements are often done using saline or phantom solutions to replace the tissue.[38-48]

In vivo experiments or short series on animals (canine, ovine and porcine hearts) were done to investigate feasibility, efficacy and safety of microwave applications. Short and long term histopathological examinations were performed. Microwave energy was used to ablate av-junction, accessory pathways, aconitine induced atrial tachycardias, atrial flutter and ventricular tachycardias.[48-69]

Radiofrequency and microwave experiments are often performed side-by-side in order to directly compare the two methods.

Results can be roughly summarized as follows:

1. The primary mechanism of tissue injury for both microwave and radiofrequency appears to be thermal.
2. Microwave ablation has the potential to directly heat a greater volume of tissue than radiofrequency ablation.
3. Temperature as a function of depth decreases considerably slower for microwave ablation compared to radiofrequency ablation.
4. At comparable surface temperatures deeper lesions would be created by microwave ablation. Lesion size, in deeper tissue, can continue to increase for a few seconds after microwave application.
5. At comparable power and application duration deeper lesions would be created by microwave ablation.
6. Microwave can produce an ablation without requiring a perfect contact. It penetrates necrotic tissue and old scars.[70]
7. Pathologically microwave and radiofrequency lesions are comparable. Acutely they demonstrate considerable haemorrhage, chronically they become a dense fibrous scar and are well circumscribed.
8. Ablations performed on animal hearts were reported as successful. No transvalvular, vascular, other structural damage or coagulum formation were observed under usual circumstances.

Radiofrequency power is delivered as a conduction current that is concentrated at contact points and edges. Hence there are high current areas that can result in hot spots. Furthermore, the radiofrequency energy is essentially absorbed within the first millimeter of tissue. Microwave power is delivered as a field that is generated in a more uniform manner. With a correctly designed antenna, there are no high-concentration field areas. Since the microwave power is absorbed deeper in the tissue, a microwave ablation device can generate a deeper lesion at a given power and size. Microwave devices create a given lesion volume with less power, lower and smother temperature profile and without areas with concentrated power absorption. Considering all of these aspects, the likelihood of thrombus generation is thus reduced for microwave application.

2.2   The Lynx device

The AFx Microwave Surgical Ablation Device Lynx is designed to allow the application of microwave power to different tissue types during surgical procedures (Figure 14). It is used to produce linear lesions on the endocardial surface of both atria. The antenna is mounted at the end of a malleable shaft to allow precise microwave application at the targeted site. Surrounding the antenna is a shield to direct the power through the defined window into the tissue to be ablated as well as create a layer of thermal protection for other tissues nearby. A thermocouple is embedded near the antenna section to record temperature internal to the device and to prevent catastrophic overheating of the antenna section during an ablation procedure. The proximal end of the malleable shaft is mounted into a handle.   A cord extends from the handle to the connector allowing the Lynx to connect to the generator system outside the sterile field.

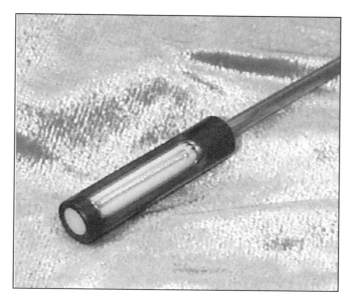

Figure 14. Intraoperative tool.

The generator is a 2450 MHz Magnetron with controls for power, application duration and temperature (Figure 15). It provides variable power outputs from 35 to 75 watts in 5-watt increments, but is set for 40 - 45 watts power and 20 - 30 sec duration for application of endocardial ablations (Table1). This generates a consistent 3 to 5 mm lesion depth, sufficient for transmural ablations of the atrial myocardium. Lesion length and width correspond to antenna length and antenna area width and are approximately 2 cm and 4 mm respectively. Shorter times and powers result in lesions that may be too shallow for transmurality, and higher time and power result in increased width of lesion without any benefit in assuring transmurality (Figure 16). Since the power delivery is highly related to the antenna design, this data is specific to the Lynx device. The antenna is applied directly to the tissue to be ablated – lesions can be connected in order to obtain a long linear lesion line without any gap.

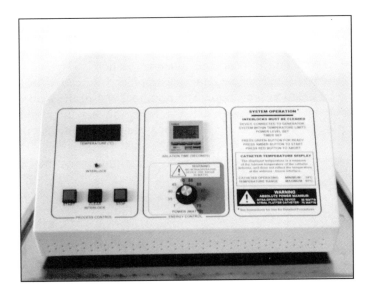

Figure 15. Microwave generator.

Table 1: Average lesion depth (mm) of three ablations at the shown power and duration.

	33.4 Watts	37.8 Watts	42.2 Watts
20 Seconds	2.50	2.733	3.366
25 Seconds	3.25	3.366	3.433
30 Seconds	4.10	4.233	4.800

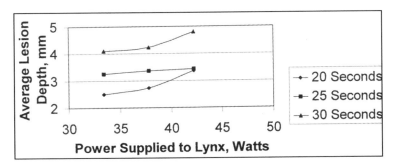

Figure 16. Lesion depth as a function of power and duration.

3. INTRAOPERATIVE MICRO-WAVE ABLATION IN OPEN HEART SURGERY

The original Maze procedure achieved high success rates with respect to primary success in restoring sinus rhythm as well as the absence of recurrences. Hence, the Maze concept for treatment of AF has proved its viability, but simplification of the operative procedure is of paramount importance. Several ablation alternatives to the classic cut and sew technique have been proposed and clinically used as there are cryoablation technique,[71,72] radiofrequency or cooled RF ablation,[73-75] as well as the application of microwave devices.[76,77] Lynx is the first microwave surgical tool that is being clinically testet (Figure 17).

3.1 The MICRO-STAF and MICRO-PASS trials

Since December 1998 the additional concomitant microwave ablation for curative treatment of chronic AF has been performed in two groups of patients: patients who received mitral valve replacement / reconstruction (MICRO-STAF: **MICRO**wave Application in **S**urgical **T**reatment of **A**trial **F**ibrillation) and patients who received coronary artery bypass grafting (MICRO-PASS: **MICRO**wave Application for the Treatment of Atrial Fibrillation in B**ypass**-Surgery). Besides the indication for mitral valve repair (MVR) or coronary artery bypass grafting (CABG) the most essential inclusion criterion was documented chronic AF longer than 6 months. For the complete list of inclusion and exclusion criteria see reference 77. Further, verbal and written informed consent had to be given by the patients. Ethic approval for the additional rhythmological intervention was received by the Freiburg Ethic Commission.

The main aim was to proof the feasibility of intraoperative microwave application and to establish and maintain sinus rhythm in the particular patient group and to finally achieve the restitution of atrial function.

The antenna was applied directly to the tissue to be ablated and the generator set to apply a power of 40 watts over 25 sec. The lesions were approximately 2 cm in length and subsequent lesions could be connected visually (Figure 18).

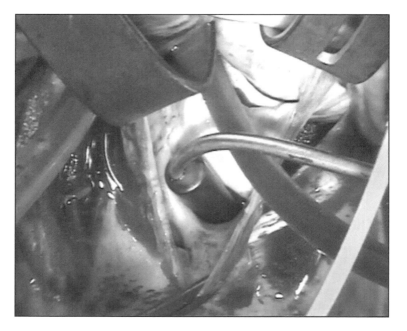

Figure 17. Intraoperative Lynx device.

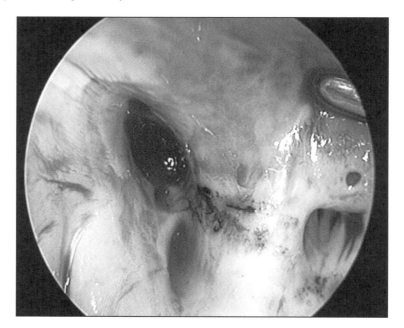

Figure 18. Microwave lesion. See also Color Plate 2.

After left atriotomy (via Watson groove) and establishing bloodlessness continuous leftatrial ablation lines were induced as follows: The microwave probe was introduced into the left atrium and the procedure started under visual guidance at the posterior mitral valve annulus and about three applications were applied so that the first complete lesion line ended 1 cm deep in the lower left pulmonary vein. Then, the next lesion line started at the same depth and contralateral the first lesion line towards the upper left pulmonary vein. After one or two further lesions the line ended at about 1 cm deep in the upper left pulmonary vein. The next lesion line started from the upper left pulmonary vein and reached the upper right pulmonary vein after about 5 lesions. The procedure was completed with two or three further applications that extended from the upper right pulmonary vein into the lower right pulmonary vein (Figure 19). Energy applications had to be adapted to the variations of the pulmonary veins. The antiarrhythmic intervention was complete at this point in patients with CABG.

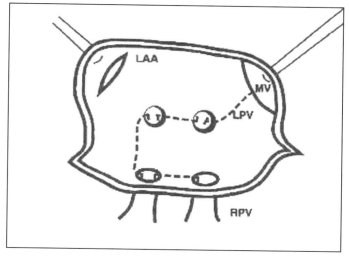

Figure 19. Left atrium lesion line. LAA, left atrial appendix; MV, mitral valve; LPV, left pulmonary vein; RPV, right pulmonary vein.

In patients with MVR the rhythmological intervention was finished after right atrial atriotomy sparing the septum and the electric isolation of the isthmus with about three further applications that extended a lesion line in the isthmus area from the septal leaflet of the tricuspid valve to the inferior vena cava. Finally CABG or mitral valve reconstruction/ replacement was performed respectively. All patients received anticoagulation therapy (INR 3.0 - 3.5). Postoperative rhythm was controlled daily. Follow-up examinations were scheduled for postoperative days 1-9, 10, 30, 90, 180 and 360. In case of recurrence of AF patients received a low dose Sotalol therapy, and electric cardioversions before day 90. Rhythm was evaluated using the results of rest and Holter ECG, mechanical atrial function in dependence on atrial A-wave detection in a transthoracic Doppler study. For complete list of planned examinations see Table 4.

Up to now 29 patients (7 men, 22 women, age 65.4 ± 7.0 years) with MVR and 18 patients (11 men, 7 women, age 70.0 ± 4.5 years) with CABG have received intraoperative microwave applications. Mean duration of AF and mean leftventricular ejection fraction was similar in both groups, about 6 years and 60 %. Left atrial size (parasternal view) was 54.5 ± 7.0 mm for patients with MVR and 46.7 ± 4.4 mm for patients with CABG.

The time needed for the antiarrhythmic intervention was 18.0 ± 7.5 min in the Micro-Staf group, and 15.5 ± 5.3 min in the Micro-Pass group. The corresponding numbers of energy applications were 18.2 ± 3.5 and 15.4 ± 2.8. One patient with MVR received a dual chamber pacemaker due to sinus bradycardia. There was one perioperative death due to unexpected additional aortic dissection and implantation of a conduitgraft, and one apoplexy with neurological remission due to an exulcerated aortic plaque with a floating thrombus in the Micro-Pass group. Neither of the two events was in relation to the additional intraoperative intervention. Up to now no documented cases of pulmonary vein stenosis exist. All patients were planned for pulmonary vein angiography at 1 year follow up. Tables 2 and 3 show current data regarding rhythm for follow-up days 30, 180 and 360.

Table 2: Micro-Staf I Study. Follow-up

Follow-up Day	30	180	360
Valid Data	29	24	13
Sinus rhythm	22 (75.9%)	15 (62.5%)	8 (61.5%)
AF	7 (24.1%)	4 (16.7%)	3 (23.1%)
Atypical atrial flutter	0	5 (20.8%)	2 (15.4%)

Table 3: Micro-Pass I Study. Follow-up.

Follow-up Day	30	180	360
No. of patients	17	11	6
Sinus rhythm	13 (76.5%)	8 (72.7%)	4 (66.7%)
AF	2 (11.8%)	0	0
Atypical atrial flutter	2 (11.8%)	3 (27.3%)	2 (33.3%)

A transmitral and transtricuspidal flow (A-wave in transthoracic Doppler study) was detected in all patients with stable sinus rhythm. A typical example of an atypical atrial flutter is shown in Figure 20. This could be related to left atrial scar reentry – the patients are planned for left atrial mapping.

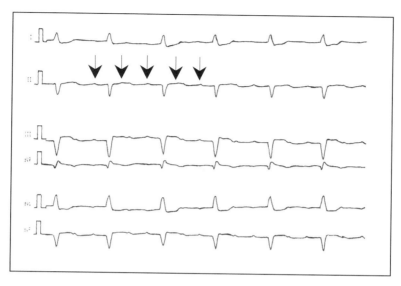

Figure 20a. ECG recording of aypcial atrial flutter. ↓, P-wave

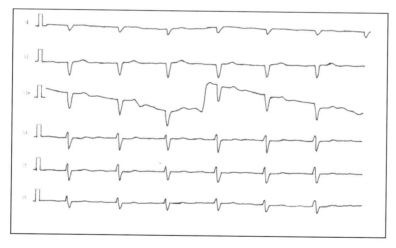

Figure 20b. ECG recording of atypical atrial flutter.

The prospective randomized multicenter trials Micro-Staf II and Micro-Pass II aim to confirm the results of these pilot studies (Table 4), and the first patient has been included in February 2000.

Table 4: Micro-Staf II /Micro-Pass II Study design.

| | | Random-ization | MVR or CABG + Microwave ablation | | | | |
| | | | MVR or CABG | | | | |

Day	-28-1	1-9	10	30	90	180	360
Anamnesis	X		X	X	X	X	X
Quality of Life	X					X	X
Rest ECG	X	daily	X	X	X	X	X
Ergometry	X			X	X	X	X
Holter ECG	X		X	X	X	X	X
Echocardiography	X		X	X	X	X	X
TEE	X						X
EPS							X

COMMENTS

The microwave surgical tool is easy to use and safe. This type of energy seems to be especially appropriate for the intraoperative use.

Potential advantages of microwave energy application and the described line concept are:

- less traumatic treatment procedure compared with the Maze-operation as extensive incisions and sutures are not required
- reduction of the time spend on an antiarrhythmic operation
- maintenance of atrial contraction of the left atrial appendage as well as the left atrial posterior wall of the left atrium
- long isolation lesions with few applications
- visual check of continuity and connection of the lesion lines.

The intraoperative microwave energy application with limited linear lesions can terminate chronic AF in patients undergoing open heart surgery.

Further investigations will focus on epicardial application of microwave energy for a curative treatment of AF.

REFERENCE

1. Kannel WB, Abbot RD, Savage DD, et al. Epidemiologic features of chronic atrial fibrillation: the Framingham study. N Engl J Med 1982; 306:1018-102.
2. Bruchfield GM, Hammermeister KE, Steinrauf HK et al. Left atrial dimension and risk of embolism in patients with a prosthetic heart valve. J Am Coll Cardiol 1990; 15:32-41.
3. Allessie MA, Lammers WJEP, Bonke FIM, Hollen IM. Experimental evaluation of Moe's multiple wavelet hypothesis of atrial fibrillation. In: Zipes DP, Jalife J, editors. Cardiac electrophysiology and arrhythmias. Orlando, Florida: Grune & Stratton, 1985: 265-75.
4. Cox JL, Boineau JP, Schuessler RB et al. Modification of the maze procedure for atrial flutter and fibrillation. I. Rationale and surgical results. J Thorac Cardiovasc Surg 1995; 110:473-84.
5. Cox JL, Schuessler RB, D'Agostino HJ Jr, et al. The surgical treatment of atrial fibrillation, III. Development of a definitive surgical procedure. J Thorac Cardiovasc Surg 1991; 101:569-83.
6. Cox JL, Sundt TM III. The surgical management of atrial fibrillation. Annu Rev Med 1997; 48:511-23.
7. Sundt TM III, Camillo CJ, Cox JL. The maze procedure for cure of atrial fibrillation. Cardiol Clin 1997; 15:739-48.
8. Kobayashi J, Kosakai Y, Nakano K et al. Improved success rate of the maze procedure in mitral valve disease by new criteria for patients selection. Eur J Cardio-thorac Surg 1998; 13:247-52.
9. Kosakai Y, Kawaguchi AT, Isobe F et al. Cox maze procedure for chronic atrial fibrillation associated with mitral valve disease. J Thorac Cardiovasc Surg 1994; 108(6):1049-
10. Kosakai Y, Kawaguchi A, Isobe F, et al. Modified maze procedure for patients with atrial fibrillation undergoing simultaneous open heart surgery. Circulation 1995; 92(Suppl. II):II-359-II-364.
11. Sueda T, Nagata H, Shikata H, et al. Simple left atrial procedure for chronic atrial fibrillation associated with mitral valve disease. Ann Thorac Surg 1996; 62:1796-800.
12. Sueda T, Nagata H, Orihashi K, et al. Efficacy of a simple left atrial procedure for chronic atrial fibrillation in mitral valve operations. Ann Thorac Surg 1997; 63:1070-5.
13. Kamata J, Kawazoe K, Izumoto H, et al. Predictors of sinus rhythm restoration after Cox maze procedure concomitant with other cardiac operations. Ann Thorac Surg 1997; 64:394-8.
14. Izumoto H, Kawazoe K, Kitahara H, Kamata J. Operative results after the Cox/maze procedure combined with a mitral valve operation. Ann Thorac Surg 1998; 66:800-4.
15. Hindricks G, Kottkamp H, Hammel D, Mergenthaler J, Borggrefe M, Scheld HH, and Breithardt G. Radiofrequency ablation of atrial fibrillation: early clinical experience with a catheter-guided intraoperative approach. Eur Heart J [Suppl], 18. 1997. Ref Type: Abstract
16. Kottkamp H, Hindricks G, Hammel D et al. Intra-operative Radiofrequency Ablation of Chronic Atrial Fibrillation: A Left Atrial Curative Approach by Elimination of Anatomic "Anchor" Reentrant Circuits. J Cardiovasc Electrophysiol 1999; 6:772-9.
17. Zarse M, Deharo JC, and Allessie MA. Radiofrequency ablation of anatomical atrial circuits in a rabbit model of atrial fibrillation. Circulation 94[Suppl. I], I-676. 1996. Ref Type: Abstract
18. Melo J, Adragao PR, Neves J, Ferreira M, Rebocho M, Teles R, and Morgado F. Electrosurgical Treatment of Atrial Fibrillation with a New Intraoperative Radiofrequency Ablation Catheter. Thorac.Cardiovasc.Surg. 47[Suppl. III], 370-372. 1999. Ref Type: Abstract
19. Haines DE, Watson DD. Tissue heating during radiofrequency catheter ablation: a thermodynamic model and observation in isolated perfused and superfused canine right ventricular free wall. Pacing Clin Electrophysiol 1989; 12(6):962-76.
20. Liem LB. Newer Modalities in Cardiac Arrhythmia Ablation: The Role of Microwave Energy. Cardiac Arrthythmia and Electrophysiology. Stanford University Medical Center, 1999.

21. Liem LB, Mead RH, Shenasa M, Kernoff R. In vitro and in vivo results of transcatheter microwave ablation using forward-firing tip antenna design. Pacing Clin Electrophysiol 1996 Nov.; 19(11 Pt 2):2004-8.

22. Lin JC. Catheter microwave ablation therapy for cardiac arrhythmias. Bioelectromagnetics 1999; Suppl 4:120-32:120-32.

23. Lin JC, Wang YJ. The cap-choke catheter antenna for microwave ablation treatment. IEEE Trans Biomed Eng 1996 June; 43(6):657-60.

24. Mazzola F, Huang SKS, and Lin, J. C. Determinants of lesion size using a 4-milimeter split-tip antenna electrode for microwave catheter ablation. Pacing Clin.Electrophysiol. 17[4 Pt II], 814. 1994. Ref Type: Abstract

25. Shetty S, Ishii TK, Krum DP et al. Microwave applicator design for cardiac tissue ablations. J Microw Power Electromagn Energy 1996; 31(1):59-66.

26. Avitall B, Khan M, Krum D et al. Physics and engineering of transcatheter cardiac tissue ablation. J Am Coll Cardiol 1993 Sept.; 22(3):921-32.

27. Haines DE. Current and future modalities of catheter ablation for the treatment of cardiac arrhythmias. J Invasive Cardiol 1992 July; 4(6):291-9.

28. Haugh C, Davidson ES, Estes NA, III, Wang PJ. Pulsing microwave energy: a method to create more uniform myocardial temperature gradients. J Interv Card Electrophysiol 1997 Feb.; 1(1):57-65.

29. Haugh, C., Estes NAM, Manolis AS, and Wang, P. J. Pulsing microwave energy: a method to create more uniform temperature gradients in depth. Pacing Clin.Electrophysiol. 17[4 pt II], 831. 1994. Ref Type: Abstract

30. Liem LB. Progress in cardiac arrhythmia ablation: potential for broader application and shorter procedure time. J Cardiothorac Vasc Anesth 1997 Dec.; 11(7):895-900.

31. Nath S, Haines DE. Biophysics and pathology of catheter energy delivery systems. Prog Cardiovasc Dis 1995 Jan.; 37(4):185-204.

32. Wang PJ, Yong PG. New Energy Sources for Ablation. In: Singer I., editor. Interventional Electrophysiology. Baltimore: Williams & Wilkins, 1997: 445-68.

33. Wellens HJ, Sie HAT, Smeets JL et al. Surgical treatment of atrial fibrillation. J Cardiovasc Electrophysiol 1998; 9(8):S151-S154.

34. Nevels RD, Arndt GD, Raffoul GW et al. Microwave catheter design. IEEE Trans Biomed Eng 1998 July; 45(7):885-90.

35. Stauffer PR, Suen SA, Satoh, T., and et al. Comparative thermal dosimetry of interstitial microwave and radiofrequency-LCF hyperthermia. Int.J.Hyperthermia 5[3], 307-318. 1989. Ref Type: Abstract

36. Whayne, J. G. and Haines, D. E. Computer modeling of microwave antenna designs using the finite element analysis method. Pacing Clin.Electrophysiol. 16[4 Pt II], 921. 1993. Ref Type: Abstract

37. Khebir A, Youheir K, Savard P. Modeling a microwave catheter antenna for cardiac ablation. IEEE MTT-S 1995;299-302.

38. Ahmad A, Estes NAM, Manolis AS, and Wang, P. J. Does microwave heating in saline predict the 3-dimensional heating pattern in myocardium. J.Am.Coll.Cardiol. 35A. 1994. Ref Type: Abstract

39. Gu Z, Rappaport CM, Wang PJ, VanderBrink BA. A 2 1/4-turn spiral antenna for catheter cardiac ablation [In Process Citation]. IEEE Trans Biomed Eng 1999 Dec.; 46(12):1480-2.

40. Haines, D. E. and Whayne, J. G. What is the radial temperature profile achieved during microwave catheter ablation with a helical cord antenna in canine myocardium? J.Am.Coll.Cardiol. 19, 99A. 1992. Ref Type: Abstract

41. Sealy WC, Gallagher JJ, Kasell J. His bundle interruption for control of inappropriate ventricular responses to atrial arrhythmias. Ann Thorac Surg 1981; 32(5):429-38.

42. Wang, P. J., Haugh, C. J., Schoen FJ, and et al. Left ventricular thrombus formation after high power microwave ablation: implications for temperature and power regulation. Circulation 88[4 Pt 2], I-354. 1993. Ref Type: Abstract

43. Wang, P. J., Ahmad A, Lenihan T, and et al. Developing and testing a feedback control system for microwave ablation: in vitro and in vivo results. Pacing Clin.Electrophysiol. 17[4 Pt II], 782. 1994. Ref Type: Abstract

44. Whayne JG, Nath S, Haines DE. Microwave catheter ablation of myocardium in vitro. Assessment of the characteristics of tissue heating and injury. Circulation 1994 May; 89(5):2390-5.

45. Whayne, J. G. and Haines, D. E. Comparison of thermal profiles produced by new antenna designs for microwave catheter ablation. Pacing Clin.Electrophysiol. 15, 580. 1992. Ref Type: Abstract

46. Whayne, J. G., Nath, S., and Haines, D. E. The effect of antenna design and microwave frequency on tissue temperature profiles during microwave catheter ablation invitro. Circulation 86[I], 192. 1992. Ref Type: Abstract

47. Wonnell TL, Stauffer PR, Langberg JJ. Evaluation of microwave and radio frequency catheter ablation in a myocardium-equivalent phantom model. IEEE Trans Biomed Eng 1992 Oct.; 39(10):1086-95.

48. Yang X, Watanabe I, Kojima T et al. Microwave ablation of the atrioventricular junction in vivo and ventricular myocardium in vitro and in vivo. Effects of varying power and duration on lesion volume. Jpn Heart J 1994 Mar.; 35(2):175-91.

49. Adragao P, Parreira L, Morgado F et al. Microwave ablation of atrial flutter [In Process Citation]. Pacing Clin Electrophysiol 1999 Nov.; 22(11):1692-5.

50. Beckman, K. J., Lin, J. C., Wang Y, and et al. Production of reversible and irreversible atrioventricular block by microwave energy. Circulation 76, IV-405. 1987. Ref Type: Abstract

51. Coggins D, Chin M, Wonnell, T., and et al. Efficacy of microwave energy for ventricular ablation. Pacing Clin.Electrophysiol. 14, 703. 1991. Ref Type: Abstract

52. Cohen TJ, Coggins D, Chin, M. C., and et al. Microwave ablation of ventricular myocardium: the effects of varying duration on lesion volume. Circulation , II-711. 1991. Ref Type: Abstract

53. Cohen TJ, Coggins DL, Chin, M. C., and et al. Microwave ablation of atrial myocardium: the effects of varying duration on lesion volume. Circulation 86[4], I-784. 1992. Ref Type: Abstract

54. Huang SKS, Lin, J. C., Mazzola F, and et al. Percutaneous microwave ablation of the ventricular myocardium using a 4-mm split-tip antenna electrode: a novel method for potential ablation of ventricular tachycardia. J.Am.Coll.Cardiol. 34A. 1994. Ref Type: Abstract

55. Ikeda T, Sugi K, Enjoji Y et al. Relation between the size of lesions and arrhythmias produced by microwave catheter ablation with a special electrode device. Jpn Circ J 1994 Mar.; 58(3):214-21.

56. Langberg JJ, Wonnell T, Chin MC et al. Catheter ablation of the atrioventricular junction using a helical microwave antenna: a novel means of coupling energy to the endocardium. Pacing Clin Electrophysiol 1991 Dec.; 14(12):2105-13.

57. Liem LB, Mead RH. Microwave linear ablation of the isthmus between the inferior vena cava and tricuspid annulus. Pacing Clin Electrophysiol 1998 Nov.; 21(11 Pt 1):2079-86.

58. Lin JC, Hariman RJ, Wang YJ, Wang YG. Microwave catheter ablation of the atrioventricular junction in closed-chest dogs. Med Biol Eng Comput 1996 July; 34(4):295-8.

59. Lin JC, Beckman KJ, Hariman RJ et al. Microwave ablation of the atrioventricular junction in open-chest dogs. Bioelectromagnetics 1995; 16(2):97-105.

60. Lin, J. C., Wang Y, and Hariman, R. J. Microwave catheter ablation of the canine atrioventricular junction. J.Am.Coll.Cardiol. 16, 357A. 1993. Ref Type: Abstract

61. Pires LA, Huang SKS, Lin JC. Comparison of radiofrequency (RF) versus microwave (MW) energy catheter ablation of the bovine ventricular myocardium. Pacing Clin Electrophysiol 1994; 17(4 Pt II):782.

62. Rho TH, Ito M, Pride HP et al. Microwave ablation of canine atrial tachycardia induced by aconitine. Am Heart J 1995 May; 129(5):1021-5.

63. Ruder M, Mead, R. H., Baron K, Radin M, and Higgins S. Microwave ablation: in vivo data. Pacing Clin.Electrophysiol. 17[4 Pt II], 781. 1994. Ref Type: Abstract

64. Tardif JC, Groeneveld PW, Wang PJ et al. Intracardiac echocardiographic guidance during microwave catheter ablation. J Am Soc Echocardiogr 1999 Jan.; 12(1):41-7.

65. Wagshal AB, Huang S, Lin, J. C., and et al. Use of a newly-designed microwave antenna for catheter ablation of the atrioventricular junction. J.Am.Coll.Cardiol. 82A. 1994. Ref Type: Abstract

66. Wang PJ, Schoen FJ, Aronovitz M, Haugh, C., Gadhoke A, and Estes NAM. Microwave catheter ablation under the mitral annulus: a new method of accessory pathway ablation. Pacing Clin.Electrophysiol. 16[4 Pt II], 866. 1993. Ref Type: Abstract

67. Wang PJ, Gadhoke A, Schoen FJ, and et al. Microwave catheter ablation via the coronary sinus: the need for power and temperature regulation. Pacing Clin.Electrophysiol. 17[4 Pt II], 813. 1994. Ref Type: Abstract

68. Watanabe I, Nakai T, Yanagawa S et al. Catheter ablation of canine ventricular myocardium. The use of repetitive short time constant capacitive shocks to increase lesion volume. Jpn Heart J 1997; 38(1):107-15.

69. Watanabe H, Hayashi J, Sugawara M et al. Experimental application of microwave tissue coagulation to ventricular myocardium. Ann Thorac Surg 1999 Mar.; 67(3):666-71.

70. Dany Bérubé. Traitement des arythmies cardiaques par ablation micro-onde, Philosophiae doctor thesis. Biomedical engineering institute 1998.

71. Liem BL, Mead RH. Microwave linear ablation of the isthmus between the inferior vena cava and tricuspid annulus. Pacing Clin Electrophysiol 1998; 21:2079-86.

72. Sie HT, Ramdat Misier AR, and et al. Radiofrequency ablation of atrial fibrillation in patients undergoing mitral valve surgery; first experience. Circulation 94[8], I-675. 1996. Ref Type: Abstract

73. Elvan A, Pride HP, Eble JN, et al. Radiofrequency catheter ablation of the atria reduces inducibility and duration of atrial fibrillation in dogs. Circulation 1995; 91:2235-44.

74. Khargi K. The potential role of the cooled tip radiofrequency ablation catheter in the Cox-Maze III procedure. Thorac. Cardiovasc. 1999; 47 (Suppl.). J Thorac Cardiovasc Surg 47, 373. 1999. Ref Type: Abstract

75. Kottkamp H, Hindricks G, Hammel D et al. Intraoperative radiofrequency ablation of chronic atrial fibrillation: A left atrial curative approach by elimination of anatomic "anchor" reentrant circuits. 1999; 10:772-780. J Cardiovasc Electrophysiol 1999; 10:772-80.

76. Spitzer SG, Richter P, Knaut M, Schuler S. Treatment of atrial fibrillation in open heart surgery--the potential role of microwave energy. Thorac Cardiovasc Surg 1999 Aug.; 47 Suppl 3:374-8:374-8.

77. Knaut M, Spitzer SG, Karolyi L. et al. Intraoperative Microwave Ablation for Curative Treatment of Atrial Fibrillation in Open Heart Surgery - The MICRO-STAF and MICRO-PASS Pilot Trial. Thorac Cardiovasc Surg 1999; 47(Suppl):379-84.

Part V

Future Perspective

Chapter 33

THE FUTURE OF CATHETER MAPPING AND ABLATION

Eugene Downar
Toronto General Hospital, Toronto, Ontario, Canada

Over the past decade spectacular advances have been achieved in the field of catheter mapping and ablation. The range of arrhythmias for which curative treatment can be offered is ever widening and the success rate climbing. Furthermore initial fears that indiscriminate empiric ablation would spell the end of the science of electrophysiology have proven to be groundless. In fact the opposite has occurred. With the explosion of clinical invasive electrophysiology major new insights in to the mechanisms of arrhythmias in the human heart have been gained. In many instances the pathophysiology of clinical arrhythmias has had to be completely revised and rewritten.

It is all the more impressive that most of the achievements have been attained without any major change in the basic technique of catheter mapping and ablation. Linear electrode catheters are guided fluroscopically by standard X-ray equipment. An exploring electrode catheter identifies a target usually through point by point mapping. Standard RF energy is delivered through the exploring electrode. Each of these basic components of the procedure has marked innate restrictions, which limit the scope and facility of what can be achieved with standard catheter ablation approach.

Fluoroscopy provides great visualization of the catheters but very little information on cardiac anatomy and how the catheters relate to that anatomy. It is further limited to two dimensions. Point by point mapping with a single exploring electrode is time consuming and requires electrical and hemodynamic stability. Standard RF delivery systems tend to produce punctuate lesions and are difficult to deploy so as to produce linear transmural lesions when needed.

L. Bing Liem and E. Downar (eds.), Progress in Catheter Ablation, 533-536.

Many of the contributors to this book describe exciting new technologies designed to overcome some of the limitations of current techniques.

The challenges for the future lie in five main areas: -

Improved visualization of detailed cardiac anatomy.

On-line demonstration of the position of electrodes in relationship to that anatomy.

Projection of excitation (timing and voltage) on to the anatomic detail.

Access to regions other than the endocardium e.g. intramural myocardium and epicardium surfaces.

Delivery of specific ablation lesions tailored to specific arrhythmias.

Ideally catheter ablation should deliver the most succinct lesion that will disrupt an arrhythmogenic mechanism without producing unnecessary collateral injury. Such a lesion should be based on accurate mapping, which can only be facilitated by a detailed depiction of the anatomy involved. Additional benefits of being able visualize cardiac anatomy include: -

Identification of specific structures being sought e.g. coronary sinus os, pulmonary vein orifices, crista terminalis.

Recognition of abnormal lesions of scar, mural thrombus, anatomic anomalies such as diverticuli and frank congenital malformations.

Identification of trabeculae, chordae and other structures thwarting the manipulation of an exploring catheter in to a desired region.

Accurate delineation of the cardiac surface of the chamber being mapped to identify any significant mismatch between that chamber and an electrode array or derived 3-D shell from electro-anatomic mapping.

Safety issues such as may be involved the guidance of multiple transeptal sheaths in distorted anatomy.

Currently available fluoroscopic techniques offer useful video mixing of angiographic loops with live fluoroscopy. This can provide some anatomic feedback during catheter manipulation but only in one plane. Spin acquisition during angiography can provide 3-D images of angiograms of comparatively static regions such as cerebral vessels. Cardiac motion provides a challenge to adapting this technique to the heart. It is likely however that before long 3-D angiograms will be available for video mixing. When spatially synchronized it will be possible to guide catheters under fluoroscopic control within the 3-D projection of the previously acquired angiogram.

Accurate 3-D shells of intra-cardiac space can be acquired by electro-anatomic mapping system. Unfortunately anatomic detail in such depictions is sparse. In addition there is the inconvenience of having to work with two separate workstations showing two separate images; one fluoroscopic the other electro-anatomic. There is no reason why the two images could not be spatially "nested" and viewed together as an integrated image in multiple projections. This will provide a larger anatomic context for the electro-anatomic image. By providing fluoroscopic feedback of the exploring catheter's position it should shorten the learning period to acquire expertise in electro-anatomic mapping.

Intracardiac echocardiography is the one technique, which currently provides most the detailed anatomic information at the time of an electrophysiological study. It can readily identify potential target structures such as the crista terminalis and pulmonary veins that may otherwise be difficult to visualize. It can also enhance the safety of transseptal procedures and monitor catheter – tissue contact during ablation.

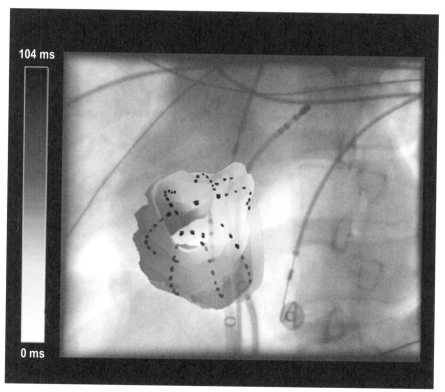

Figure 1. 4-D Map of ventricular activation during sinus rhythm superimposed on fluoroscopic image. Intracardiac echocardiograms (obtained with ICE™ catheter) of right ventricular cavity with a basket catheter (EPT Constellation™) in place were used to reconstruct the right ventricular endocardial surface. Local electrograms from the basket catheter were used to obtain color map of endocardial activation sequence (see color code at side). The combined electroanatomic image is then superimposed on the fluoroscopic image of the basket catheter in the corresponding obliquity after correcting for scale.

We have been able to do 3-D echo reconstructions of the ventricles with basket catheters in place. The activation data from the basket array can be integrated with the 3-D echo images. This information can be further integrated with fluoroscopic images of the basket at the time of the mapping. In this way it is possible to obtain "4-D" maps of ventricular activation and to display this on the fluoroscopy screen (see Figures 1 and 2). Although this can only be achieved retrospectively at present, it is not difficult to imagine that such information will be available at the time of a catheter ablation procedure in the not too distant future.

Magnetic resonance imaging offers perhaps the most detailed cardiac images and includes details of intramural tissue. Although at present MRI has not played any major role in facilitating catheter mapping this will probably soon change. Already it is possible to obtain incredibly detailed 3-D MRI angiograms using Gadolinium. Such images of for example, pulmonary vein anatomy, when integrated with fluoroscopic images will provide powerful tools for facilitating catheter mapping and ablation. Direct MRI-guided electrophysiological intervention is an exciting prospect whose future may not be that distant.

Finally it is hard to imagine an EP intervention laboratory of the future that would not provide improved access to the epicardial surface. Mini thoracotomy procedures may be routine in such a laboratory and may offer an easy access for laser and cryoablation of specific arrhythmias.

In contemplating the future it is interesting to consider the past. Hippocrates in 400 BC stated:

"Those diseases that medicines do not cure are cured by the knife. Those that the knife does not cure are cured by fire. Those that the fire does not cure must be considered incurable".

In some ways this aphorism is remarkably prescient as far as recent arrhythmia management is concerned. However current sentiment among EP interventionists sees failure to cure by fire as a reason to redouble effort to find a curative ablation procedure. Judging by the results of the recent past, future prospects are indeed exciting.

Chapter 34

A RETROSPECTIVE MUSING ON SURGERY FOR CARDIAC ARRHYTHMIAS

Gerard M. Guiraudon
London Health Science Center, London, Ontario and The University of Ottawa Heart Institute, Ottawa,Ontario, Canada.

INTRODUCTION

Because of its short life, surgery for cardiac arrhythmias is a good model of the accelerated evolutions in therapeutic interventions. This paper is, it should be said, for the sake of a certain objectivity, a recount of the philosophical view of both an active witness and participant. Arrhythmia surgery was the last field in clinical cardiology to be included in the surgical fold. In those golden years, cardiac surgery was or seemed the only effective intervention to treat cardiac disorders. Cardiac arrhythmias with their unpredictability and electrical storms were left aside because the common wisdom was that the plumbing techniques would not correct electrical short circuits.

Surgery is a branch of the tree of basic and clinical knowledge. The surgeon has to assimilate the concepts and translate the pathophysiology into interventional rationale and surgical techniques. Surgery is the final pathway on the road to treat the disease, but the map is set by physicians and scientists.

1. THE TARGET, THE BULLET, THE GUN. THE QUEST FOR A DEFINITION OF SURGERY

Planning a therapeutic action implies reconciling three parts: the target, the bullet, and the gun. Although that concept applies to all interventions, it is well evidenced by instrumental interventions. Surgical approaches to cardiac arrhythmias offer many comprehensive examples.[1-3]

L. Bing Liem and E. Downar (eds.), Progress in Catheter Ablation, 537-560.
© 2001 *Kluwer Academic Publishers. Printed in the Netherlands.*

1.1   The Target

The target is the "anatomical substrate" defined by the currently accepted pathophysiology of the problem or symptoms to be treated. The accessory atrioventricular (AV) pathway is the target of interventions to eliminate the symptoms associated with Wolff-Parkinson-White (WPW) syndrome because it is one of the necessary links for the reentrant loop to occur and the necessary conditions for cardiac arrhythmias to occur. The definition of "target" varies over time with progress in pathophysiology and/or approaches. At one time the entire AV node was the target to treat AV nodal reentrant tachycardias. Neutralization of the target was associated with loss of AV node function and complete heart block with its dependency on permanent pacing.[4,5] A better understanding of anatomy and pathophysiology allowed description of a more discrete target: the intranodal limbs (pathways) of the reentrant loops. The neutralization of one of these small discrete target allowed "ablation" of the target with preservation of the AV nodal function.[6] Therefore the target should be constantly revisited and made smaller and more discrete to allow disabling of target and   pathophysiological mechanism with preservation of function. The definition and/or choice of targets requires lengthy development to be exhaustive. It is the most critical component of any therapeutic strategy.

1.2   The Bullet

The bullet is the agent aimed at neutralizing the target using traditional cutting or ablation with various forms of energy (radio frequency electric current, cryoablation, microwave energy, etc), Modification of target instead of "destruction "is a preferred alternative, when feasible etc. The target can be neutratized using two critical concepts which were identifies early in our experince:the concept of ablation[7] and the concept of exclusion[8] when anatomy or physiology make ablation either hazardous or incomplete. The bullet should focus on the target and only neutralize he target to avoid collateral damage. "Ablation" of the tiny accessory AV pathway using appropriate technique is a good illustration of discrete Target-specific ablation.

1.3   The Gun

The gun is the way the bullet is delivered on target. The choice of the delivery system depends on many factors. The two most important being the target and the bullet. The three factors of the triad interfere on each other: the change of one could allow the change and improvement of one or the other or both. However there may be more than one way of delivery to choose. The AV accessory pathway can be "accessed" using a variety of routes and bullets. We will describe the surgical approach to the AV accessory pathway, as an example, because this experience was critical in conceptualizing the triad principle and consequently in realizing that surgery was only one of many routes a therapeutic bullet can be delivered by.[3]

Surgical Route

To access the accessory pathway that is located mostly within the atrioventricular groove near the AV annulus, the initial "classical" surgical approach was similar to the surgical approach used for mitralvalve or tricuspid valve surgery.[9,10] Because the accessory pathway was located in the vicinity of the atrio-ventricular annulus , it was deemed suitable to use to approach the AV annulus, the approach used to insert a atrio-ventricular valve. Unfortunately the approach required a number of traumatic ancillary steps: general anaesthesia with tracheal intubation, median sternotomy, epicardial mapping used as a guide to localize the accessory pathway, cardiopulmonary bypass, aortic clamping with concomitant myocardial preservation techniques, and right or left atriotomy to expose the AV annulus of interest. When the "target" was accessed, the bullet could be delivered, that is, dissection of the AV groove and separation of the atrial and ventricular myocardium to eliminate the accessory pathway connection. A complex endocardial approach was used to access the AV sulcus, which is, by nature, an epicardial structure.

Each step of the surgical chain of delivery is associated with inherent risks (mortality or morbidity). The overall "surgical risk" is the summation of all "elementary risks."[1,2]

Review of the surgical technique in the late seventies, using the triad concept, showed that minor risk is associated with the bullet (dissection of the AV groove) while the major risks are associated with the surgical delivery, i.e: cardiopulmonary bypass[11] and aortic clamping.[12] This applies for most surgically delivered therapies , which are deemed a necessary evil. To reduce surgical risk is to amend or eliminate the key steps in delivery associated with the greater risk.

The morbidity of surgery for the Wolf-Parkinson-White syndrome reduced, not by changing the target, but by changing the impact of bullet on the targeted region, and dramatically modifying the "gun."[13,14] The epicardial approach used epicardial dissection of the AV sulcus in the region of interest without the need to open the heart. The heart could be kept beating, without significant hemodynamic compromise. Cardiopulmonary bypass and cross-clamping of the aorta, with their inherent adverse effects, could be eliminated. The surgical delivery was simpler; patients could be extubated in the operating room and bypass the intensive care unit. They had an easier, quicker and gentler recovery with the same degree of efficacy (ablation of the accessory pathway). The efficacy determined by rational choices of target and bullet not by guns.

1.3.1   Catheter Route

As experience with management and exploration of the WPW syndrome progressed, it became apparent that catheters that precisely localize accessory pathways by recording their electrical potential, could concomitantly deliver the bullet "on target" using electrical energy via the catheters. Investigators embarked successfully in the development of the catheter delivery that was already used for AV nodal ablation. A new bullet:radio-frequency [RF] energy replaced DC shocks energy. DC shocks[15] were a bomb of mass destruction compare to the size of target (bullet side effects) while RF energy allowed a safe delivery of target specific bullet on target using an endocardial catheter[16,17] with minimal side effects In July 1990, RF catheter ablation of the accessory pathway associated with the WPW syndrome could be successfully used in most patients, avoiding the surgical delivery.. After 10 years of pregnant dedication and skill by pioneers the catheter technique took charge and offered safer one-day curative intervention. A much greater number of patients could benefit from a cure, not because the therapy was more effective, but because it was much less invasive. History of interventions shows that adverse events are the most powerful adverse factors to promoting a novel therapy. Development of catheter techniques, in cardiology, had illustrated this tenet over and over again at each " passage" from surgical delivery to catheter delivery.[18]

1.3.2   Other Routes

There are other routes to delivering other bullets, namely drugs, or other energies. Discussion of these approaches is not part of our purpose, but their roles and options should be kept in mind. A target-specific drug with the ability to permanently neutralize the target is the "magic" bullet and the ultimate goal.

1.4   Side Effects

Side effects are effects associated with therapeutic interventions that do not affect the target. Most side effects are unwanted, but some are, in very rare instances, beneficial.[19] This definition shows that surgery is mainly a "side effect" associated with major morbidity and mortality. Paradoxically, the "surgical side effects" are so well accepted without due examination that their characteristics are ignored. Besides the cost in human suffering, there is a costly industry dedicated to treat surgical side effects: the intensive care unit (ICU), step-down unit, rehabilitation programs, etc. The cost is very high at the economic and human level. There is no unavoidable curse that makes the approach of a given target surgical. Only our inability to revisit the target and design new bullet keep that therapy in the surgical domain. "Surgery" should be used only as a temporary and necessary delivery system, while every efforts are made to design a better delivery. To use a moto outside our field, the surgery should be part of the solution, not of the problem.

The current development and acceptance of other less invasive deliveries in cardiac surgery is bringing further evidences, if they were needed that the delivery system : the gun is the key determinant of morbidity.[20,21]

1.5   Patients' Outcome

Patients' outcome is the summation of (1) effects of therapy on target; (2) magnitude and nature of side effects; and (3) patient improvement and satisfaction, not to mention the premier factor: cost. Because surgery is a dramatic way of delivering a therapy, it is the main determinant of postoperative "complications," hospital length of stay, duration of recovery, and return to an active life.[22] In the management of cardiac patients, surgery has an overall impact that is disproportionate to the number of patients involved. Cardiac surgery is the primary target for planners, administrators, payers, and state legislators[23] to improve care delivery and outcomes. Operative therapy must deliver a very special bullet that is associated with high efficacy, prolonged palliation or cure, minimal unwanted effects, and excellent outcome if it is to compete successfully with other alternative instrumental interventions. Failure to comply with the above principle may produce stillborn or retarded surgical techniques.

Claude Bernard Legacy: Surgical Interventions as an Experiment

The target/bullet/gun concept showed that therapy and pathophysiology and anatomy are closely interrelated and therapeutic approaches may be designed in the best interest of patients and science: i.e. a therapeutic experiment. This revisited scientific surgical attitude gives the intellectual equipment and impetus to work along two lines of thoughts: #1 To design surgical approaches as an experiment without compromising safety and efficacy to make scientific observations, increase our body of knowledge and improve interventionnal techniques. It should be considered unethical to miss an opportunity to learn while cutting. #2 To revisit and improve surgical technique in each dimension of the triad and achieve the same efficacy on target without excessive risks. This line of research was the beginning of the so-called, for a better phrase, minimally invasive surgery. Decreasing the surgical risks is a complex task. Its main target is to eliminate the use of aortic cross-clamping and myocardial preservation and the heart-lung machine. The evolution of the surgery for the WPW syndrome is a good illustration of this novel attitude.

2.   THE EPICARDIAL VIEW: THE WPW STORY

In the seventies electrophysiologists were concerned with the significant morbidity and mortality associated with the accepted endocardial approach, pioneered by W.C. Sealy and J.J. Gallagher.[9,10] That technique was similar to the one used for valvular surgery and carried a risk acceptable, indeed, for patients with severe valvular diseases and a poor prognosis without surgical correction but much less acceptable for patients with the Wolff-Parkinson-White syndrome, albeit some of them were identified at high risk of sudden cardiac death. Common wisdom suggested that the risk of therapy should be consistent with the risk associated with the natural history of the disease.

Meeting that goal required revisiting the each elements of the triad and including the experimental aspect of the new technique took.

2.1   Anatomy of the Target

Review of accessory pathway anatomy[24] suggested strongly that the vast majority of pathways were located within the atrioventricular sulcus close to the atrio- ventricular annulus or at a distance. Data were few but were consistent. Unfortunately the surgical dissection of the accessory pathway using the endocardial approach did not provide reliable insights into the anatomy of the pathways. The location of the pathways within the sulcus implied that a intervention limited to the sulcus without entering the heart would suffice.

2.2   Modifying the Bullet

This principle established, a technique was to be developed to address the feasibility of epicardial dissection the atrio-ventricular sulcus and its associated hazards. The following issues were addressed in the experimental laboratory:

-Coronary arteries can be preserved intact by careful dissection, and by avoiding using certain ablative technique, such as cryoablation or radiofrequency energy (RF) in a way that coronary arteries could be permanently damaged.[25]

-Atrial wall insertion on the AV annulus is a fragile spot. Close dissection can be dangerous and be replaced by transmural cryoablation, which was a documented a safe technique to neutralize the para-annular myocardium.[26]

-Physiology of coronary sinus, great cardiac vein and afferent epicardial cardiac veins was studied. It was documented that permanent interruption (ligation) of epicardial cardiac veins and/or great cardiac veins was not associated with permanent myocardial damage. These veins could be ligated to repair an accidental injury. Only the coronary sinus itself could no be ligated without myocardial damage.[27]

At the end of the study it was documented that the atrio-ventricular sulcus could be dissected and that all potential attachments of the accessory pathway could be either divided or cryoablated.

2.3   Modifying the Gun; the Delivery System

Dissection of the AV sulcus on the beating heart implies a good stable, safe and reliable exposure of AV sulcus in the region of interest, without the need for cardio-pulmonary bypass i.e. without hemodynamic compromise. If these conditions are met, the surgery can be delivered using only a median sternotomy. Exposure and dissection of the sulcus requires a dramatic change in mentality to accept that the heart can be manipulated and dislocated under specific conditions without hemodynamic compromise. The thoracic incision is to be modified to ease exposing selected parts of the heart.

As far as dislocating the heart is concerned, it has to be understood that dislocation itself does not produce cardiac dysfunction and hypotension. Dislocation is not per se associated with impaired venous return, AV valve dysfunction or ventricular systolic dysfunction. Careful observation showed that dislocation, especially manual dislocation, is always associated with a certain degree of ventricular compression, which is associated with impaired ventricular filling and consequent low ventricular output and hypotension.

Techniques to dislocate the heart were described to expose the various regions: The posteroseptal region was exposed by dislocating the right ventricle upward using a rigid pledgetted U-suture and by deflecting the diaphragm downward using a large stay suture. An excellent and safe exposure was obtain to satisfaction.[28] It took a little longer to described a good exposure off pump for the free wall: the sling exposure[14] All those changes and improvements were part of a continuum of observation into practical and scientific concepts.

2.4   Virtual Reality Check

The most critical moment in developing a new technique is the quantum leap into clinical application: The crossing of the unknown. "Le passage a l'acte."

Indeed the team had to go through mental readiness for preparation of first clinical cases. This process is the most demanding step in developing a new surgical technique. It consists, to quote Pascal the scientist, to seat in a room and do nothing. This capsule definition of intelligence by Pascal characterizes well the intellectual process of doing and redoing over and over again the surgery in virtual reality to become familiar with all the details, to discover the possible incidents, variants and complications, to come up with adequate solutions to all anticipated problems, to write down a comprehensive surgical manual and to arrive the day of the first clinical case with considerable virtual but solid experience. This mental training process allows bridging the divide between the concept and its experimental verification in the laboratory and the human application. If the new technique cannot be performed in virtual reality to satisfaction, it cannot be done in real life. Description of this mental preparation period is not in the editorial requirements of scientific papers, because either it is deemed to go without saying or, more likely, it belongs to philosophy of science. In our experience it is the unavoidable, sine qua none, condition for successful creation and development of novel techniques.

2.5   **Epistemologic Return**

Development of a new technique should adhere to the tenets of latest scientific knowledge and practice,   but   also   should be designed as an experiment to contribute to knowledge using scientific method, but without compromising patient care in term of safety and effectiveness. Expected better patients outcome should be documented as well. The epicardial approach was used as a research tool and allowed surgery to contribute insights into the functional anatomy of accessory pathways and into the concept of mini-invasive surgery on the beating heart:

Functional Anatomy and variant of the AV Accessory Pathways: Discrete dissection of the AV groove on the beating heart was used as a investigatory procedure in addition to intra-operative epicardial cardiac mapping. Fine dissection allowed us to precisely determine the time when the accessory pathway conduction was interrupted by gentle discrete dissection. But more importantly when the AV pathway conduction persisted in the area of interest during dissection, it was assumed that either the dissection was incomplete or the pathway location was not where expected. Some surgical approaches for variant pathways were planned pre-operatively (Mahaim pathways) or intra-operatively, when intra operative evidences pointed out another location. Time was spent out of the operative room reviewing all data and planning a variant revisited approach.

Functional anatomy and location of the common pathways were described.[29] Their locations in relation with special anatomical landmark determined. The Right ventricular free wall pathway were found either deep, almost sub endocardial and difficult to access epicardially or superficial in the inferior segment (visible in rare instances). The left free wall pathways were mostly para-annular. The sub-varieties of anteroseptal,[30] posteroseptal[31] and the wrongly labelled left-anteroseptal were described, as our knowledge of cardiac anatomy and understanding of function and anatomy of AV pathways progressed. Variant pathways were identified: the AV nodal-His bundle-like so-called Mahaim' fibers;[32] the coronary sinus diverticulum;[33] the intra-membranous septum pathways associated with aberrant pre-excitation.[34,35] Etc.....

These were exciting times: surgery only was curing patients, a novel twist of fate in cardiac surgery, but also was contributing to science and preparing the next generation of less invasive delivery system: the endocardial catheter. Catheter ablation was developing concurrently and was greatly benefiting of the 'surgical' description of the AV pathway anatomy. In July 1990 the catheter ablation technique took charge and surgery was history. The catheter, that was the tool providing the basis to interventional electrophysiology, reclaimed the entire ownership of the field that was temporarily sublet to surgery. The surgery had already overplayed its role for too long.

"Minimally Invasive Surgery": The epicardial approach for the Wolf Parkinson White syndrome was the first routine "off pump surgery" to replace an accepted "on pump, open heart" technique. During the same period off pump CABG surgery was being developed.[20,21] Acceptance for surgical the technique seem arrhythmia specific. In the early eighties, cardiologists accepted and promoted the "off pump" technique while many surgeons were reluctant. The minimally invasive approaches, which were pioneered in the eighties were to develop later in the nineties and are widely accepted now.

3.   THE ARRHYTHMOGENIC RIGHT VENTRICULAR DYSPLASIA: THE "GLOBAL APPROACH"

The story of the ARVD and its associated ventricular tachycardias is unique, because it was recognized and successfully treated using ventriculotomies guided by epicardial mapping on the first two cases.[7] Recognized means that the cardiac pathology was identified as an unknown entity. Successfully means that in the short term ventricular tachycardias were controlled. These were the first surgical cases that documented that ventricular tachycardias could be interrupted using electrophysiologically guided direct surgery. These surgical, kind of serendipituous, successes allowed to have more cases referred and to get the clinical material to progress in the pathophysiology of the disease.

Surgical therapy preceded knowledge of the disease, and was carried out without regards to the triad principle. This is not an isolated case in the story of surgery for arrhythmias. Success, bailing out ignorance, justifies a warrant to pursuit positive experience. ARVD is now a well described and understood disease, with exceptional indication for surgical correction, albeit it has served as a unique model for developing surgery for ventricular arrhythmias.[36-40]

3.1 Mapping as a Target. The WPW Connection

A that time in 1973, surgery for the Wolff-ParkinsonWhite syndrome was the unique model. Mapping was an reliable guide and seemed to do the thinking for the surgeon.

Ventricular tachycardia (VT's) associated with ARVD were deemed associated with a re-entrant mechanism. It was speculated that using the same guide (cardiac mapping) and the same principle (incision at critical early site), the re-entrant loop could be "definitely interrupted." Actually, VT were interrupted by a simple ventriculotomy at "the site of earliest ventricular activation determined by epicardial mapping, aping WPW surgery, albeit with slightly different underlying concepts. Ventricular re-entrant mechanism was associated with slow conduction, manifested by delayed activation potential recorded outside the normal duration of QRS during the entire cardiac cycle (diastolic activation). These "late potentials" were the substrate for the necessary slow component of continuous re-entrant activation associated with the tachycardia mechanism. The areas where delayed activation was recorded led to the concept of arrhythmogenic anatomical substrate, which was to become a very productive concept consistent with the "target" principle.

These mapping data defined two target zones:[41,42] the earliest ventricular activation localized the exit site of the actual reentrant circuit, where the reentrant activation activates the rest of the ventricles . Areas of delayed activations localized the area of cardiac pathology associated with electrophysiologic disturbances, meanly slow conduction. These areas were recognized as the anatomical arrhythmogenic substrate (although the phrase was an oxymoron), part of which was necessary to the reentrant loop to occur. This initial naive and simplistic view has sustained the test of time , but with many sophisticated improvements.

3.2 Cardiac Pathology

The pathology was quite unique. There was a large ballooning right ventricle, with dyskinetic area, at the infundibulum, apex and inferior wall. The fatty infiltration gave a yellow-purplish color to the myocardium. . Microscopic examination showed myocardial fibers disappearing without a trace and being replaced by fat (apostosis is now the documented mechanism). It was clearly a new pathological entity. Surgical experience and surgical pathology documented that adiposis could be circumscribed to the right ventricular free wall (RVFW), or involve the entire ventricular myocardium, namely the left ventricle.

3.3   **Is Bigger Better. The Right Ventricular Free Wall**

In 1981, review of 12 surgical cases established that ventriculotomies were not successful in permanently interrupting the tachycardia, because the entire RVFW was arrhythmogenic.[43] Patients with left involvement could experience cardiac failure. The conclusion was that, in patients in whom ARVD is limited to the RVFW, the RVFW should be the surgical **target** and should be entirely neutralized. At first, this seemed an unrealistic target, but issues were addressed in a comprehensive manner. The RVFW disconnection concept which was described was a kind of intellectual fluke or the product of a split intellect, because at the time less surgery was advocated for the WPW syndrome, a bullet of massive "destruction" of cardiac physiology was being used.   The right ventricular free wall exclusion was similar to AV nodal ablation for atrio-ventricular nodal reentrant tachycardia where disabling the tachycardia mechanism was associated with inherent disabling of atrio-ventricular nodal function. Right ventricular free wall disconnection was described after the following concerns were addressed.[44]

Anatomical feasibility.   Study of the functional anatomy of the right ventricle showed that it could be disarticulated and reimplanted. The tricuspid valve system could be preserved. In most mammals, but not in humans, the papillary muscles attach to the septum. This evolutionary trick allows the RVFW to dilate without concomitant tricuspid valve dysfunction.   In humans, the papillary muscle is re-attached to the septum, if feasible. Despite complex trabeculation and tricuspid valve apparatus, the RVFW could be detached without injury to major structures and re-implanted.

Right ventricular physiology. Physiologic studies supported the concept that the entire circulation could be supported by the left ventricle alone, under given conditions:normal low pulmonary resistance. Pathological models, such as tricuspid atresia, and Fontan's operation were more indirect evidences. A series of total disconnections of the right ventricular free wall were carried out in the dog. It was documented that the RVFW could be disconnected with preservation of some degree of RV systole associated with major paradoxical septum motion, no evidence of cardiac failure and long term survival.[45]

Indications for RVFW disconnection.   We speculated that the ideal candidate will be an ARVD without evidence of LV involvement. But there was an inherent limitation - the difficulty of documenting that the LV is intact. It is actually easier to document pathology than normalcy.   Left ventricular angiogram and ejection fraction were used as markers.

Virtual reality preparation was most difficult because of the uniqueness of the pathophysiology of the surgical design.

The surgery. Shortly after completion of preparedness, two patients with ARVD and quasi-incessant resistant VT were referred from Newfoundland: an ARVD nest. The surgery went according to the virtual reality plan. Patient did well post-operatively. It was very rewarding to see that the experimental construct sustained the clinical test.

Although the RVFW disconnection seemed a surgical step too far, it documented that the concept was valid. Across the north American continent, one patient or so every year was to benefit from it. Over the years we learned to select the best candidates, based essentially on left ventricular function tests.[21]. The time and effort to treat a handful of patients were not wasted. RFVW disconnection not only contributed to the understanding of ARVD, but became, and still is, a remarkable experimental model to study cardiac physiology, with unexpected clinical applications.[46,47]

4.   VENTRICULAR TACHYCARDIAS AFTER ACUTE MYOCARDIAL INFARCTION: THE ELUSIVE TARGET

Concomitantly an approach to VT after acute myocardial infarction based on similar premises was attempted. It was anticipated that epicardiac mapping would be an effective guide in localizing the reentrant mechanism; and that interrupting VT would prolong life. These assumptions were made without a correct appreciation of the magnitude of myocardial scarring and associated left ventricular dysfunction. And that left ventricular function is the single most independent marker of survival in patients with ventricular arrhythmias.

Epicardial mapping failed to provide reliable guidance, but at least pointed out that the substrate was endocardial, and the endocardium should be mapped. Unfortunately, failure to interrupt the tachycardia was blamed on mapping instead of the mapper (blaming the messenger), and there was no consensus to proceeding with endocardial mapping, at least at our institution.[48]

Surgical pathology documented that ischemic lesions were mostly endocardial. In fact there was a discrete anatomical landmark to infarct scar, not epicardially, but endocardially: the endocardial fibrosis, as a landmark, was rediscovered from total oblivion.

However, initial difficulties were productive and allowed to design the first direct surgical approach to ventricular tachycardias after acute myocardial infarction. The Encircling Endocardial Ventriculotomy (EEV) which was based on electrophysiologic and mapping data, but did require mapping guidance at the time of surgery.[8] Fortunately, Mark Josephson in Philadelphia, would describe a more discrete endocardial approach based on intraoperative endocardial mapping.[52]

Mapping was still used to localize an area, not to pinpoint a small discrete segment. Mapping was a guide for regional localization of the mechanism and delineated a target far greater than needed to disable the mechanism. Consequently the bullet was too large, was associated with collateral damage and attained efficacy with compromising left ventricular function, because every collateral damage on target beyond the arrhythmogenic scar had potential adverse effects on ventricular function and surgical risks.

Surgery for VT after acute myocardial infraction did not achieve wide acceptance. The number of patients operated on every year remained minuscule compared to the size of the patient population. Surgery fared poorly in clinical trials, because of safety (high mortality and morbidity) and even in studies with no surgical mortality.[50,51]

The failed development of surgery for ventricular tachycardias determined by: Inadequate match between target and bullet, with excessive collateral damage and the inherent outwards effects of the delivery system (gun) on left ventricular function. Mainly, to cite a few, ventriculotomy, aortic cross-clamping and myocardial preservation.

The ischemic anatomical arrhythmogenic substrate was elusive, changing with vicarious substrates and buried into a large arrhythmogenic scar (the border zone of the aneurysm). The size of the tissue involved is often underestimated, as evidenced by the fact that the greater the mass of scar tissue, the greater the arrhythmogenic potential.[52] Consequently, the target was never discrete and/or well defined. Intraoperative mapping, with limited time and technology, produced only crude guidance, pinpointing the discrete substrate in rare cases.

While safety was asking for discrete small ablation, efficacy was asking for the largest ablation of targeted substrate. But, for reasons of safety (myocardial preservation), surgical technique was forced to compromise effectiveness, i.e. instead of matching the bullet (amount of neutralized arrhythmogenic myocardium) with the target (comprehensive delineation of substrate), the target was matched with a smaller but apparently safer bullet. This compromise between efficacy and function was never well determined because its impact on outcome was dwarfed by the effects of side effects of surgical delivery (cardiopulmonary bypass, aortic cross-clamping, aneursymectomy), which seemed to almost nullify the benefits of arrhythmia surgery. Cardiac mapping was never able to delineate a discrete target to deliver a discrete bullet.[53]

The results were aggravated by the fact that patients with life threatening ventricular arrhythmias have severe left ventricular dysfunction. The surgery could not be safely offered to the ones who needed it the most.

During the same period, Michel Mirowski[54] was developing the implantable cardioverter defibrillators (ICD) which allowed to document, because of its dramatically reduced side effects, that control of ventricular tachycardias prolong life in patients with left ventricular dysfunction: MADIT,[55] AVID[56] trials. An another example of side effects of delivery (gun) nullifying the beneficial effect of the bullet.

The conclusion is clear. Pacing and pumping are two sides of the same coin, with equal value, but pacing (rhythm) cannot be restored at the expense of pumping.

5.   ATRIAL FIBRILLATION: THE ATRIAL FIBRILLATION STORY

The history of surgical approach to atrial fibrillation has specific traits. The surgical approach for non-valvular atrial fibrillation, which was labelled lone atrial fibrillation, was described before a mechanism was documented and before the condition was recognized as a malady. In other world before the medical community at large recognized the problem and implicitly searched for solutions. The development of surgery for atrial fibrillation did not meet the therapeutic triad criteria, with its logical and comprehensive path.

5.1   The Epistemological Gap or the Crave for Action

In the early eighties, when the first surgical technique, the Corridor operation was described there was a need for a documented mechanism for atrial fibrillation. The random reentrant mechanism suggested by G Moe[57] and confirmed in animal studies by M Allessie[58] was an accepted model to explained the activation pattern during atrial fibrillation. But no claims were made and no evidences were produced to establish random reentry as the underlying mechanism. . The concept of a focal initiating or perpetuating mechanism was supported by indirect evidences such as atrial fibrillation triggered by focal tachycardias (WPW, Flutter, AVNRT) and theoretical and intellectual wisdom. Consequently, a valid target could not be identified without a documented mechanism Without a target the triad concept was void. This purely empirical situation did not discourage the drive for action.

5.2   Scientific Premises were Moot

The natural history and various clinical presentations of non-valvular atrial fibrillation had not been studies as yet. Its labeling as "lone " was telling. This was an electrocardiographic curiosity that did not require medical attention. There was only two studies which showed that lone atrial fibrillation was benign and not associated with any increased risk compare with the rest of the population in terms of life expectancy and incidence of stroke.[59,60] Therefore any intervention was an aggravation. It did not seem that there was a need, at that time, to embark in designing and implementing a surgical approach for lone atrial. But there were some theoretical reasons for actions.

#1 The perceived need for a curative intervention available for every cardiac arrhythmia.

#2 The intellectual impact of therapeutic interventions that have historically stimulated interest in the disease under consideration, as illustrated by the WPW syndrome story. Therapeutic interventions when successful become good incentives for good research.

#3 Despite the current accepted attitude of neglected benignity there were empirical evidences that patients with lone atrial fibrillation could be very problematic with severe symptoms and complication such as post-tachycardia syndrome and/or stroke.

5.3   The Rationale was Empirical

Anatomy and pathology, which has been for other arrhythmias a remarkable guide, did not provide specific lesions that could suggest a discrete arrhythmogenic substrate or mechanism.[61-63]

The rationale was elaborated on the following assumptions.

#1 In normal heart the role of atrial contraction is negligible because the normal ventricle is a sucking pump with a very active filling.[64] This assumption made the preservation or restoration of atrial contraction a second priority.

#2 Atrial chronotropic function was deemed critical to achieve normal hemodynamics, albeit some contemporary studies suggested that patients with lone atrial fibrillation had normal exercise responses on the treadmill test.[65]

#3 The rationale was to target the random reentry activation for want of a definite target. It was documented that atrial fibrillation requires a critical mass of atrial tissue to sustain.[57,58]   Exclusion of atrial tissue associated with concomitant reduction of not excluded tissue, associated with either fragmentation or channelling was the gist of the general rationale. It was anticipated that an intervention based on atrial exclusion and incisions would prevent the triggering mechanism from inducing atrial fibrillation and that (this was more speculative) that the perpetuation of the sinus rhythm will have a preventive effect on atrial fibrillation.

4 There was very good empirical evidences that the left atrium was the site of fibrillating mechanism and should be either excluded or ablated.

#5 The risk of stroke was never underestimated based on experience with mitral valve surgery-associated atrial fibrillation. A left atrial appendectomy was a necessary adjunct without known untoward effects.[19,66]

5.4   The Corridor Operation

The Corridor concept[67] was developed in the early eighties after discarding the simpler concept of left atrial exclusion that we contemplated in the seventies. The Corridor consisted of a strip of right atrium and septum harbouring the sinus node and the atrioventricular node-His bundle system. Experience with epicardial approach to the WPW syndrome provided guidance for surgical dissections of the anteroseptal region, septum and posteroseptal regions. Anteroseptal dissection suggested that division of the sinus node artery or devascularization of the sinus node were compatible with preservation of its function. Post-operative sinus node dysfunction was thought to be more likely associated with pre-existing sinus node dysfunction: a known feature of the natural history of atrial fibrillation.

The results of the Corridor operation were consistent with its concept and rationale. Sinus rhythm was restored and patients were asymptomatic. Clinical experience was insufficient in number to assess the impact on outcome. Long term studies showed deterioration of results over time.[68-70]

5.5   Success as a Rationale

In the following years a new operation was developed: the Maze Operation.[71-73]   It was based on the same body of empirical knowledge and incorporated the Corridor experience. It intended to preserve some degree of left atrial function, to obtain a more physiologic surgical design. Through trials and errors, and successive modifications a surgical technique, the Maze operation, was described. The last version gave satisfactory results in term of arrhythmia control and preservation of the left atrial function on echocardiographic recording. No surgical series was large enough to document significant effects on outcome, beside arrhythmia control.

5.6   Gun Control or Less Surgery

Because surgical delivery is associated with very significant side effects, the Maze operation was never used to address the entirety of the patients population, mimicking the fate of surgery for the WPW syndrome, when open heart technique was the only option.[9,10] The number of patients referred for an intervention is essentially determined by the magnitude of its side effects and grows as the delivery becomes less invasive: From open heart technique to closed beating heart technique; from closed heart to catheter technique.

5.7   The Growth in Knowledge and Experience

During the nineties a number of very interesting and critical events took place.

At the surgical level it was shown that surgery for atrial fibrillation was a kind of overkill. Less incisions, exclusion and channeling, reduced empirically, yielded similar results, although no conclusions regarding the underlying mechanism could be drawn. It confirmed the empirical nature of interventions. Sueda operation,[74] left atrial isolation,[75] fragmentation,[76] spiral operation,[77] to cite a few.   Surgery for atrial fibrillation was more and more associated with mitral valve surgery. Simpler techniques were used, in order to obtain a satisfactory efficacy associated with low surgical risk in selected patients. Melo,[78] in Portugal, pioneered and developed these techniques. At, the same time, he attempted to analyze the complex problematic symptoms and described a practical scoring system to express adequately the crux of the matter.[79]

Analysis of surgical results was not informative: Success could not document that the empirical rationale was true. Failure could only suggest that either the surgical technique has not been performed adequately, or that the surgical rationale did control the entire spectrum of mechanisms. An other speculation was that the failure was an electrical illusion and that in fact the surgery has uncover either a new arrhythmia or an arrhythmia scrambled by atrial fibrillation; Suggesting the daring hypothesis that atrial fibrillation may prevent the study of atrial fibrillation. Two of our patients after having a spiral operation, which is aimed at channelling the entire atria, presented with very fast regular atrial tachycardia post-operatively, which in retrospect were focal pulmonary vein tachycardias. Success, defined as the absence of atrial fibrillation and restoration of sinus rhythm, was not informative either. Surgical techniques were not designed as a surgical experiment and no valid knowledge could be obtained. The entire experience was an epistemologic disappointment. The Corridor as well as the left atrial exclusion were the only techniques, which confirmed that the site of the "mechanism ' was most likely located in the left atrium.[68,70,75]

The conclusion was that surgical techniques were to complex and/or extensive to yield valid data regarding the underlying mechanism. Review of results of each technique was not informative to address the following concerns: Which part of surgical action is effective in disabling the mechanism, which part is pro-arrhythmic in design or if "imperfect," which parts are useless to say the least, and last but not least what are the side effect of incision beyond their intended effects on the target. Experience with ventriculotomies and atrial incisions provided good evidences that an incision is not a simple line and may be associated with severe regional effects..

Further study of pathology of non-valvular atrial fibrillation provided no clues or avenue.[80]

5.8   Surgical Side Effects Scrambling the Interpretation of Results: The Triumph of the Gentle Catheter

The critical quantum leap was to come from the electrophysiological laboratory in Bordeaux under the leadership of Michel Haissaguerre,[81] with an surprising intellectual twist, using catheter ablation. Because interventionists did not have, at that time, a better rationale than their surgical counterparts, it was elected, as a practical attitude, to reproduce with the catheter, the surgical technique, but without the side effects. This attitude was consistent with the history of science. Every scientific hypothesis is initially based on empirical observations. Empiricism is indispensable to science: it feeds it with good food for thoughts to verify. This attitude was to be proved very productive:

It was documented that lines of block can interrupt atrial fibrillation, defined as the chaotic activation, consistent with random reentry,[82,83] but without validating the speculated mechanism.

Incomplete or non-continuous line of block could have severe side effects and become the substrate for fast reentrant circuit activation to develop after ablation. This fast flutter-like tachycardia could produce symptoms, worse than the pre-existing atrial fibrillation.[84] Treatment of this flutters were very difficult and time consuming because it was difficult to localize the gaps.

The real breakthrough was to come, when it was documented that interruption of the chaotic activation allowed the initiating/ perpetuating mechanism to be identified: Focal reentry tachycardias within the adventitia of pulmonary veins were uncovered after control of atrial fibrillation and were identified as the long awaited initiating factor. The light was set on at the end of the blazing catheter. The anatomical substrate for pulmonary vein tachycardias was the myocardial fibres that are normally present within the adventitia of not only the pulmonary veins but all the veins opening into a cardiac chamber. For the first time, beside atrial fibrillation associated with triggering tachycardias, such as AVRT associated with the WPW syndrome, or AVNRT, or atrial flutter, **an initiating and potentially perpetuating mechanism** of atrial fibrillation was identified. This finding was consistent with the identification of a new form of paroxysmal atrial fibrillation associated with premature atrial contraction.

The entire field was to be revisited with a scientific basis.

5.9   Basic Science Confirmation

Simultaneously, basis science was making major contribution. By using new technology to study atrial fibrillation. J. Jaliffe team in Syracuse NY and M. Allessie team in Maastrisch, the Netherlands and many other in the field were to documented a number of critical concepts: Mapping of atrial fibrillation show fast stable reentrant circuit, suggesting a focal initiating and perpetuating mechanism. In our laboratory, C. Morrillo documented in an animal model that cryoablation of that area interrupted the atrial fibrillation.[85] Random reentrant activation was documented to have to critical characteristics suggesting the presence of a focal perpetuating focus:

#1 Atrial fibrillation begets atrial fibrillation.[86] Continuous reactivation of atrial fibrillation make the atrial lasting longer and induce atrial remodelling that enhance perpetuation of atrial fibrillation (atrial electrophysiological remodelling). #2 Mapping large atrial segments of atrial fibrillation in a sheep model documented that more wavelets enter the area than exit the area. This shows that the multiple wavelets activation requires to be continuously reactivated.[87-89]

The later was the confirmation of the focal discovery in humans.

5.10   The End of a Story and the Beginning of a New One

A mechanism for atrial fibrillation has been documented: It may not be the only one, but its focal nature is consistent with intellectual speculation that a multi-focal tachycardia is hard to conceptualize. Commonly the atrial tachycardia is a fast reentrant atrial tachycardia localized in the adventitial of the pulmonary veins, with a variable prevalence for each pulmonary vein, albeit the tachycardia can be localize anywhere is the atrial wall. This mechanism does not exclude other mechanisms, but renders them unlikely. A sustained random reentry made self-sustained after long lasting reactivation cannot be excluded.

The empirical story ends here, and the rational story starts. The never ending process of investigating goes on. There is no end to the story.

This paper is dedicated to George, Colette and all, patients and physicians, who were supporting beyond belief.

REFERENCES

1.   Guiraudon GM. Musing while Cutting. J. Card. Surg. 1998; 13:156-162.
2.   Guiraudon GM, Klein GJ, Van Hemel N. et al: Atrial Flutter: Lessons from surgical interventions (musing on atrial flutter mechanism). PACE 1996; 19 (Pt. II): 1933-1938.
3.   Guiraudon GM: Surgical treatment of Wolff-Parkinson-White syndrome- A retrospectroscopic view. Ann Thorac Surg 1994; 58: 1254-1261.
4.   Meijler FL, Janse J: Morphology and electrophysiology of the mammalian atrioventricular node. Physiol Rev 1988; 68: 608-647.
5.   Harrison L. Gallagher JJ, Kasell J, et al: Cryosurgical ablation of the AV node - His bundle: A new method for producing AV block. Circulation 1977; 55: 463-470.
6.   Guiraudon GM, Klein GJ, Sharma AD, et al: Skeletonization of the atrioventricular node surgical alternative for AV nodal reentrant tachycardia: Experience with 32 patients. Ann Thorac Surg 1990; 49: 565-573.

7. Guiraudon G, Frank R, Fontaine G. Interet des cartographies dans le traitement chirurgical des tachycardies ventriculaires rebelles recidivantes. Nouv Presse Med 1974; 3: 321.

8. Guiraudon G, Fontaine G, Frank R. et al. Encircling endocardial ventriculotomy: a new surgical treatment for life-threatening ventricular tachycardias resistant to medical treatment following myocardial infarction. Ann Thorac Surg 1978; 26: 438-444.

9. Sealy WC, Hatter BG, Blumenschein SD, et al. Surgical treatment of Wolff Parkinson White syndrome. Ann Thorac Surg 8:1, 1969

10. Gallagher JJ,Kassell J, Sealy WC, et al. Epicardial mapping in the Wolff Parkinson White syndrome. Circulation 1978;57:854

11. Kirklin JW: The science of cardiac surgery. Eur J Cardiothorac Surg 1990; 4: 63-71.

12. Buckberg GD: Myocardial protection: An overview. Semin Thorac Cardiovasc Surg. 1993; 5: 98-106.

13. Guiraudon GM, Klein GJ, Sharma AD, et al: Closed heart technique for Wolff-Parkinson-White syndrome: Further experience and potential limitations. Ann Thorac Surg 1986; 42: 651-657

14. Guiraudon GM, Klein GJ, Yee R, et al: Surgical epicardial ablation of left ventricular pathway using sling exposure. Ann Thorac Surg 1990; 50: 968-971.

15. Warin JF, Haissaguerre M, Lemetayer P, et al: Catheter ablation of accessory pathways with a direct approach: Results in 35 patients. Circulation 1988; 78: 800-815.

16. Scheiman MM, Morady F, Hess DS, et al: Catheter-induced ablation of atrioventricular junction to control refractory supraventricular arrhythmias. JAMA 248: 851-55, 1982

17. Gallagher JJ, Swenson RH, Kassell JH, et al: Catheter technique for closed chest ablation of the atrioventricular conduction system. N Engl J Med 306:194-00, 1982

18. Guiraudon GM, Guiraudon CM, Klein GJ, et al: Operation for the Wolff-Parkinson-White syndrome in the catheter ablation era. Ann Thorac Surg 1994; 57: 1084-1088.

19. Guiraudon, GM, Klein GJ: Left atrial appendectomy for stroke prevention in patients with atrial fibrillation. Do we need more evidences to apply it? (Abstract) Arch Mal Coeur Vaiss 1998; 91 (Suppl III): 128.

20. Ankeney JL: To use or not to use the pump oxygenator in coronary bypass operations. Ann Thorac Surg 1975; 10: 108-109.

21. Buffolo E. Andrade JCS, Succi J, et al: Direct myocardial revascularization without cardio-pulmonary bypass. J. Thorac Surg 1985; 33: 26-29.

22. Eugene H, Blackstone MD: Outcome analysis using hazard function methodology. Ann Thorac Surg 1996; 61: 52-57.

23. Hannah EL, Kilburn H Jr, O'Donnell JF, et al: Adult open heart surgery in New York State: An analysis of risk factors and hospital mortality rates. JAMA 1990; 264: 2768-2774.

24. Anderson RH, Becker AE, Brechenmacher C, Ventricular preexcitation : A proposed nomenclature for its substrate. Eur J Cardiol 31: 27, 1975

25. Klein GJ, Harrison L, Ideker RE, et al. Reaction of myocardium to cryosurgery;electrophysiology and arrhythmogenic potential. Circulation 1979;59:364-72

26. Klein GJ, Guiraudon GM, Perkins DG, Jones DL, Yee R, Jarvis E. Surgical correction of the Wolff Parkinson White syndrome in the closed heart using cryosurgery: a simplified approach. JACC 1984;1;405-49

27. Morell Tp, McLellan DG, Guiraudon GM. Coronary sinus ligation in the dog. Value of the mid cardiac vein. Clinical and investigative medicine, suppl 11,5D:45, 1988

28. McLellan DG, Guiraudon GM, Morell TP, Guiraudon CM. Does partial ligation make complete ostial coronary sinus ligation feasible? Clinical and investigative Medicine Suppl, 23,5:48,1989

29. Guiraudon GM, Klein GJ, Sharma AD, Surgical Ablation of posterior septal accessory pathways in the Wolff Parkinson White syndrome by a closed heart technique.J Thorac Cardiovasc Surg 92: 406,1986

30. Guiraudon GM, Klein GJ, Sharma A, Yee R. regional subclassification of accessory pathways in the Wolff Parkinson White syndrome based on dissection and electrophysiology. PACE 1989;12;657

31. Guiraudon GM, Klein GJ, Sharma AD, Surgical approach to anterior septal accessory pathways in 20 patients with the Wolff Parkinson White syndrome . Eur J Cardiothorac Surg 2: 201, 1988

32. Klein GJ, Guiraudon GM, Kerr CR, et al "Nodoventricular" accessory pathways: evidence for a distinct accessory AV pathway with AV node-like properties. J Am Coll Cardiol 11: 1035, 1988

33. Guiraudon GM, Guiraudon CM, Klein GJ, et al. The coronary sinus diverticulum- a pathological entity associated with the Wolff Parkinson White syndrome. Am J Cardiol c62: 733, 1988

34. Teo WS, Guiraudon GM, Klein GJ, et al. Hypothesis testing as an approach to the analysis of complex tachycardias.- an illustrative case of a preexcitation variant. PACE 14:1427-61, 1991

35. Guiraudon GM, Klein GJ, Yee R. Surgery for Wolff Parkinson White and supraventricular tachycardias. In Tachycardias : mechanism and management. Josephson ME, Wellens HJJ (eds)pp 297-312, Futura publishing, Mount Kisco, NY 1993

36. Fontaine G, Guiraudon GM, Frank R, et al Stimulation studies and epicardial mapping in ventricular tachycardia: study of mechanism and selection for surgery. In Kulbertus HE(ed): Reentrant Arrhythmias. Lancaster, MTP Press 1977,pp 334-50

37. Fontaine G, Guiraudon G, Frank R, et al. Arrhythmogenic right ventricular dysplasia: A previously unrecognized syndrome [abstract]. Circulation 59(suppl II)65,1979.

38. Marcus FI, Fontaine G, Guiraudon G, et al Right ventricular dysplasia: a report of 24 cases. Circulation 65: 384-99, 1982

39. Frank R, Fontaine G, Vedel J, Mialet G, Sol C, Guiraudon G, Grosgogeat Y. Electrophysiology de 4 cas de dysplasie ventriculaire droite arythmogene. Arch. Mal.. Coeur. 1978; 71; 973

40. Fontaine G, Guiraudon G,Frank R, Fillette F, Tonet J, Grosgogeat Y. Correlation between latest potentials in sinus rhytm and earliest activation during chronic ventricular tachycardi.. In; Medical and surgical mangement of tachycardias. Bircks WE, Loogen F, Schulte HD,Seipel(eds). Springer verlag.Publisher Heidelberg, 1980, pp138-54

41. Fontaine g,Guiraudoon GM,Frank R, Fillette F,Cabrol C, Grosgogeat Y. Surgical managementof ventricular tachycardia unrelated to myocardial ischemia or infarction. Am J Cardiol. 1982;49:397-410

42. Guiraudon G, Fontaine G, Frank R, et al:Is the reentry concept a guide to the surgical treatment of chronic ventricular tachycardia? In Bircks W, Loongen F, Schulte HD, Seipel L(eds); Medical and surgical management of tachyarrhythmias. New York, Springer-Verlag, 1980,pp 155-72

43. P Guiraudon G, Fontaine G, Frank R. et al. Surgical treatment of ventricular tachycardia guided by ventricular mapping in 23 patients without coronary artery disease. Ann Thorac Surg 1981; 32: 439-450.

44. Guiraudon GM, Klein GJ, Gulamhusein SS, et al. Total disconnection of the right ventricular free wall: surgical treatment of right ventricular tachycardia associated with right ventricular dysplasia. Circulation 1983; 67: 463-470.

45. Jones DL, Guiraudon GM, Klein GJ. Total disconnection of the right ventricular free wall; physiological consequences in the dog. Am Heart J 1984;107: 1169-77

46. Guiraudon GM, Klein G, Guiraudon C, et al. Long term prognosis of patients with right ventricular free wall disconnection for arrhythmogenic right ventricular dysplasia: left ventricular ejection fractions as a marker of outcome. PACE 1996; 19(Pt II): 628.

47. Guiraudon GM, Guiraudon CM, Klein GJ. Surgical approaches. In Arrhythmogenic right ventricular cardiomyopathy/dysplasia. Nava A, Rossi L, Thiene G, (eds) pp392-98.1997, Elsevier publisher.

48. Guiraudon GM, Fontaine G, Frank R, Vedel J, Escande G, Cabrol C.New concepts in the surgical management of ventricular tachycardia. In Advances in the mangement of arrhythmias. Kelly DT (ed) Telectronics Sydney Publisher 1978. p225

49. Josephson ME, Harden AH, Horowitz LN. Endocardial excision: a new surgical technique for the treatment of recurrent ventricular tachycardia. Circulation 1979; 60: 1430-1439.

50. Van Hemel NM, Kingma JH, Defauw JJAM, Hoogteijling van Dusseldrop E et al. Continuation of antiarrhythmic drugs, or arrhythmia surgery after multiple drug failures: a randomized trial in the treatment of postinfarction ventricular tachycardia. Eur Heart J ; 1986; 17:564-73

51. Guiraudon GM, Thakur RK, Klein GJ, Yee R, Guiraudon CM, et al. Encircling endocardial cryoablation for ventricular tachycardia after myocardial infarction: experience with 33 patients. Am Heart J 1994; 128: 982-89

52. Guiraudon GM, Klein GJ,Guiraudon CM.Ventricular tacchycardias. Antiarrhythmic surgery: the legacy. In: Fighting sudden cardiac death: a worldwide challenge. Aliot E, Clementy J, Prystowsky EN (editors) Futura Publishing , Amonk NY, 2000.

53. Eugene Downar E, Saito J, Doig JC, Chen TC, Sevaptsidis E, Masse S, Kimber S, Mickleborough L. Endocardial mapping of ventricular tachycardia in the intact human ventricle. III. Evidence of multiuse reentry with spontaneous and induced block in portions of reentrant path complex. JACC 1995;25:1591-600

54. In memoriam; Michel Mirowski, M.D. 10/14/24-3/26/90. Pacing Clin electrophysiol 1991;14;864-966

55. P Moss AJ, Hall WJ, Cannom DS, et al. Improved survival with an implanted defibrillator in patients with coronary disease at high risk for ventricular arrhythmia: Multicenter automatic defibrillator implantation trial investigators. N. Engl J. Med. 1996; 335: 1933-1940.

56. Antiarrhythmics versus implantable defibrillators investigators. A comparison of antiarrhythmic-drug therapy with implantable defibrillators in patients resuscitated from near-fatal ventricular arrhythmias. N. Engl. J. Med. 1997; 337: 1576-1583.

57. Moe GK,: on the multiple wavelet hypothesis of atrial fibrillation. Arch Int Pharmacody Ther, 140:183-88, 1962

58. Allessie MA, Lammers WJEP, Bonke FIM. Experimental evaluation of Moe's multiple wavelet hypothesis of atrial fibrillation. In Zipes DP, Jalife J,(eds) Cardiac Electrophysiology and arrhythmias. Grune & Stratton , New York, 1985, PP 265-75

59. Kopecky SL, Gersh BJ, McGoon MD, et al. The natural history of lone atrial fibrillation. A population-based study over 3 decades. N Engl J Med 317:669-74, 1987

60. Brand FN, Abbott RD, Kannel WB, et al. Characteristics and prognosis of lone atrial fibrillation. 30 years follow up in the Framingham Study. JAMA 254:3449-53, 1985

61. James TN. Diversity of histopathologic correlates of atrial fibrillation. In kulbertus HE, Olson SB, Schlepper M (eds) Atrial fibrillation. Astra Publishers, Modudal, Sweden, 1982,p 13

62. Frustaci A, Caldarulo M, Buffon A et al. Cardiac biopsy in patients with 'primary' atrial fibrillation: evidence of occult myocardial diseases. Chest 1991;2: 303

63. Guiraudon CM, Ernst NM, Guiraudon GM, et al. The pathology of drug resistant lone atrial fibrillation in eleven surgically treated patients. In Kingma van Hemel NM, Lie Ki, (eds) Atrial fibrillation: a treatable disease? Kluwer academic Publishers, Boston, 1992, p41

64. Robinson TF, Factor SM, Sonnenblick EH. The heart as a suction pump. Scientific American 1986;254, 6;84

65. Ruffy R. Atrial fibrillation. In Cardiac Electrophysiology, from cell to bedside. Second edition. Zipes DP, Jalife J (eds)WB Saunders 1995,pp682-90

66. Blackshear JL, Odell Ja. Appendage obliteration to reduce stroke in cardiac surgical patients with atrial fibrillation. Ann Thor surg 1996;61: 755-5

67. Guiraudon GM, Campbell CS, Jones DL, et al Combined sino-atrial node atrioventricular isolation: a surgical alternative to His bundle ablation in patients with atrial fibrillation Circulation.1985;72(suppl 2):III-220.

68. Leitch JW, Klein G, Yee R, et al. Sinus node atrioventricular node isolation: long-term results with the Corridor operation for atrial fibrillation. J. Am Coll Cardiol 1991; 17,4:970.

69. Defauw JJAM , Guiraudon GM, van Hemel NM, Vermeulen FEE, Kingma JH, de Bakker JMT. Surgical therapy of atrial fibrillation with the 'Corridor' operation. Ann Thorac Surg 1992,53: 564-71

70. Van Hemel NM, Defauw JJAM, Kingma JH, et al .Long term results of the" Corridor" operation for atrial fibrillation. Br Heart J 1994;71: 170

71. Cox JL, Boineau JP, Schuessler RB, et al. Successful surgical treatment of atrial fibrillation: Review and clinical update. JAMA 1991; 266: 1976-1980

72. Cox JL, Boineau JP, Schuessler RB, et al. Five years experience with the Maze procedure for atrial fibrillation. Ann Thorac Surg 1993; 56:814-24.

73. Cox Jl, Schuessler RB, Cain ME, et al. Surgery for atrial fibrillation, Sem Thorac Cardiovasc Surg 1989;1:67-73

74. Sueda T, Nagata H, Orihashi K, Morita S, Okada K, Sueshiro M, Hirai S, Matsuura Y. efficacy of a simple left atrial procedure for chronic atrial fibrillation in mitral valve operations. Ann Thorac Surg 1997; 63:1070-5

75. Graffinia A, Ressia L, Pagnani F, et al. Left atrial isolation for the treatment of atrial fibrillation due to mitral valve disease. Hemodynamic evaluation. N Trend in Arrhythmia IX 1993;4:1069.

76. Shyu KG, Cheng J-J, Cheng J-J, et al. Recovery of atrial function after atrial compartment operation for chronic atrial fibrillation ihn mitral valve disease. JACC 1994;24:392-98

77. Guiraudon GM, Klein GJ, Guiraudon CM, Yee R. Surgical approaches to supraventricular tachycardias. Singer I, Barold SS, Camm AJ (eds). Nonpharmacological Therapy of Arrhythmias for the 21st Century: The State of the Art. Futura Publishing Co., Armonk, NY, 1998.

78. Melo JQ, Neves J, Adragao P, Ribeiras R, Ferreira MM, Bruges L, Canada M, Ramos T. When and how to report results of surgery on atrial fibrillation. Eur. J Cardiothoracic Surg. 1997; 12:739-745.

79. Melo J, Adragao PR, Neves J,Ferreira M, rebocho M, Teles R, Morgado F. Electrosurgical treatment of atrial fibrillation with a new intraoperative radiofrequency ablation catheter. Thorac Cardiovasc Surg 1999;47:suppl 3:370-2

80. Guiraudon CM, ErnstNM, klein GJ, et al .the pathology of intractable "primary" atrial fibrillation. Circulation 1992; *6(suppl I)4:I-662

81. Haissaguerre M, Jais P, Shah DC, Takahashi A, Hocini M, Quiniou G, Garrigue S, Mouroux AE, Le Metayer P, Clementy J.: Spontaneous initiation of atrial fibrillation by ectopic beats originating in the pulmonary veins. New Engl. .J. Med. 1998, 339: (10) 659-666.

82. Avitall B, hare J, Mughall, et al. Ablation ofb atrial fibrillation in a dog model JACC 1994;23 suppl ; 276A. Abstract.

83. Schwaz J, Pellersels G, Fisher B, et al. A catheter -based approach to atrial fibrillation in humans. Circulation 1994;(suppl 4):I-335. Abstract

84. Haissaguerre M, Jais P, Shah DC, et al. Right and left radiofrequency catheter therapy of paroxysmal atrial fibrillation. J cardiovasc Electrophysiology 1996;7:1132-44

85. Morillo CA, Klein GJ, Jones DL, Guiraudon CM. Chronic rapid atrial pacing: Structural, functional, and electrophysiological characteristics of a new model of sustained atrial fibrillation. Circulation 1995;91:1958-95

86. Wijffels MC, Kirchhof CJ,DOrland R, Allessie MA. Atrial fibrillation begets atrial fibrillation: a study in awake chronically instrumented goats. Circulation 1995;92:1954-68

87. Pertsov AM Jalife J. Three dimentional Vortex-like reentry. in Cardiac electrophysiology ' from cell to bedside . Zipes DP, Jalife J. (eds)WB Saunders Publisher Philadelphia 1995,pp 403-10

88. Chen J, Mandapati R, Berenfeld O, Skanes AC, Gray AC, Jalife J. Dynamics of wavelets and their role inatrial fibrillation in the isolated sheep heart. Cardiovasc Res2000;48:220-32

89. Mandapati R, Skanes A, Chen J, Berenfeld O, Jalife J. Stable microreentrant souirces as a mechanism of atrial fibrillation in the isolated sheep heart .Circulation 2000;101:194-9

SUGGESTED READING

1. De Bono Edward. Lateral thinking, Creativity step by step. Harper & Row Publisher, N.Y.; 1970.

2. Erasmus Desiderius. The Praise of Folly. Translated by C.H. Miller. Yale University Press; 1979.
3. Plato. Symposium and the Death of Socrates. Translated by T. Griffith. Wordsworth Classics of World Literature; 1997.
4. Bernard Claude. An introduction to the study of experimental Medicine. (1865) Dover Publications Inc, New York, NY.1957
5. Grinnell Frederick. The Scientific Attitude, 8th Edition. The Guilford Press; 1992.
6. Popper KR. The myth of the framework. Edited by Notturno. Routledge, 1994.
7. Kuhn TS. The structure of scientific revolutions. University of Chicago Press; 1962.

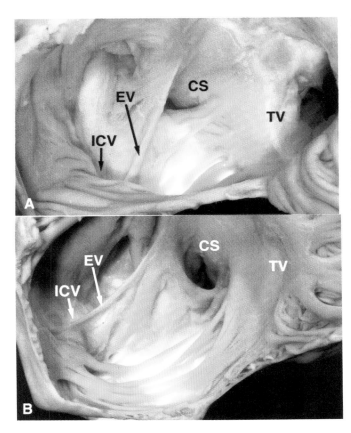

Plate 1. Examples of a so-called non-uniform muscular trabecular alignment in the tricuspid cavo isthmus; specimens oriented and labelled as in Figure 1 (Chapter 3). (A) shows a few relatively large (trans-illuminated) fibrous parts between the muscular trabeculae; (B) shows a multitude of such "defects." Note that non-uniformity is particular outspoken in the area adjoining the os of the coronary sinus. See chapter 3 Figure 3.

Plate 2. Microwave lesion from the Lynx device. See chapter 32 Figure 18.

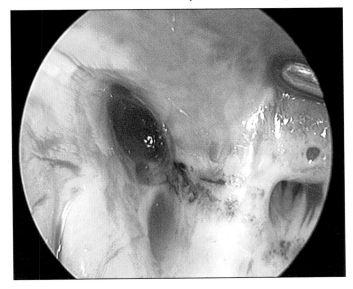

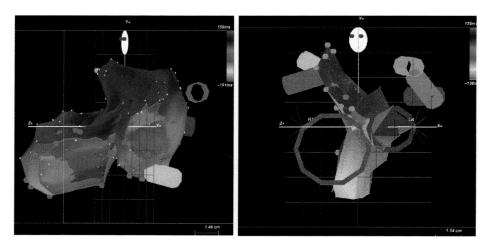

Plate 3 (left). Reconstruction of both atrial levels in a patient after a double switch procedure in order to correct a congenitally corrected transposition of the great arteries and an atrial tachycardia. On the atrial level, a Senning type surgery was performed, displaying the pulmonary venous atrium on the picture's left side. Here, course of the tachycardia around the "right sided" mitral annulus can be suspected from the activation map, as a homogeneous display of the complete time span of the window of interest (equivalent to complete color range) is distributed around the mitral annulus, and relatively latest activation (purple) meets relatively earliest activation (red), termed "head meets tail". See chapter 12 Figures 1 and 2. **Plate 4** (right). Reconstruction of the systemic venous atrium in a patient after Senning type atrial switch procedure for d-transposition of the great arteries. In case of a macro-reentry tachycardia, an incomplete display of the full color range (blue, light blue and green are missing) gives evidence for an incomplete reconstruction of the tachycardias circuit within that chamber. Differential interpretations are: 1. Chamber just as bystander of the tachycardia, 2. Chamber just as part of the circuit, compete in conjunction with the opposite chamber.

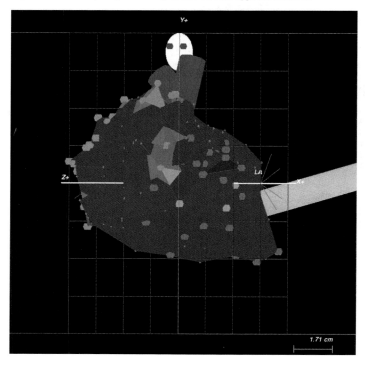

Plate 5. 3-D electro-anatomical reconstruction of the right atrium of a patient after Fontan surgery (LAO projection, propagation map mode). Yellow tube shows rough course of the coronary sinus, gray and brown tubes show transition to and course of the pulmonary trunk. Blue dots mark areas with doubled potentials (line of electrical block), gray dots mark areas with loss of electrical signals (scars), brown dots mark occurrence of A and V signals (area of the right sided atrioventricular junction at atretic tricuspid annulus), yellow dots where solely V signals were detected. See chapter 12 Figure 3.

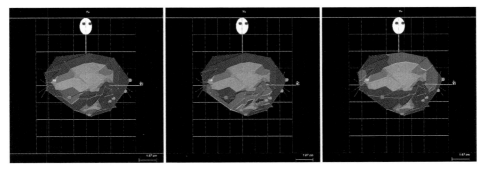

Plate 6. Partial reconstruction in a patient after Fontan procedure (RAO projection) showing two scars (gray fields) at the lateral atrial wall confining an area of vital myocardium, identified before for being critical for the maintenance of a reentry tachycardia. In preparation of an ablation line, aiming to combine both scars, propagation through this area was visualized by pacing in its close proximity (yellow marker: position of transient screw electrode). Figures a (left) – c (right) display electrical conduction trough the designated area before ablation was started. See chapter 12 Figure 4.

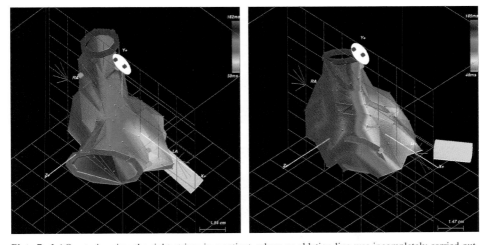

Plate 7. LAO-anterior view the right atrium in a patient, where an ablation line was incompletely carried out, attempting a complete block between the insertion of the superior caval vein (green ring) and the anterior aspect of the tricuspid annulus (brown ring). Pacing was carried out close to the ostium of the coronary sinus displaying a homogeneous propagation from the pacing site towards the attempted ablation line. Note the difference between site of latest activation before the ablation line was completed, purple color located at the lateral free atrial wall (a) and after successful block of the targeted area, purple color located adjacent to the ablation line, opposite to the pacing site (b). See chapter 5 Figure 5.

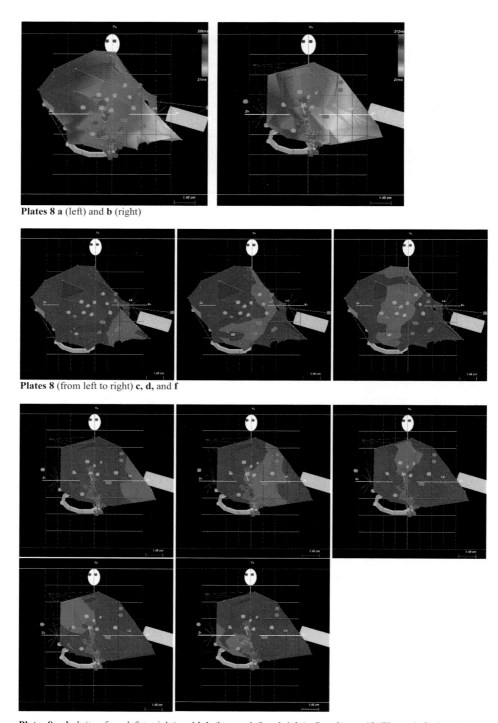

Plates 8 a (left) and **b** (right)

Plates 8 (from left to right) **c, d,** and **f**

Plates 8 g, h, i, (top from left to right) and **j, k** (bottom left and right). See chapter 12 (Figure 6) for legend.

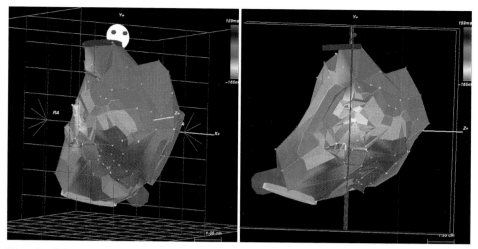

Plates 9 a (left) and **b** (right)

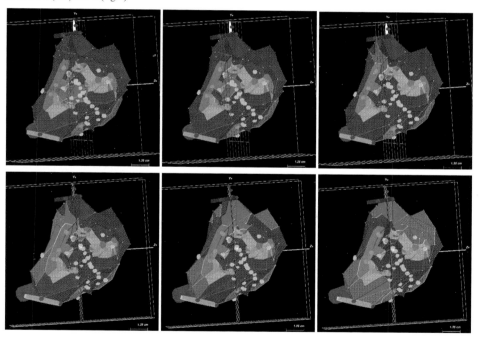

Plates 9 d, e, and **g** (top from left top right) and **h, i, j** (bottom from left to right). See chapter 12 Figure 7.

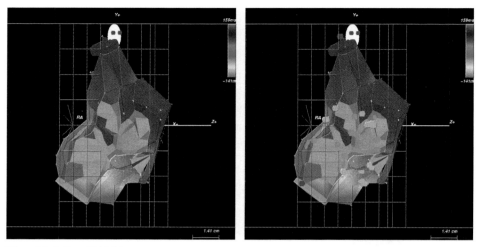

Plates 9 k (left) and **l** (right)

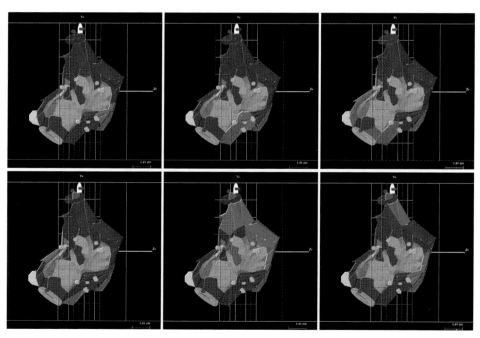

Plates 9 m, n, and **o** (top from left to right) and **p, q, t** (bottom from left to right). See chapter 12 (Figure 7) for legend.

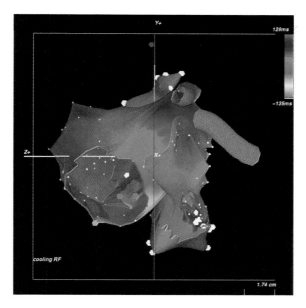

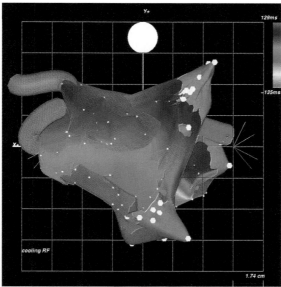

Plates 10 a (top, left lateral view) and **b** (bottom, posterior-anterior view) show reconstruction of both the pulmonary venous atrium (right side on plate 10 a) and the systemic venous atrium (left side on plate 10 a) in the activation map mode while reentry tachycardia. Tricuspid annulus is depicted by the brown ring, the mitral annulus by the red ring, tube display entrance of pulmonary veins into the pulmonary venous atrium. Grey areas on systemic venous atrium depict connection to superior and inferior caval vein, on pulmonary venous atrium scar resulting from lateral atriotomy. See Chapter 12 Figures 8 a and b.

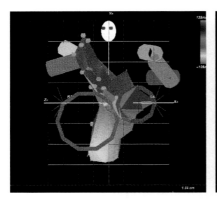
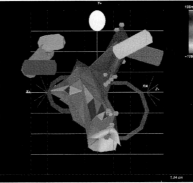

Plates 11 a (LAO view) and **b** (posterior anterior view) show reconstruction of the systemic venous atrium in the activation map mode during atrial reentry tachycardia. Red ring depicts mitral annulus, gray ring the tricuspid annulus. Tube display course of pulmonary veins close to the pulmonary venous atrium (not to be seen on this pictures). Blue dots mark areas with splitted local electrograms, orange dot at site of His bundle recording, yellow dots at site of fractionated local electrograms. See chapter 12 Figures 9 a and b.

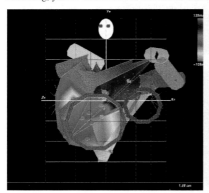
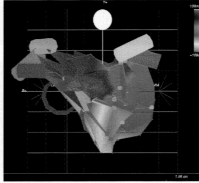

Plates 11 c (LAO view) and **d** (posterior anterior view) show the pulmonary venous atrium during tachycardia, brown dots mark areas with doubled local signals. See chapter 12 Figures 9 c and d.

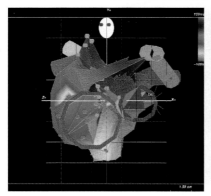
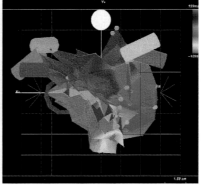

Plates11 e (LAO view) and **f** (posterior anterior view) display both reconstructed atriums while tachycardia. Course of the reentry circuit was similar to the Mustard case (see above), as like the ablation strategy that has been carried out successfully. See chapter 12 Figures 9 e and f.

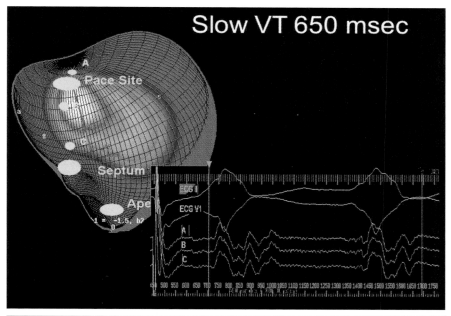

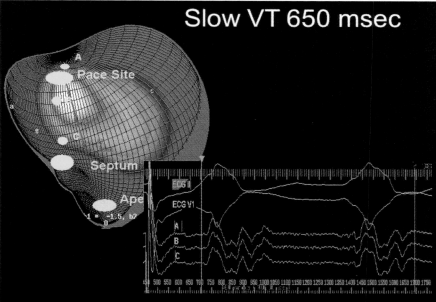

Plate 12. Shown is an example of concealed entrainment during a ventricular tachycardia that has a cycle length of 650 msec. The top panel shows the isopotential map at the time of the onset of the last entrained QRS complex, immediately following pacing (from the site marked Pace Site) which resulted in concealed entrainment. The pacing stimulus can be seen at the beginning of the electrograms. The bottom panel shows the isopotential map of the ventricular tachycardia at the onset of the QRS complex, which identifies the exit site of the ventricular tachycardia reentry circuit. Note that the exit site of the entrained ventricular beat has a similar exit site as that of the native ventricular tachycardia, as would be expected after concealed entrainment. The septum and apex are marked. See chapter 15 Figure 6.

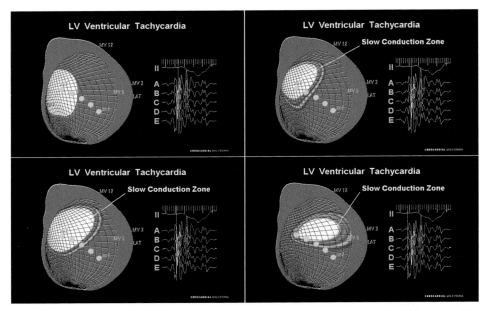

Plate 13. An example of ventricular tachycardia is shown. The isopotential map at the time of the onset of the QRS is shown in the upper left corner. Each of the next three panels show a presystolic isopotential map at progressively earlier times relative to the onset of the QRS complex during ventricular tachycardia: –10 msec (upper right corner), -20 msec (lower left corner), and –30 msec (lower right corner). Note progressive activation from the base to the apex of the left ventricle. Lat=lateral wall, MV3=3 o'clock on the mitral annulus in the lateral anterior oblique view, MV5=5 o'clock, and MV12=12 o'clock, sept=septal wall. The closed yellow circles represent the recording sites of the virtual electrograms A through E. See chapter 15 Figure 7.

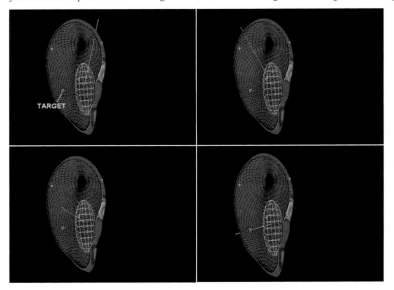

Plate 14. An example of the locator signal being used to guide the roving catheter to a target site. The green line originates from the center of the balloon (denoted by the yellow wire mesh) and meets the endocardial reconstruction to denote the position of the roving catheter at the endocardium. From left to right and top to bottom, the roving catheter is steered to the target site. See chapter 15 Figure 8.

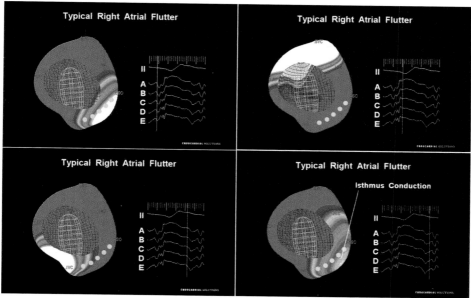

Plate 15. Isopotential maps are shown during the circuit typical counter-clockwise atrial flutter. Each map denotes the endocardial activation at different times. The virtual electrograms are also displayed from the right atrial isthmus with the time of each activation map denoted by the vertical time line. The bottom right panel shows the endocardial activation during conduction through the low right atrial isthmus. The yellow wire mesh denotes the noncontact balloon. The closed yellow circles represent the recording sites of the virtual electrograms A through E. See chapter 15 Figure 9.

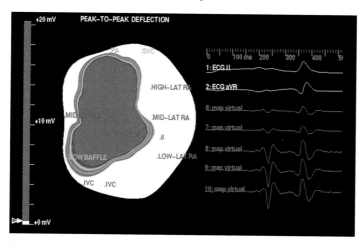

Plate 16. Peak voltage map of a Fontan atrium (atriopulmonary connection). Right atrial geometry is displayed in a right posterior oblique plane. Peak voltages are measured from >3000 sites on the endocardial surface during a single cycle (of sinus rhythm in this example). Areas with peak voltages >0.4mV are displayed in purple and areas <0.4mV are displayed in white. Virtual unipolar electrograms are displayed alongside, with the sites from which they are recorded indicated by the numbered position on the geometry. This example demonstrates that the majority of atrial mass in the chronic Fontan atrium consists of diseased, hypertrophied myocardium plus inert surgical material. Only a small area of the posterior wall displays electrical potentials of significant value. Electrograms recorded from the white area are small, fractionated or absent. During isopotential mapping activation was seen to spread over the purple area. The remainder of the atrium was electrically silent. See chapter 16 Figure 1.

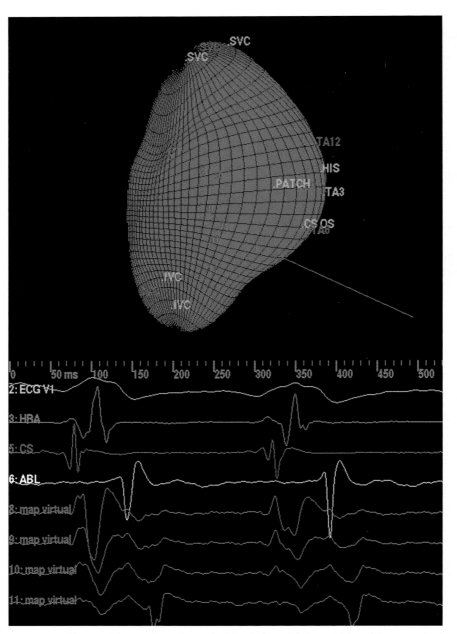

Plate 17. Double potentials around an atriotomy incision during atrial flutter: Right atrial geometry is viewed in a right anterior oblique plane. Virtual electrograms in channels 8-10 are recorded from the sites labeled on the map, along the presumed atriotomy incision on the lateral right atrial wall. The position of the ablation catheter tip is indicated by the locator signal (green line). Double potentials are seen in the virtual electrograms, indicating that the incision acts as a line of conduction block. Labels in green are on the near side of the geometry. Labels in yellow are on the far side and seen through the geometry. SVC, superior vena cava; IVC, inferior vena cava; CS OS, coronary sinus ostium; TA, tricuspid valve annulus; CT, crista terminalis. See chapter 16 Figure 2.

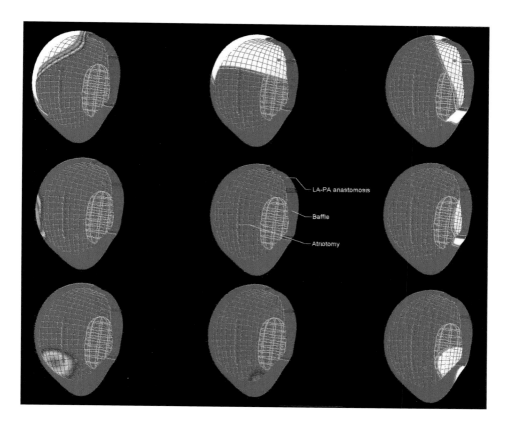

Plate 18. Fontan (atriopulmonary connection): Right atrial geometry is shown in a left lateral plane. The medial wall has been clipped away to allow an internal view of the structure. The left atrial roof to pulmonary artery anastomosis plus the pericardial baffle that helps direct flow from the IVC to the anastomosis have been drawn on the geometry. The lateral wall atriotomy scar is also depicted. The yellow frame depicts the position of the MEA. The colored areas represent negative endocardial potentials (depolarization) against the purple background. Macroreentry is visualised moving around the atrium in an anti-clockwise fashion. The atriotomy acts as a central barrier to conduction. As the activation wavefront descends anterior to the atriotomy is becomes low amplitude with reduced velocity. A radiofrequency linear lesion between the lower atriotomy and inferior vena cava terminated tachycardia. See chapter 16 Figure 4.

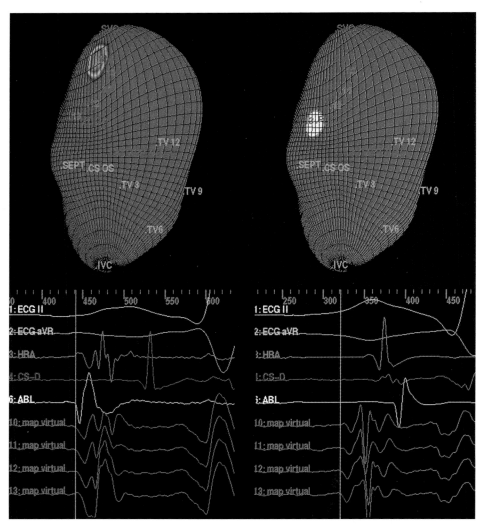

Plate 19. Focal atrial tachycardia. An external view of right atrial geometry in a right anterior oblique plane. Negative potentials (depolarization) are depicted as colors against a purple background. Contact and virtual electrograms are shown. Virtual unipolar electrograms (channels 10–13) are taken from the points on the geometry marked by the appropriate numbers. The yellow vertical line indicates the point in time that corresponds to the isopotential map. A) Sinus rhythm. The site of earliest activation is the high right atrium/SVC junction (i.e. the sinus node complex). This coincides with the onset of the surface P wave. The high right atrial catheter (HRA) and ablation catheter (ABL) are also positioned close to the sinus node. The virtual unipolar electrograms confirm that activation begins at number 10 and spreads in a caudal direction. The earliest electrogram has a QS configuration. B) Automatic atrial tachycardia. The site of earliest activation is on the mid lateral wall within the crista terminalis. Activation in the high right atrial and ablation catheters occurs later in the cycle. The earliest activation in the virtual electrograms is now in number 13, with activation spreading in a cranial direction. Labels in green are on the near side of the geometry. Labels in yellow are on the far side and seen through the geometry. SVC, superior vena cava; IVC, inferior vena cava; SEPT, atrial septum; CS OS, coronary sinus ostium; TV, tricuspid valve; SN, sinus node. See chapter 16 Figure 5.

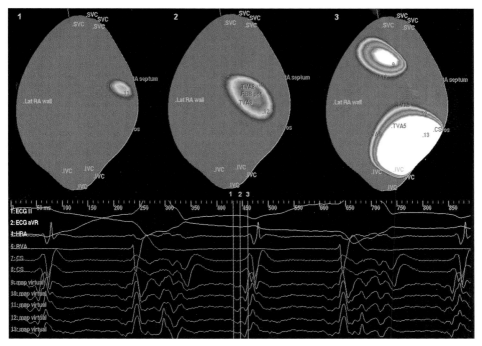

Plate 20. Accessory pathway and Ebstein's anomaly: 3 frames from a single cycle of tachycardia are shown. Right atrial geometry is depicted in a left anterior oblique view. Negative endocardial potentials (depolarization) are indicated by the colors on the isopotential map against a purple background. Contact and virtual electrograms are shown below. The virtual electrograms (channels 9-13) are taken from the corresponding sites labeled on the right atrial geometry. The vertical yellow lines correspond to the points in time that are displayed on the isopotential maps. 1) Earliest right atrial activation. A small, low amplitude area of depolarization is seen on the anteromedial septum. 2) Activation moves in an anterior direction towards the tricuspid valve annulus, still low amplitude. This is depicted as a small negative potential in the virtual electrograms. 3) Global activation begins and spreads around the tricuspid valve annulus and over the right atrial endocardial surface. This corresponds with a larger, steeper QS complex in the virtual electrograms. In this case, tracking activation back to the earliest site facilitated successful ablation without harm coming to the conduction system (note the presence of a right bundle branch potential within the activation route). Labels in green are on the near side of the geometry. Labels in yellow are on the far side and seen through the geometry. SVC, superior vena cava; IVC, inferior vena cava; CS os, coronary sinus ostium; TVA, tricuspid valve annulus; RBB pot, right bundle branch potential. See chapter 16 Figure 7.

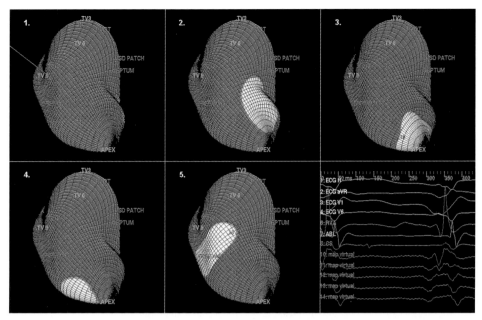

Plate 21. Fallots VT: Right ventricular geometry view from a cranially orientated left anterior oblique plane. Virtual electrograms (channels 10-14) are recorded from the anterosuperior free wall along the site of the presumed ventriculotomy incision. The appropriately numbered labels on the geometry indicate the recording sites. Frames 1 and 2 show activation spreading up the apical septum from inferior to superior. The VSD patch prevents activation heading towards the base of the septum. Frames 3 and 4 show how the ventriculotomy acts as a barrier, with the wavefront having to turn around the apical end of the incision. Frame 5 shows activation now able to depolarize the free wall from apex to base. This line of block is confirmed by the presence of double potentials in the virtual electrograms along the site of the ventriculotomy. The position of the ablation catheter (ABL) is indicated by the locator signal (green line) in frame 1. Labels in green are on the near side of the geometry. Labels in yellow are on the far side and seen through the geometry. TV, tricuspid valve annulus; RVOT, right ventricular outflow tract. See chapter 16 Figure 9.

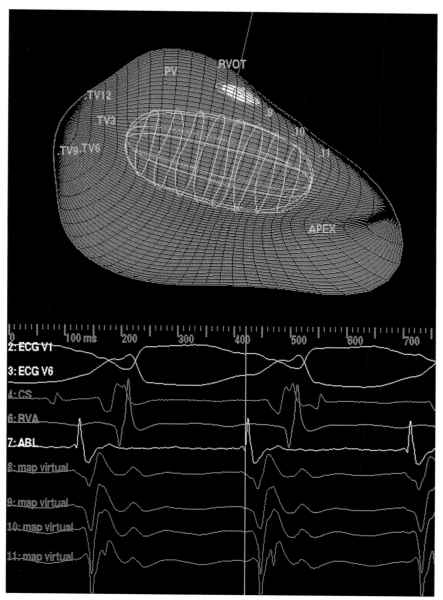

Plate 22. Right ventricular outflow tract tachycardia. Right ventricular geometry is displayed in a right anterior oblique view with the free wall clipped away to provide an internal view of the septum, medial outflow tract and inferior wall. The yellow frame indicates the MEA position. Contact and virtual electrograms are displayed below. The virtual electrograms (channels 8-11) are taken from the numbered sites on the geometry. The vertical yellow line indicates the point in time displayed on the isopotential map. Earliest systolic activation is shown occurring 20 msec before the onset of the surface QRS. The site is indicated by the white spot of color (negative potential) on the isopotential map. The virtual electrogram from this point (channel 8) shows the earliest activation and a QS morphology. The green line on the geometry represents the locator signal, which has guided the ablation catheter tip to this site. The bipolar contact electrogram is shown in channel 7. TV, tricuspid valve; PV, pulmonary valve; RVOT, right ventricular outflow tract. See chapter 16 Figure 10.

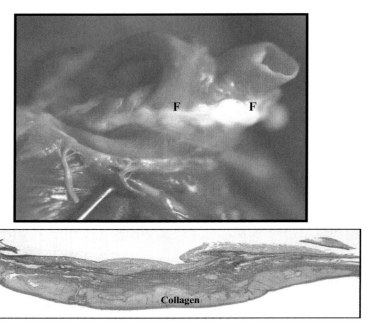

Plate 23. Histopathology of the Afib ablation linear lesions created with the 4-mm ring type ablation catheter. F = fibrous tissue. See chapter 22 Figure 18.

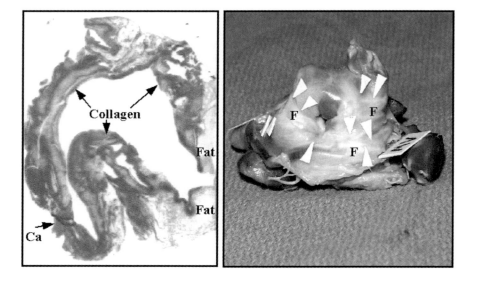

Plate 24. Histopathology of the Afib ablation linear lesions created with the 12-mm coil electrodes. Ca = calcium, F = fibrous tissue. See chapter 22 Figure 19.

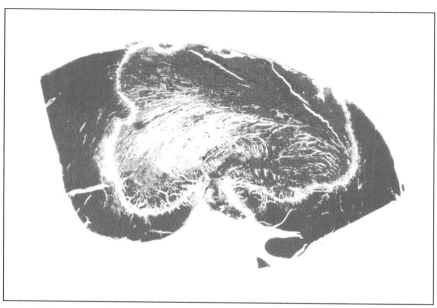

Plate 25. A fully transmural photocoagulation lesion of 14 mm depth (approximately 2.5 cm³) was obtained in 40 seconds at a wavelength of 1064 nm. The duration of power application was 40 seconds. Note the relative sparing of the endocardial surface in normal myocardium due to cooling from circulating blood in contact with the endocardial surface. See chapter 25 Figure 1.

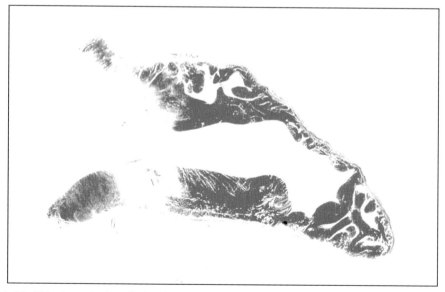

Plate 26. This shows the 2 week chronic lesion of the isolated left atrial appendage whose acute electrical isolation was shown in Figure 3. On re-study 2 weeks later electrical entrance and exit block was confirmed. A 2-3 mm wide area of fibrosis surrounded the entire atrial appendage. See chapter 25 Figure 4

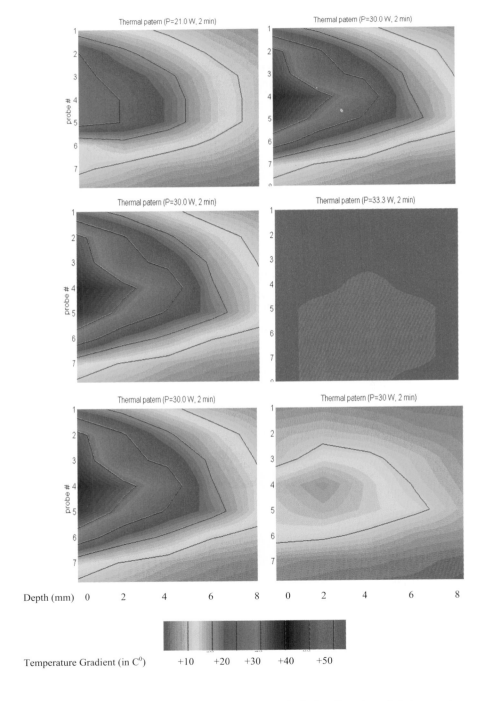

Plate 27. The effect on thermal distribution of power magnitude (top figures); angle between antenna and tissue (parallel, middle left; and 30 degrees, middle right) and antenna contact (complete contact, lower left; 1-mm distance, lower right). See chapter 26 Figures 3, 4, and 5.

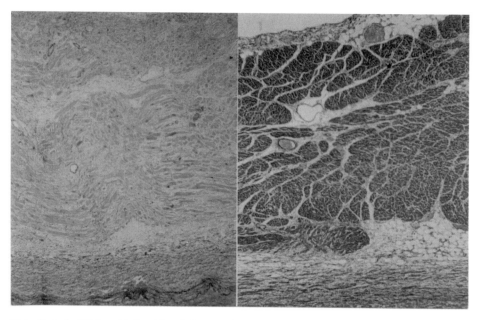

Plate 28. Left: Thickened left atrial wall from a mitral patient. Right: Atrial wall from a 60 years old normal subject. Note the adipose tissue at the endocardium/myocardium interface (elastic van Gieson × 40). See chapter 31 Figure 3.

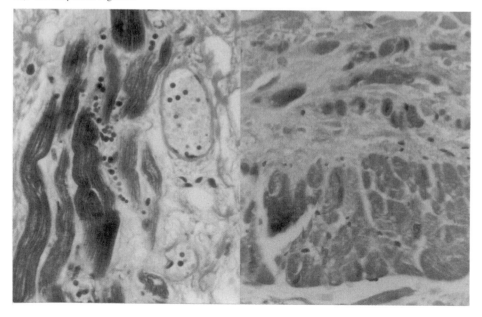

Plate 29. Left: Myocardium from a mitral patient with interstitial fibrosis and myocite hyperplasia. Right: The effect on the myocardium from a mitral patient of an endocardial radiofrequency application (Gomori's trichrome × 400). See chapter 31 Figure 4.

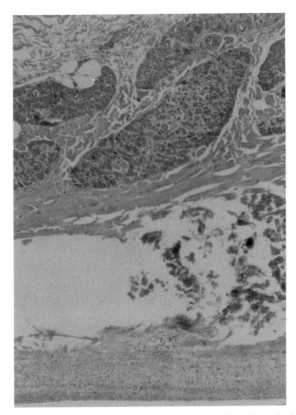

Plate 30. Transmural lesion induced by an endocardial RF application at 70° C in a mitral patient. Note the loss of tissue at the endocardium/myocardium interface (Gomori's trichrome × 40). See chapter 31 Figure 5.

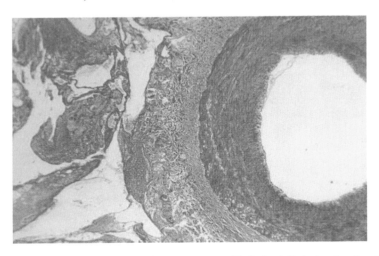

Plate 31. RF application at 70° C over the right coronary artery. The lesion is limited to the adventitia sparing the media and the endotelium. (Gomori's trichrome ×100). See chapter 31 Figure 6.

Index

A

B

C

S

T

U

V

W

Developments in Cardiovascular Medicine

109. J.P.M. Hamer: *Practical Echocardiography in the Adult.* With Doppler and Color-Doppler Flow Imaging. 1990   ISBN 0-7923-0670-8
110. A. Bayés de Luna, P. Brugada, J. Cosin Aguilar and F. Navarro Lopez (eds.): *Sudden Cardiac Death.* 1991   ISBN 0-7923-0716-X
111. E. Andries and R. Stroobandt (eds.): *Hemodynamics in Daily Practice.* 1991   ISBN 0-7923-0725-9
112. J. Morganroth and E.N. Moore (eds.): *Use and Approval of Antihypertensive Agents and Surrogate End-points for the Approval of Drugs affecting Antiarrhythmic Heart Failure and Hypolipidemia.* Proceedings of the 10th Annual Symposium on New Drugs and Devices (1989). 1990   ISBN 0-7923-0756-9
113. S. Iliceto, P. Rizzon and J.R.T.C. Roelandt (eds.): *Ultrasound in Coronary Artery Disease.* Present Role and Future Perspectives. 1990   ISBN 0-7923-0784-4
114. J.V. Chapman and G.R. Sutherland (eds.): *The Noninvasive Evaluation of Hemodynamics in Congenital Heart Disease.* Doppler Ultrasound Applications in the Adult and Pediatric Patient with Congenital Heart Disease. 1990   ISBN 0-7923-0836-0
115. G.T. Meester and F. Pinciroli (eds.): *Databases for Cardiology.* 1991   ISBN 0-7923-0886-7
116. B. Korecky and N.S. Dhalla (eds.): *Subcellular Basis of Contractile Failure.* 1990   ISBN 0-7923-0890-5
117. J.H.C. Reiber and P.W. Serruys (eds.): *Quantitative Coronary Arteriography.* 1991   ISBN 0-7923-0913-8
118. E. van der Wall and A. de Roos (eds.): *Magnetic Resonance Imaging in Coronary Artery Disease.* 1991   ISBN 0-7923-0940-5
119. V. Hombach, M. Kochs and A.J. Camm (eds.): *Interventional Techniques in Cardiovascular Medicine.* 1991   ISBN 0-7923-0956-1
120. R. Vos: *Drugs Looking for Diseases.* Innovative Drug Research and the Development of the Beta Blockers and the Calcium Antagonists. 1991   ISBN 0-7923-0968-5
121. S. Sideman, R. Beyar and A.G. Kleber (eds.): *Cardiac Electrophysiology, Circulation, and Transport.* Proceedings of the 7th Henry Goldberg Workshop (Berne, Switzerland, 1990). 1991
                                                                             ISBN 0-7923-1145-0
122. D.M. Bers: *Excitation-Contraction Coupling and Cardiac Contractile Force.* 1991   ISBN 0-7923-1186-8
123. A.-M. Salmasi and A.N. Nicolaides (eds.): *Occult Atherosclerotic Disease.* Diagnosis, Assessment and Management. 1991   ISBN 0-7923-1188-4
124. J.A.E. Spaan: *Coronary Blood Flow.* Mechanics, Distribution, and Control. 1991   ISBN 0-7923-1210-4
125. R.W. Stout (ed.): *Diabetes and Atherosclerosis.* 1991   ISBN 0-7923-1310-0
126. A.G. Herman (ed.): *Antithrombotics.* Pathophysiological Rationale for Pharmacological Interventions. 1991   ISBN 0-7923-1413-1
127. N.H.J. Pijls: *Maximal Myocardial Perfusion as a Measure of the Functional Significance of Coronary Arteriogram.* From a Pathoanatomic to a Pathophysiologic Interpretation of the Coronary Arteriogram. 1991   ISBN 0-7923-1430-1
128. J.H.C. Reiber and E.E. v.d. Wall (eds.): *Cardiovascular Nuclear Medicine and MRI.* Quantitation and Clinical Applications. 1992   ISBN 0-7923-1467-0
129. E. Andries, P. Brugada and R. Stroobrandt (eds.): *How to Face "the Faces' of Cardiac Pacing.* 1992
                                                                             ISBN 0-7923-1528-6
130. M. Nagano, S. Mochizuki and N.S. Dhalla (eds.): *Cardiovascular Disease in Diabetes.* 1992
                                                                             ISBN 0-7923-1554-5
131. P.W. Serruys, B.H. Strauss and S.B. King III (eds.): *Restenosis after Intervention with New Mechanical Devices.* 1992   ISBN 0-7923-1555-3
132. P.J. Walter (ed.): *Quality of Life after Open Heart Surgery.* 1992   ISBN 0-7923-1580-4
133. E.E. van der Wall, H. Sochor, A. Righetti and M.G. Niemeyer (eds.): *What's new in Cardiac Imaging?* SPECT, PET and MRI. 1992   ISBN 0-7923-1615-0
134. P. Hanrath, R. Uebis and W. Krebs (eds.): *Cardiovascular Imaging by Ultrasound.* 1992
                                                                             ISBN 0-7923-1755-6
135. F.H. Messerli (ed.): *Cardiovascular Disease in the Elderly.* 3rd ed. 1992   ISBN 0-7923-1859-5
136. J. Hess and G.R. Sutherland (eds.): *Congenital Heart Disease in Adolescents and Adults.* 1992
                                                                             ISBN 0-7923-1862-5
137. J.H.C. Reiber and P.W. Serruys (eds.): *Advances in Quantitative Coronary Arteriography.* 1993
                                                                             ISBN 0-7923-1863-3

Developments in Cardiovascular Medicine

138. A.-M. Salmasi and A.S. Iskandrian (eds.): *Cardiac Output and Regional Flow in Health and Disease.* 1993
ISBN 0-7923-1911-7
139. J.H. Kingma, N.M. van Hemel and K.I. Lie (eds.): *Atrial Fibrillation, a Treatable Disease?* 1992
ISBN 0-7923-2008-5
140. B. Ostadel and N.S. Dhalla (eds.): *Heart Function in Health and Disease.* Proceedings of the Cardiovascular Program (Prague, Czechoslovakia, 1991). 1992
ISBN 0-7923-2052-2
141. D. Noble and Y.E. Earm (eds.): *Ionic Channels and Effect of Taurine on the Heart.* Proceedings of an International Symposium (Seoul, Korea, 1992). 1993
ISBN 0-7923-2199-5
142. H.M. Piper and C.J. Preusse (eds.): *Ischemia-reperfusion in Cardiac Surgery.* 1993 ISBN 0-7923-2241-X
143. J. Roelandt, E.J. Gussenhoven and N. Bom (eds.): *Intravascular Ultrasound.* 1993 ISBN 0-7923-2301-7
144. M.E. Safar and M.F. O'Rourke (eds.): *The Arterial System in Hypertension.* 1993 ISBN 0-7923-2343-2
145. P.W. Serruys, D.P. Foley and P.J. de Feyter (eds.): *Quantitative Coronary Angio- graphy in Clinical Practice.* With a Foreword by Spencer B. King III. 1994
ISBN 0-7923-2368-8
146. J. Candell-Riera and D. Ortega-Alcalde (eds.): *Nuclear Cardiology in Everyday Practice.* 1994
ISBN 0-7923-2374-2
147. P. Cummins (ed.): *Growth Factors and the Cardiovascular System.* 1993 ISBN 0-7923-2401-3
148. K. Przyklenk, R.A. Kloner and D.M. Yellon (eds.): *Ischemic Preconditioning: The Concept of Endogenous Cardioprotection.* 1993
ISBN 0-7923-2410-5
149. T.H. Marwick: *Stress Echocardiography.* Its Role in the Diagnosis and Evaluation of Coronary Artery Disease. 1994
ISBN 0-7923-2579-6
150. W.H. van Gilst and K.I. Lie (eds.): *Neurohumoral Regulation of Coronary Flow.* Role of the Endothelium. 1993
ISBN 0-7923-2588-5
151. N. Sperelakis (ed.): *Physiology and Pathophysiology of the Heart.* 3rd rev. ed. 1994 ISBN 0-7923-2612-1
152. J.C. Kaski (ed.): *Angina Pectoris with Normal Coronary Arteries: Syndrome X.* 1994
ISBN 0-7923-2651-2
153. D.R. Gross: *Animal Models in Cardiovascular Research.* 2nd rev. ed. 1994 ISBN 0-7923-2712-8
154. A.S. Iskandrian and E.E. van der Wall (eds.): *Myocardial Viability.* Detection and Clinical Relevance. 1994
ISBN 0-7923-2813-2
155. J.H.C. Reiber and P.W. Serruys (eds.): *Progress in Quantitative Coronary Arteriography.* 1994
ISBN 0-7923-2814-0
156. U. Goldbourt, U. de Faire and K. Berg (eds.): *Genetic Factors in Coronary Heart Disease.* 1994
ISBN 0-7923-2752-7
157. G. Leonetti and C. Cuspidi (eds.): *Hypertension in the Elderly.* 1994 ISBN 0-7923-2852-3
158. D. Ardissino, S. Savonitto and L.H. Opie (eds.): *Drug Evaluation in Angina Pectoris.* 1994
ISBN 0-7923-2897-3
159. G. Bkaily (ed.): *Membrane Physiopathology.* 1994 ISBN 0-7923-3062-5
160. R.C. Becker (ed.): *The Modern Era of Coronary Thrombolysis.* 1994 ISBN 0-7923-3063-3
161. P.J. Walter (ed.): *Coronary Bypass Surgery in the Elderly.* Ethical, Economical and Quality of Life Aspects. With a foreword by N.K. Wenger. 1995
ISBN 0-7923-3188-5
162. J.W. de Jong and R. Ferrari (eds.), *The Carnitine System.* A New Therapeutical Approach to Cardiovascular Diseases. 1995
ISBN 0-7923-3318-7
163. C.A. Neill and E.B. Clark: *The Developing Heart: A "History' of Pediatric Cardiology.* 1995
ISBN 0-7923-3375-6
164. N. Sperelakis: *Electrogenesis of Biopotentials in the Cardiovascular System.* 1995 ISBN 0-7923-3398-5
165. M. Schwaiger (ed.): *Cardiac Positron Emission Tomography.* 1995 ISBN 0-7923-3417-5
166. E.E. van der Wall, P.K. Blanksma, M.G. Niemeyer and A.M.J. Paans (eds.): *Cardiac Positron Emission Tomography.* Viability, Perfusion, Receptors and Cardiomyopathy. 1995 ISBN 0-7923-3472-8
167. P.K. Singal, I.M.C. Dixon, R.E. Beamish and N.S. Dhalla (eds.): *Mechanism of Heart Failure.* 1995
ISBN 0-7923-3490-6
168. N.S. Dhalla, P.K. Singal, N. Takeda and R.E. Beamish (eds.): *Pathophysiology of Heart Failure.* 1995
ISBN 0-7923-3571-6
169. N.S. Dhalla, G.N. Pierce, V. Panagia and R.E. Beamish (eds.): *Heart Hypertrophy and Failure.* 1995
ISBN 0-7923-3572-4

Developments in Cardiovascular Medicine